QSPR/QSAR Studies by Molecular Descriptors

QSPR/QSAR Studies by Molecular Descriptors

Mircea V. Diudea
Editor

Nova Science Publishers, Inc.
Huntington, New York

Senior Editors: Susan Boriotti and Donna Dennis
Office Manager: Annette Hellinger
Graphics: Wanda Serrano
Information Editor: Tatiana Shohov
Book Production: Latoya Clay, Cathy DeGregory and Lynette Van Helden
Circulation: Anna Cruz, Ave Maria Gonzalez, Ron Hedges, Andre Tillman

Library of Congress Cataloging-in-Publication Data

QSPR/QSAR studies by molecular descriptors / Mircea V. Diudea, editor
p. cm.
Includes index.
ISBN 1-56072-859-0
1. QSAR (Biochemistry) 2. Drugs--Design. I. Diudea, Mircea V.
RM301.42.Q285 2000 CIP
615'.19--dc21 00-048980

227 Main Street, Suite 100
Huntington, New York 11743
Tele. 631-424-6682Fax 631-424-4666
e-mail: Novascience@earthlink.net
Web Site: http://www.nexusworld.com/nova

Printed in the United States of America

CONTENTS

Chapter 1

A Personal View About Topological Indices For QSAR / QSPR

Alexandru T. Balaban
Polytechnic University, Organic Chemistry Department,
Bucharest, Romania

1. A Personal Introductory Note

The introduction will start with a few personal reminiscences about how it felt in the sixties and seventies to work on graph-theoretical problems, in comparison with the present-day situation. My interest in enumerating all possible monocyclic aromatic compounds containing the three and only three allowed types of sp^2-hybridized atoms (with two, one, or zero electrons in the non-hybridized orbital forming the π-electron delocalized system) was my first enumeration problem that could be solved by graph-theoretical methods with a mathematician friend, Silviu Teleman.[1] The next problem is still unsolved: the enumeration of all possible benzenoids with a given number of rings, equivalent to the "hexagonal-cell animals" problem. Following the advice of Silviu Teleman, I started a correspondence with Frank Harary, which led to him visiting me in Bucharest, and then making joint progress for this enumeration.[2] Another unsolved problem that occupied me at that time was that of valence isomers of annulenes, equivalent to the enumeration of cubic graphs. A step-by-step procedure was found,[3] followed by a book summarizing what was known on such valence isomers,[4] but the mathematically elegant solution published later [5] was not of much help to chemists who wished to have formulas for cubic multigraphs, still a difficult enterprise.[6]

Working in this area at that time was like driving a car before Ford had made cars available to many middle-class Americans: one drove along the existing dusty country roads with practically no traffic, but in exchange, what liberty one had for traveling around and for discovering new marvelous landscapes! I published many papers in the series "Chemical Graphs", detecting (and often solving) various interesting problems, without any competition. The first book on *Chemical Applications of Graph Theory* appeared in 1976.[7] To cite Coleridge,

"And there were gardens bright with sinuous rills
Where blossomed many an incense-bearing tree;
And here were forests ancient as the hills,
Enfolding sunny spots of greenery."

One had the privilege of working on anything that sparkled one's imagination, e. g. finding that some reaction graphs were related to trivalent "g-cage graphs",[8] i. e. graphs having a given minimal size g of their circuits and the minimal number of vertices, such as the Petersen graph which is the 5-cage (this discovery of reaction graphs opened the door to the quest for yet unknown larger cages, such as the 10-cage [9] and the 11-cage;[10] no serious work has yet been done to this day on cages with $g > 12$). To return to Coleridge, one had then the sentiment of his Ancient Mariner:

"The fair breeze blew,
The white foam flew,
The furrow followed free.
We were the first
That ever burst
Into that silent sea..."

My involvement with topological indices started fairly late, in 1979, with centric graphs, as will be discussed in detail further below, and brought back the collaboration with Zeno Simon and his coworkers which had started when he was in Bucharest, before he had moved to Timisoara.[11-13] He had developed his MSD method, which in a later version became the MTD method (Minimal Steric/Topological Difference), and had as objective the finding of Quantitative Structure-Activity Relationships (QSAR) between chemical structures and their biological activities.[14,15] The problem was to find appropriate molecular descriptors, and this led to topological indices in a jointly published book.[16]

The present-day situation in chemical applications of graph theory has changed markedly. Continuing the traffic analogy, one drives at high speed on highways, freeways and turnpikes, there are now lots of cars, and sometimes there are collisions. Happily, there are also many friends scattered around the globe. I have collaborated with many scientists and students in Romania and abroad, and I have published several monographs in this field [4,7,16-19] and numerous papers under various 'series titles' such as "Chemical Graphs", "Design of Topological Indices" (initiated by my former graduate student, Ovidiu Ivanciuc) or "Molecular Topology" in collaboration with professor Mircea Diudea, who teaches a course on chemical topology in Cluj to undergraduate students. He also collaborated with Dr. Ivanciuc in publishing a textbook on this topic.[20] I must also mention the research group in Timisoara where, in addition to Professor Simon, other mathematical chemists are active, namely Prof. D. Ciubotariu and Dr. M. Medeleanu. It is gratifying to see that all my former collaborators have now their own projects which they pursue independently, but occasionally we still collaborate. After 1989, when I spent alternate semeters in Romania and in the USA, there were enhanced opportunties for continuing or initiating collaborations with theoretical chemists from foreign countries: Professors D. Bonchev and O. Mekenyan from Bulgaria who developed their OASIS program, Professors D. J. Klein and W. A. Seitz from the Texas A & M University, and Prof. S. C. Basak from the Natural Resources Research Institute, University of Minnesota-Duluth. Even earlier, in 1987, with an international team totaling 14 mathematical chemists, we had published a consolidated report on the enumeration of benzenoids.[21]

2. Local Vertex Invariants and Topological Indices: Brief Overview

In the following paragraphs, several LOcal Vertex Invariants (LOVIs) and Topological Indices (TIs) will be reviewed. It must be said from the beginning that this cannot be an exhaustive review because of space limitations, therefore a certain bias and subjectivity are unavoidable, and apologies are offered for the omissions, because ... the traffic on the QSAR / QSPR highway is nowadays very dense...

The central problem in QSPR / QSAR is to convert chemical structures into mathematical molecular descriptors that are relevant to the physico-chemical property or to the mechanism of the biological activity. It was shown by Katritzky and Gordeeva [22] that for QSPR (Quantitative Structure-Property Relationship) studies, topological indices are among the best descriptors, but for QSAR studies they have to be complemented with other parameters such as the hydrophobicity (introduced by Hansch and his coworkers [23-26]) which is involved in molecular transport across biological membranes.

For molecules with N non-hydrogen atoms, represented as constitutional (molecular) hydrogen-depleted graphs (in which these atoms are represented by points or vertices, and covalent bonds by lines or edges connecting these points), chemical constitution can be easily encoded as an adjacency matrix **A**. The entries a_{ij} for this matrix are 1 for two adjacent atoms i and j (i. e. atoms which are connected by a covalent bond) and 0 otherwise. The result is a symmetrical matrix with N rows and N columns. The sum (v_i) over row i or column i is the degree of vertex i; for instance, as the customary nomenclature of organic chemistry calls it, a quaternary carbon atom (connected to four other non-hydrogen atoms) has degree $v_i = 4$; similarly, a secondary carbon atom has degree $v_i = 2$.

A more detailed topological information is provided by the distance matrix **D**, whose entries d_{ij} represent topological distances between vertices i and j, that is the number of bonds along the shortest path between these vertices. Matrix **D** can be deduced from **A** and vice-versa. Thus, **A** and **D** both have zeroes along the main diagonal and the same entries 1, but all off-diagonal zeroes in **A** are replaced in **D** by integers that are larger than 1. Sums of entries along row i or column i in **D** are called distance-sums (distasums), s_i.

Both matrices, **A** and **D**, contain all the necessary information for molecular constitution. This means that there is a one-to-one correspondence between the hydrogen-depleted graph and each of these two matrices. On their basis topological indices have been devised, as will be shown further below. It had been conjectured that the eigenvalues or the characteristic polynomial of **A** or **D** could characterize uniquely a chemical graph, but this conjecture was proved to be unfounded by Balaban and Harary [27] (and later reafirmed by Herndon,[28] in a rebuttal of another attempt to redeem the characteristic polynomial).

The molecular constitution can thus be encoded in matrix form (either adjacency matrix **A**, or distance matrix **D**). Irrespective of the arbitrary labeling of vertices, the sums over row i or column i of these two matrices, v_i and d_i, respectively, are local vertex invariants (LOVIs). The degree v_i of vertex i in organic molecules can be an integer from 1 to 4, but there is no limit for the distasum d_i. From these or related LOVIs one can obtain global molecular descriptors, called topological indices (TIs), via mahematical operations such as summation, summation of squares, summation of products over edge endpoints, etc.

Other symmetrical matrices with integer entries that have found use in defining TIs are (i) the detour matrix (entries are the longest paths between vertices i and j) which is identical to **D** for acyclic graphs, but different from **D** for cyclic graphs; [29-36] and (ii) the reverse Wiener matrix whose entries are differences between the largest distance (called the graph diameter) and the topological distance between vertices i and j.[37] The detour matrix was introduced into the chemical literature independently by the Bucharest group [29] and the Zagreb group [30] (the former used the name "maximum path matrix of a molecular graph"); calculations of largest distances (longest paths), however, are c.p.u. intensive.

For all three isomers of pentane, namely n-pentane **1**, isopentane (2-methylbutane) **2**, and neopentane (2,2-dimethylpropane) **3**, two types of LOVIs, namely the vertex degrees and distasums, are indicated on Fig. 1. Also on Fig. 1 one may see the least branched and most branched isomers of heptane, namely n-heptane (**4**), and 2,2,3-tetramethylbutane (**5**), respectively. It may be seen that nonequivalent vertices have the same LOVI (vertex degree 2) in graphs **1** and **4**, and this is also true for nonequivalent endpoints (vertices of degree 1) in **2** and **5**. However, distasums discriminate all such nonequivalent vertices. It will be noted that for any hydrogen-depleted acyclic graph with N vertices, differences between distasums for endpoints and for the vertices to which they are attached are equal to N – 2.

Figure 1

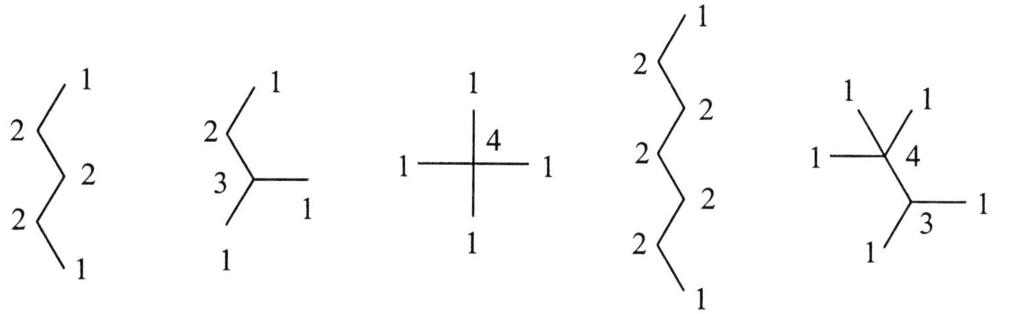

1 **2** **3** **4** **5**

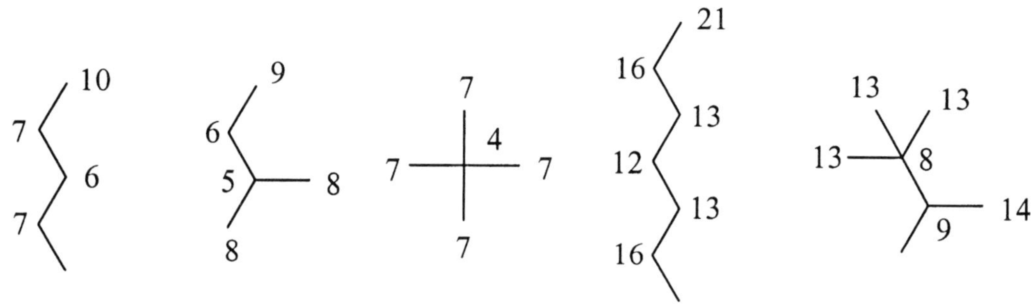

3. First-Generation Topological Indices

The simplest (first-generation) TIs are *integer numbers* obtained from *integer LOVIs*.[38] The history of TIs starts with Wiener [39] and Platt,[40] who independently came with the idea of correlating properties with molecular constitution. One of the first and still useful TIs was proposed by H. Wiener as the half-sum of all entries in **D** or of all distasums, and Hosoya [41] named the result Wiener's index or Wiener number:

$$W = (\Sigma_i \Sigma_j d_{ij}) / 2 = (\Sigma_i s_i) / 2$$

For the three pentane isomers **1** - **3** (Fig. 1), W values are 20, 18, and 16, respectively. Two TIs are said to be *degenerate* if they have the same value, although they correspond to different (non-isomorphic) graphs. No TI proposed so far is free of degeneracy but some TIs have higher and some have lower degeneracy. Index W has a high degeneracy: thus for alkanes, the degeneracy starts with two pairs of heptane constitutional isomers: W = 46 for 2,2- dimethylpentane and 2,3-dimethylpentane, and W = 48 for 2,4-dimethylpentane and 3-ethylpentane.

Extensions of the Wiener index were proposed for various purposes; the detour index is one of these extensions;[31,36] the hyper-Wiener index, the Szeged index and the three-dimensional Wiener index will be mentioned below. The Wiener matrix continues to be the source of novel graph invariants.[42] Computational methods have been described for obtaining the Wiener index for benzenoid graphs,[43,44] or infinite polymeric chains,[45-47] and relationships between W and the graph Laplacian have been published.[48]

Platt's first-neighbor index f is obtained by summing for each edge the number of its adjacent edges.[40] This index is related to Gordon and Scantlebury's index N_2 by the relationship $f = 2N_2$ (N_2 indicates in how many ways one may superimpose on the hydrogen-depleted graph a path of length 2, i. e. a propane subgraph C–C–C).[49] Also this index has a high degeneracy which starts with constitutional isomers of heptanes in the alkane series: $N_2 = 7$ for 2,3- dimethylpentane and 2,4-dimethylpentane. For a long linear alkane chain, the ratio $N / [2(N-1)]$ tends towards 1/2 when $N \rightarrow \infty$.

Hosoya's index [41] Z is the sum (from zero to N / 2) of nonadjacent numbers of edges, i. e. the number of ways in which k edges of the graph may be chosen so that no two of these edges are adjacent. For k = 1 we obtain for this nonadjacent number of ways the actual number of edges, and by definition for k = 0 we obtain 1.

Two other first-generation TIs, advocated by the Zagreb group,[50] are the sum of squares of vertex degrees, and the sum of products over all edges i–j:

$$M_1 = \Sigma_i v_i^2$$

$$M_2 = \Sigma_{ij} v_i v_j$$

Centric indices for acyclic graphs were proposed in 1979 by summing squares of numbers (δ_i^2) of vertices pruned stepwise from the periphery towards the graph center which is either one vertex or a pair of adjacent vertices.[51]

$$B = \Sigma_i (\delta_i^2)$$

A normalized centric index can be defined relative to the least branched (linear alkane) and to the most branched graphs with the same number of vertices (star-graph).[51] The centric index B has also high degeneracy starting with heptane constitutional isomers: B = 21 for all three dimethylpentanes (2,2-, 2,3- and 2,4-dimethylpentane) because all of them have the same lopping (pruning) sequence: 1,2,4. This idea of centric indices was later generalized together with Bonchev and Mekenyan for cyclic graphs,[52] and together with Basak et al. for substituents.[53]

The Schultz index [54,55] was introduced as MTI (molecular topological index) based on the row matrix sum $\mathbf{v}[\mathbf{A} + \mathbf{D}]$ where $\mathbf{v}$ is the vertex degree; two pairs of octane isomers share the same MTI value: MTI = 242 for 2,2,4-trimethylpenane and 3-ethyl-2-methylpentane; MTI = 260 for 3-ethylhexane and 2,2-dimethylhexane. It was found that W and MTI are almost collinear.[56]

The Szeged index (Sz) was introduced by Gutman by analogy with the Wiener index, but extending to cyclic graphs one of the definitions of W for acyclic graphs.[57-59] One counts in different sets the numbers n_1 and n_2 of vertices closer to one or the other endpoint of each edge, disregarding equidistant vertices. Then $Sz = \Sigma\, n_1 \times n_2$ for all pairs of endpoints. Procedures based on "cuts in benzenoid graphs" for computing their Szeged indices were developed.[59]

A somewhat related TI is the hyper-Wiener index R introduced by Randić [42,60] and developed by Lukovits,[61] and later by Klein, Lukovits and Gutman.[62] For acyclic graphs, any pair of vertices gives rise to two disconnected subgraphs if the unique path connecting these two vertices, and any side-chains attached to this path, are deleted. The sum of products of the number of vertices in these two subgraphs over all distinct pairs is the hyper-Wiener index. Generalizations to acyclic graphs and computing algorithms were developed. This index measures the "expansiveness"of a graph. There is a simple relationship between R and W, namely $2R = W + D_2$, where the last term is the second moment of distance, related to the mean square distance (D) to be mentioned in the next section.

The Rücker index is based on counts of all walks from vertex i to vertex j (edges in a walk may occur more than once);[63] powers of **A** allow a fairly easy calculation of the numbers of walks.

4. Second-Generation Topological Indices

Second-generation TIs are *real numbers* based on *integer LOVIs*. One of the most successful TIs, the molecular connectivity (χ), was proposed by Milan Randić in 1975 as the sum (over all edges i–j in the graph) of the reciprocal square root of products of vertex degrees for edge endpoints (this is a sum of "weighted edges"):[64]

$$\chi = \Sigma_{ij}\, (v_i\, v_j)^{-1/2}$$

Randić's index has a lower degeneracy than first-generation indices. For the series of alkanes, the first degeneracy appears for two pairs of constitutionally isomeric octanes: 3-methylheptane and 4-methylheptane share the same value of $\chi = 3.8081$; 3,4-dimethylhexane and 3-ethyl-2-methylpentane share the value $\chi = 3.7187$.

Kier, Hall, Randić and coworkers then generalized this idea for longer paths than edges (which can be considered as paths of length L = 1 in the graph).[65] The three carbon atoms in a propane graph form a path of lengh L = 2, an n-butane graph is a path of length L = 3, and so on. An isobutane graph is a cluster (star-graph) on 4 vertices. Thus, we have a sum of "weighted paths", yielding connectivity indices of higher order L:

$$^{L}\chi = \Sigma_{ijk\ldots}(v_i\, v_j\, v_{jk}\, .\,.\,.)^{-1/2}$$

Two monographs by Kier and Hall [66,67] presented many successful QSAR data using their extended connectivities; a third book describes their electrotopological state index.[68,69] All these indices have recently been reviewed as book chapters.[19b-d]

For taking into account the nature of atoms symbolized by vertices, Kier and Hall proposed the use of "valence connectivity indices".[70] These are calculated with formulas similar to Randić's formula, but products of edge endpoint (or path vertex) invariants are no longer of vertex degrees but of weights (valence delta values δ_i) given by:

$$\delta_i = (Z_i^v - H_i)/(Z_i - Z_i^v - 1)$$

where Z_i^v indicates the number of valence electrons in atom i, Z is its atomic number, and H_i is the number of hydrogen atoms attached to atom i.

Kappa indexes and a flexibility index developed by Kier[71] are calculated as ratios relative to structures that correspond to the least branched (linear chain) and most branched (star graph) molecule with the same number A of non-hydrogen atoms. For paths ^LP_i of length L one has:

$$^L\kappa = 2(^LP_{max} \times {}^LP_{min}) / (^Lp_i)^2$$

As mentioned earlier, an edge is a path of length L = 1. The nature of atoms is introduced by means of a corrective factor α which is derived from the covalent radius of an atom relative to that of an sp^3-hybridized carbon. Thus when L = 2, one obtains for $^2\kappa_\alpha$:

$$^2\kappa_\alpha = (A + \alpha - 1)(A + \alpha - 2)^2 / (^2P_i + \alpha)^2$$

Later, Kier introduced a flexibility index,[72] defined as $\phi = {}^1\kappa_\alpha \times {}^2\kappa_\alpha / A$. For a linear alkane, $\phi = A - 1$, i. e. the count of $C(sp^3) - C(sp^3)$ bonds.

The mean square root distance derived from all topological distances (denoted by i in the next formula) is defined as:[73]

$$D = [(\Sigma_i i^2) / (\Sigma_i i)]^{1/2}$$

If i denotes only the distances between endpoints, the above formula defines a related index D_1 which correlates with octane numbers of alkanes even better than D. There is no degeneracy of D for octanes, but a pair of isomeric octanes have the same D_1 value.

All TIs depend both on molecular branching and molecular size. For some TIs it is possible to reconstruct the molecular constitution from the value of its TI if its degeneracy is not too high; this solution of the "inverse problem" allows one to make predictions in QSAR.[74,75]

Starting with 1982, I developed the average distance connectivity index (J) based on distasums,[76] in order to reduce the degeneracy of previous indices, because distasums (unlike vertex degrees) are seldom identical for nonequivalent vertices in non-isomorphic graphs, as it was seen in Fig. 1. One sums "weighted average topological distances" for all edges i–j:

$$J = [q / (\mu + 1)]\Sigma_{ij} (d_i d_j)^{-1/2}$$

The numbers q of graph edges, and μ of cycles in the graph are introduced into the above formula in order to avoid the automatic increase of J with graph size and cyclicity. Indeed, for an infinite linear carbon chain it was demonstrated [77] that J = π = 3.14159... The first degeneracy for J in the alkane series appears among the 355 constitutionally isomeric dodecanes, e. g. for the two isomers 2,3,3,6- and 2,2,5,5-tetramethyloctane.[78] The nature of atoms can be taken into account by means of parameters based on their relative atomic numbers, electronegativities, or covalent radii, with respect to those of carbon atoms.[79-81]

Table 1 displays for the alkanes from Fig. 1 two properties (boiling point, NBP in °C; and PON, posted octane number), and a few of the first- and second-generation TIs.

The resistance distance matrix has as entries numbers that correspond to electrical resistances between vertices i and j if each edge in the graph is a resistor of one ohm.[82] For acyclic graphs this matrix is identical to **D**, but for cyclic graphs its entries are rational fractions, not integers. One has defined a TI with low degeneracy, called the Kirchhoff number, based on this matrix.[83]

Table 1. Physico-Chemical Properties and Selected TIs of Alkanes Presented in Fig. 1

Alkane:	1	2	3	4	5
NBP	36.5	27.9	9.5	98.4	80.9
PON	62.5	91.35	82.85	0	106.7
W	20	18	16	56	42
D	2.236	1.949	1.673	3.055	2.035
D_1	4	2.708	2	6	2.646
J	2.191	2.54	3.024	2.447	3.541
χ	2.414	2.27	2	3.414	2.943

Another symmetrical matrix with rational numbers as entries is the reciprocal distance matrix: its entries are reciprocals of the topological distances. It was developed independently in Bucharest [84] and Zagreb,[85] and we agreed to call the TI obtained on the basis of this matrix the Harary Index.[84,85] Its degeneracy is slightly lower than that of the W index.

A different approach to lowering the high degeneracy of some TIs such as the Wiener index was to make use of Shannon's formula which uses base-two logarithms in information theory. The first such "information-theoretic indices" were proposed by Bonchev and Trinajstić,[86-88] and by Basak and coworkers.[89-91] The former types of indices consider separately the information on each class of summands. They were reviewed thoroughly in Bonchev's book.[87] Konstantinova described informational indices, related to the former ones; one of these indices has a very low degeneracy, which was checked on benzenoid systems.[92]

Basak's indices take into account all atoms in the constitutional formula (hydrogens also being included), and one considers the information content provided by various classes of atoms. There are three types of Basak informational indices: IC (mean information content or complexity of a hydrogen-filled graph, with vertices grouped into equivalence classes having r vertices; the equivalence is based on the nature of atoms and bonds, in successive neighborhood groups); CIC (complementary information content); and SIC (structural information content), and they are not intercorrelated with other TIs. In the following formula, the summation spans the range from i = 1 to i = r:

$$IC_r = -\Sigma_i\, p_i \log_2 p_I$$

$$SIC = IC / \log_2 N$$

$$CIC = \log_2 N - IC$$

The probability that a randomly selected vertex occurs in the i-th equivalence class is denoted by p_i.

A recent paper describes the superpendentic index ($\int^P$),[93] based on the pendent matrix, which is a submatrix of **D** obtained by retaining only the columns corresponding to pendent vertices, i. e. endpoints (vertices of degree 1). The index $\int^P$ is defined as:

$$\int^P = [\Sigma_i \Sigma_j P_{(ij)}]^{0.5}$$

where $P_{(ij)}$ is the length of the shortest path between vertices i and j, and the first sum indicates the maximum value(s) in each row (with two equal maximal values, their sum is taken) while the second sum is for all columns. This index correlates satisfactorily with the bioactivity for antiulcer activity (inhibitor of gastric H^+, K^+ - ATPase enzyme).

Bertz employed line graphs (graph derivatives of progressively increasing orders) for new TIs and developed a mathematical approach for defining branching.[94,95] Later, Estrada developed this idea and proposed an edge connectivity index which correlates well with molar volumes and other physico-chemical properties of alkanes.[96,97]

5. Third-Generation Topological Indices

Third-generation TIs are based on new, *real-number LOVIs* and, of course, the *TIs must also be real numbers*. Since the set of integers, although infinite, is smaller than the set of real numbers, such TIs have less chance to be degenerate than the previous ones. One has to invent such real-number LOVIs and then to validate them; usually the validation for LOVIs is by intramolecular comparison in linear, branched or cyclic graphs, and for the corresponding TIs by intermolecular comparison within a series of isomeric alkanes and cycloalkanes.

A matrix such as **A** or **D** can be converted into a system of linear equations whose unknowns are real-number LOVIs and whose coefficients are the matrix entries supplemented by two column vectors which can convey chemical or topological information; one vector replaces the zeroes on the main diagonal, and the other vector provides the free terms of the equations.[98] The result is a "triplet TI" denoted by the components of the triplet, namely the matrix, the main diagonal vector, and the free term vector. Then the LOVIs may be assembled into a TI by various operations. Thus, AZV triplet LOVIs summed over all vertices yield the "AZV topological index" which correlates well some physical properties of alkane hydrocarbons. The combinatorial nature of the triplet combinations and assembly operations affords a large variety of TIs that may be adapted to different databases.

Another type of LOVI results by applying information theory for topological distances *at the vertex level*, providing informational LOVIs; then a formula similar to Randić's index assembles such LOVIs into four types of TIs denoted by letters U, V, X, or Y.[99]

The adjacency matrix **A** considers only nearest-neighbor interactions and is identical to the Hückel matrix in quantum chemistry; on the other hand, the LOVIs derived from the distance matrix **D** place the largest weight on the more distant vertices. Chemical interactions, however, are strongest between adjacent atoms, but more remote atoms also exert an influence that is gradually decreasing with the distance, as shown by the through-bond inductive effect. Reciprocal distances mentioned earlier take only partly into account such effects.[84,85,100] A different idea is to devise "regressive distances" or "regressive vertex degrees" by means of non-symmetrical layer matrices [101] whose entries in row i represent sums of topological distances or degrees, respectively, for vertices in shells around vertex i; an exponentially decreasing factor multiplies each successive shell. The results are indices that change slightly the distasum or the vertex degree, respectively, according to the molecular topology. With Professor Diudea we developed this idea,[102,103] and then he published further studies in this area,[104,105] including several studies on TIs of dendrimers where he has a pioneering role.[106,107]

Extremal eigenvalues and corresponding eigenvectors of matrices **A** or **D** can also be used as TIs and LOVIs, respectively. [108-111] It was shown by Burden that two such eigenvalue may characterize subgraphs.[112]

Galvez and his coworkers developed charge indices denoted by G_k and J_k starting from a matrix resulted by multipling the adjacency matrix with the inverse square distance matrix. These indices can correlate the charge distribution in molecules, and may be used for correlations with dipole moments in unsaturated and aromatic hydrocarbons.[113]

Diudea and coworkers constructed a non-symmetrical N×N matrix (the Cluj matrix) which can be used for developing new TIs.[114-117] When using reciprocal distance values, highly discriminating numerical invariants are obtained.

So far, the lowest degeneracy appears to be that of EAID indices proposed by Hu and Xu, using a more complicated procedure based on the layer matrix.[118] Next in line comes probably Hall and Kier's total topological index τ based on the topological state invariant;[119] index τ was found by Hu and Xu to present degeneracies starting with alkanes with 20 carbon atoms and with cyclic multigraphs with 8 vertices.[120]

Newer ideas for TIs are the adaptation of TIs to the corresponding data base: Ivanciuc and Balaban explored the optimal molecular descriptor for a data base by allowing the exponent in the formulas for χ or J to differ from $-1/2$;[121,122] Randić's approach is by computing for each data base a new type of molecular connectivity χ "optimal index" in which the adjacency matrix has on its main diagonal variable parameters that have to be optimized for each type of atom in the molecules present in the data base.[123]

6. Fourth-Generation Topological Indices

Fourth-generation TIs are those that include information on *stereochemical features* of molecules. Since a whole chapter of a recently published book was devoted to 3D molecular modeling,[18a] this section will be brief. This type of TIs is now being developed, and so far has achieved only limited success for diasteromers and enantiomers.[124-127]

Diastereomers may be modeled by geometrical distances (instead of topological ones) introduced into the distance matrix. This approach was championed by Randić and Razinger [124] (who first developed topographic indices using a notation similar to that employed earlier for the periphery codes of benzenoids [125]), by Pogliani (who described a *cis/trans* connectivity X_{ct} descriptor),[126] and by Xu et al.[127] Zefirov and his coworkers added interesting suggestions and comments to topographic indices.[128] However, a more elegant solution proposed by Lekishvili is the use of complex numbers which characterize a plane.[129] As a personal opinion, perhaps the use of quaternions would be indicated for 3D structures. A notation used in the enumeration of staggered alkane rotamers may be employed for characterizing acyclic and cyclic staggered conformations.[130]

Enantiomers are more difficult to be distinguished topologically, but progress has been made by Schultz [131] and by Galvez and his coworkers. [132]

Three-dimensional Wiener indices, introduced by Trinajstić and coworkers, are patterned after Wiener numbers, but the entries in the corresponding matrix are geometrical distances (in Ångstroms) between atoms i and j.[133]

7. Topological Indices: Intercorrelations and Physical Meaning

One should be aware that there are intercorrelations among TIs,[134-136] therefore one should either eliminate collinearly correlated TIs using the available statistical packages available for principal component analysis,[137] or one should use Randić's orthogonalization procedure for intercorrelated parameters.[138-140]

Basak and coworkers emphasized a four-step hierarchy in QSAR / QSPR approaches: the first rung of the ladder consists in topostructural information, next come topochemical features, and at the top levels one has geometrical and quantum-chemical data. Many physico-chemical properties can be correlated satisfactorily with the first two levels; for specific properties, however, it is necessary to include the next type(s) which involve more elaborate and time-consuming calculations, as well as more parameters (hence the experimental data base must be larger in order to accomodate these parameters for obtaining statistical significance).[141,142] In a study on clustering of TIs using a set of 139 hydrocarbons (alkanes, alkylbenzenes, polycyclic aromatics) and a set of 1037 diverse chemicals form the US EPA ASTER system, it was observed [143] that the first and main principal component includes TIs that are size-related (such as W, the lower connectivity indices, Zagreb indices, or triplet indices with Z or N on the main diagonal); the second cluster contains path connectivities of intermediate and longer order; in the next clusters, information content indices are grouped together, and J-type indices are also grouped together.

Reviews about TIs [144-149] emphasize the fact that although TIs do not have a precise physical meaning, they are measures for "topological shape" i. e. the degree of branching or cyclicity, and they correlate well with molecular volume or surface area. Some of the TIs have been designed to account for the flexibility and geometrical shape (Kier's ϕ and κ, respectively). Some other TIs can model infinite linear polymers with their electrical or thermal properties, as shown by Bonchev et al. (who used a normalized Wiener index for infinite graphs) and by Katritzky, as will be shown below.

Molecular shape is a vast topic, which has been addressed in several ways. Here only Mezey's approach, based on rigorous quantum-chemical calculations, will be mentioned.[18b,150]

8. Topological Indices in QSPR Studies

The great advantage of TIs is their ease of calculation for any imagined structure at low "c.p.u. cost". Many QSPR studies with TIs have been published, and they can be found in reviews [144-149] and in treatises on applications of chemical graph theory.[88] For facilitating the computation of TIs several commercially available programs such as CODESSA,[151-152] POLLY,[153] or MOLCONN are available.[154]

From all physical properties characterizing the 17 million substances indexed till now, the boiling point at normal pressure (NBP) for relatively small molecules has been the object of numerous QSPR studies because it presents a fairly regular dependence on structure: in the absence of hydrogen bonding, the NBP increases with molecular weight, and for equal molecular weights it decreases with increasing branching. From the very beginning, Wiener, Platt, Hosoya and other authors have tested the validity of their new TIs by using them for correlating alkane structures with their NBPs. Data bases for NBPs and other physical properties have been published by several authors in their QSPR studies.[155-157] Numerous publications for various alkanes (usually up to the decanes) report a standard deviation for the calculated NBPs of a few degrees,[155-158] and Randić's optimal descriptors even to 1-2 °C.[123]

For industrially important chemicals, TIs (sometimes together with other molecular descriptors) allow a satisfactory correlation with predictive capacity.[159-162] More interesting for organic and biochemical studies are molecules with various heteroatoms which also give good agreement with calculated NBPs when the appropriate descriptors are used: haloalkanes C_1 - C_4 among which the chlorofluorocarbons (CFCs), fluorocarbons, and hydrochlorofluorocarbons are the most important for the greenhouse effect and the depletion of the ozone layer (especially the CFCs);[163-166] acyclic [167,168] or cyclic molecules with oxygen and sulfur heteroatoms devoid of hydrogen bonds,[169] and various organic compounds such as carbonyl derivatives (esters, aldehydes, ketones).[170a] Interestingly, acyclic saturated and unsaturated mono- and di-nitriles also allow good QSPR correlations for their NBPs with one exception: the largest observed jump from one molecule to the next homolog occurs for the pair oxalonitrile (cyanogen) and malononitrile:[170b] the addition of a single methylene group increases the NBP from –22 °C to + 219 °C for these two homologs; the explanation resides in the linear structure of the former molecule with zero dipole moment, and in the V-shaped structure of the latter molecule with a dipole moment of 3.58 Debyes.

For a more general approach, correlations between alkane structure and critical data or vapor pressures allow a more comprehensive approach.[171-176] For instance, with calculated data for the parameters in the Antoine equation, one is able to predict the boiling point at any presure.[174]

A multitude of various physical properties can be satisfactorily described by TIs alone with linear, multilinear, or non-linear equations; such properties are: molar volume at 20 °C, heat of vaporization at 25 °C, critical pressure, surface tension at 20 °C, melting point, heat capacity, Gibbs energy, formation enthalpy, refractive index, and density.[155-157] Katritzky and coworkers published impressive correlations for empirical solvent polarity scales,[177] and for the glass transition temperature of polimers.[178] The aqueous solubility of organic compounds,[179-182] values of ^{13}C-NMR chemical shifts,[183] and even the melting points of substituted benzene derivatives [184] are amenable to such QSPR studies (melting points depend so much on geometry and intermolecular forces that they can be correlated with structure only in congeneric systems).

Artificial neural networks (ANNs) and genetic algorithms are often employed when the correlations are non-linear. Zefirov and his coworkers reported that one can sometimes use ANNs for direct predictions of properties.[185] Many other physico-chemical and biochemical data were correlated with computer programs which combine TIs with other descriptors, such as geometrical parameters obtained by molecular mechanics calculations, quantum-chemical data, numerical descriptors, and (as will be shown below in the case study for peptides) simple numerical descriptors. The most active groups that have developed such programs are headed by Katritzky (CODESSA program), Jurs, Basak (POLLY program), and Klopman (CASE program). The various properties can be found in the bibliography provided, which is detailed but still not exhaustive.

Among the chemical properties which are known to depend strongly on structure are the octane numbers of alkanes, cycloalkanes, alkenes, and aromatics.[186,187]

9. Topological Indices in Biological and Environmental QSAR Studies

Some of the first biological QSAR studies with TIs were reviewed extensively in the two books of Kier and Hall,[39,40] using mainly their generalized path/cluster/valence connectivity indices, and will not be repeated here. A few reviews describing biomedical QSAR studies have been published more recently.[188-191]

The presence of "bay regions" in polycyclic aromatic hydrocarbons such as benzo[a]pyrene is a necessary but insufficient condition for carcinogenic activity. A complete enumeration of such hydrocarbons can be accomplished with the aid of computer programs.[192,193] The book "Modeling of Cancer Genesis and Prevention" [193] and several studies on QSAR of retinoids and arotinoids contribute with further examples on using the weighted index J for correlating chemical structures with their anticancer activities.[194-196]

A few other QSAR studies using TIs will be mentioned: antileukemic compounds,[197] the aqueous solubility of drugs and their intestinal absorption,[198,199] the biological activity of benzamidines,[200] and the antimicrobial activity of a series of compounds.[201]

Closely related to bioactivity studies are QSAR data applied in environmental science. Only a few reviews[202,203a] and a book [203] dedicated to this topic will be mentioned, but several journals publish regularly QSAR applications of TIs in environmental problems: *SAR and QSAR in Environmental Research*, and *Environmental Toxicology and Chemistry.*

10. A Case Study of a Recent QSAR for Immunosuppressive Peptides

An eloquent example for the usefulness of TIs is provided by a recent report published by Lahana and his coworkers.[204] The bioactivity of the lead compound (an immunosuppressive peptide for skin and heart allograft survival in mice) was increased about 100 times by a computer-assisted design using 13 molecular descriptors. These descriptors were independent of three-dimensional factors and therefore were very fast to be computed. Four of these descriptors were TIs: three Kier-Hall indices (ϕ, $^2\kappa_\alpha$, and χ^v) and Balaban's J index. Other parameters were the calculated lipophilicity (log P), the ellipsoidal and molar volumes, the molar refractivity, and the dipole moment. The remaining four descriptors were simple numerical data for the numbers of atoms (oxygen, nitrogen) or groups (ethyl, hydroxyl). With 35 natural and non-natural aminoacids that could occupy the 7 positions of the relevant portion of the decapeptidic chain, the virtual combinatorial library would have numbered 64 billion structures; a first filter based on the lipophilicity reduced the number of aminoacids to six (one non-natural and five natural amino acids). All the resulting $6^7 \cong 280{,}000$ structures were calculated in order to ascertain whether their 13 descriptors fitted into the favorable domains previously determined from the learning set of about 20 active and inactive compounds. Only 26 peptides passed this test, i. e. one in about 10,000, and they were analyzed by molecular dynamics simulations in order to compare the similarity between their conformational space and that of the active peptides. The five peptides that passed this last filter were synthesized and tested *in vivo*; one of these was about 100 times more active than the best peptide known till then.

The conclusion that one may draw from this approach confirms Katritzky and Gordeeva's favorable assessment of the value of TIs used together with other descriptors for QSAR studies,[22] and contradicts criticisms about using TIs in QSAR. If TIs proved their utility for peptides whose stereochemistry is so important, then *a fortiori* they should work (together with other descriptors) for peptidomimetics or any other smaller molecules in drug design.

Another spectacular use of the J and χ indices was described by Colombian scientists: the secondary structure of transfer RNAs could be correlated with the biosynthetic amino acid pathways, confirming Wong's coevolution theory of the genetic code with the emergence of new amino acids in primitive living organisms.[205]

11. The Future of Topological Indices: A Personal Opinion

A revolution in experimental drug design has recently happened with the advent of combinatorial libraries that can be synthesized in thousands per day by means of robotics and tested by means of fluorescent, immunochemical and radioactive techniques. This high-throughput method is useful after a lead compound has been found, and one has to optimize its structure by systematic variation of substituents attached to the molecular scaffold. The optimization aims at maximizing the therapeutic ratio, i. e. at increasing the beneficial activity and decreasing the toxicity or other unwanted side-effects.

The preceding case study indicates that because of the combinatorial aspects involved in multiple substitution, a first screening of virtual combinatorial libraries is quite profitable in terms of reducing the number of substances to be prepared and tested. Because TIs can be computed for any imaginable structure in a very short time, they are bound to be used increasingly in the future, as in the case study examined in the preceding section. Of course, other molecular descriptors that are essential for defining the biological activity will probably have to be included.

12. References

1. Balaban, A. T., An Attempt for the Systematization of Monocyclic Aromatic Compounds (in Roumanian), *Studii si cercetari chim., Acad. R. P. Romania*, **1959**, *7*, 257-295.
2. Balaban, A. T.; Harary, F., Chemical Graphs. IV. Dihedral Groups and Monocyclic Aromatic Compounds, *Rev. Roum. Chim.*, **1967**, *12*, 1511-1515.
3. Balaban, A. T., Valence Isomerism of Cyclopolyenes (Chemical Graphs.I), *Rev. Roum. Chim.*, **1966**, *11*, 109-112; Idem, Chemical Graphs. VIII. Valence Isomerism and General Cubic Graphs, *ibid.*, **1970**, *15*, 463-485.
4. Balaban, A. T.; Banciu, M.; Ciorba, V., *Annulenes, Benzo-, Hetero-, Homo-Derivatives and Their Valence Isomers*, Boca Raton, Florida, 1986, vols. 1-3.
5. Harary, F.; Palmer, E. M., *Graphical Enumeration*, Academic Press, New York, **1973**, p. 174.
6. Balaban, A. T.; Vancea, R.; Motoc, I.; Holban, S., Chemical Graphs. 43. Fortran IV Program for Computing the Numbers of General Cubic Graphs on *p* Vertices, *J. Chem. Inf. Comput. Sci.* **1986**, *26*, 72-76.
7. Balaban, A. T., editor, *Chemical Applications of Graph Theory*, Academic Press, London, **1976**.
8. Balaban, A. T.; Farcasiu, D.; Banica, R., Chemical Graphs. II. Graphs of Multiple 1,2-Shifts in Carbonium Ions and Related Systems, *Rev. Roum. Chim.*, **1966**, *11*, 1205-1227.
9. Balaban, A. T., A Trivalent Graph of Girth Ten, *J. Comb. Theory*, **1972**, *12* **B**, 1-5.
10. Balaban, A. T., Trivalent Graphs of Girth Nine and Eleven, and Relationships Between Cages, *Rev. Roum. Math. Pures Appl.*, **1973**, *18*, 1033-1043.
11. Balaban, A.T.; Simon, Z., Aromaticity Constants, *Tetrahedron*, **1962**, *18*, 315-321.
12. Simon, Z.; Balaban, A. T., Relative Stability of Isomeric Aromatic Monocyclic Systems Appreciated by M.O. Methods, *Rev. Chim. Acad. Romania*, **1962**, *7*, 550-560; Idem, Energy Levels of Pyrylium Salts with *para*-Substituted Phenyl Groups, *ibid.*, **1964**, *9*, 339-349.
13. Balaban, A. T.; Simon, Z., Aromaticity. V. Stability of Monocyclic Aromatic Compounds, *Rev. Roum. Chim.*, **1965**, *10*, 1059-1092.
14. Simon, Z.; Chiriac, A.; Holban, S.; Ciubotariu, D.; Mihalas, G. I., *Minimum Steric Difference: the MTD Method for QSAR Studies*, Research Studies Press, Letchworth, and Wiley, New York, **1984**.
15. Chiriac, A.; Ciubotariu, D.; Simon, Z. editors, *QSAR-MTD Method*, Mirton Publ., Timisoara, 1996 (in Romanian).(a) Chapter 1 by Simon, Z.; Oprea, T., Receptor-Effector Interaction, pp. 1-15. (b) Chapter 7 by T. Oprea, 3D-QSAR, Theoretical Aspects of the CoMFA Method, pp. 221-231.
16. Balaban, A. T.; Chiriac, A.; Motoc, I.; Simon, Z., *Steric Fit in QSAR*, Lecture Notes in Chemistry No. 15, Springer, Berlin, **1980**.
17. Ivanciuc, O.; Balaban, A.T., Graph Theory in Chemistry, in *Encyclopedia of Computational Chemistry*, Schleyer, P. v. R.; Allinger, N. L.; Clark, T.; Gasteiger,

J.; Kollman, P. A.; Schaefer III, H. F.; Schreiner, P. R., editors, Wiley, Chichester, **1998**, pp. 1169-1190.

18. Balaban, A. T., editor, *From Chemical Topology to Three-Dimensional Geometry*, Plenum Publishing Corporation, New York,1997. (a) Chapter 1 by Balaban, A.T. From Chemical Graphs to 3D Molecular Modeling", pp. 1-24. (b) Chapter 2 by Mezey, P. G., Descriptors of Molecular Shape in 3D", pp. 25-42. (c) Chapter 3 by Mekenyan, O.; Veith, G. D., 3D Molecular Design: Search for Active Conformers in QSAR, pp. 43-72. (d) Chapter 4 by Basak, S. C.; Grunwald, G. D.; Niemi, G. J., Use of Graph-Theoretic and Geometric Molecular Descriptors in Structure-Activity Relationships, pp. 73-116. (e) Chapter 6 by Randić, M.; Razinger, M., On Characterization of 3D Molecular Structure, pp. 159-236.
19. Devillers, J.; Balaban, A. T., editors, *Topological Indices and Related Descriptors in QSAR and QSPR*, Gordon and Breach, Reading, UK, 1999. (a) Chapter 2 by Balaban, A. T.; Ivanciuc, O., Historical Development of Topological Indices; (b) Chapter 7 by Kier, L. H.; Hall, L. B., Molecular Connectivity Chi Indices for Database Analysis and Structure-Property Modeling; (c) Chapter 10 by Kier, L. H.; Hall, L. B., The Kappa Indices for Molecular Modeling of Molecular Shape and Flexibility; (d) Chapter 11 by Kier, L. H. Hall, L. B., The Electrotopological State: Structure Modeling for QSAR and Database Analysis; (e) Chapter 12 by Basak, S. C., Information-Theoretic Indices of Neighborhood Complexity and Their Application; (f) Chapter 12 by Devillers, J., Autocorrelation Descriptors for Modeling (Eco)Toxicological Endpoints; (g) Chapter 13 by Dubois, J. E.; Doucet, J. P.; Panaye, A.; Han, B. T., DARC Site Topological Correlations: Ordered Structural Descriptors and Property Evaluation; (h) Chapter 14 by Basak, S. C.; Gute, B. D.; Grunwald, G. D., A Hierarchical Approach to the Development of QSAR Models Using Topological, Geometrical and Quantum Chemical Parameters.
20. Diudea, M. V.; Ivanciuc, O., *Molecular Topology* (in Romanian language), Comprex Publ., Cluj, **1998**.
21. Balaban, A. T.; Brunvoll, J.; Cioslowski, J.; Cyvin, B. N.; Cyvin, S. J.; Gutman, I.; He Wenchen; He Wenjie; Knop, J.V.; Kovacevic, M.; Müller, W.R.; Szymanski, K.; Tosic, R.; Trinajstić, N., Enumeration of benzenoid and coronoid hydrocarbons, *Z. Naturforsch.*, **1987**, *42c*, 863-870.
22. Katritzky, A. R.; Gordeeva, E. V., Traditional Topological Indices *vs.* Electronic, Geometrical and Combined Molecular Descriptors in QSAR/QSPR Research, *J. Chem. Inf. Comput. Sci.*, **1993**, *33*, 835-857.
23. Hansch, C.; Sammes, P. G.; Taylor, J. B., editors, *Comprehensive Medicinal Chemistry*. Ramsden, C. A., editor of vol. 4, *Quantitative Drug Design*, Pergamon Press, Oxford, 1990. (a) Chapter 18.6 by Taylor, P. J., Hydrophobic Properties of Drugs, pp. 241-290. (b) Chapter 18.7 by Leo, A. J., Methods of Calculating Partition Coefficients, pp. 295-320. (c) Chapter 21.1 by Fujita, T., The Extrathermodynamic Approach to Drug Design, pp. 497-560.
24. Hansch, C.; Leo, A., *Exploring QSAR: Fundamentals and Applications in Chemistry and Biology*, ACS Professional Reference Book, Am. Chem. Soc., Washington, DC, 1995; Hansch, C.; Leo, A.; Hoekman, D., *Exploring QSAR: Hydrophobic,*

Electronic, and Steric Constants, ACS Professional Reference Book, Am. Chem. Soc., Washington, DC, 1995; Hansch, C.; Fujita, T., editors, *Classical and Three-Dimensional QSAR in Agrochemistry*, Am. Chem. Soc., Washington, DC, 1995.
25. Hansch, C.; Maloney, P. P.; Fujita, T.; Muir, R. M., Correlation of Biological Activity of Phenoxyacetic Acids with Hammett Substituent Constants and Partition Coefficients, *Nature*, **1962**, *194*, 178-180.
26. Fujita, T.; Iwasa, J.; Hansch, C., A New Substituent Constant, pi, Derived from Partition Coefficients, *J. Am. Chem. Soc.* **1964**, *86*, 5175-5179; Hansch, C.; Clayton, J. M., Lipophilic Character and Biological Activity of Drugs. II. The Parabolic Case, *J. Pharm. Sci.* **1973**, *62*, 1-21.
27. Balaban, A. T.; Harary, F., The Characteristic Polynomial Does Not Uniquely Determine the Topology of a Molecule, *J. Chem. Doc.* **1971**, *11*, 258-259.
28. Herndon, W. C., The Characteristic Polynominal Does Not Uniquely Determine Molecular Topology, *J. Chem. Doc.* **1974**, *14*, 150-151.
29. Ivanciuc, O.; Balaban, A.T., Design of Topological Indices. Part 8. Path Matrices and Derived Molecular Graph Invariants, *Math. Chem. (MATCH),* **1994**, *30*, 141-152.
30. Amić, D.; Trinajstić, N., On the Detour Matrix, *Croat. Chem. Acta*, **1995**, *68*, 53-62.
31. Lukovits, I., The Detour Index, *Croat. Chem. Acta*, **1996**, *69*, 873-882; Lukovits, I.; Razinger, M., On the Calculation of the Detour Index, *J. Chem. Inf. Comput. Sci.* **1997**, *37*, 283-286.
32. Trinajstić, N.; Nikolić, S.; Lucic, B.; Amić, D.; Mihalić, Z., The Detour Matrix in Chemistry, *J. Chem. Inf. Comput. Sci.* **1997**, *37*, 631-638.
33. Rücker, G.; Rücker, C. Symmetry-Aided Computation of the Detour matrix and the Detour Index. *J. Chem. Inf. Comput. Sci*, **1998**, *38*, 710-714.
34. Nikolić, S.; Trinajstić, N.; Mihalić, Z., The Wiener Index: Development and Applications, *Croat. Chem. Acta*, **1995**, *68*, 105-129.
35. Zhu, H.; Klein, D. J.; Lukovits, I., Extensions of the Wiener Number, *J. Chem. Inf. Comput. Sci.* **1996**, *36*, 420-428.
36. Nikolić, S.; Trinajstić, N.; Juric, A.; Mihalić, Z., The Detour Matrix and the Detour Index of Weighted Graphs, *Croat. Chem. Acta*, **1996**, *69*,1577-1591.
37. Balaban, A. T.; Mills, D.; Basak, S. C., Reverse Wiener Indices, *Croat. Chim. Acta,* in press.
38. Balaban, A. T., Using Real Numbers as Vertex Invariants for Third-Generation Topological Indices, *J. Chem. Inf. Comput. Sci.* **1992**, *32*, 23-28; Idem, Local vs. Global (i. e. Atomic vs. Molecular) Numerical Modeling of Molecular Graphs, *ibid.*, **1994**, *34*, 398-402; Idem, Real-Numbe Local (Atomic) Invariants and Global (Molecular) Topological Indices, *Rev. Roum. Chim.*, **1994**, *39*, 245-257.
39. Wiener, H., Structural Determination of Paraffin Boiling Points, *J. Am. Chem. Soc.* **1947**, *69*, 17-20.
40. Platt, J. R., Prediction of Isomeric Differences in Paraffin Properties, *J. Phys. Chem.* **1952**, *56*, 328-336.
41. Hosoya, H., Topological Index. A Newly Proposed Quantity Characterizing the Topological Nature of Structural Isomers of Saturated Hydrocarbons. *Bull. Chem.*

Soc. Jpn., **1971**, *44*, 2332-2339; Hosoya, H.; Gotoh, M.; Murakami, M.; Ikeda, S., Topological Index and Thermodynamic Properties. Part 5. How Can We Explain the Topological Dependency of Thermodynamic Properties of Alkanes with the Topology of Graphs ? *J. Chem. Inf. Comput. Sci.* **1999**, *39,* 192-196.

42. Randić, M.; Guo, X.; Oxley, T.; Krishnapriyan, H. J., Wiener Matrix: Source of Novel Graph Invariants, *J. Chem. Inf. Comput. Sci.* **1993**, *34*, 709-716.
43. Dobrynin, A. A., New Congruence Relations for the Wiener Index of Cata-Condensed Benzenoid Hydrocarbons, *J. Chem. Inf. Comput. Sci.* **1998**, *38,* 405-409.
44. Chepoi, V.; Klavzar, S., The Wiener Index and the Szeged Index of Benzenoid Systems in Linear Time, *J. Chem. Inf. Comput. Sci.* **1997**, *37,* 752-755.
45. Bonchev, D.; Mekenyan, O., A Topological Approach to the Calculation of the π-Electron Energy and Energy Gap of Infinite Conjugated Polymers, *Z. Naturforsch.*, **1980**, *35a*, 739-747.
46. Bonchev, D.; Mekenyan, O.; Polansky, O. E., A Topological Approach to the Predicting of the Electron Energy Characteristics of Conjugated Infinite Polymers. II. PPP-Calculations, *Z. Naturforsch.*, **1981**, *36a*, 643-646.
47. Balaban, T. S.; Balaban, A. T.; Bonchev, D., A Topological Approach to the Predicting of the Electron Energy Characteristics of Infinite Polymers. VI. Rational Formulas for the Normalized Wiener Index and a Comparison with Index J (to be published).
48. Chan, O.; Lam, T. K.; Merris, R., Wiener Number as an Immanant of the Laplacian of Molecular Graphs, *J. Chem. Inf. Comput. Sci.* **1997**, *37,* 762-765.
49. Gordon, M.; Scantlebury, G. R., Nonrandom Polycondensation: Statistical Theory of the Substitution Effect, *Trans. Faraday Soc.*, **1964**, *60*, 604-621.
50. Gutman, I.; Ruscic, B.; Trinajstić, N.; Wilcox, Jr., C. F., Graph Theory and Molecular Orbitals. XII. Acyclic Polyenes, *J. Chem. Phys.* **1975**, *62*, 3399-3405.
51. Balaban, A. T., Chemical Graphs. Part 35. Five New Topological Indices for the Branching of Tree-Like Graphs, *Theor. Chim. Acta*, **1979**, *5*, 239-261.
52. Bonchev, D.; Balaban, A. T.; Mekenyan, O., Generalization of the Graph Centre Concept and Derived Topological Indices, *J. Chem. Inf. Comput. Sci.* **1980**, *20*, 196-213 .
53. Balaban, A. T.; Bertelsen, S.; Basak, S. C., New Centric Topological Indexes for Acyclic Molecules (Trees) and Substituents (Rooted Trees), and Coding of Rooted Trees, *Math. Chem. (MATCH),* **1994**, *30*, 55-72.
54. Schultz, H. P., Topological Organic Chemistry. Part 1. Graph Theory and Topological Indices of Alkanes, *J. Chem. Inf. Comput. Sci.* **1989**, *29*, 227-228.
55. Schultz, H. P.; Schultz, E. B.; Schultz, T. P., Topological Organic Chemistry. Part 2. Graph Theory, Matrix Determinants and Eigenvalues, and Topological Indices of Alkanes, *J. Chem. Inf. Comput. Sci.* **1990**, *30*, 27-29.
56. Gutman, I., A Formula for the Wiener Number of Trees and Its Extension to Graphs Containing Cycles, *Graph Theory Notes New York*, **1994**, *27*, 9-15.
57. Klavzar, S.; Gutman, I., A Comparison of the Schultz Molecular Topological Index with the Wiener Index, *J. Chem. Inf. Comput. Sci.* **1996**, *36*, 1001-1003.

58. Khadikar, P. V.; Deshpande , N. V.; Kale, P. P.; Dobrynin, A.; Gutman, I.; Dömöter, G., The Szeged Index and an Analogy with the Wiener Index, *J. Chem. Inf. Comput. Sci.* **1995**, *35*, 547.
59. Klavzar, S.; Gutman, I., An Algorithm for the Calculation of the Szeged Index of Benzenoid Hydrocarbons, *J. Chem. Inf. Comput. Sci.* **1995**, *35*, 1011-1014.
60. Randić, M., Novel Molecular Description for Structure-Property Studies, *Chem. Phys. Lett.*, **1993**, *211*, 478-483.
61. Lukovits, I.; Linert, W., A Novel Definition of the Hyper-Wiener Index for Cycles, *J. Chem. Inf. Comput. Sci.* **1994**, *34*, 899-902.
62. Klein, D. J.; Lukovits, I.; Gutman, I., On the Definition of the Hyper-Wiener Index for Cycle-Containing Structures, *J. Chem. Inf. Comput. Sci.* **1995**, *35,* 50-52.
63. Rücker, G; Rücker, C., Counts of All Walks as Atomic and Molecular Descriptors, *J. Chem. Inf. Comput. Sci.* **1993**, *33*, 683-695.
64. Randić, M., On Characterization of Molecular Branching, *J. Am. Chem. Soc.* **1975**, *97*, 6609-6615.
65. Kier, L. B.; Hall, L. H.; Murrray, W. J.; Randić, M., Molecular Connectivity. Part 1. Relationship to Nonspecific Local Anesthesia, *J. Pharm. Sci.*, **1975**, *64*, 1971-1974; Kier, L. B.; Murrray, W. J.; Randić, M.; Hall, L. H., Molecular Connectivity. Part 5. Connectivity Series Concept Applied to Density, *J. Pharm. Sci.*, **1976**, *65*, 1226-1230.
66. Kier, L. B.; Hall L. H., *Molecular Connectivity in Chemistry and Drug Research*, Academic Press, New York, 1976.
67. Kier, L. B.; Hall L. H., *Molecular Connectivity in Structure-Activity Studies*, Research Studies Press, Letchworth, **1986**.
68. Kier, L. B.; Hall L. H., *The Electrotopological State*, Academic Press, New York, **1999**.
69. Hall, L. H.; Kier, L. B., Electrotopological State Indices for Atom Types: A Novel Combination of Electronic, Topological, and Valence State Information. *J. Chem. Inf. Comput. Sci.*, **1995**, *35*, 1039-1045.
70. Kier, L. B.; Hall L. H., Molecular Connectivity. Part 7. Specific Treatment of Heteroatoms, *J. Pharm. Sci.* **1976**, *65*, 1806-1809.
71. Kier, L. B., A Shape Index from Molecular Graphs, *Quant. Struct. Act. Relat.* **1985**, *4*, 109-116.
72. Kier, L. B., An Index of Molecular Flexibility from Kappa Shape Attributes. *Quant. Struct.-Act. Relat.* **1989**, *8*, 221-224.
73. Balaban, A. T., Topological Indices Based on Topological Distances in Molecular Graphs, *Pure Appl. Chem.* **1983**, *55*, 199-206.
74. Zefirov, N. S.; Palyulin, V. A.; Radchenko, Yu. V. Problem of Generation of Structures with Given Properties - Solution of the Inverse Problem for the Case of the Centric Balaban Index, *Dokl. Akad. Nauk SSSR*, **1991**, *316*, 921-924.
75. Skvortseva, M. I.; Baskin, I. I.; Slovokhovotova, O. L.; Palyulin, V. A.; Zefirov, N. S., Inverse Problem in QSAR/QSPR Indices for the Case of Topological Indices Characterizing Molecular Shape (Kier Indices), *J. Chem. Inf. Comput. Sci.* **1993**, *33*, 630-634.

76. Balaban, A. T., Highly Discriminating Distance-Based Topological Index, *Chem. Phys. Lett.* **1982**, *80*, 399-404.
77. Balaban, A. T.; Ionescu-Pallas, N; Balaban, T. S., Asymptotic Values of Topological Indices J and J' (Average Distance Sum Connectivities) for Infinite Acyclic and Cyclic Graphs, *Math. Chem. (MATCH),* **1985**, *17*, 121-146.
78. Balaban, A. T.; Quintas, L. V., The Smallest Graphs, Trees, and 4-Trees, with degenerate Topological Index J, *Math. Chem. (MATCH),* **1983**, *14*, 213-233.
79. Balaban, A. T., Chemical Graphs. Part 48. Topological Index J for Heteroatom-Containing Molecules Taking into Account Periodicities of Element Properties, *Math. Chem. (MATCH),* **1986**, *21*, 115-122.
80. Ivanciuc, O; Ivanciuc, T.; Balaban, A. T., Design of Topological Indices. Part 10. Parameters Based on Electronegativity and Covalent Radius for the Computation of Molecular Graph Descriptors for Heteroatom-Containing Molecules. *J. Chem. Inf. Comput. Sci.,* **1998**, *38*, 395-401.
81. Balaban, A. T.; Filip, P., Computer Program for Topological Index J (Average Distance Sum Connectivity), *Math. Chem. (MATCH),* **1984**,*16,* 163-190.
82. Klein, D. J.; Randić, M., Resistance Distance, *J. Math. Chem.*, **1993**, *12*, 81-95.
83. Bonchev, D.; Balaban, A. T.; Liu, X.; Klein, D. J., Molecular Cyclicity and Centricity of Polycyclic Graphs. Part 1. Cyclicity Based on Resistance Distances and Reciprocal Distances, *Int. J. Quantum Chem.*, **1994**, *50*, 1-20.
84. Ivanciuc, O.; Balaban, T. S.; Balaban, A. T., Design of Topological Indices. Part 4. Reciprocal Distance Matrix, Related Local Vertex Invariants and Topological Indices, *J. Math. Chem.* **1993**, *12*, 309-318.
85. Plavšić, D.; Nikolić, S.; Trinajstić, N.; Mihalić, Z., On the Harary Index for Characterization of Chemical Graphs, *J. Math. Chem.* **1993**, *12*, 235-250.
86. Bonchev, D.; Trinajstić, N., Information Theory, Distance Matrices, and Molecular Branching, *J. Chem. Phys.*, **1977**, *67*, 4517-4533.
87. Bonchev, D., *Information-Theoretic Indices for Characterization of Chemical Structure*, Research Studies Press, Letchworth, **1993**.
88. Trinajstić, N., *Chemical Graph Theory*, 2nd Ed., CRC Press, Boca Raton, Florida, 1992, pp. 225-273.
89. Basak, S. C., Use of Molecular Complexity Indices in Predictive Pharmacology and Toxicology, *Med. Sci. Res.*, **1967**, *15*, 605.
90. Basak, S. C.; Magnuson, V. R., Determining Structural Similarity of Chemicals Using Graph-Theoretic Indices, *Discrete Appl. Math.* **1988**, *19*, 17-44.
91. Raychaudhury, C.; Ray, S. K.; Roy, A. B.; Ghosh, J. J.; Basak, S. C., Discrimination of Isomeric Structures Using Information Theoretic Topological Indices, *J. Comput. Chem.*, **1984**, *5*, 581-588.
92. Konstantinova, E. V., The Discrimination Ability of Some Topological and Information Distance Indices for Graphs of Unbranched Hexagonal Systems, *J. Chem. Inf. Comput. Sci.* **1996**, *36,* 54-57.
93. Gupta, S; Singh, M; Madan, A.K., Superpendentic Index: A Novel Topological Descriptor for Predicting Biological Activity, *J. Chem. Inf. Comput. Sci.* **1998**, *38,* 450-456.

94. Bertz, S. H., The Bond Graph, *J. Chem. Soc. Chem. Commun.*, **1981**, 818-820.
95. Bertz, S. H., Branching in Graphs and Molecules, *Discr. Appl. Math.* **1988**, *19*, 65-83 (reprinted in *Applications of Graphs in Chemistry and Physics*, eds. Kennedy, J. W.; Quintas, L. V.), North-Holland, Amsterdam, **1988**, pp. 65-83).
96. Estrada, E., Edge Adjacency Relationships and a Novel Topological Index Related to Molecular Volume, *J. Chem. Inf. Comput. Sci.*, **1995**, *35*, 31-33; Idem, Edge Adjacency Relationships in Molecular Graphs Containing Heteroatoms; a New Topological Index Related to Molecular Volume, *J. Chem. Inf. Comput. Sci.*, **1995**, *35*, 701-707.
97. Gutman, I.; Estrada, E., Topological Indices Based on the Line Graph of the Molecular Graph, *J. Chem. Inf. Comput. Sci.*, **1996**, *36*, 541-543; Estrada, E.; Gutman, I., A Topological Index Based on Distances of Edges of Molecular Graphs, *J. Chem. Inf. Comput. Sci.*, **1996**, *36*, 850-853; Estrada, E.; Guevara, N.; Gutman, I., Extension of Edge Connectivity Index. relationships to Line Graph Indices and QSPR Applications, *J. Chem. Inf. Comput. Sci.*, **1998**, *38*, 428-431.
98. Filip, P. A.; Balaban, T. S.; Balaban, A. T., A New Approach for Devising Local Graph Invariants: Derived Topological Indices with Low Degeneracy and Good Correlational Ability, *J. Math. Chem.* **1987**, *1*, 61-83.
99. Balaban, A. T.; Balaban, T. S., New Vertex Invariants and Topological Indices of Chemical Graphs Based on Information on Distances, *J. Math. Chem.* **1991**, *8*, 383-397.
100. Diudea, M. V., Indices of Reciprocal Property or Harary Indices, *J. Chem. Inf. Comput. Sci.* **1997**, *37*, 292-299.
101. Diudea, M. V., Layer Matrices in Molecular Graphs, *J. Chem. Inf. Comput. Sci.* **1994**, *34*, 1064-1071.
102. Diudea, M. V.; Minailiuc, O.; Balaban, A. T., Molecular Topology. Part 4. Regessive Vertex Degrees (New Graph Invariants) and Derived Topological Indices, *J. Comput. Chem.* **1991**, *12*, 527-535.
103. Balaban, A. T.; Diudea, M. V., Real Number Vertex Invariants: Regressive Distance Sums and Related Topological Indices, *J. Chem. Inf. Comput. Sci.* **1993**, *33*, 421-428.
104. Diudea, M. V., Wiener and Hyper-Wiener Numbers in a Single Matrix, *J. Chem. Inf. Comput. Sci.* **1996**, *36*, 535-540.
105. Diudea, M. V.; Randić, M., Matrix Operator, W(M_1, M_2, M_3), and Schultz-Type Indices, *J. Chem. Inf. Comput. Sci.* **1997**, *37*, 1095-1100.
106. Diudea, M., Wiener Matrix of Dendrimers, *Math. Chem. (MATCH),* **1995**, *32*, 71-83.
107. Diudea, M.; Parv, B., Molecular Topology. Part 25. Hyper-Wiener Index of Dendrimers, *J. Chem. Inf. Comput. Sci.* **1995**, *35*, 1015-1018.
108. Lovasz, L.; Pelikan, J., On the Eigenvalues of Trees, *Period. Math. Hung.*, **1973**, *3*, 175-182.
109. Balaban, A. T.; Ciubotariu, D.; Medeleanu, M., Topological Indices and Real Vertex Invariants Based on Graph Eigenvalues or Eigenvectors, *J. Chem. Inf. Comput. Sci.* **1991**, *31*, 517-523.

110. Gutman, I.; Markovic, S., Benzenoid Graphs with Maximum Eigenvalues, *J. Math. Chem.*, **1993**, *13*, 213-215.
111. Medeleanu, M.; Balaban, A. T., Real-Number Vertex Invariants and Schultz-Type Indices Based on Eigenvectors of Adjacency and Distance Matrices, *J. Chem. Inf. Comput. Sci.* **1998**, *38*, 1038-1047.
112. Burden, F. R., Molecular Identification Number for Substructure Searches, *J. Chem. Inf. Comput. Sci.* **1989**, *29*, 225-227.
113. Galvez, J.; Garcia, R.; Salabert, M. T.; Soler, R., Charge Indexes. New Topological Descriptors. *J. Chem. Inf. Comput. Sci.*, **1994**, *34*, 520-525.
114. Diudea, M. V.; Horvath, D.; Graovac, A., Molecular Topology. Part 15. 3D Distance Matrices and Related Topological Indices, *J. Chem. Inf. Comput. Sci.* **1995**, *35*, 129-135.
115. Diudea, M. V.; Parv, B.; Gutman, I., Detour-Cluj Matrix and Derived Graph Invariants, *J. Chem. Inf. Comput. Sci.* **1997**, *37*, 1101-1108.
116. Diudea, M. V., Cluj Matrix Cj_u: Source of Various Graph Descriptors. *Math. Chem. (MATCH),* **1997**, *35*, 169-183; Cluj Matrix Invariants, *J. Chem. Inf. Comput. Sci.* **1997**, *37*, 300-305.
117. Diudea, M. V.; Gutman, I. Wiener-Type Topological Indices. *Croat.Chem.Acta.* **1998**, *71*, 21-51.
118. Hu, C.; Xu, L., On Highly Discriminating Molecular Topological Index, *J. Chem. Inf. Comput. Sci.* **1996**, *36*, 82-90.
119. Hall, L. H.; Kier, L. B., Determination of Topological Equivalence in Molecular Graphs from the Topological State, *Quant. Struct.-Act. Relat.*, **1990**, *9*, 115-131.
120. Hu, C.; Xu, L., On Hall and Kier's Topological State and Total Topological Index, *J. Chem. Inf. Comput. Sci.* **1994**, *34*, 1251-1258.
121. Ivanciuc, O.; Ivanciuc, T.; Cabrol-Bass, D.; Balaban, A. T., Investigation of Alkane Branching (and Resulting Partial Ordering) with Topological Indices. *Commun. Math. Comput. Chem. (Match),* **2000**, *42*, 155-180.
122. Randić, M.; Hansen, P.J.; Jurs, P.C., Search for Useful Graph Tehoretical Invariants of Molecular Structure, *J. Chem. Inf. Comput. Sci.* **1991**, *28*, 60-68.
123. Randić, M.; Basak, S. C., Optimal Molecular Descriptors Based on Weighted Path Numbers, *J. Chem. Inf. Comput. Sci.* **1999**, *39*, 261-266.
124. Randić, M.; Razinger, M., Molecular Topographic Indices, *J. Chem. Inf. Comput. Sci.* **1995**, *35*, 140-147.
125. Balaban, A. T., Chemical Graphs. Part 12. Configurations of Annulenes, *Tetrahedron,* **1971**, *7*, 6115-6131.
126. Pogliani, L., On a Graph-Theoretical Characterization of cis/trans Isomers, *J. Chem. Inf. Comput. Sci.* **1994**, *34*, 801-804.
127. Xu, L.; Wang, H. Y.; Su, Q., A Newly Proposed Topological Index for Discrimination of Cis/Trans Isomers. *Comput. Chem.*, **1992**, *16*, 187.
128. Zefirov, N. S.; Tratch, S. S., Sme Notes on Randić -Razinger's Approach to Characterization of Molecular Shapes, *J. Chem. Inf. Comput. Sci.* **1997**, *37*, 900-912
129. Lekishvili, G., On the Characterization of Molecular Stereostructure: 1. Cis-Trans Isomerism, *J. Chem. Inf. Comput. Sci.*, **1997**, *37*, 924-928.

130. Balaban, A. T., Chemical Graphs. Part 27. Enumeration and Codification of Staggered Conformations of Alkanes. *Rev. Roum. Chim.*, **1976**, *21*, 1049-1071.
131. Schultz, H. P.; Schultz, E. B.; Schultz, T. P., Topological Organic Chemistry. Part 9. Graph Theory and Molecular Topological Indices of Stereoisomeric Organic Compounds, *J. Chem. Inf. Comput. Sci.* **1991**, *35*, 864-870.
132. Julian-Ortiz, J. V.; Alapent, C. G.; Rios-Santaorina, I.; Garcia-Domenech, R., *J.* Galvez, Prediction of Properties of Chiral Compounds by Molecular Topology, J. *Molec. Graph. Model.* **1998**, *16*, 14-18.
133. Bogdanov, B.; Nikolić, S.; Trinajstić, N., On the Three-Dimensional Wiener Number, *J. Math. Chem.*, **1989**, *3*, 299-309; Idem, On the Three-Dimensional Wiener Number: A Comment, *ibid.*, **1990**, *5*, 305-306.
134. Motoc, I.; Balaban, A. T., Topological Indices: Intercorrrelations, Physical Meaning, Correlational Ability, *Rev. Roum. Chim.* **1981**, 26, 593-600.
135. Motoc, I.; Balaban, A. T.; Mekenyan, O.; Bonchev, D., Topological Indices: Inter-Relations and Composition, *Math. Chem. (MATCH),* **1982**,13, 369-404.
136. Pogliani, L., From Molecular Connectivity Indices to Semiempirical Connectivity Terms: Recent Trends in Graph Theoretical Descriptors, **Chem. Rev. 2000**, *100*, 3827-3858.
137. "SAS/STAT User's Guide", Release 6.03 edition (1988). SAS Institute, Inc., Box 8000, Cary, NC 27511.
138. Randić, M., Orthogonal Molecular Descriptors, *New J. Chem.* **1991**, *15*, 517-525; Idem, Resolution of Ambiguities in Structure-Property Studies by the Use of Orthogonal Molecular Descriptors, *J. Chem. Inf. Comput. Sci.* **1991**, *31*,311-320.
139. Amić, D.; Davidovic- Amić, D.; Trinajstić, N., Calculation of Retention Times of Anthocyanins with Orthogonalized Topological Indices, *J. Chem. Inf. Comput. Sci.* **1995**, *35*,136-139.
140. Šoškić, M.; Plavšić, D.; Trinajstić, N., 2-Difluoromethylthio-4,6-bis(monoalkyl-amino)-1,3,5-triazines as Inhibitors of Hill Reaction: A QSAR Study with Orthogonal Descriptors, *J. Chem. Inf. Comput. Sci.* **1996**, *36,* 146-150.
141. Basak, S. C.; Gute, B. D.; Grunwald, G. D. Use of Topostructural, Topochemical, and Geometric Parameters in the Prediction of Vapor Pressure: A Hierarchical QSAR Approach, *J. Chem. Inf. Comput. Sci.* **1997**, *37*, 651-655.
142. Basak, S. C., Magnuson, V. R., Niemi, G. J., Regal, R. R., Determining Structural Similarity of Chemicals Using Graph-Theoretic Indices, *Discrete Appl. Math.* **1988**, *19*, 17-44.
143. Basak, S.; Balaban, A.T.; Grunwald, G. D.; Gute, B. D., Topological Indices: Their Nature and Mutual Relatedness, *J. Chem. Inf. Comput. Sci.* **2000**, *40*, 891-898.
144. Balaban, A. T.; Motoc, I.; Bonchev, D.; Mekenyan, O., Topological Indices for Structure-Activity Correlations, in *Steric Effects in Drug Design*, editors Charton, M.; Motoc, I., *Top. Curr. Chem.* **1983**, *114*, 21-55.
145. Randić, M., Topological Indices, in *Encyclopedia of Computational Chemistry*, Schleyer, P. v. R.; Allinger, N. L.; Clark, T.; Gasteiger, J.; Kollman, P. A.; Schaefer III, H. F.; Schreiner, P. R., editors, Wiley, Chichester, **1998**, pp. 3018-3032.

146. Rouvray, D. H., Search for Useful Topological Indexes in Chemistry, *Am. Sci.* **1973**, *61*, 729-735; Idem, Uses of Graph Theory, *Chem. Brit.*, **1974**, *10*, 11-15; Idem, Should We Have Designs of Topological Indexes ? in *Chemical Applications of Topology and Graph Theory*, ed. King, R. B. (*Stud. Phys. Theor. Org. Chem.* **1983**, *28*, 159-177), Elsevier, Amsterdam.
147. Stankevich, M. I.; Stankevich, I. V.; Zefirov, N. S., Topological Indexes in Organic Chemistry, *Usp. Khim.*, **1988**, *57*, 337-366; *Russ. Chem. Rev. (Engl. Transl.)*, **1988**, *57*, 191-208; Baskin, I. I.; Skvortsova, M. I.; Stankevich, I. V.; Zefirov, N. S., On Basis of Invariants of Labeled Molecular Graphs, *J. Chem. Inf. Comput. Sci.*, **1995**, *35*, 527-531.
148. Randić, M., On Characterization of Chemical Structure, *J. Chem. Inf. Comput. Sci.* **1997**, *37*, 672-687; Idem, On Characterization of Cyclic Structures, *ibid.*, 1063-1071.
149. Randić, M.; Hansen, P. J.; Jurs, P. C., Search for Useful Graph Theoretical Invariants of Molecular Structure, *J. Chem. Inf. Comput. Sci.* **1988**, *28*, 60-68.
150. Mezey, P., *Shape in Chemistry: An Introduction to Molecular Shape and Topology*, VCH Publishers, New York, **1993**.
151. Katritzky, A. R.; Lobanov, V. S.; Karelson, M., *CODESSA Manual*, University of Florida: Gainesville, Fl, **1995**.
152. Karelson, M.; Lobanov, V. S.; Katritzky, A. R., Quantum-Chemical Descriptors in QSAR/QSPR Study, *Chem. Rev.* **1996**, *96*, 1027-1043.
153. Basak, S. C.; Harris, D. K.; Magnuson, V. R., *POLLY 2.3* (Copyright of the University of Minnesota, **1988**).
154. Hall, L. H., *MOLCONN and MOLCONN2*, Hall Associates Consulting, 2 Davis Street, Quincy, MA 02170.
155. Seybold, P. G.; May, M.; Bagal, U. A., Molecular Structure-Property Relationships, *J. Chem. Educ.,* **1987**, *64*, 575-581.
156. Needham, D. E.; Wei, I.; Seybold, P. G., Molecular Modeling of the Physical Properties of Alkanes, *J. Am. Chem. Soc.*, **1988**, *110*, 4186-4194.
157. Gakh, A. A.; Gakh, E. G.; Sumpter, B. G.; Noid, D. W. Neural Network-Graph Theory Approach to the Prediction of the Physical Properties of Organic Compounds. *J. Chem. Inf. Comput. Sci.*, **1994**, *34*, 832-839.
158. Liu, S; Cao, C.; Li, Z., Approach to Estimation and Prediction for Normal Boiling Point (NBP) of Alkanes Based on a Novel Molecular Distance-Edge (MDE) Vector. *J. Chem. Inf. Comput. Sci.*, **1998**, *38*, 387-394.
159. Egolf, L. M.; Wessel, M. D.; Jurs, P. C., Prediction of Boiling Points and Critical Temperatures of Industrially Important Organic Compounds from Molecular Structure, *J.Chem. Inf. Comput. Sci.* **1994**, *38*, 639-645.
160. Wessel, M. D.; Jurs, P. C., Prediction of Bormal Boiling Points for a Diverse Set of Industrially Important Organic Compounds from Molecular Structure, *J. Chem. Inf. Comput. Sci.* **1995**, *35*, 841-850.
161. Katritzky, A. R.; Mu, L.; Lobanov, V. S.; Karelson, M. Correlation of Boiling Points with Molecular Structure. 1. A Training Set of 298 Diverse Organics and a Test Set of 9 Simple Organics. *J. Phys. Chem.* **1996**, *100*, 10400-10407.

162. Katritzky, A. R.; Lobanov, V. S.; Karelson, M. Normal Boiling Points for Organic Compounds: Correlation and Prediction by a Quantitative Structure-Property Relationship. *J. Chem. Inf. Comput. Sci.* **1998**, *38*, 28-41.
163. Balaban, A. T.; Kier, L. B.; Joshi, N., Correlations between Chemical Structure and Normal Boiling Points of Halogenated Alkanes C_1 - C_4. *J. Chem. Inf. Comput. Sci.* **1992**, *32*, 233-237.
164. Balaban, A. T.; Basak, S. C.; Colburn, T.; Grunwald, G. D. Correlation between Structure and Normal Boiling Points of Haloalkanes C_1 - C_4 Using Neural Networks. *J. Chem. Inf. Comput. Sci.* **1994**, *34*, 1118-1121.
165. Murray, J. S.; Lane, P; Politzer, P. Special Relationships of Fluorinated Methane / Ethane Boiling Points and Heats of Vaporization to Molecular Properties. *Theochem.*, **1995**, *342*, 15-21.
166. Gakh, A. A.; Gakh, E. G.; Sumpter, B. G.; Noid, D. W.; Trowbridge, L. D., Estimation of the Properties of Hydrofluorocarbons by Computer Neural Networks, *J. Fluorine Chem.*, **1995**, *73*, 107-111.
167. Balaban, A. T.; Joshi, N.; Kier, L. B.; Hall, L. H. Correlations between Chemical Structure and Normal Boiling Points of Acyclic Ethers, Peroxides, Acetals, and Their Sulfur Analogues. *J. Chem. Inf. Comput. Sci.* **1992**, *32*, 237-244.
168. Ivanciuc, O.; Ivanciuc, T.; Balaban, A. T., Quantitative Structure-Property Relationship Study of Normal Boiling Points for Halogen-/Oxygen-/Sulfur-Containing Organic Compounds Using the CODESSA Program, *Tetrahedron*, **1998**, *54*, 9129-9142.
169. Stanton, D. T.; Jurs, P. C., Computer Assisted Prediction of Normal Boiling Points of Furans, Tetrahydrofurans, and Thiophenes. *J. Chem. Inf. Comput. Sci.* **1991**, *31*, 301-310.
170. (a) Balaban, A. T.; Mills, D.; Basak, S. C. Correation Between Structure and Normal Boiling Points of Acyclic Carbonyl Compounds, *J. Chem. Inf. Comput. Sci.* **1999**, *39*, 000-000; (b) Idem, Normal Boiling Points of 1,ω-Alkanedinitriles: the Highest Increment in a Homologous Series, (ibid.,) **1999**, *39*, 769-774.
171. Wang, S.; Milne, G. W. A. Graph Theory and Group Contributions in the Estimation of Boiling Points. *J. Chem. Inf. Comput. Sci.*, **1994**, *34*, 1242-1250.
172. Mihalić, Z.; Nikolić, S.; Trinajstić, N. Comparative Study of Molecular Descriptors Derived from the Distance Matrix. *J. Chem. Inf. Comput. Sci.*, **1992**, *32*, 28-37.
173. Basak, S. C.; Gute, B. D.; Grunwald, G. D. A Comparative Study of Topological and Geometrical Parameters in Estimating Normal Boiling Point and Octanol/Water Partition Coefficient. *J. Chem. Inf. Comput. Sci.* **1996**, *36*, 1054-1060.
174. Balaban, A. T.; Feroiu, V., Correlation Between Structure and Critical Data or Vapor Pressures of Alkanes by Means of Topological Indices. *Reports Molec. Theory*, **1990**, *1*, 133-139.
175. Turner, B. E.; Costello, C. L.; Jurs, P. C., Prediction of Critical Temperatures and Pressures of Industrially Important Organic Compounds from Molecular Structure. *J. Chem. Inf. Comput. Sci.*, **1998**, *38*, 639-645.

176. Katritzky, A. R.; Lobanov, V. S.; Karelson, M.; Murugan, R.; Grendze, M. J.; Toomey, J. E., Jr. Comprehensive Descriptors for Structural and Statistical Analysis. I. Correlations Between Structure and Physical Properties of Substituted Pyridines, *Rev. Roum. Chim.*, **1996**, *41*, 851-867.
177. Katritzky, A. R.; Mu. L.; Karelson, M., QSPR Treatment of the Unified Nonspecific Solvent Polarity Scale, *J. Chem. Inf. Comput. Sci.*, **1997**, *37*, 756-761.
178. Katritzky, A. R.; Rachwal, P.; Law, K. W.; Karelson, M.; Lobanov, V. S., Prediction of Polymer GlassTransition Temperatures Using a General Quantitative Structure-Property Relationship Treatment. *J. Chem. Inf. Comput. Sci.*, **1996**, *36*, 879-884.
179. Nelson, T. M.; Jurs, P. C., Prediction of Aqueous Solubility of Organic Compounds, *J. Chem. Inf. Comput. Sci.* **1994**, *34*, 601-609.
180. Sutte, J. M.; Jurs, P. C., Prediction of Aqueous Solubility for a Diverse Set of Heteroatom-Containing Organic Compounds Using a Quantitative Structure-Property Relationsip, *J. Chem. Inf. Comput. Sci.* **1996**, *36*, 100-107.
181. Katritzky, A. R.; Mu. L.; Karelson, M., A QSPR Study of the Solubility of Gases and Vapors in Water, *J. Chem. Inf. Comput. Sci.*, **1996**, *36*, 1162-1168.
182. Katritzky, A. R.; Wang, Y.; Sild, S.; Tamm, T.; Karelson, M., QSPR Studies on Vapor Pressure, Aqueous Solubility, and the Prediction of Water-Air Partition Coefficients, *J. Chem. Inf. Comput. Sci.*, **1998**, *38*, 720-725.
183. Mitchell, B. E.; Jurs, P. C., Computer Assisted Simulation of ^{13}C Nuclear Magnetic Spactra of Monosaccharides, *J. Chem. Inf. Comput. Sci.* **1996**, *36,* 58-64.
184. Katritzky, A. R.; Maran, U.; Karelson, M.; Lobanov, V. S., Prediction of Melting Points for the Substituted Benzenes: A QSPR Approach, *J. Chem. Inf. Comput. Sci.*, **1997**, *37*, 913-919.
185. Baskin, I. I.; Palyulin, V. A.; Zefirov, N. S., A Neural Device for Searching Direct Correlations between Structures and Properties of Chemical Compounds, *J. Chem. Inf. Comput. Sci.* **1997**, *37*, 715-721.
186. Balaban, A. T.; Motoc, I., Chemical Graphs. Part 36. Correlations Between Octane Numbers and Topological Indices of Alkanes, *Math. Chem. (MATCH),* **1979**, *5*, 197-218.
187. Balaban, A. T.; Kier, L. B.; Joshi, N., Structure-Property Analysis of Octane Numbers for Hydrocarbons (Alkanes, Cycloalkanes, Alkenes), *Math. Chem. (MATCH),* **1992**, *28*, 151-164.
188. Balaban, A. T., QSAR and Computational Methods in Drug Discovery, in *Encyclopedia of Analytical Chemistry*, (Meyers, R.A., Ed.), Wiley, Chichester, **2000**, vol.8, pp. 7288-7311
189. H. van de Waterbeemd, editor, *Chemometric Methods in Drug Design* (Methods and Principles in Medicinal Chemistry, vol. 2), VCH Publishers, New York, 1995.
190. Sabljic, A.; Trinajstić, N., Quantitative Structure-Activity Relationships; the Role of Topological Indices, *Acta Pharm. Jugosl.*, **1981**, *31*, 189-214.
191. Trinajstić, N.; My, M. A.; Gargas, M. J., On the Quantitative Structure-Activity Relationship in Drug Research, *Acta Pharm. Jugosl.*, **1986**, *36*, 267-279.
192. Balaban, A. T.; Niculescu-Duvaz, I.; Simon, Z., Topological Aspects in QSAR for Biologically-Active Molecules, *Acta Pharm. Jugosl.*, **1987,** *37*, 7-36.

193. Voiculetz, N.; Balaban. A. T.; Niculescu-Duvaz, I.; Simon, Z., *Modeling of Cancer Genesis and Prevention*, CRC Press, Boca Raton, Florida, **1990**.
194. Balasubramanian, K.; Kauffman, J. J.; Koski, W. S.; Balaban, A. T., Graph Theoretical Characterization and Computer Generation of Certain Carcinogenic Benzenoid Hydrocarbons and Identification of Bay Regions, *J. Comput. Chem.*, **1980**, *1*, 149-157.
195. Bermudez, C. I.; Daza, E. E.; Andrade, E., Characterization and Comparison of *Escherichia coli* Transfer RNAs by Graph Theory based on Secondary Structure, *J. theor. Biol.* **1999**, *197*, 193-205.
196. Balaban, A. T.; Catana, C.; Dawson, M.; Niculescu-Duvaz, I., Applications of Weighted Topological Index J for QSAR of Carcinogenesis Inhibitors (Retinoic Acid Derivatives), *Rev. Roum. Chim.*, **1990**, *35*, 1005-1008.
197. Bonchev, D.; Mountain, C. F.; Seitz, W. A.; Balaban, A. T., Modeling the Anticancer Action of Some Retinoid Compounds by Making Use of the OASIS Method, *J. Med. Chem.* **1993**, *36*, 1562-1569; Bonchev, D.; Seitz, W. A.; Mountain, C. F.; Balaban, A. T., Modeling the Anticarcinogenic Action of Retinoids by Making Use of the OASIS Method. Part 3. Inhibition of the Induction of Ornithine Decarboxylase by Arotinoids. *J. Med. Chem.* **1993**, *36*, 1562-1569.
198. Gough, J. D.; Hall, L. H., Modeling Antileukemic Activity of Carboquinones with Electrotopological State and Chi Indices, *J. Chem. Inf. Comput. Sci.* **1999**, *39*, 356-361.
199. Wessel, M. D.; Jurs, P. C.; Tolan, J. W.; Muskal, S. M., Prediction of Human Intestinal Absorption of Drug Compounds from Molecular Structure, *J. Chem. Inf. Comput. Sci.* **1998**, *38,* 726-735.
200. Huuskonen, J.; Salo, M.; Taskinen, J., Aqueous Solubility of Drugs Based on Molecular Topology and Neural Network Modeling, *J. Chem. Inf. Comput. Sci.* **1998**, *38,* 450-456.
201. Basak, S. C.; Gute, B. D.; Ghatak, S., Prediction of Complement-Inhibitory Activity of Benzamidines Using Topological and Geometric Parameters, *J. Chem. Inf. Comput. Sci.* **1999**, *39*, 255-260.
202. García-Domenech, R.; J. V. de Julián-Ortiz, Antimicrobial Activity Characterization in a Heterogeneous Group of Compounds, *J. Chem. Inf. Comput. Sci.* **1998**, *38,*445-449.
203. Sabljic, A., Quantitative Modeling of Soil Sorption for Xenobiotic Chemicals, *Environ. Health Prospect.*, **1989**, *83*, 179-190.
204. Karcher, W.; Devillers, J., editors, *Practical Applications of QSAR in Environmental Chemistry and Toxicology*, Kluwer Academic Publishers, Dordrecht, 1990. (a) Karcher, W.; Devillers, J., SAR and QSAR in Environmental Chemistry and Toxicology: Scientific Tool or Wishful Thinking?, pp. 1-12. (b) Dearden, J. C., Physico-Chemical Descriptors, pp. 25-60. (c) Sabljic, A., Topological Indices and Environmental Chemistry, pp. 61-82. (d) Basak, S. C., A Nonempirical Approach to Predicting Molecular Properties Using Graph-Theoretic Invariants, pp. 83-104.

205. Grassy, G.; Calas, B.; Yasri, A.; Lahana, R.; Woo, J.; Iyer, S.; Kaczorek, M.; Floc'h, R.; Buelow, R., Computer-Assisted Rational Design of Immunosuppressive Compounds, *Nature Biotechnology*, **1998**,*16*, 748 - 752.

Chapter 2

WIENER-TYPE GRAPH INVARIANTS

István Lukovits
Chemical Research Center, Hungarian Academy of Sciences,
H-1525 Budapest, P.O.Box 17, Hungary.

1. INTRODUCTION

The Wiener index[1] W is a graph invariant, which is equal to the sum of all distances between the vertices of the underlying graph:

$$W = 1/2\sum_{ij} d_{ij}$$

where d_{ij} denotes the (topological) distance between vertices i and j. Note that the graph theoretical expressions "graph", "vertex" and "edge" are synonymous with the well known notions "structural formula", "atom" and "chemical bond", respectively. As an example, let's consider the computation of W for cyclobutane (Fig. 1.). Hydrogen atoms will not be considered, therefore methane corresponds to a single vertex, ethane to two vertices joined by a single edge, etc. Therefore, $d_{12} = 1$, $d_{13} = 2$ and $d_{14} = 1$, $d_{23} = 1$, $d_{24} = 2$, $d_{34} = 1$ and $W_{cyclobutane} = 1 + 2 + 1 + 1 + 2 + 1 = 8$. The second column of Table 1. lists Wiener indices of several alkanes.

Since it has been proposed before fifty years, W became one of the most often investigated (and applied) graph theoretical indices, because of its interesting mathematical properties and its usefulness in studies on quantitative structure-property relationships (QSPR). W was used to explain the variation in boiling points, molar volumes, refractive indices, heats of isomerization and heats of vaporization of alkanes[1]. Later on correlation between the heats of formation, atomization, isomerization and vaporization, density, critical pressure, surface-tension, viscosity, melting points, partition coefficients, chromatographic retention indices and the Wiener index for various kinds of molecules were demonstrated[2]. W was also used to relate pharmacological potencies of drugs to their structure[3]. Relationships between W and intermolecular forces have also been demonstrated.[4] It is now assumed that W is a measure of the "compactness" of the molecule[2]. Several reviews[2,5-11] on topological indices and W were published, and the reader is encouraged to consult at least some of these.

Fig. 1. Hydrogen Suppressed Graph of Cyclobutane

Table 1. Wiener-Type Indices of Hydrocarbons

Molecule	W	w	Sz	R	P
Methane	0	0	0	0	0
Propane	4	4	4	4	4
Cyclopropane	3	6	3	2	9
N-butane	10	10	10	10	10
Isobutane	9	9	9	9	9
Cyclobutane	8	16	16	5	24

Because of the success of the Wiener index in QSPR studies, a great number of graph invariants related to W were proposed[12-18]. Table 2 lists several invariants related to W. There is a subgroup of invariants, which are equivalent with W for acyclic structures, but differ from W in cyclic structures. In this paper expression "Wiener-type indices" will be used to denote just these invariants. The aim of this paper is to review the definition and computation of several Wiener-type indices.

Table 2. Indices Related to W

Name of Index	Author	Reference
Wiener	Wiener	1
Resistance distance	Klein, Randić	24
Detour	Amić, Trinajstić	20
	Ivanciuc, Balaban	21
	John	22
Szeged	Gutman	19
Laplacian	Trinajstić et al.	25
All-path	Lukovits	23
Hyper-Wiener	Randić	12
Cluj Matrix invariants	Diudea	13
Harary	Plavšić et al.	17
Expanded Wiener number	Tratch et al.	18
Hyper-Szeged	Diudea	14
Hyper-detour	Lukovits	16

2. Wiener-Type Indices

Besides the "sum of distances" approach, there is another formula which may be used to calculate W. The formula, proposed by Wiener[1] himself, may be obtained as follows: remove a single edge e from an acyclic graph T. As a result of this operation we obtain two acyclic graphs T_1 and T_2, the number of vertices of the resulting graphs is N_1 and N_2, respectively, and $N_1 + N_2 = N$, where N denotes the number of vertices in T. W may be obtained by using the following formula:

$$W = \Sigma\, N_1 \times N_2$$

where the summation has to be performed for all edges e. This formula is valid for acyclic graphs only, but for these structures definitions based on the "sum of products" and the "sum of distances" are equivalent. The "Szeged index" (Sz) proposed by Gutman[19] was obtained by a modification of the "sum of products" rule. To calculate Sz the following algorithm should be used: 1. Remove edge e from graph G. 2. Determine N_1, which is equal to the number of vertices being closer to the vertex on the "left hand side" (including the vertex itself) than to the vertex on the "right hand side" of e. Vertices being at equal distances from e, are not considered. A similar definition applies for N_2. 3.

Repeat procedure for all edges e and add up the contributions. For acyclic graphs the numerical value of Sz and W are identical, but for cyclic structures or cycle-containing graphs Sz and W are usually - but not necessarily – not equal. As an example let's consider the computation of $Sz_{cyclobutane}$ (Fig. 1). Remove edge (1,2), then $N_1 = 2$ and $N_2 = 2$, and $N_1 \times N_2 = 4$. Because of symmetry reasons the contribution of the other edges is also four, and therefore $Sz_{cyclobutane} = 16$.

Expression "shortest path" is not relevant for acyclic graphs, because between any pair of vertices there is a single path in T. Replacement of formula "shortest path" by expression "longest path" in eq. 1 yields a numerical value of the graph invariant that is identical with W for acyclic graphs, but is different for cyclic structures. The name of the new invariant, that was proposed independently by several authors[20-22], is the detour index (w). w may be obtained by replacing distance d_{ij} (eq. 1) by formula "the length of the longest path between vertices i and j", Δ_{ij}:

$$w = 1/2 \sum_{ij} \Delta_{ij}$$

For cyclobutane (Fig. 1): $\Delta_{12} = 3$, $\Delta_{13} = 2$, $\Delta_{14} = 3$, $\Delta_{23} = 3$, $\Delta_{24} = 2$ and $\Delta_{34} = 3$, therefore $w = 3 + 2 + 3 + 3 + 2 + 3 = 16$.

Expression "shortest path" in eq. 1 could also be replaced by formula "sum of lengths of all paths between vertices i and j". By using this modified definition numerical value of the resulting graph invariant (the all-path index, P) would also be identical with W for acyclic graphs, since there is only a single path between any pair of vertices i and j. P may be defined by the following equation[23]:

$$P = 1/2 \sum_{i,j} \sum_{\pi_{ij}} |\pi_{ij}|$$

where π_{ij} denotes a path between vertices i and j, and $|\pi_{ij}|$ denotes the length of such path. For cyclobutane (Fig. 1) between any pair of vertices two paths exist, and for each pair, $\Sigma |\pi_{ij}| = 4$. There are six pairs of vertices altogether, and therefore $P_{cyclobutane} = 24$.

Two additional Wiener-type invariants should be mentioned, the "resistance-distance" (R) by Klein and Randić[24], and the "Laplacian index" by Trinajstić et al.[25] Resistance distance is obtained if the edges of any graph are replaced by unit resistors, and the resistance between all pairs of vertices are added:

$$R = 1/2 \sum_{ij} R_{ij}$$

where R_{ij} denotes the "resistance" between vertices i and j, provided that adjacent vertices are connected by unit resistors. The Laplacian index is the sum of positive eigenvalues of the Laplacian matrix, and this invariant is equal to W in acyclic graphs, but will be different from it for cycle-containing structures. It has been shown that the

Laplacian index and the resistance-distance are equivalent if acyclic graphs are considered.[26] Table 1. lists the numerical values of W, w, Sz, R, and P of several acyclic and cyclic alkanes.

3. On The Numerical Values of Wiener-Type Invariants

The "inverse QSPR" problem, namely to reconstruct G from a number of its invariants, has not been solved thus far. However, for definite subclasses of graphs, G can be reconstructed by systematically generating numerical values of invariants of G. In this procedure the *first* step is to determine the size of the graph (i.e. the number of its vertices) for which the reconstruction should be attempted. The *second* step is to determine the maximal and minimal values of the index under consideration. The extremal values of the Wiener index,[27,28] the hyper-Wiener index,[29] resistance distance,[30] detour,[20] Szeged,[31] and "all-path"[23] have been published. Table 3 lists the minimal and maximal values of W, w, Sz, R, and P related graphs containing 23 vertices. It can be seen that the range of P is much greater than the range of any other Wiener-type index. Therefore, P may be more discriminative for cycle-containing structures than W, w, Sz, or R. The *third* step is to generate the numerical values of the respective index based on the formulas (see next section).

Table 3. Extremal Values of Wiener-Type Indices of Graphs Containing 23 Vertices

Invariant	Minimum		Maximum	
	Type of graph	Value	Type of graph	Value
W	complete	253	chain	2024
w	star	484	complete	5566
Sz	complete	253	complete bipartite	17424
R	complete	22	chain	2024
P	star	484	complete	6101663744

Derivation of formulas, used to obtain the numerical values of W for various types of structures, have been reviewed earlier.[32-35] Formulas of the detour index, [16, 20, 22] "all-path", [23] Szeged, [36] and resistance distance[30] have been obtained for several subsets of structures. The formulas obtained for W, w, R are third-order polynomials in terms of the number of atoms. It was shown[31] that Sz may be a fourth order polynomial in N, while P increases exponentially (Tab. 3) with N.[23]

Besides of formulas, algorithms were also proposed to obtain the numerical value of various Wiener-type indices. Žerovnik[37] devised a method to obtain Sz, while two independent algorithms were proposed to obtain w.[38, 39]

4. Structure-Property Relationships

The Wiener index became popular in part because of its "ability" to explain the variation in the various physical-chemical properties of acyclic, saturated hydrocarbons.[1] The derivation of the different variants of W is a consequence of the success of W, although quite few actual structure-property relationships were obtained by using Wiener-type invariants. Regression equations involving Sz as independent variable was used to investigate polychlorinated biphenyls.[40] The detour index was used to explain the variation in the boiling points of alkanes.[16, 41]

5. References

1. Wiener, H. Correlation of Heats of Isomerization and Differences in Heats of Vaporization of Isomers among the Paraffin Hydrocarbons. *J. Am. Chem. Soc.* **1947** *69*, 2636-2638.
2. Gutman, I.; Yeh, Y.N.; Lee, S.L.; Luo, Y.L. Some Recent Results in the Theory of the Wiener Number. *Indian J. Chem.* **1993**, *32A*, 651-661.
3. Lukovits, I. Decomposition of the Wiener Topological Index. Application to Drug-Receptor Interactions, *J. Chem. Soc. Perkin Trans. II.* **1988**, 1667-1671.
4. Gutman, I.; Potgieter, H. Wiener Index and Intermolecular Forces. *J. Serb. Chem. Soc.* **1997**, *62*, 185-192.
5. Nikolić, S.; Trinajstić, N.; Mihalić; Z. The Wiener Index: Development and Applications. *Croat. Chem. Acta*, **1995**, *68*, 105-129.
6. Mihalić, Z.; Nikolić, S.; Trinajstić, N. Comparative Study of Molecular Descriptors Derived from the Distance Matrix. *J. Chem. Inf. Comput. Sci.* **1992**, *32*, 28-37.
7. Rouvray, D. The Value of Topological Indices in Chemistry. *Commun. Math. Chem. (MATCH)* **1975**, *1*, 125-134.
8. Randić, M. Chemical Structure – what is "She"? *J. Chem. Ed.* **1992**, *69*, 713-718.
9. Zhu, H. Y, Klein, D. J, Lukovits, I. Extensions of the Wiener Number, *J. Chem. Inf. Comput. Sci.* **1996**,. *36*, 420-428.
10. Diudea, M. V., Gutman, I. Wiener-Type Topological Indices. *Croat. Chem. Acta*, **1998**, *71*, 21-51.
11. Klein, D. J. Graph Geometry, Graph Metrics, & Wiener. *Commun. Math. Chem. (MATCH)*, **1997**, *35*, 7-27.
12. Randić, M. Novel Molecular Descriptor for Structure-Property Studies. *Chem. Phys. Lett.* **1993**, *211*, 478-483.
13. Diudea, M. V. Cluj Matrix Invariants. *J. Chem. Inf. Comput. Sci.* **1997**, *37*, 300-305.
14. Diudea, M. V.; Minailiuc, O. M.; Katona, G.; Gutman, I. Szeged Matrices and Related Numbers. *Commun. Math. Chem. (MATCH)*, **1997**, *35*, 129-143.
15. Gutman, I., Estrada, E. Topological Indices Based on the Line Graph of the Molecular Graph. *J. Chem. Inf. Comput. Sci.* **1996**, *36*, 541-543.
16. Lukovits, I. The Detour Index, *Croat. Chem. Acta* **1996**, *69*, 873-882.

17. Plavšić, D., Nikolić, S., Trinajstić, N., Mihalić Z. On the Harary Index for the Characterization of Chemical Graphs. *J. Math. Chem.* **1993**, *12*, 235-250.
18. Tratch, S. S.; Stankevich, M. I.; Zefirov, N. S. Combinatorial models and algorithms in chemistry. The expanded Wiener number. - A novel topological index. *J. Comput. Chem.* **1990**, *11*, 899-908.
19. Gutman, I. A Formula for the Wiener Number of Trees and its Extension to Graphs Containing Cycles, *Graph Theory Notes, New York,* **1994**, *27*, 9-15.
20. Amić, D, Trinajstić, N. On the Detour Matrix. *Croat. Chem. Acta*, **1995**, *68*, 53-62.
21. Ivanciuc, O., Balaban, A. Design of Topological Indices. 8. Path Matrices and Derived Molecular Graph Invariants. *Commun. Math. Chem.* (*MATCH*) **1994**, *30*, 141-152.
22. John, P. Über die Berechnung der Wiener Index für ausgewaehlte Delta-dimensionale Gitterstrukturen. *Commun. Math. Chem.* (*MATCH*) **1995**, *32*, 207-219.
23. Lukovits, I. An All-Path Version of the Wiener Index. *J. Chem. Inf. Comput. Sci.* **1998**, *38*, 125-129.
24. Klein, D. J., Randić, M. Resistance distance. *J. Math. Chem.* **1993**, *12*, 81-95.
25. Trinajstić, N.; Babić, D.; Nikolić, S.; Plavšić, D.; Amić, D.; Mihalić, Z. The Laplacian Matrix in Chemistry. *J. Chem. Inf. Comput. Sci.* **1994**, *34*, 368-376.
26. Gutman, I., Mohar, B. The Quasi-Wiener and the Kirchoff Indices Coincide. *J. Chem. Inf. Comput. Sci.* **1996**, *36*, 982-985.
27. Entringer, R. C., Jackson, D. E., Snyder, D. A. Distance in graphs. *Czech. Math. J.* **1984**, *8*, 1-21.
28. Bonchev, D.; Trinajstić, N. Information Theory, Distance Matrix and Molecular Branching. *J. Chem. Phys.* **1977**, *67*, 4517-4533.
29. Gutman, I., Linert, W., Lukovits, I., Dobrynin, A. A. Trees with Extremal Hyper-Wiener Index: Mathematical Basis and Chemical Applications. *J. Chem. Inf. Comput. Sci.* **1997**, *37*, 349-354.
30. Lukovits, I.; Nikolić, S.; Trinajstić, N. Resistance Distance in Regular Graphs. *Int. J. Quantum. Chem.* **1999**, *71*, 217-225.
31. Dobrynin, A. A., Graphs Having the Maximal Value of the Szeged Index. *Croat. Chem. Acta*, **1997**, *70*, 819-825.
32. Gutman, I. A new Method for the Calculation of the Wiener Number of Acyclic Molecules. *J. Mol. Struct.* (*Theochem*), **1993**, *285*, 137-142.
33. Lukovits, I. General Formulas for the Wiener Index, *J. Chem. Inf. Comput. Sci.* **1991**,.*31*, 503-507.
34. Lukovits, I. Wiener Index: Formulas for Non-homeomerphic Graphs. *Croat. Chem. Acta*. **1998**, *71*, 449-458.
35. Dobrynin, A. A. A New Formula for the Calculation of the Wiener Index of Hexagonal Chains. *Commun. Math. Chem.* (*MATCH*), **1997**, *35*, 75-90.
36. Dobrynin, A. A.; Gutman, I. Szeged Index of Some Polycyclic Bipartite Graphswith Circuits of Different Size. *Commun. Math. Chem.* (*MATCH*), **1997**, *35*, 117-128.
37. Žerovnik, J. Computing the Szeged index. *Croat. Chem. Acta*, **1996**, *69*, 837-843.
38. Lukovits, I.; Razinger, M. On Calculation of the Detour Index. *J. Chem. Inf. Comput. Sci.* **1997**, *37*, 283-286.

39. Trinajstić, N., Nikolić, S., Mihalić, Z. On Computing the Molecular Detour Matrix, *Int. J. Quantum Chem.* **1997**, *65*, 415-419.
40. Karmarkar, Sn.; Karmarkar, Sa.; Joshi, S.; Das, A.; Khadikar, P. Novel Application of Wiener vis-a-vis Szeged Indices in Predicting Polychlorinated Biphenyls in the Environment. *J. Serb. Chem. Soc.* **1997**, *62*, 227-234.
41. Rücker, G.; Rücker, C. Symmetry Aided Computation of the Detour Matrix and the Detour Index. *J. Chem. Inf. Comput. Sci.* **1998**, *38*, 710-714.

Chapter 3

On Calculation of Molecular Descriptors Based on Various Graphical Bond Orders[†]

Dejan Plavšić and Ante Graovac
The Ruđer Bošković Institute, P.O.B. 180, HR-10002 Zagreb,
The Republic of Croatia

1. Introduction

Molecular structure is one of the basic concepts of chemistry since properties and behavior of molecules follow from their structures.[1-6] In particular, properties of a molecule are a consequence of a complicated interplay of its topology (atomic connectivity), metric characteristics (bond lengths, valence and torsional angles) and detailed dynamics of electrons and nuclei.[7, 8] Finding out how various molecular features depend on molecular structure is one of the central fields of research of chemistry and particularly the main subject of QSPR (quantitative structure-property relationship) and QSAR (quantitative structure-activity relationship) studies.[9-25] Among different approaches to QSPR/QSAR, the structure-explicit approach based on graph theoretical methods is especially interesting and attractive due to its effectiveness and simplicity.

Within many congeneric series of chemical compounds the variations of molecular metric and electronic structure are small. Consequently, one can approximate that in such series changes of many of molecular properties are conditioned only by topology. Molecular topology is conventionally represented by a (molecular) graph being essentially a nonnumerical mathematical object.[16, 23, 26] To model quantitatively a topology-property/activity relationship in a series of molecules, it is necessary to quantify the structural information contained in their molecular graphs. First a graph G is transformed into a more convenient mathematical representation (matrix, polynomial, etc.) and then by an algorithm the structural information contained in G is converted into

---

† Dedicated to Professor Tomaž Pisanski on the occasion of his 50th birthday.

a graph invariant - a scalar numerical characteristic of *G* which has the same value for any graph isomorphic to *G*. The number of graph invariants that can be constructed is unlimited but chemically interesting are only those graph invariants encoding structural factors predominantly influencing the molecular properties. These invariants are usually called molecular descriptors or topological (graph theoretical) indices.[16]

The representation of a molecule (or molecular graph) by a single number (molecular descriptor) entails a considerable loss of information concerning the molecular structure. Therefore, to diminish the loss of information an intensive search for novel molecular descriptors that would improve the graph theoretical characterization of molecular structure has been undertaken in three main directions.[27, 28] The first direction is a construction of ad hoc molecular descriptors and generalization of the existing molecular descriptors, the second, the design of novel polynomials as a source of new molecular descriptors, and the third direction, the creation of novel graph matrices and generalization of the existing ones whose selected invariants could be used as novel molecular descriptors.

Thus far a large number of graph invariants has been put forward in the hope that they encode chemically relevant information. Unfortunately, the investigations of their features and in particular their applications and roles in topology-property/activity studies of molecules have been carried out only for a small number of invariants. One of the reasons why only a small number of the proposed molecular descriptors have been tested is the lack of efficient algorithms for their calculation. To reveal the real value and use of a graph invariant in chemistry, the invariant has to be tested on a great number of large and diverse sets of compounds. Clearly, this requires numerous calculations of the invariant that can be easily and quickly carried out only by an efficient algorithm.

2. Molecular Descriptors X'/X

Randić has recently put forward and preliminarily tested novel and interesting composite bond-additive graph invariants, X'/X, constructed from already known molecular descriptors, X.[27-34] The invariant X'/X of a molecular graph *G* is the sum over all its edges of graphical bond orders based on the molecular descriptor X (see § 3. for details). The preliminary testing of the invariants X'/X based on the connectivity index χ,[35] the Wiener number W,[36] the hyper-Wiener number R,[32] the total number of paths P,[30] the Balaban index J[37] and the Hosoya index Z,[38] was carried out by examining heptane and octane isomers. To wit, a fairly large number of their physicochemical properties was modeled in the framework of the single- and two-variable linear regression models. The preliminary testing had pointed out all the aforementioned invariants X'/X as "promising" molecular descriptors, however the additional studies of these X'/X descriptors were not carried out. The primary cause was the complexity of the algorithms for their calculation being all based on the computation of the corresponding molecular descriptor X of *G* and of all its spanning subgraphs *G-e*. For *G* having *N* vertices and *R* rings (the number of rings *R* in a molecule equals the cyclomatic number[16] of the corresponding molecular graph) the total number of the G-e spanning subgraphs is N+R-1. Hence, one needs to develop novel, simple, and efficient algorithms for calculation of the molecular descriptors X'/X. The desirable algorithms would be those based on analytical expressions that make possible to calculate the X'/X descriptors directly from structural characteristics (like number of vertices, edges and paths, valencies of vertices, etc.) of G. In the following sections we give a survey of the recently obtained explicit formulae[39-45] for calculation of a number of molecular descriptors X'/X.

3. Definitions

3.1. Graphical Bond Order X_e/X

The graphical bond order X_e/X of an edge e in a molecular graph G is defined by the expression[29, 34]

$$X_e/X = \frac{X(G-e)}{X(G)} , \tag{1}$$

where X(G) and X(G-e) denote the X descriptor of G and its spanning subgraph G-e, respectively. G-e is derived from G by erasing the edge e. The quantity X_e/X can be interpreted as a relative "contribution" of the edge e to (the X descriptor of) G. Since G is connected, its spanning subgraph G-e is connected if and only if G contains at least one ring and the edge e is one among the edges making up the ring(s). If G-e is disconnected it consists of two components, G_1 and G_2. Depending on the kind of the selected descriptor X, contributions of G_1 and G_2 are either added up,

$$X(G-e) = X(G_1) + X(G_2) \tag{2}$$

or multiplied,

$$X(G-e) = X(G_1)\, X(G_2) . \tag{3}$$

In case of the connectivity index χ, the total number of paths P, the Wiener number W or the hyper-Wiener number R the contributions of components of G-e are given by Eq. (2), while for, e.g., the Hosoya index Z, Eq. (3) is applied. (Note, that in a modification of Z suggested by Randić[28, 29] Eq. (2) is applied.)

3.2. Molecular Descriptor X'/X

The X'/X descriptor, X'/X=(X'/X)(G), of a molecular graph G is defined as the sum of graphical bond orders X_e/X of all edges of G,[29, 34]

$$X'/X = \sum_e X_e/X = \frac{1}{X(G)} \sum_e X(G-e) \; . \tag{4}$$

4. Explicit Formulae for Calculation of Molecular Descriptors X'/X

A closer inspection of Eq. (4) points out that the search for explicit formulae which would enable us to calculate X'/X descriptors of a molecular graph G directly from G, can be reduced to seeking for analytical expressions for X(G-e) in which only structural characteristics of G appear.

4.1. Explicit Formula for Calculation of Molecular Descriptor χ'/χ

Twenty five years ago Randić introduced the connectivity index χ.[35] The χ index, χ=χ(G), of a molecular graph G is defined as

$$\chi = \sum_{e_{ij}} (v_i v_j)^{-1/2} \; , \tag{5}$$

where v_i and v_j are the valencies of vertices i and j in G making up the edge e_{ij} . The summation goes over all edges of G. In particular, χ of the trivial graph, K_1, having a single vertex, equals zero by definition.

The connectivity index has a very widespread application not only in chemometrics and in QSPR/QSAR in particular, but also in the biological sciences as well as in the physical sciences. To illustrate the outstanding importance of the connectivity index, let us just mention that χ is the only topological index to have had two entire books devoted to it and its applications.[9, 10]

The χ'/χ descriptor is constructed from the connectivity index χ and is defined by the expression[29, 34]

$$\chi'/\chi = \frac{1}{\chi(G)} \sum_e \chi(G-e) \; , \tag{6}$$

where $\chi(G)$ and $\chi(G\text{-}e)$ stand for the χ index of G and $G\text{-}e$, respectively, and the summation goes over all edges of G.

The first and at the same time the crucial step in the construction of an explicit formula for χ'/χ enabling us to calculate χ'/χ directly from G, is to find out an analytical expression for $\chi(G\text{-}e)$. The derivation of such an analytical expression[43] shall be stated. Suppose that G has N vertices and R rings and let i and j be adjacent vertices in G with valencies v_i and v_j, respectively. Erasing of the edge e_{ij} from G creates the spanning subgraph $G\text{-}e_{ij}$ and changes the valencies of i and j to v_i -1 and v_j -1, respectively, while the valencies of all other vertices remain unchanged. An edge of $G\text{-}e_{ij}$ being neither incident with the vertex i nor with the vertex j makes a contribution to $\chi(G\text{-}e_{ij})$ identical to its contribution to $\chi(G)$. In $G\text{-}e_{ij}$ there are $N+R-v_i-v_j$ edges with this property, and their total contribution to $\chi(G\text{-}e_{ij})$ is given by

$$\chi(G)-(v_i v_j)^{-1/2}-\sum_{\substack{e_{im}\\ m\neq j}}(v_i v_m)^{-1/2}-\sum_{\substack{e_{jn}\\ n\neq i}}(v_j v_n)^{-1/2},$$

where v_m and v_n represent the valencies of vertices m and n being adjacent to the vertices i and j, respectively. The summation in the third (fourth) term runs over all edges of G incident with the vertex i (j) except the edge e_{ij}. The remaining v_i+v_j -2 edges of $G\text{-}e_{ij}$ are incident either with the vertex i or with the vertex j. Their total contribution to $\chi(G\text{-}e_{ij})$ equals

$$\sum_{\substack{e_{im}\\ m\neq j}}\left[(v_i-1)v_m\right]^{-1/2}+\sum_{\substack{e_{jn}\\ n\neq i}}\left[(v_j-1)v_n\right]^{-1/2}.$$

In general, one can write

$$\chi(G-e_{ij})=\chi(G)-(v_i v_j)^{-1/2}-\sum_{\substack{e_{im}\\ m\neq j}}(v_i v_m)^{-1/2}-\sum_{\substack{e_{jn}\\ n\neq i}}(v_j v_n)^{-1/2}+\sum_{\substack{e_{im}\\ m\neq j}}\left[(v_i-1)v_m\right]^{-1/2}+\sum_{\substack{e_{jn}\\ n\neq i}}\left[(v_j-1)v_n\right]^{-1/2}. \tag{7}$$

Dividing $\chi(G\text{-}e_{ij})$ by $\chi(G)$ one gets the graphical bond order, $\chi_{e_{ij}}/\chi$, of the edge e_{ij} of G. Now that we have knowledge of the analytical expression for $\chi(G\text{-}e)$, the next step is adding up χ's of all the $N+R$-1 spanning subgraphs $G\text{-}e$ of G. By noting that

$$\sum_{e_{ij}}\left[\sum_{\substack{e_{im}\\ m\neq j}}(v_i v_m)^{-1/2}+\sum_{\substack{e_{jn}\\ n\neq i}}(v_j v_n)^{-1/2}\right]=\sum_{e_{ij}}(v_i+v_j-2)(v_i v_j)^{-1/2} \tag{8}$$

and

$$\sum_{e_{ij}}\left\{\sum_{\substack{e_{im}\\ m\neq j}}\left[(v_i-1)v_m\right]^{-1/2}+\sum_{\substack{e_{jn}\\ n\neq i}}\left[(v_j-1)v_n\right]^{-1/2}\right\}=\sum_{e_{ij}}\frac{v_i\left[(v_i-1)v_j\right]^{1/2}+v_j\left[(v_j-1)v_i\right]^{1/2}}{v_i v_j}, \tag{9}$$

the sought-after explicit formula for the χ'/χ descriptor immediately follows:

$$\chi'/\chi = N + R + \frac{1}{\chi(G)}\sum_{e_{ij}}\frac{v_i\left[(v_i-1)v_j\right]^{1/2}+v_j\left[(v_j-1)v_i\right]^{1/2}-(v_i+v_j)(v_i v_j)^{1/2}}{v_i v_j} \tag{10}$$

This formula is well defined for every connected graph with N 2 vertices. The application of the formula is illustrated in Figure 1 for the hydrogen-suppressed graph of 1-(2-propyl)-2-methyl-benzene.

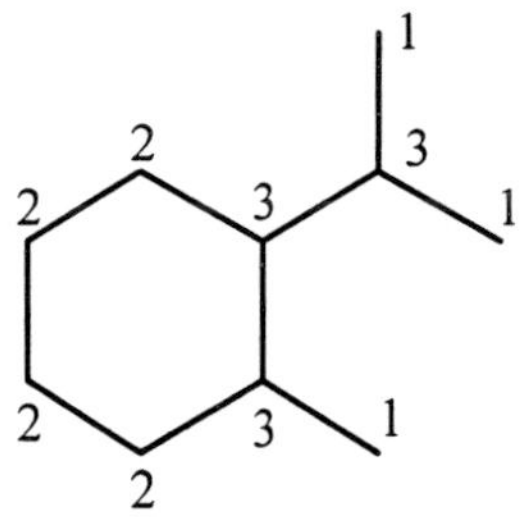

$$\chi'/\chi = 10 + 1 + \frac{1}{4.7152}\left[3\,\frac{3\cdot 2^{1/2} - 4\cdot 3^{1/2}}{1\cdot 3} + 3\,\frac{4\cdot 2^{1/2} - 4\cdot 2}{2\cdot 2} + 2\,\frac{2\cdot 3^{1/2} + 3\cdot 2 - 5\cdot 6^{1/2}}{2\cdot 3} + 2\,\frac{6\cdot 6^{1/2} - 6\cdot 3}{3\cdot 3}\right] = 9.7053$$

Figure 1. Calculation of the molecular descriptor χ'/χ of the hydrogen--suppressed graph of 1-(2-propyl)-2-methyl-benzene. The number at each site represents its graph-theoretical valency.

In some special cases Eq. (10) takes a rather simple form, e.g., for the path graph with N vertices, P_N,

$$\chi'/\chi = \frac{(N-4)(N-3)+4\left[2^{1/2}(N-3)+1-\mathrm{k}\right]}{N-3+2(2^{1/2}+\mathrm{k})} \; ; \; N \geq 2 \, , \tag{11}$$

where the parameter k takes the following values,

$$\mathrm{k} = \begin{cases} 3/2 - 2^{1/2} & \text{for } N = 2 \\ 0 & \text{for } N > 2 \end{cases} \tag{12}$$

and for the cycle graph with N vertices, C_N,

$$\chi'/\chi = N - 3 + 8^{1/2} \; ; \; N \geq 3 . \tag{13}$$

4.2. Explicit Formulae for Calculation of Molecular Descriptor P'/P

A novel structure-explicit graph matrix, the **P** matrix, has recently been put forward.[30] The **P** matrix, **P**=**P**(G), of a molecular graph G with N vertices is the square symmetric matrix of order N whose entry in the i-th row and j-th column is given by the expression

$$(\mathbf{P})_{ij} = \begin{cases} \mathrm{P}(G - e_{ij})/\mathrm{P}(G) & \text{if the vertices i and j are adjacent} \\ 0 & \text{otherwise} \end{cases} \tag{14}$$

where P(G) and P(G-e_{ij}) denote the total numbers of paths P in G and G-e_{ij}, respectively. "Otherwise" means that either the vertices i and j are not adjacent or i=j. Since each edge is assigned a weight given by P(G-e)/P(G), the **P** matrix can also be considered as the weighted adjacency matrix.

The P'/P descriptor was originally introduced as the **P** matrix invariant equal to the sum of all entries in the upper or lower triangle of **P**. This descriptor can also be defined quite generally and independently of the **P** matrix by the expression,[34]

$$\mathrm{P'/P} = \frac{1}{\mathrm{P}(G)} \sum_{e} \mathrm{P}(G-e) \, , \tag{15}$$

where the summation goes over all edges of G.

For an arbitrary molecular graph, what means a graph containing ring(s) as well, it is not possible to construct a closed formula for the P'/P descriptor. However, it is possible to construct explicit formulae for P'/P of some special types of graphs, e.g., connected undirected acyclic graphs (trees), cycle graphs, etc.

The derivation of three explicit formulae for computing the P'/P descriptor of a tree graph T directly from T [40] shall be stated. Suppose T is a tree with N vertices. By deletion of the edge e_{ij}, T breaks into two components, whose numbers of vertices equal $n_i(e_{ij})$ and $n_j(e_{ij})=N-n_i(e_{ij})$, respectively. Owing to the existence of bijective mapping from the set of all pairs of vertices of T to the set of paths connecting them (the uniqueness of paths in T), P(T) can be expressed by means of N only,

$$\mathrm{P}(T)=\binom{N}{2}. \tag{16}$$

In keeping with Eqs. (1) and (2) the graphical bond order, $\mathrm{P}_{e_{ij}}/\mathrm{P}$, of the edge e_{ij} in T is given by

$$\begin{aligned}\mathrm{P}_{e_{ij}}/\mathrm{P} &= \frac{(\mathrm{n}_i(e_{ij}))^2-\mathrm{n}_i(e_{ij})+(N-\mathrm{n}_i(e_{ij}))^2-(N-\mathrm{n}_i(e_{ij}))}{N^2-N}\\ &=1-2\frac{\mathrm{n}_i(e_{ij})(N-\mathrm{n}_i(e_{ij}))}{N^2-N}.\end{aligned} \tag{17}$$

To get the desired formula for the P'/P descriptor of T one has to add up P_e/P 's of all N-1 edges of T,

$$\mathrm{P'/P}=N-1-\frac{2}{N^2-N}\sum_{e_{ij}}\mathrm{n}_i(e_{ij})(N-\mathrm{n}_i(e_{ij})). \tag{18}$$

The application of this formula is illustrated in Figure 2 for the hydrogen-suppressed graph of 2,4-dimethyl-hexane.

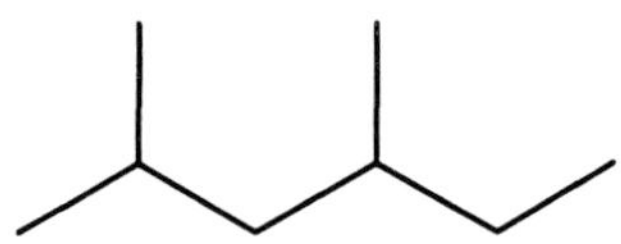

$$\mathrm{P'/P}=8-1-\frac{2}{64-8}\left[4\cdot 1\cdot 7+3\cdot 5+4\cdot 4+6\cdot 2\right]=4.4643$$

Figure 2. Calculation of the molecular descriptor P'/P of the hydrogen-suppressed graph of 2,4-dimethyl-hexane.

We give now a brief outline of the derivation of the two alternative explicit formulae for P'/P of T. If two paths x and y in T are in relation $x \subseteq y$ then it is said that the path x is "internal" with respect to the path y and the path y is "external" with respect to the path x.[46, 47] The quantity $n_i(e_{ij})(N-n_i(e_{ij}))$ can be interpreted as the number of paths in T being "external" with respect to the edge e_{ij}. A path of topological (graph theoretical) length r in T contains r "internal" edges and therefore it appears as the "external" path with respect to edges of T exactly r times. Consequently, the following relations hold:

$$\sum_{e_{ij}} n_i(e_{ij})(N - n_i(e_{ij})) = \sum_{r} r\,P(r) = \sum_{i<j} d(i,j) \,, \tag{19}$$

where P(r) stands for the total number of paths of the length r in T and d(i, j) for the distance between vertices i and j in T. The first summation runs over all edges of T, the second summation goes over all path lengths in T, i.e., from the length 1 (of an edge) up to the length of the longest path in T, and the third summation is over all pairs of vertices of T.

Plainly, the first alternative explicit formula is

$$P'/P = N - 1 - \frac{2}{N^2 - N}\sum_{i<j} d(i,j) \,. \tag{20}$$

The general analytical expression for the number of paths of length r in T reads as follows:[40]

$$P(r) = \sum_{m=0}^{r-2+g} (-1)^{m+h}(r - m - 1) \sum_{\substack{d(i,j)=m \\ i<j}} v_i v_j + (-1)^{r+1}\left(\frac{r-1}{2}\sum_i v_i^2 + N - 1\right) , \tag{21}$$

where v_i is the valency of the vertex i. The parameters g and h take the following values:

$$g = \begin{cases} 1 & \text{for } r = 1 \\ 0 & \text{for } r \geq 2 \end{cases} \tag{22}$$

and

$$h = \begin{cases} 1 & \text{for } r = \text{odd} \\ 0 & \text{for } r = \text{even} \,. \end{cases} \tag{23}$$

One should note that

$$\sum_{d(i,j)=0} v_i v_j = \sum_i v_i^2 \ . \qquad (24)$$

It is worthwhile to mention that the number of paths, P(r), of a given length, r 3, in T can also be calculated recursively,[40]

$$P(r) = \sum_{\substack{d(i,j)=r-2 \\ i<j}} v_i v_j - 2P(r-1) - P(r-2) \ , \qquad (25)$$

where the initial conditions are given by

$$P(1) = N - 1 \qquad (26)$$

and

$$P(2) = \frac{1}{2}\sum_i v_i^2 - N + 1 \ . \qquad (27)$$

The second alternative explicit formula for P'/P of T is obtained by combining Eqs. (18), (19) and (21), and reads as follows

$$P'/P = (N-1) - \frac{2}{N^2 - N}\sum_{r=1}^{r \le N-1} r \left[\sum_{m=0}^{r-2+g} (-1)^{m+h}(r-m-1) \sum_{\substack{d(i,j)=m \\ i<j}} v_i v_j + (-1)^{r+1}\left(\frac{r-1}{2}\sum_i v_i^2 + N - 1\right) \right] . \qquad (28)$$

The parameters g and h take the values from Eqs. (22) and (23).

In case of the path graph and the cycle graph with N vertices, the corresponding expressions for P'/P are rather simple,

$$P'/P = \frac{2}{3}(N-2) \ ; \quad N \ge 2 \qquad (29)$$

and

$$P'/P = \frac{N}{2} \ ; \quad N \ge 3 \ , \qquad (30)$$

respectively.

4.3. Explicit Formula for Calculation of Molecular Descriptor R'/R

The first molecular descriptor, the path number, was put forward in 1947 by Wiener.[36] The path number, nowadays referred to as the Wiener number, W, was originally defined as the number of bonds between all pairs of atoms in an acyclic molecule. Later Hosoya defined W in the framework of graph theory as the sum of topological distances between all pairs of vertices of a connected undirected graph G.[38] If G is a tree T then W can be expressed as

$$\mathrm{W} = \sum_{e_{\mathrm{ij}}} \mathrm{n_i}(e_{\mathrm{ij}})\mathrm{n_j}(e_{\mathrm{ij}}) \,, \tag{31}$$

where $\mathrm{n_i}(e_{\mathrm{ij}})$ and $\mathrm{n_j}(e_{\mathrm{ij}})=N-\mathrm{n_i}(e_{\mathrm{ij}})$ represent the numbers of vertices of the two components of T-e_{ij}, and the summation goes over all edges of T.

Fifty years after the Wiener number had been introduced, Randić generalized Eq. (31) and put forward a new molecular descriptor of acyclic molecules, the hyper-Wiener number R.[32] The R descriptor, R=R(T), of a tree graph T is defined by the expression

$$\mathrm{R} = \sum_{p_{\mathrm{rs}}} \mathrm{n_r}(p_{\mathrm{rs}})\mathrm{n_s}(p_{\mathrm{rs}}) \,, \tag{32}$$

where p_{rs} stands for the path connecting vertices r and s in T, $\mathrm{n_r}(p_{\mathrm{rs}})$ and $\mathrm{n_s}(p_{\mathrm{rs}})$ denote the numbers of vertices of T lying on one side of the path p_{rs}, closer to the vertex r, and on the other side of the path p_{rs}, closer to the vertex s, respectively. The summation runs over all paths in T. By definition for the trivial path p_{ii} the $\mathrm{n_i}(p_{\mathrm{ii}})$ equals zero.

Randić also introduced the composite bond-additive molecular descriptor R'/R constructed from the hyper-Wiener number R. The R'/R descriptor, R'/R=(R'/R)(T), of a connected undirected acyclic graph T is defined as[32, 34]

$$\mathrm{R'/R} = \frac{1}{\mathrm{R}(T)} \sum_{e} \mathrm{R}(T-e) \,, \tag{33}$$

where R(T) and R(T-e) denote the R descriptor of T and T-e, respectively, and the summation runs over all edges of T.

The "standard" algorithm for calculation of R'/R of T based on Eqs. (33), (32) and (2), demands the knowledge of all paths in T, all the spanning subgraphs T-e of T and all their paths as well as the calculation of the hyper-Wiener number R of T and of all its spanning subgraphs T-e.[34] The question arises can one construct an analytical expression for R'/R enabling us to calculate R'/R in a much simpler way directly from T. The answer is affirmative since such an expression has recently been found out.[44] Its derivation will be stated.

Let T be a tree with N vertices (see Figure 3) and let i and j be adjacent vertices in T and e_{ij} the edge connecting them. Suppose that $P(T)$ is the set of all paths of T. In relation to i, j and e_{ij} the set $P(T)$ can be partitioned into four disjoint subsets:

$P_1(T)$ - consisting of paths p_{uv} being "external" with respect to the edge e_{ij}, $p_{uv} \supseteq e_{ij}$;

$P_2(T)$ - consisting of paths p_{ai} containing the vertex i as a terminal vertex but $e_{ij} \not\subset p_{ai}$, and of their "internal" paths of the type p_{af} , $p_{af} \subset p_{ai}$;

$P_3(T)$ - consisting of paths p_{bj} containing the vertex j as a terminal vertex but $e_{ij} \not\subset p_{bj}$, and of their "internal" paths of the type p_{bg} , $p_{bg} \subset p_{bj}$; and

$P_4(T)$ - consisting of all other paths of T.

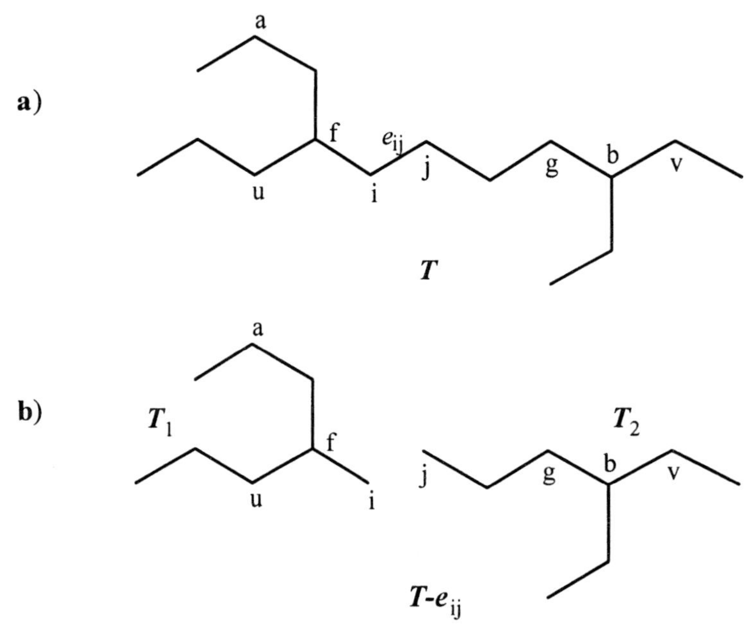

Figure 3. a) A tree graph T. An edge of T is denoted by e_{ij}. b) The spanning subgraph T-e_{ij} of T with components T_1 and T_2.

The removal of e_{ij} from T entails breaking of T into two components, T_1 and T_2 , whose vertex sets are V(T_1) and V(T_2), respectively, as well as the disappearance of all "external" paths with respect to the edge e_{ij}. Consequently, the set of all paths in T-e_{ij}, $P(T\text{-}e_{ij})$, equals $P_2(T) \cup P_3(T) \cup P_4(T)$, and if the set $P(T\text{-}e_{ij})$ is partitioned in a similar fashion as the path set $P(T)$, then $P_1(T\text{-}e_{ij}) = \varnothing$ and $P_k(T\text{-}e_{ij}) = P_k(T)$, k=2-4.

A contribution of a path p_{ai}, $p_{ai} \in P_2(T\text{-}e_{ij})$, to $R(T\text{-}e_{ij})$ can be expressed as the difference between its contribution to $R(T)$, $n_a(p_{ai})n_i(p_{ai})$, and $n_a(p_{ai})n_j(e_{ij})$. The quantity $n_a(p_{ai})n_j(e_{ij})$ represents that part of the contribution of p_{ai} to $R(T)$ arising from vertices of T that after the erasure of e_{ij} create $V(T_2)$. An "internal" path p_{af} of the path p_{ai} makes a contribution to $R(T\text{-}e_{ij})$ equal to $n_a(p_{af})(n_f(p_{af})\text{-}n_j(e_{ij}))$. Contributions of the paths belonging to $P_3(T\text{-}e_{ij})$ to $R(T\text{-}e_{ij})$ can be expressed in a similar way. Paths being the elements of $P_4(T\text{-}e_{ij})$ make identical contributions to $R(T\text{-}e_{ij})$ and $R(T)$.

The difference between $R(T)$ and $R(T\text{-}e_{ij})$ is given by the expression,

$$R(T) - R(T - e_{ij}) = \sum_{p_{uv} \in P_1(T)} n_u(p_{uv})\, n_v(p_{uv}) + n_j(e_{ij}) \sum_{a \in V(T_1)} \sum_{c \in p_{ai}} n_a(p_{ac}) + n_i(e_{ij}) \sum_{b \in V(T_2)} \sum_{d \in p_{bj}} n_b(p_{bd}) \;, \tag{34}$$

where the summation in the first term goes over all elements of $P_1(T)$, and in the second (third) term the summation runs over all vertices of the path p_{ai} (p_{bj}) and over all vertices making the vertex set $V(T_1)$ ($V(T_2)$). The first term on the right-hand side of Eq. (34) refers to contributions of all "external" paths with respect to the edge e_{ij}. The second (third) term represents the difference of the contributions of all paths being the elements of the set $P_2(T)$ ($P_3(T)$) before and after erasing e_{ij} from T.

Dividing Eq. (34) by $R(T)$ and by noting that

$$\sum_{c \in p_{ai}} n_a(p_{ac}) = d(a,i)\, n_a(p_{ai}) \tag{35}$$

and

$$\sum_{d \in p_{bj}} n_b(p_{bd}) = d(b,j)\, n_b(p_{bj}) \;, \tag{36}$$

where d(a, i) and d(b, j) stand for the distances between the vertices a and i and between the vertices b and j, respectively, one gets the graphical bond order, $R_{e_{ij}}/R$, of the edge e_{ij} of T,

$$R_{e_{ij}}/R = 1 - \frac{1}{R(T)}\left(\sum_{p_{uv}\in P_1(T)} n_u(p_{uv})n_v(p_{uv}) + n_j(e_{ij})\sum_{a\in V(T_1)} d(a,i)n_a(p_{ai}) + n_i(e_{ij})\sum_{b\in V(T_2)} d(b,j)n_b(p_{bj})\right) . \tag{37}$$

The graphical bond orders of other edges of T are found by appropriate partitions of the set P(T) and by following similar procedures.

By adding up graphical bond orders of all N-1 edges of T one obtains the R'/R descriptor of T,

$$R'/R = N - 1 - \frac{1}{R(T)}\sum_{e_{ij}}\left(\sum_{p_{uv}\in P_1(T)} n_u(p_{uv})n_v(p_{uv}) + n_j(e_{ij})\sum_{a\in V(T_1)} d(a,i)n_a(p_{ai}) + n_i(e_{ij})\sum_{b\in V(T_2)} d(b,j)n_b(p_{bj})\right) . \tag{38}$$

It is not difficult to see that

$$\sum_{e_{ij}}\sum_{p_{uv}\in P_1(T)} n_u(p_{uv})n_v(p_{uv}) = \sum_{p_{rs}\in P(T)} d(r,s)n_r(p_{rs})n_s(p_{rs}) , \tag{39}$$

and due to the uniqueness of paths in T, the second and the third term in parentheses on the right-hand side of Eq. (38) can be expressed as:

$$n_j(e_{ij})\sum_{a\in V(T_1)} d(a,i)n_a(p_{ai}) = \sum_{a\in V(T_1)} (d(a,j)-1)n_a(p_{aj})n_j(p_{aj}) \tag{40}$$

and

$$n_i(e_{ij})\sum_{b\in V(T_2)} d(b,j)n_b(p_{bj}) = \sum_{b\in V(T_2)} (d(b,i)-1)n_b(p_{bi})n_i(p_{bi}) . \tag{41}$$

By noting that

$$\sum_{e_{ij}}\left[\sum_{a\in V(T_1)} (d(a,j)-1)n_a(p_{aj})n_j(p_{aj}) + \sum_{b\in V(T_2)} (d(b,i)-1)n_b(p_{bi})n_i(p_{bi})\right] = \sum_{p_{rs}\in P(T)} 2(d(r,s)-1)n_r(p_{rs})n_s(p_{rs}) \tag{42}$$

and combining Eq. (38) with Eqs. (39)-(42) one gets a more compact expression for R'/R of *T*,

$$\mathrm{R'/R} = N + 1 - \frac{3 \sum_{p_{rs} \in P(T)} \mathrm{d(r,s)} \mathrm{n_r}(p_{rs}) \mathrm{n_s}(p_{rs})}{\sum_{p_{rs} \in P(T)} \mathrm{n_r}(p_{rs}) \mathrm{n_s}(p_{rs})} , \tag{43}$$

where the summations run over all paths of *T*. The quantity $\mathrm{d(r, s)n_r}(p_{rs})\mathrm{n_s}(p_{rs})$ represents the length d(r, s) of the path p_{rs} multiplied by the number of "external" paths with respect to the path p_{rs}. By analysis of "external" and "internal" paths of a given path in *T*, it has been shown that[47]

$$\sum_{p_{rs} \in P(T)} \mathrm{n_r}(p_{rs}) \mathrm{n_s}(p_{rs}) = \frac{1}{2} \sum_{r<s} \mathrm{d(r,s)(d(r,s)+1)} , \tag{44}$$

where the summation goes over all pairs of vertices of *T*. The nominator of the fraction on the right-hand side of Eq. (43) can be expressed by means of distances only,

$$\sum_{p_{rs} \in P(T)} \mathrm{d(r,s)} \mathrm{n_r}(p_{rs}) \mathrm{n_s}(p_{rs}) = \frac{1}{6} \sum_{r<s} \mathrm{d(r,s)(d(r,s)+1)(d(r,s)+2)} . \tag{45}$$

Combining Eq. (43) with Eqs. (44) and (45) one gets the sought-after formula for calculation of the R'/R descriptor of *T*,

$$\mathrm{R'/R} = N + 1 - \frac{\sum_{r<s} \mathrm{d(r,s)(d(r,s)+1)(d(r,s)+2)}}{\sum_{r<s} \mathrm{d(r,s)(d(r,s)+1)}} . \tag{46}$$

This formula renders us possible to calculate the R'/R descriptor directly from *T*, just from the knowledge of the number of vertices in *T* and distances between them.

Although the formula has been derived for connected acyclic structures, it is well defined for connected cycle-containing structures as well. Therefore it is quite reasonable to accept Eq. (46) as a novel general definition of the molecular descriptor R'/R. Furthermore, R'/R defined in this manner fits in well with the recently redefined hyper-Wiener number R.[47] The application of the formula is illustrated in Figure 4 for the hydrogen-suppressed graph of 1-(2-propyl)-2-methyl-benzene.

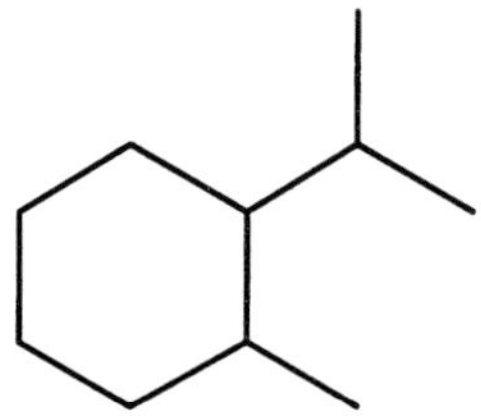

$$\text{R}'/\text{R} = 10+1-\frac{10\cdot 1\cdot 2\cdot 3+13\cdot 2\cdot 3\cdot 4+12\cdot 3\cdot 4\cdot 5+8\cdot 4\cdot 5\cdot 6+2\cdot 5\cdot 6\cdot 7}{10\cdot 1\cdot 2+13\cdot 2\cdot 3+12\cdot 3\cdot 4+8\cdot 4\cdot 5+2\cdot 5\cdot 6} = 5.6494$$

Figure 4. Calculation of the molecular descriptor R'/R of the hydrogen-suppressed graph of 1-(2-propyl)-2-methyl-benzene.

In some special cases Eq. (46) takes a rather simple form, e.g., for P_N,

$$\text{R}'/\text{R} = \frac{2}{5}(N-2)\;;\quad N \geq 2 \tag{47}$$

and for C_N, the expression depends on the parity of N,

$$\text{R}'/\text{R} = \begin{cases} \dfrac{5N-7}{8} & \text{for } N = 2\text{m}+1\;;\; \text{m} \in \mathbf{N} \\[2ex] \dfrac{5N-7}{8} - \dfrac{9}{8(N+1)} & \text{for } N = 2\text{m}+2\;;\; \text{m} \in \mathbf{N}\;. \end{cases} \tag{48}$$

4.4. Explicit Formula for Calculation of Molecular Descriptor Z'/Z

Hosoya noticed the chemical significance of certain combinatorial properties of molecular graphs, in particular the importance of independent sets of edges.[38] A set S of edges of a (molecular) graph G is independent if no two edges of S are adjacent in G. Two distinct edges of G are adjacent if they are incident with a common vertex. The number of independent sets of k edges of G is denoted by a(G, k). The related generating function is known as the Z-counting polynomial Q(G; x),[38]

$$\text{Q}(G;\text{x}) = \sum_{\text{k}=0}^{[N/2]} \text{a}(G,\text{k})\,\text{x}^{\text{k}}\;, \tag{49}$$

where N is the number of vertices of G, and $[N/2]$ stands for the integer part of $N/2$. The empty set and all singleton sets are independent, hence $\text{a}(G,0)=1$ and $\text{a}(G,1)$ equals the number of edges of G. Hosoya also introduced a graph invariant, the Z index, equal to the total number of independent sets of edges of G,[38]

$$Z = Z(G) = \sum_{k=0}^{[N/2]} a(G,k) \; . \tag{50}$$

Clearly, the Z index equals the value of the Z-counting polynomial for x=1,

$$Z = Q(G;1) \; . \tag{51}$$

Recently Randić has introduced the new composite molecular descriptor Z'/Z constructed from the Z index.[29, 34] The Z'/Z descriptor, Z'/Z=(Z'/Z)(G), of a molecular graph G is defined by the expression,

$$Z'/Z = \frac{1}{Z(G)} \sum_{e} Z(G-e) \; , \tag{52}$$

where Z(G) and Z(G-e) stand for the Z index of G and G-e, respectively, and the summation goes over all edges of G. If G-e is disconnected then the contributions of its components are given by Eq. (3).

The search for a formula making calculation of Z'/Z directly from G possible is reduced to finding out an analytical expression for the sum $\sum Z(G-e)$ in which only quantities related to G appear. The straight way to obtain such an expression is to express $\sum Z(G-e)$ by means of Z(G).[39, 41, 42] Let G be a molecular graph with N vertices and R rings. The basic recursion relation for Z(G) is

$$Z(G) = Z(G - e_{ij}) + Z(G - e_{ij} - A(e_{ij})) \; , \tag{53}$$

where $A(e_{ij})$ is the set of edges adjacent to the edge e_{ij}. The first term on the right-hand side of Eq. (53) equals the number of independent sets of edges of G that do not contain the edge e_{ij}. The number of the remaining independent sets of G, clearly, equals $Z(G\text{-}e_{ij}\text{-}A(e_{ij}))$, and all of them contain the edge e_{ij}. Hence, one can write,

$$Z(G - e_{ij} - A(e_{ij})) = \sum_{k=1}^{[N/2]} a(G,k,e_{ij}) \; , \tag{54}$$

where a(G, k, e_{ij}) represents the number of independent sets of k edges of G containing the edge e_{ij}. Combining Eqs. (53) and (54) with the identity[48]

$$\sum_{e_{ij}} a(G,k,e_{ij}) = k\, a(G,k)\ , \tag{55}$$

one obtains the relationship between $\sum$ Z(G-e) and Z,

$$\sum_{e_{ij}} Z(G - e_{ij}) = (N + R - 1)Z - \sum_{k=1}^{[N/2]} k\, a(G,k)\ , \tag{56}$$

and the sought-after formula for calculation of Z'/Z directly from G,

$$Z'/Z = (N + R - 1) - \frac{\sum_{k=1}^{[N/2]} k\, a(G,k)}{\sum_{k=0}^{[N/2]} a(G,k)}\ . \tag{57}$$

The application of this formula is illustrated in Figure 5 for the hydrogen-suppressed graph of 1-(2-propyl)-2-ethyl-benzene.

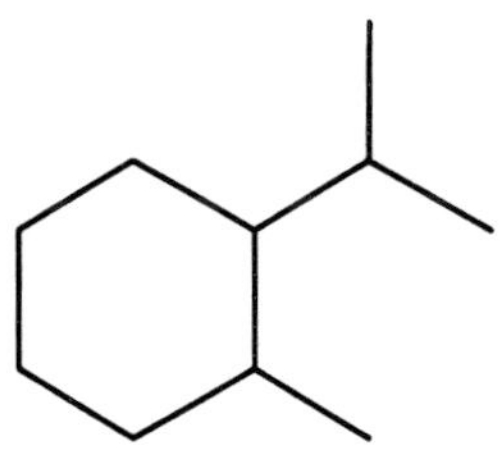

$$Z'/Z = 10 + 1 - 1 - \frac{10 + 2\cdot 32 + 3\cdot 37 + 4\cdot 11}{1 + 10 + 32 + 37 + 11} = 7.4835$$

Figure 5. Calculation of the molecular descriptor Z'/Z of the hydrogen--suppressed graph of 1-(2-propyl)-2-methyl-benzene.

Since the nominator of the fraction on the right-hand side of Eq. (57) is just the derivative of Q(G;x) for x=1, Q'(G;1), Eq. (57) can also be written as

$$Z'/Z = (N + R - 1) - \frac{Q'(G;1)}{Q(G;1)}\ . \tag{58}$$

To compute the Z'/Z descriptor of an arbitrary molecular graph it is necessary and sufficient to have knowledge of the number of vertices and the number of rings as well as the number of independent sets of k edges of the graph. Evidently, the first two demands are trivial, but the third, if one thinks about an explicit analytical expression for computing $a(G,k)$'s is not possible to fulfill in general. However, it is possible to derive explicit formulae for $a(G,k)$'s for some special classes of graphs. Formulae for the first few $a(G,k)$'s of a tree graph T read as follows[39]

$$a(T,2)=\frac{1}{2}\sum_{e_{ij}} a(T,2,e_{ij}) = \frac{1}{2}\sum_{e_{ij}} \left[a(T,1)-(v_i+v_j-1)\right]$$
$$=\frac{1}{2}\left[N(N-1)-\sum_{i} v_i^2\right], \tag{59}$$

$$a(T,3)=\frac{1}{3}\left[(N-1)(a(T,2)+N+1)+\sum_{i} v_i^3-(N+2)\sum_{i} v_i^2+3\sum_{e_{ij}} v_i v_j\right], \tag{60}$$

and

$$a(T,4)=\frac{1}{4}\Bigg[(N-1)(a(T,3)+a(T,2)+2N+3)-\sum_{i} v_i^4+(N+3)\sum_{i} v_i^3-$$
$$(a(T,2)+3N+7)\sum_{i} v_i^2-4\sum_{\substack{p_{rs}\\ d(r,s)=2}} v_r v_s+(3N+13)\sum_{e_{ij}} v_i v_j-4\sum_{e_{ij}} v_i v_j(v_i+v_j)\Bigg], \tag{61}$$

where v_i is the valency of vertex i, and p_{rs} denotes the path of length two with terminal vertices r and s.

In case of the path graph P_N, the analytical expressions for $a(P_N,k)$ and the Z'/Z descriptor are rather simple,

$$a(P_N,k)=\binom{N-k}{k} \quad ; \quad 0\le k\le [N/2] \tag{62}$$

and

$$Z'/Z = (N-1) - \frac{\sum_{k=1}^{[N/2]} k \binom{N-k}{k}}{\sum_{k=0}^{[N/2]} \binom{N-k}{k}} , \tag{63}$$

respectively.

The Z'/Z descriptor of the cycle graph C_N can be computed by using the expression,

$$Z'/Z = \frac{N\, Z(P_N)}{Z(C_N)} , \tag{64}$$

and the following recursions

$$Z(C_N) = Z(P_N) + Z(P_{N-2}) \;\; ; \;\; N \geq 3 \tag{65}$$

and

$$Z(P_N) = Z(P_{N-1}) + Z(P_{N-2}) \;\; ; \;\; N \geq 3 \; . \tag{66}$$

Since $Z(P_N)$ equals the N-th Fibonacci number, F_N, (the initial conditions for the Fibonacci recursion: $F_N = F_{N-1} + F_{N-2}$, are $F_0 = F_1 = 1$) the expression for $Z(P_N)$ is given by the Binét formula. The explicit formula for Z'/Z of C_N then reads as follows

$$Z'/Z = \frac{N\left[\left(\frac{1+5^{1/2}}{2}\right)^{N+1} - \left(\frac{1-5^{1/2}}{2}\right)^{N+1}\right]}{5^{1/2}\left[\left(\frac{1+5^{1/2}}{2}\right)^{N} + \left(\frac{1-5^{1/2}}{2}\right)^{N}\right]} . \tag{67}$$

5. Concluding Remarks

The X'/X descriptor of a molecular graph *G* was introduced by Randić as the sum of graphical bond orders X_e/X of all edges of *G*. A review of our recent results on various molecular descriptors X'/X is given in this chapter. We have shown that instead of calculation of all X_e/X 's one can compute the molecular descriptor X'/X directly from structural characteristics (like number of vertices, edges and paths, valencies of vertices, the number of independent sets of edges, etc.) of *G*. This has been explicitly illustrated for X'/X where X stands for the connectivity index χ, the total number of paths P, the hyper-Wiener number R, and the Hosoya index Z.

6. Acknowledgments

We are grateful to Dr. Milan Šoškić (Zagreb) for useful comments. This work was supported by the Ministry of Science and Technology of the Republic of Croatia, the Croatian-Slovenian project "Discrete Mathematics in Chemistry", and the collaborative project of the Hungarian Academy of Sciences and the Croatian Academy of Sciences and Arts.

7. References

1. Turro, N. J. Geometric and Topological Thinking in Organic Chemistry. *Angew. Chem. Int. Ed. Engl.* **1986**, 25, 882-901.
2. Seybold, P. G.; May, M.; Bagal, U. A. Molecular Structure - Property Relationships. *J. Chem. Educ.* **1987**, 64, 575-581.
3. Randić, M. The Nature of Chemical Structure. *J. Math. Chem.* **1990**, 4, 157- 184.
4. Mekenyan, O.; Basak, S. C. Topological Indices and Chemical Reactivity. In *Graph Theoretical Approach to Chemical Reactivity*; Bonchev, D., Mekenyan, O., Eds.; Kluwer: Dordrecht, Netherlands, 1994., Chapter 8, pp 221-239.
5. Milne, G. W. A. Mathematics as a Basis for Chemistry. *J. Chem. Inf. Comput. Sci.* **1997**, 37, 639-644.
6. Randić, M. On Characterization of Chemical Structure. *J. Chem. Inf. Comput. Sci.* **1997**, 37, 672-687.
7. Szabo, A.; Ostlund, N. S. *Modern Quantum Chemistry. Introduction to Advanced Electronic Theory*; 1st revised ed.; McGraw-Hill: New York, 1989.
8. McWeeny, R. *Methods of Molecular Quantum Mechanics*; 2nd ed.; Academic Press: London, 1992.
9. Kier, L. B.; Hall, L. M. *Molecular Connectivity in Chemistry and Drug Research*; Academic Press: New York, 1976.
10. Kier, L. B.; Hall, L. M. *Molecular Connectivity in Structure-Activity Analysis*; Research Studies Press Ltd.: Letchworth, England, 1986.

11. Trinajstić, N.; Randić, M.; Klein, D. J. On the Quantitative Structure-Activity Relationship in Drug Research. *Acta Pharm. Jugosl.* **1986**, 36, 267-279.
12. Rouvray, D. H. Predicting Chemistry from Topology. *Sci. Am.* **1986**, 254(3), 36- 43.
13. Rouvray, D. H. The Limits of Applicability of Topological Indices. *J. Mol. Struct. (Theochem)* **1989**, 185, 187-201.
14. Basak, S. C.; Niemi, G. J.; Veith, G. D. Predicting Properties of Molecules Using Graph Invariants. *J. Math. Chem.* **1991**, 7, 243-272.
15. Randić, M. Resolution of Ambiguities in Structure-Property Studies by Use of Orthogonal Descriptors. *J. Chem. Inf. Comput. Sci.* **1991**, 31, 311-320.
16. Trinajstić, N. *Chemical Graph Theory*; 2nd revised ed.; CRC Press: Boca Raton, FL, 1992.
17. Randić, M.; Mihalić, Z.; Nikolić, S.; Trinajstić, N. Graph-Theoretical Correlations - Artifacts or Facts? *Croat. Chem. Acta* **1993**, 66, 411-434.
18. Katritzky, A. R.; Gordeeva, E. Traditional Topological Indices *vs* Electronic, Geometrical, and Combined Molecular Descriptors in QSAR/QSPR Research. *J. Chem. Inf. Comput. Sci.* **1993**, 33, 835-857.
19. Hansch, C.; Leo, A.; Hoekman, D. *Exploring QSAR;* American Chemical Society, Washington, DC., 1995.
20. Karelson, M.; Lobanov, V. S.; Katritzky, A. R. Quantum-Chemical Descriptors in QSAR/QSPR Studies. *Chem. Rev.* **1996**, 96, 1027-1043.
21. Šoškić, M.; Plavšić, D.; Trinajstić, N. 2-Difluoromethylthio-4,6-bis(monoalkylamino)-1,3,5-triazines as Inhibitors of Hill Reaction: A QSAR Study with Orthogonalized Descriptors. *J. Chem. Inf. Comput. Sci.* **1996**, 36, 146-150.
22. Bögel, H.; Dettmann, J.; Randić, M. Why is the Topological Approach in Chemistry so Successful? *Croat. Chem. Acta* **1997**, 70, 827-840.
23. Balaban, A. T., Ed.; *From Chemical Topology to Three-Dimensional Geometry*; Plenum Press: New York, 1997.
24. Katritzky, A. R.; Karelson, M.; Lobanov, V. S. QSPR as a Means of Predicting and Understanding Chemical and Physical Properties in Terms of Structure. *Pure Appl. Chem.* **1997**, 69, 245-248.
25. Plavšić, D.; Trinajstić, N.; Amić, D.; Šoškić, M. Comparison between the Structure-Boiling Point Relationships with Different Descriptors for Condensed Benzenoids. *New J. Chem.* **1998**, 22, 1075-1078.
26. Gutman, I.; Polansky, O. E. *Mathematical Concepts in Organic Chemistry*; Springer-Verlag: Berlin, 1986.
27. Randić, M. In Search of Structural Invariants. *J. Math. Chem.* **1992**, 9, 97-146.
28. Randić, M.; Trinajstić, N. In Search for Graph Invariants of Chemical Interest. *J. Mol. Struct.* **1993**, 300, 551-571.
29. Randić, M. Search for Optimal Molecular Descriptors. *Croat. Chem. Acta* **1991**, 64, 43-54.
30. Randić, M. Generalized Molecular Descriptors. *J. Math. Chem.* **1991**, 7, 155- 168.
31. Randić, M. Comparative Regression Analysis. Regressions Based on Single Descriptors. *Croat. Chem. Acta* **1993**, 66, 289-312.

32. Randić, M. Novel Molecular Descriptor for Structure-Property Studies. *Chem. Phys. Lett.* **1993**, 211, 478-483.
33. Randić, M. Hosoya Matrix - A Source of New Molecular Descriptors. *Croat. Chem. Acta* **1994**, 67, 415-429.
34. Randić, M.; Mihalić, Z.; Nikolić, S.; Trinajstić, N. Graphical Bond Orders: Novel Structural Descriptors. *J. Chem. Inf. Comput. Sci.* **1994**, 34, 403-409.
35. Randić, M. On Characterization of Molecular Branching. *J. Am. Chem. Soc.* **1975**, 97, 6609-6615.
36. Wiener, H. Structural Determination of Paraffin Boiling Points. *J. Am. Chem. Soc.* **1947**, 69, 17-20.
37. Balaban, A. T. Highly Discriminating Distance-Based Topological Index. *Chem. Phys. Lett.* **1982**, 89, 399-404.
38. Hosoya, H. Topological Index. A Newly Proposed Quantity Characterizing the Topological Nature of Structural Isomers of Saturated Hydrocarbons. *Bull. Chem. Soc. Jpn.* **1971**, 44, 2332-2339.
39. Plavšić, D.; Šoškić, M.; Landeka, I.; Gutman, I.; Graovac, A. On the Relation between the Path Numbers ^1Z, ^2Z and the Hosoya Z Index. *J. Chem. Inf. Comput. Sci.* **1996**, 36, 1118-1122.
40. Plavšić, D.; Šoškić, M.; Landeka, I.; Trinajstić, N. On the Relation between the P'/P Index and the Wiener Number. *J. Chem. Inf. Comput. Sci.* **1996**, 36, 1123- 1126.
41. Plavšić, D.; Šoškić, M.; Žaković, Z.; Gutman, I.; Graovac, A. Extension of the **Z** Matrix to Cycle-Containing and Edge-Weighted Molecular Graphs. *J. Chem. Inf. Comput. Sci.* **1997**, 37, 529-534.
42. Gutman, I.; Plavšić, D.; Šoškić, M.; Landeka, I.; Graovac, A. On the Calculation of the Path Numbers ^1Z, ^2Z and the Hosoya Z Index. *Croat. Chem. Acta* **1997**, 70, 941-954.
43. Plavšić, D.; Šoškić, M.; Lerš, N. On the Calculation of the Molecular Descriptor χ'/χ. *J. Chem. Inf. Comput. Sci.* **1998**, 38, 529-534.
44. Plavšić, D. On the Definition and Calculation of the Molecular Descriptor R'/R. *Chem. Phys. Lett.* **1999**, 304, 111-116.
45. Plavšić, D.; Lerš, N.; Sertić-Bionda, K. On the Relation between W'/W Index, Hyper-Wiener Index and Wiener Number. *J. Chem. Inf. Comput. Sci.* **2000**, 40, 000-000.
46. Mohar, B.; Pisanski, T. How to Compute the Wiener Index of a Graph. *J. Math. Chem.* **1988**, 2, 267-277.
47. Klein, D. J.; Lukovits, I.; Gutman, I. On the Definition of the Hyper-Wiener Index for Cycle-Containing Structures. *J. Chem. Inf. Comput. Sci.* **1995**, 35, 50-52.
48. Gutman, I. Some Analytical Properties of the Independence and Matching Polynomials. *Commun. Math. Chem. (MATCH)* **1992**, 28, 139-150.

Chapter 4

MODELING THE SOLUBILITY OF ALIPHATIC ALCOHOLS IN WATER. GRAPH CONNECTIVITY INDICES *VERSUS* LINE GRAPH CONNECTIVITY INDICES

Sonja Nikolić and Nenad Trinajstić
The Ruđer Bošković Institute, HR-10001 Zagreb,
The Republic of Croatia
Dragan Amić and Drago Bešlo
Faculty of Agriculture, The Josip Juraj Strossmayer University,
HR-31001 Osijek, The Republic of Croatia
Subhash C. Basak
Natural Resources Research Institute, University of Minnesota,
Duluth, MN 55811, USA

1. INTRODUCTION

In this chapter we report on modeling the aqueous solubility of aliphatic alcohols. We are interested in aliphatic alcohols because they are toxic materials and thus represent dangerous environmental pollutants. The toxic action of alcohols on the higher organisms, presumably through the phenomenom of narcosis, depends on their solubility in water. The lower alcohols: methanol, ethanol and propanol, mix with water in any ratio, while this is not the case with other aliphatic alcohols, especially higher ones.

Recently in the area of structure-property modeling based on topological indices[1] appeared several reports, e.g.,[2,3] which, if supported, will open up a new perspective for this kind of chemical modeling. The most interesting to us for the present purpose are the following two papers: In the first Estrada and Rodriguez[4] have shown that the edge-connectivity index produces the best single-variable QSPR[5] models for five out of seven physicochemical properties of octanes and in the second Gutman *et al.*[6] have reported that the use of line graphs significantly improves the predictive power of topological indices. We tested both of these results on modeling the aqueous solubility of aliphatic alcohols, because there is a number of structure-water solubility models for alcohols in the literature[7,8] to which the obtained models could be compared. We also tested the result that in some cases the optimum exponent of the (valence) vertex- and edge-connectivity indices is not -0.5.[9]

Since we completely agree with the following statement by Katritzky, Karelson and Lobanov:[10] "*As scientists, today we are increasingly urged to do science of relevance to society. QSPR allows us to carry out science that will undoubtedly help us to make production of new molecules useful in all facets of life and society more cheaply, more efficiently, and in a more environmentally friendly manner. At the same time, it offers the highest intellectual challenges for the development of meaningful relationships, novel theories, and deeper understanding into the molecular nature of the world in which we live.*", we believe that the QSPR modeling will become the tool of choice for many physical, organic, inorganic, analytical, medicinal, environmental, industrial, pharmaceutical, etc. chemists in times to come. There are already very encouraging results published using the so-called "in silico"[11] approach to the rational design of therapeutic compounds.[12] Therefore, it seems to us worthwhile to search for the most reliable "in silico" methodology to carry out the QSPR modeling. The present article describes one attempt in this direction. There are also other directions open for the exploration.[12-17] It should be also noted that throughout the article we will use the chemical graph-theoretical concepts and language[18,19] only to simplify the analysis.

Although line graphs have found so far a limited use in the structure-property-activity modeling,[6,20,21] they were described in a monograph on chemical graph theory[22] and under the name bond graphs were used for deriving the molecular complexity indices.[23] In formal graph theory,[24] the line graph is a standard concept. The line graph L(G)=L of a graph G is a graph derived from G in a such a way that the edges in G are replaced by vertices in L. Two vertices in L are adjacent if the corresponding two edges in G are incident, that is, have a vertex in common. The construction of a line graph from a tree is shown in Figure 1.

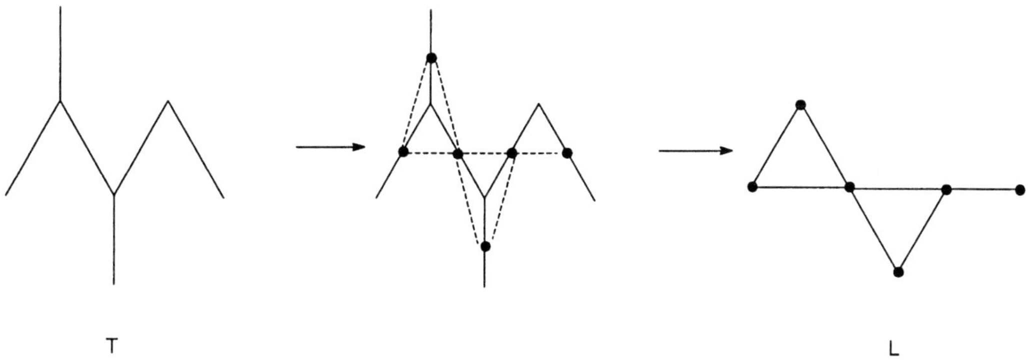

Figure 1. Construction of a line graph L from a branched tree T.

Note that the numbers of vertices V and edges E of the line graph L and the corresponding graph G are related by:

$$V(L) = E(G) \quad (1)$$

$$E(L) = (1/2)\sum_i d_1^2(G) - E(G) \quad (2)$$

where d_i (i=1,2,...,V) are degrees of vertices in G. Using

$$\sum_i d_1^2(G) = M_1 \quad (3)$$

where M_1 is called[25,26] the first Zagreb index,[27] and introducing (3) into (2) we obtain expression:

$$E(L) = (1/2)\, M_1 - E(G) \quad (4)$$

which was also given by Gutman and Estrada,[28] but without factor 1/2. From eq. (4) follows an amusing result that the M_1-index of the graph is simply equal twice the number of vertices and edges in the corresponding line graph:

$$M_1 = 2\,[E(L) + E(G)] = 2\,[E(L) + V(L)] \quad (5)$$

2. Modified Valence Vertex- and Edge-Connectivity Indices

The standard definition of the valence vertex-connectivity index is:[29]

$$\chi^{v} = \sum_{edges} \left[\delta(v_1)\delta(v_j)\right]^{-0.5} \tag{6}$$

where $\delta(v_i)$ and $\delta(v_j)$ are weights (valence-delta values) of vertices v_i and v_j making up the i-j edge in a weighted graph modeling the molecular heterosystem. The valence-delta values can be computed using the following expression:

$$\delta(v_i) = (Z_i^{v} - H_i) / (Z - Z_i^{v} - 1) \tag{7}$$

where Z_i^{v} is the number of valence electrons in the atom i, Z is its atomic number and H_i is the number of hydrogen atoms attached to i. The δ-value for oxygen atom in the bonding environment characteristic of aliphatic alcohols is 5. The δ-values for carbon atoms are 1, 2, 3 or 4 depending on the bonding environment of carbon. The computation of the valence vertex-connectivity index for 3-methyl-1-butanol is shown in Figure 2.

(1) 3-methyl-1-butanol

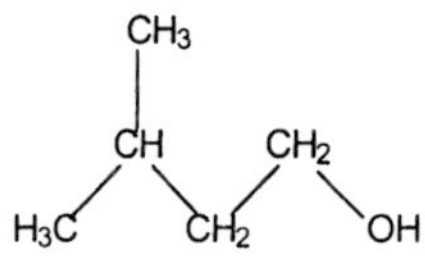

(2) Weighted tree Tw corresponding to 3-methyl-1-butanol.
Black dot denotes the position of oxygen

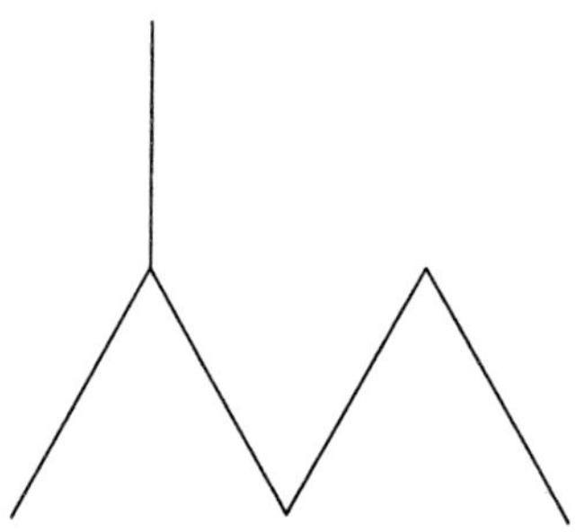

Tw

(3) Vertex-degrees in T^w

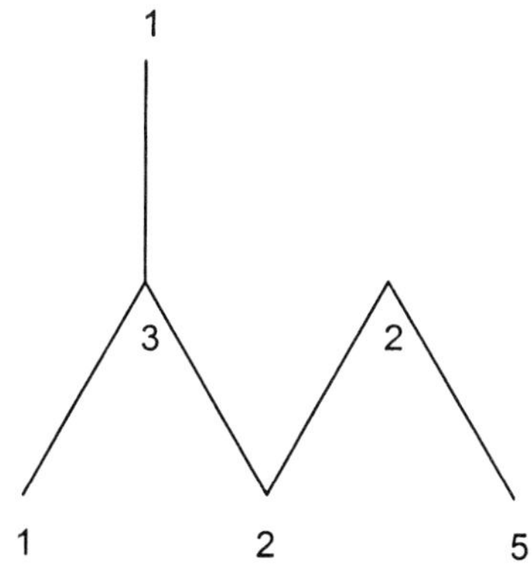

(4) Valence vertex-connectivity index

$$\chi^V(T^w) = 2\ (1\ \ 3)^{-0.5} + (2\ 2)^{-0.5} + (2\ \ 3)^{-0.5} + \ (2\ \ 5)^{-0.5} = 2.3^{\cdot}$$

Figure 2. Computation of the valence vertex-connectivity index for 3-methyl-1-butanol.

The modified valence vertex-connectivity index is defined as:[9]

$$\chi^v = \sum_{edges} \left[\delta(v_1)\delta(v_j)\right]^k \qquad k \quad 0 \tag{8}$$

where k is a variable exponent that can be varied ordinarily from -0.10 (or any smaller value) to any desired value.

The standard definition of the valence edge-connectivity index is:[30]

$$\varepsilon^v = \sum_{\substack{adjacent\\ edges}} \left[\delta(e_1)\delta(e_j)\right]^{-0.5} \tag{9}$$

where $\delta(e_i)$ and $\delta(e_j)$ are the values the weighted degrees of the edges e_i and e_j. The value of the $\delta(e)$-parameter for for the C-O bond is taken to be 0.8 as suggested by Estrada.[31] The vertex- and edge-degrees in weighted graphs are related by:

$$\delta(e) = \delta(v_i) + \delta(v_j) - \text{constant} \tag{10}$$

where the values of the constant in the case of aliphatic alcohols are: (i) 2 for CC bonds non-adjacent to C-O bond, (ii) 2.2 for CC bonds adjacent to C-O bond and (iii) 6 for the

C-O bond. As an example, the computation of the valence edge-connectivity index for 3-methyl-1-butanol is shown in Figure 3.

(1) Weighted tree T^w corresponding to 3-methyl-1-butanol. Labels stand for vertex-degrees

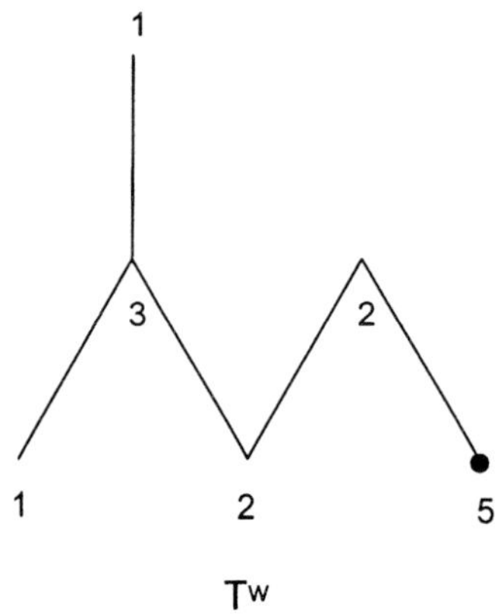

(2) Edge-degrees in T^w

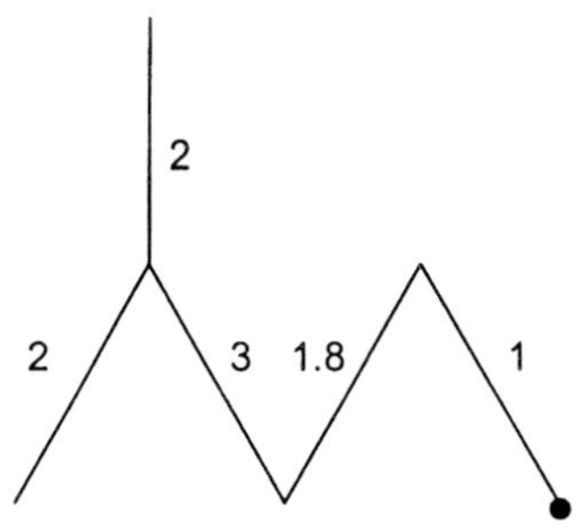

(3) Valence edge-connectivity index

$$\varepsilon^V(T^w) = (1 \quad 1.8)^{-0.5} + (1.8 \quad 3)^{-0.5} + (2 \quad 2)^{-0.5} + 2\,(2 \quad 3)^{-0.5} = 2.4$$

Figure 3. Computation of the valence edge-connectivity index for 3-methyl-1-butanol.

A simple way to assign the degrees to edges in a weighted graph is to sum up the weights of all adjacent bonds of a bond to which we wish to determine the edge-degree. This procedure is illustrated in Figure 4. In the present report we used this procedure for determining the edge-degrees in the weighted trees and corresponding weighted line graphs.

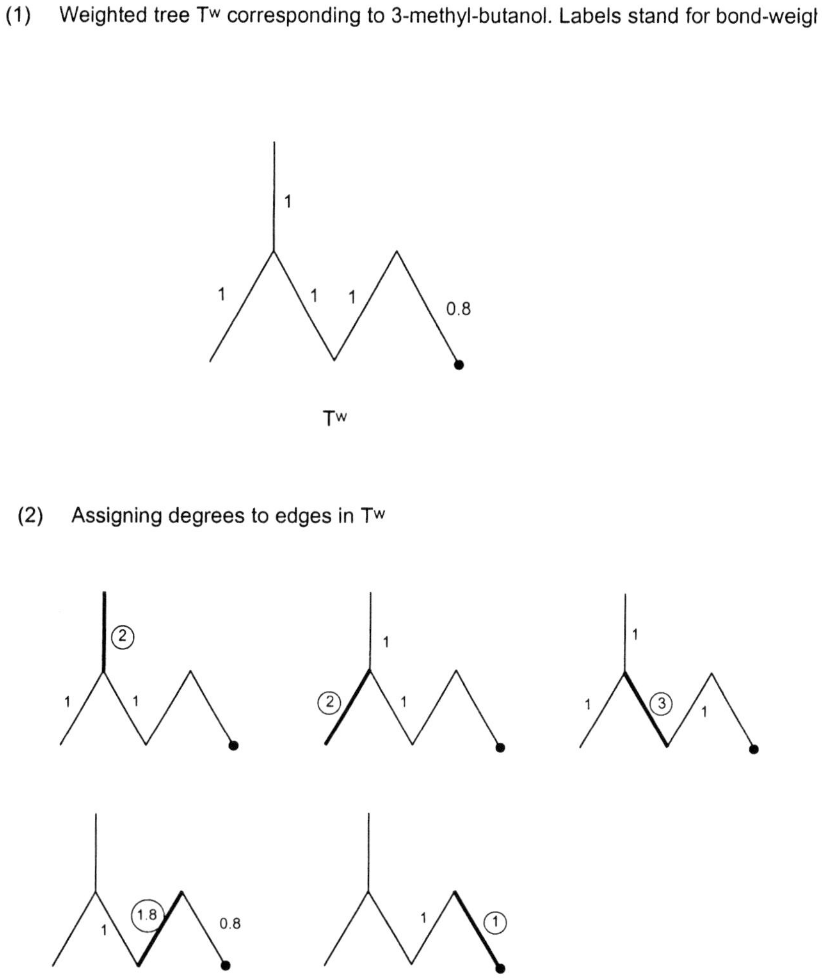

Figure 4. A simple procedure for assigning the degrees to edges in a weighted tree.

It should be noted that the edge-adjacency matrix[32] of the graph G, ${}^{E}\mathbf{A}(G)$, is identical to the vertex-adjacency matrix[32] of the line graph L of G, ${}^{V}\mathbf{A}(L)$:

$${}^{E}\mathbf{A}(G) = {}^{V}\mathbf{A}(L) \tag{11}$$

The consequence of this result is that the (valence) edge-connectivity index of G is identical to the (valence) vertex-connectivity index of the corresponding line graph L:[28]

$$\varepsilon^{v}(G) = \chi^{v}(L) \tag{12}$$

Hence, the edge-degrees of the weighted graph G^w are identical to vertex-degrees of the corresponding weighted line graph L^w. In Figure 5 is shown the construction of the weighted line graph L^w corresponding to the weighted tree T^w depicting 3-methyl-1-butanol and its vertex-degrees.

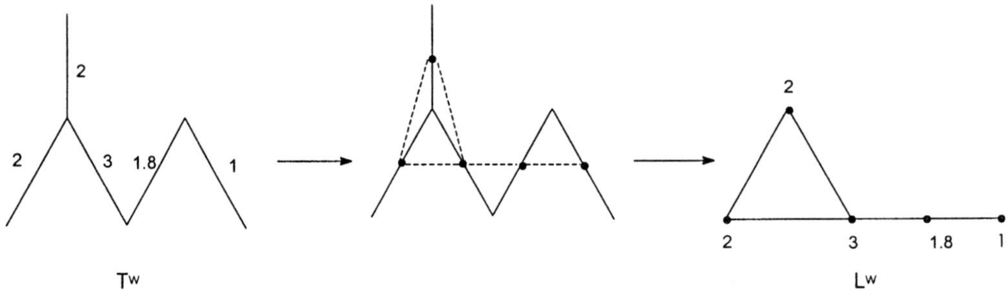

Figure 5. Construction of the weighted line graph L^w from the corresponding weighted tree T^w. The edge-valencies of T^w are identical to vertex-valencies of L^w.

In Figure 6 we show the computation of the valence edge-connectivity index for the weighted line graph corresponding to 3-methyl-1-butanol. The edge-degrees in the weighted line graph were obtained by the procedure described above and illustrated in Figure 4.

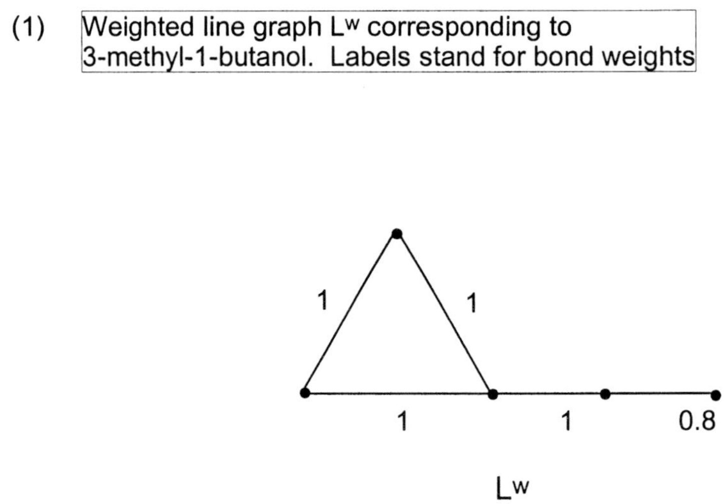

(2) Edge-deegres in L^w

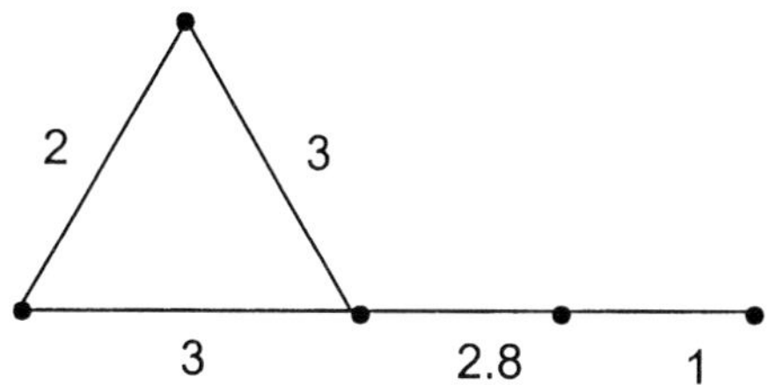

(3) Valence edge-connectivity index

$$\varepsilon^V(L^w) = (1\ \ 2.8)^{-0.5} + 2\ (2\ \ 3)^{-0.5} + 2\ (2.8\ \ 3)^{-0.5} + (3\ \ 3)^{-0.5} = 3.2$$

Figure 6. Computation of the valence edge-connectivity index for the weighted line graph L^w corresponding to 3-methyl-1-butanol.

The modified valence edge-connectivity index is defined as:

$$\varepsilon^v = \sum_{\substack{adjacent\\edges}} [\delta(v_i)\ \delta(v_j)]^k \qquad k\ \ 0 \tag{13}$$

where k is a variable exponent that can be varied ordinarily from -0.10 (or any smaller value) to any desired value.

3. Comparison Between the Structure-Solubility Models

The experimental solubilities of aliphatic alcohols in water[33,34] in terms of their natural logarithms, ln SOL, are given in Table 1.

Table 1. The Logarithm of Experimental Solubility of 54 Aliphatic Alcohols in Water

Aliphatic alcohol	ln SOL	Aliphatic alcohol	ln SOL
2-Methyl-1-propanol	0.02274	3-heptanol	-3.19418
2-Butanol	0.06579	4-heptanol	-3.19662
3-Methyl-1-butanol	-1.16796	2,2,3-Trimethyl-3-pentanol	-2.93182
2-Methyl-1-butanol	-1.05840	2-Octanol	-4.75600
2-Pentanol	-0.63488	2-Ethyl-1-hexanol	-4.99673
3-Pentanol	-0.48613	2-Nonanol	-6.31997
3-Methyl-2-butanol	-0.40497	3-Nonanol	-6.11930
2-Methyl-2-butanol	0.33861	4-Nonanol	-5.95224
3-Hexanol	-1.83258	5-Nonanol	-5.74460
3-Methyl-3-pentanol	-0.83011	2,6-Dimethyl-4-heptanol	-5.77635
2-Methyl-2-pentanol	-1.11780	3,5-Dimethyl-4-heptanol	-5.29832
2-Methyl-3-pentanol	-1.60944	2,2-Diethyl-1-pentanol	-5.57275
3-Methyl-2-pentanol	-1.63990	2-Methyl-1-octanol	-5.74460
2,3-Dimethyl-2-butanol	-0.85097	3,5,5-trimethyl-1-hexanol	-5.76992
3,3-Dimethyl-1-butanol	-2.59027	1-Dodecanol	-10.68000
3,3-Dimethyl-2-butanol	-1.41059	1-Butanol	0.09531
4-Methyl-1-pentanol	-2.28278	1-Pentanol	-1.34707
4-Methyl-2-pentanol	-1.81401	2,2-Dimethyl-1-propano	-0.64626
2-Ethyl-1-butanol	-2.78709	1-Hexanol	-2.71810
2-Methyl-2-hexanol	-2.47337	2-Hexanol	-1.99510
3-Methyl-3-hexanol	-2.26336	1-Heptanol	-4.07454
3-Ethyl-3-pentanol	-1.91732	1-Octanol	-5.40146
2,3-Dimethyl-2-pentanol	-2.00248	1-Nonanol	-6.90776
2,3-Dimethyl-3-pentanol	-1.93794	1-Decanol	-6.31997
2,4-Dimethyl-2-pentanol	-2.14558	1-Tetradecanol	-12.77171
2,4-Dimethyl-3-pentanol	-2.80181	1-Pentadecanol	-14.61402
2,2-Dimethyl-3-pentanol	-2.64367	1-Hexadecanol	-15.58747

We first searched for the optimum parameter of the valence vertex-connectivity index by varying exponent k from -0.0125 to 1.50. The standard deviation S was used as a criterion for the selection of the optimum value of k. In Figure 7 we give the change of S against k.

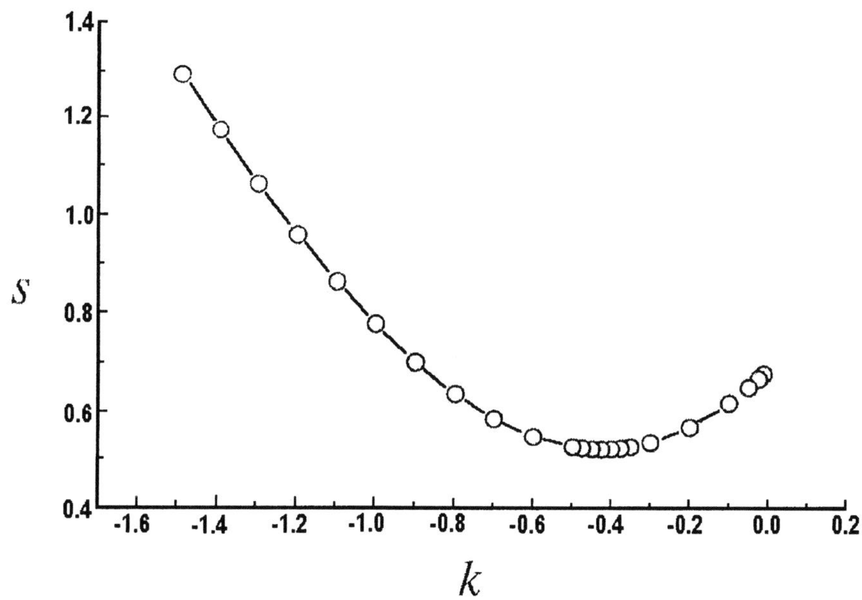

Figure 7. A plot of the standard deviation S against the exponent k in the modified valence vertex-connectivity index.

The best structure-water solubility correlation was obtained for k=-0.425. The regression equation is:

$$\ln SOL = 5.864\ (\pm\ 0.210) - 2.418\ (\pm\ 0.050)\ (\chi^{v})^{[-0.425]} \qquad (14)$$

n=54 R=0.989 S=0.526 F=2320

where $(\chi^{v})^{[-0.425]}$ is a short-hand notation for the valence vertex-connectivity indices computed using the value of -0.425 for the exponent in eq. (7). This notation will be used throughout the paper. There is only a slight improvement over the structure-water solubility model when the valence vertex-connectivity indices are computed using the standard value for the exponent, that is, k = -0.5:

$$\ln SOL = 5.814\ (\pm\ 0.211) - 2.671\ (\pm\ 0.056)\ (\chi^{v})^{[-0.5]} \qquad (15)$$

n=54 R=0.989 S=0.531 F=2279

The same approach is applied to the use of the valence edge-connectivity index. In Figure 8 we give the change of the standard deviation S against the exponent k of the valence edge-connectivity index.

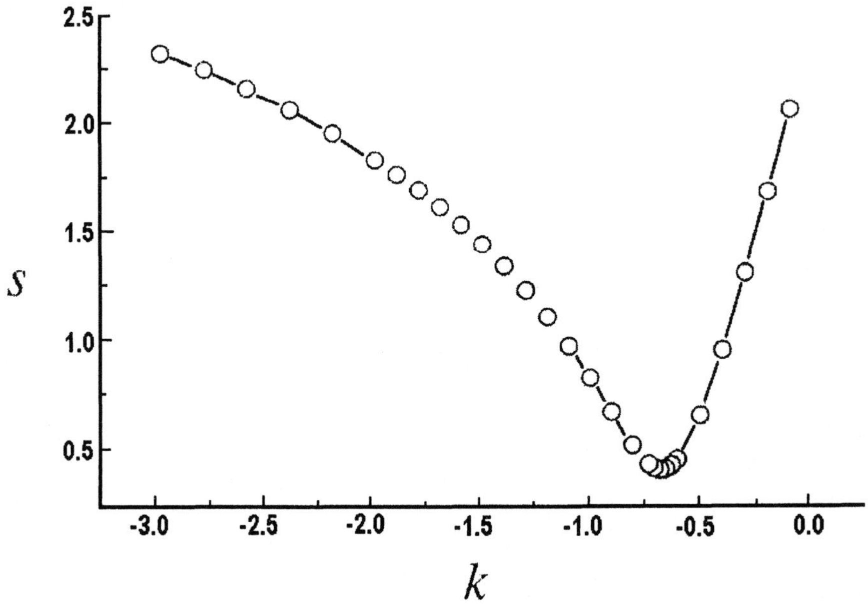

Figure 8. A plot of the standard deviation S against the exponent k in the modified valence edge-connectivity index.

The best correlation is obtained for k = -0.675:

$$\ln SOL = 5.527 (\pm 0.167) - 3.306 (\pm 0.056) (\varepsilon^{v})^{[-0.5]} \quad (16)$$

n=54 R=0.992 S=0.434 F=3426

This is a better model than the structure-water solubility model based on $(\varepsilon^{v})^{[-0.5]}$:

$$\ln SOL = 6.210 (\pm 0.282) - 2.727 (\pm 0.074) (\varepsilon^{v})^{[-0.675]} \quad (17)$$

n=54 R=0.982 S=0.680 F=1368

Eq. (17) differs from one we reported earlier (eq. (7) in ref. 7) because for three alcohols we made error in computing their weighted edge-connectivity indices (the correct values are given in brackets): 2,4-dimethyl-2-pentanol (3.5692), 2-ethyl-1-hexanol (3.8137) and 2,2-diethyl-1-pentanol (4.0931).

The same approach is also applied to the use of the valence edge-connectivity index computed for the weighted line graphs $\varepsilon^{v}(L)$. In Figure 9 we give the change of the standard deviation S against the exponent k of the valence edge-connectivity index $\varepsilon^{V}(L)$.

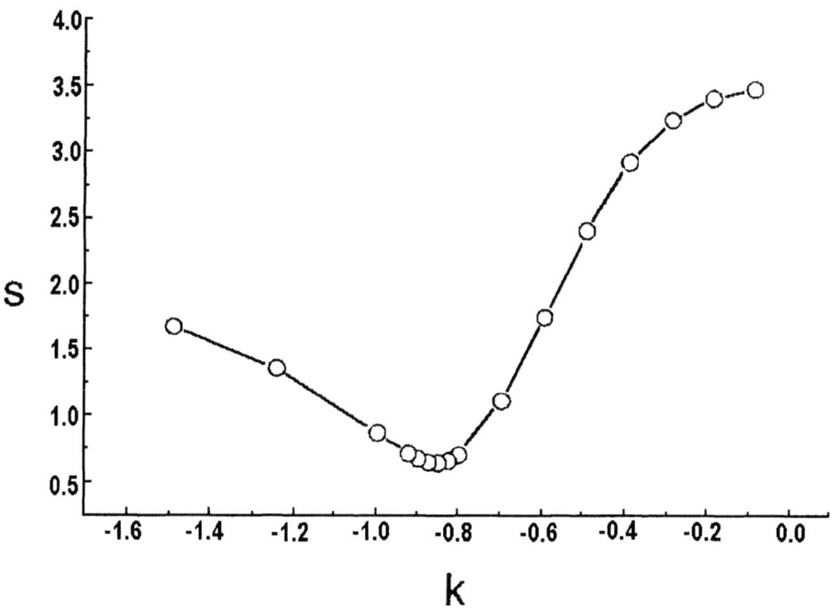

Figure 9. A plot of the standard deviation S against the exponent k in the modified valence edge-connectivity index computed for weighted line graphs corresponding to aliphatic alcohols.

The best correlation is obtained for k = -0.850:

$$\ln SOL = 4.899 (\pm 0.247) - 4.078 (\pm 0.109) [\varepsilon^{v}(L)]^{[-0.850]} \quad (18)$$

n=54 R=0.981 S=0.674 F=1392

This is a much better model than the structure-water solubility model based on the standard value of k, that is, $(\varepsilon^{v}(L))^{[-0.5]}$:

$$\ln SOL = 4.367 (\pm 1.106) - 1.942 (\pm 0.256) [\varepsilon^{v}(L)]^{[-0.50]} \quad (19)$$

n=54 R=0.725 S=2.447 F=58

It is interesting to note that the structure-water solubility model based on the valence vertex-connectivity index with k = -0.5 is better than the corresponding model the valence edge-connectivity index with k = -0.5. However, when the models with the optimum value of k are considered than the reverse is true: The model with the valence edge-connectivity index is by far superior to the model with the valence vertex-connectivity index. Actually this model, model (16), is superior to most the structure-water solubility models for aliphatic alcohols reported in the literature.[33,35]

Amidon *et al.*[33] produced three models between the water solubility of aliphatic alcohols and their surface areas. They adopted the definition of molecular surface area from Hermann:[36] A molecule is considered as a collection of spheres with each radius located at the nuclear centre. To each radius on the solute molecule (aliphatic alcohol) , a radius for the solvent (water) is added to give a surface. This approach has the convenient property of eliminating from the total surface area of a molecule those areas which are not exposed or accessible to the solvent. There is another advantage of Hermann's procedure, that is, it allows computation of the individual atom contributions to the total surface area. This permits division of the total surface area of a molecule into group contributions, e.g., hydrocarbon and hydroxyl group parts of alcohols, and the group contribution to the solubility can be estimated. Standard bond angles and bond angles were used for all aliphatic alcohols considered. Amidon *et al.*[33] have considered only 51 aliphatic alcohols, omitting those alcohols which are solid at the room temperature. Their first model relates ln SOL and the total surface area (TSA) in Å^2:

$$\ln SOL = 11.78 - 0.043\ TSA \quad (20)$$

n=51 R=974 S=0.499

Their second model relates ln SOL with the surface area of the hydrocarbon part of the aliphatic alcohol. These authors computed the hydrocarbon surface area (HYSA) by substracting the hydyroxyl group surface area (OHSA) from TSA: HYSA = TSA - OHSA. The model they obtained is:

$$\ln SOL = 8.94 - 0.0396\ HYSA \quad (21)$$

n=54 R=0.94 S=0.706

The best empirical model of Amidon *et al.*[33] relates ln SOL with the hydrocarbon surface area (HYSA) and the hydyroxyl group surface area (OHSA):

$$\ln SOL = 12.41 - 0.043\ HYSA - 0.060\ OHSA \quad (22)$$

n=51 R=0.978 S=0.462

TSA and HYSA are highly intercorrelated quantities, the value of R being 0.994. Models (20) and (22) are superior to all obtained models but model (16). This result supports views that the computed molecular surface area is an important descriptor to use in QSPR.[37]

Hall *et al.*[38] also studied the aqueous solubility of aliphatic alcohols. Their first model was derived in 1975 before Kier and Hall[29] introduced the valence vertex-connectivity index. Therefore, Hall *et al.*[38] used the vertex-connectivity index as was originally defined by Randić for hydrocarbons:[39]

$$\chi = \sum_{edges} [d(v_i)\ d(v_j)]^{-0.5} \quad (23)$$

where $d(v_i)$ is the degree of the vertex i. Hence, Hall *et al.*[38] instead of computing the vertex-connectivity index for aliphatic alcohols they computed χ for the related alkanes.

In spite of this the model they obtained is better than all models we discussed above, but model (16) (judging by the value of S):

$$\ln SOL = 6.702 - 2.666\,\chi \qquad (24)$$

n=51 R=0.978 S=0.455

Only when the empirical parameter c_{OH} which takes care about the environment of the OH group, that is, whether we deal with primary, secondary or tertiary alcohols, the two-parameter model exhibits considerable improvement over the model (16):

$$\ln SOL = 9.204 - 2.630\,\chi - 4.390\,c_{OH} \qquad (25)$$

n=50 R=0.991 S=0.289

The best two-descriptors structure-water solubility model for aliphatic alcohols so far obtained is a model with ordered orthogonal descriptors[40-42] which includes explicitly the OH group:[35]

$$\ln SOL = -3.666\,(\pm 0.037) - 2.689\,(\pm 0.479)\,\Omega^{V} - 6.336\,(\pm 0.479)\,\Omega_{OH} \qquad (26)$$

n=54 R=0.997 S=0.273 F=4479

where the symbol Ω stands for orthogonal descriptors. The published best structure-water solubility model for aliphatic alcohols (according to the S value) is a four-descriptors model with ordered orthogonal descriptors including the OH group:

$$\ln SOL = -3.666\,(\pm 0.033) - 2.689\,(\pm 0.025)\,{}^{1}\Omega^{V} - 1.225\,(\pm 0.116)\,{}^{3}\Omega^{V} - 0.650\,(\pm 0.324)\,{}^{4}\Omega^{V} + 5.747\,(\pm 0.510)\,\Omega_{OH} \qquad (27)$$

n=54 R=0.998 S=0.240 F=2897

4. Concluding Remarks

In the present work we found that in the case of structure-water solubility models for aliphatic alcohols, the valence edge-connectivity index outperforms the valence vertex-connectivity index when the optimum index-exponents were used. When the standard index-exponent of -0.5 is used, then the reverse is true. Estrada and Rodriguez[4] considered the following seven physicochemical properties of alkanes: boiling points, molar volumes, molar refractions, heats of vaporization, critical temperatures, critical pressures and superficial tensions. The edge-connectivity index produced the best single-variable models for molar volumes, molar refractions, critical temperatures, critical pressures and superficial tensions. In the case of the boiling points and heats of vaporization the vertex-connectivity index outperformed the edge-connectivity index, but in both cases the best single-variable model was based on the Hosoya Z index.[42] Since Estrada and Rodriguez[4] did not consider water solubilities, our result represents the extension of their findings.

Our findings do not support the claim by Gutman *et al.*[6] that the use of line graphs improves the predictive power of topological indices. However, we did not perform our analysis in the quite the same fashion as they did, since we did not consider higher order indices computed for line graphs. Our work supports views[43-46] that the optimum index-exponent need not be -0.5 as was suggested when the vertex-connectivity index was introduced.[39] However, from the work by Amidon *et al.*,[33] Kier and Hall,[38] and our work reported elsewhere,[7,35] emerges the following conclusion: The reliable structure-aqueous solubility models of aliphatic alcohols require the inclusion of the OH group in the set of descriptors used to build the model.

5. Acknowledgements

This work was supported, in part, by the Ministry of Science and Technology of the Republic of Croatia via Grants 00980606 (SN & NT) and 079301 (DA & DB). Part of this work was completed during the stay of SN & NT at the Center for Water and the Environment, Natural Resources Reseach Institute (NRRI), University of Minnesota, Duluth, Minnesota 55811, USA. SCB and SN & NT (during their stay at NRRI) were supported, in part, by Grants F49620-94-1-0401 and F49620-96-1-0330 from the United States Air Force.

6. References

1. Randić, M. Topological Indices. In: *The Encyclopedia of Computational Chemistry*, Schleyer, P.v.R.; Allinger, N.L.; Clark, T.; Gasteiger, J.; Kollman, P.A.; Schaefer III, H.F.; Schreiner, P.R., Eds.; Wiley: Chichester, 1998; pp. 3018-3032.
2. Burden, F.R.; Winkler, D.A. New QSAR Methods Applied to Structure-Activity Mapping and Combinatorial Chemistry. *J. Chem. Inf. Comput. Sci.* **1999**, *39*, 236-242.
3. Randić, M.; Basak, S.C. Optimal Molecular Descriptors Based on Weighted Path Numbers. *J. Chem. Inf. Comput. Sci.* **1999**, *39*, 261-266.
4. Estrada, E.; Rodriguez, L. On the Edge-Connectivity Indices in QSPR/QSAR Studies. 1. Comparison to Other Topological Indices in QSPR Studies. *J. Chem. Inf. Comput. Sci.*, **1999**, *39*, 1037-1041.
5. The term QSPR (quantitative structure-property relationship) was introduced in parallel to older term QSAR (quantitative structure-activity relationship) in Sabljic, A.; Trinajstić, N. Quantitative Structure-Activity Relationships: The Role of Topological Indices. *Acta Pharm. Jugosl.* **1981**, *31*, 189-214.

6. Gutman, I.; Popovic, Lj.; Estrada, E.; Bertz, S.H. The Line Graph Model. Predicting Physico-Chemical Properties of Alkanes. *ACH-Models in Chemistry* **1998**, *135*, 147-155.
7. For summary see Nikolić, S.; Trinajstić, N. Modeling the Aqueous Solubility of Aliphatic Alcohols. *SAR QSAR Environ. Res.* **1998**, *9*, 117-126.
8. Chenzhong, C.; Zhiliang, L., Molecular Polarizability. 1. Relationship to Water Solubility of Alkanes and Alcohols. *J. Chem. Inf. Comput. Sci.* 1998, *38*, 1-7.
9. Amić, D.; Bešlo, D.; Lucic, B.; Nikolić, S.; Trinajstić, N. The Vertex-Connectivity Index Revisited. *J. Chem. Inf. Comput. Sci.* **1998**, *38*, 819-822 and references therein.
10. Katritzky, A.R.; Karelson, M.; Lobanov, V.S. QSPR as a Means of Predicting and Understanding Chemical and Physical Properties in Terms of Structure. *Pure Appl. Chem.* **1997**, *69*, 245-248.
11. "In silico" parallels terms "in vivo" and "in vitro", implaying that the experiments are carried out on computer.
12. Grassy, G.; Calas, B.; Yasri, A.; Lahana, R.; Woo, J.; Iyer, S.; Kaczorek, M., Floc'h, R.; Buelow, R. Computer-Assisted Rational Design of Immunosuppressive Compounds. *Nature Biotechnology* **1998**, *16*, 748-752.
13. Basak, S.C.; Gute, B.D.; Drewes, L.R. Predicting Blood-Brain Transport of Drugs: A Computational Approach. *Pharm. Res.* **1996**, *13*, 775-778.
14. Balaban, A.T., Ed.; *From Chemical Topology to Three-Dimensional Geometry*. Plenum Press: New York, 1997.
15. Lucic, B.; Trinajstić, N. Multivariate Regression Outperforms Several Robust Architectures of Neural Networks in QSAR Modeling. *J. Chem. Inf. Comput. Sci.* **1999**, *39*, 121-132. The same is also valid for the QSPR modeling, see, for example, Katritzky, A.R., Chen, K.; Wang, Y.; Karelson, M.; Lucic, B.; Trinajstić, N.; Suzuki, T.; Schüürmann, G. Prediction of Liquid Viscosity for Organic Compounds by a Quantitative Structure-Property Relationship. *J. Phys. Org. Chem.*, **2000**, *13*, 80-86.; Lucic, B.; Trinajstić, N.; Sild, S.; Karelson, M.; Katritzky, A.R. A New Efficient Approach for Variable Selection Based on Multiregression: Prediction of Gas Chromatographic Retention Times and Response Factors. *J. Chem. Inf. Comput. Sci.*, **1999**, *39*, 610-621.
16. Katritzky, A.R.; Lobanov, V.S.; Karelson, M. Normal Boiling Points for Organic Compounds: Correlation and Prediction by a Quantitative Structure-Property Relationships. *J. Chem. Inf. Comput. Sci.* **1998**, *38*, 28-41.
17. Devillers, J.; Balaban, A.T., Eds.; *Topological Indices and Related Descriptors in QSAR and QSPR*. Gordon & Breach Publishers, London, 1999.
18. Trinajstić, N. *Chemical Graph Theory*, 2nd revised edition; CRC: Boca Raton, FL, 1992.
19. Ivanciuc, O.; Balaban, A.T. Graph Theory in Chemistry. In: *The Encyclopedia of Computational Chemistry*, Schleyer, P.v.R.; Allinger, N.L.; Clark, T.; Gasteiger, J.; Kollman, P.A.; Schaefer III, H.F.; Schreiner, P.R., Eds.; Wiley: Chichester, 1998; 1169-1190.
20. Diudea, M.; Horvath, D.; Bonchev, D. Molecular Topology. 14. Molord Algorithm and Real Number Subgraph Invariants. *Croat. Chem. Acta* **1995**, *68*, 131-148.

21. Estrada, E.; Guevara, N.; Gutman, I. Extension of Edge Connectivity Index. Relationships to Line Graph Indices and QSPR Applications. *J. Chem. Inf. Comput. Sci.* **1998**, *38*, 428-431.
22. Trinajstić, N. *Chemical Graph Theory*; CRC: Boca Raton, FL, 1983, Vol. I, p. 17.
23. Bertz, S.H. The Bond Graph. *J. Chem. Soc. Chem. Comm.* **1981**, 818-820.
24. Harary, F. *Graph Theory*, 2nd printing; Addison-Wesley: Reading, MA, 1971.
25. Balaban, A.T. Highly Discriminating Distance-Based Topological Index. *Chem. Phys. Lett.* **1982**, *89*, 399-404.
26. Basak, S.C.; Grunwald, G.D.; Niemi, G.J. Use of Graph-Theoretic and Geometrical Molecular Descriptors in Structure-Activity Relationships. in: *From Chemical Topology to Three-Dimensional Geometry*, Balaban, A.T., Ed., Plenum Press: New York, 1997, pp. 73-116.
27. Gutman, I.; Ruscic, B.; Trinajstić, N.; Wilcox Jr., C.F. Graph Theory and Molecular Orbitals. XII. Acyclic Polyenes. *J. Chem. Phys.* **1975**, *62*, 3399-3405.
28. Gutman, I.; Estrada, E. Topological Indices Based on the Line Graph of the Molecular Graph. *J. Chem. Inf. Comput. Sci.* **1996**, *36*, 541-543.
29. Kier, L.B.; Hall, L.H. Molecular Connectivity. VII. Specific Treatment of Heterosystems. *J. Pharm. Sci.* **1976**, *65*, 1806-1809.
30. Estrada, E. Edge Adjacency Relationships and a Novel Topological Index Related to Molecular Volume. *J. Chem. Inf. Comput. Sci.* **1995**, *35*, 31-33.
31. Estrada, E. Edge Adjacency Relationships in Molecular Graphs Containing Heteroatoms: A New Topological Index Related to Molecular Volume. *J. Chem. Inf. Comput. Sci.* **1995**, *35*, 701-707.
32. Ref. 18, Chapter 4.
33. Amidon, G.L.; Yalkowsky, S.H.; Leung, S. Solubility of Nonelectrolytes in Polar Solvents. II. Solubility of Aliphatic Alcohols in Water. *J. Pharm. Sci.* **1974**, *63*, 1858-1866.
34. Handbook of Chemistry and Physics. The 67th Edition, 3rd printing; CRC Press: Boca Raton, FL, 1987.
35. e.g., Lucic, B.; Nikolić, S.; Trinajstić, J.; Mihalić, Z. A Structure-Property Study of the Solubility of Aliphatic Alcohols in Water. *Croat. Chem. Acta* **1995**, *68*, 417-434.
36. Hermann, R.B. The Theory of Hydrophobic Bonding. II. The Correlation of Hydrocarbon Solubility in Water with Solvent Cavity Surface Area.*J. Phys. Chem.* **1972**, *76*, 2754-2759.
37. Mebane, R.C.; Schanley, S.A.; Rybolt, T.R.; Bruce, C.D. The Correlation of Physical Properties of Organic Molecules with Computed Molecular Surface Areas. *J. Chem. Educ.* **1999**, *76*, 688-693.
38. Hall, L.H.; Kier, L.B.; Murray, W.J. Molecular Connectivity. II. Relationship to Water Solubility and Boiling Point. *J. Pharm. Sci.* **1975**, *64*, 1974-1977.
39. Randić, M. On Characterization of Molecular Branching. *J. Amer. Chem. Soc.* **1975**, *97*, 6609-6615.
40. Randić, M. Orthogonal Molecular Descriptors. *New J. Chem.* **1991**, *15*, 517-525.

41. Lucic, B.; Nikolić, S.; Trinajstić, N.; Juretic, D. The Structure-Property Models Can Be Improved Using the Orthgonalized Descriptors. *J. Chem. Inf. Comput. Sci.* **1995**, *35*, 532-538.
42. Lucic, B.; Nikolić, S.; Trinajstić, N.; Juretic, D.; Juric, A. A Novel QSPR Approach to Physicochemical Properties of the α-Amino Acids. *Croat. Chem. Acta* **1995**, *68*, 435-450.
43. Hosoya, H. Topological Index. A Newly Proposed Quantity Characterizing the Topological Nature of Structural Isomers of Hydrocarbons. *Bull. Chem. Soc. Jpn.* **1971**, *44*, 2332-2339.
44. Altenburg, K. Eine Bemerkung zu dem Randicschen "Molekularen Bindungs-Index (Molecular Connectivity Index)". *Z. Phys. Chem. (Leipzig)* **1980**, *261*, 389-393.
45. Estrada, E. Graph Theoretical Invariant of Randić Revisited. *J. Chem. Inf. Comput. Sci.* **1995**, *35*, 1022-1025.
46. Nikolić, S.; Trinajstić, N.; Baucic, I. Comparison between the Vertex- and Edge-Connectivity Indices for Benzenoid Hydrocarbons. *J. Chem. Inf. Comput. Sci.* **1998**, *38*, 42-46.

Chapter 5

QSPR/QSAR BY GRAPH THEORETICAL DESCRIPTORS BEYOND THE FRONTIERS

Ernesto Estrada
[a]Department of Organic Chemistry, Faculty of Pharmacy, University of Santiago de Compostela, 15706 Santiago de Compostela, Spain
Enrique Molina
University of Camagüey, Camagüey, Cuba

"Models are to be used, not believed"
Menger, F. M.
J. Am. Chem. Soc. **107** (1985) 3105

1. INTRODUCTION

There exist some paradoxical behavior in human beings concerning the acceptance and use of novel concepts and ideas in their current lives. Almost as a norm, we have certain preferences for those well-established and traditional things. Consequently, new ideas and concepts are accepted only with some reticence. However, there are a few of these novel ideas that are accepted and incorporated to our current activities in an accelerated way. These novelties are then considered as a "new fashion" and an explosion in their uses is immediately produced.

A similar situation is also observed in the uses of molecular descriptors and approaches in QSPR/QSAR studies. Some approaches that are considered as well established and traditional are frequently employed even in cases in which they are known to produce not good results. On the other hand, certain novel schemes for QSPR and QSAR invade the literature with many examples of applications.[1]

The use of graph-theoretic molecular descriptors has become an interesting option for the generation of QSPR/QSAR models.[2-5] At present, there are many examples that prove the qualities and possibilities of these molecular descriptors in such studies. Consequently, the number of papers in which graph-theoretic molecular descriptors are used in QSPR/QSAR studies has increased, especially the so-called topological indices.[6] However, there are even some misunderstandings on the role of such molecular descriptors in chemistry and drug investigation. These misunderstandings have produced severe criticisms to their use in QSAR, and sometimes exclude them from the pool of descriptors, which are traditionally used in structure-property-activity studies.[7, 8]

The first serious attempt to put order in the definition of graph theoretical molecular descriptors was carried out by Randić in 1991.[9] This author gave a series of desired attributes that the topological indices need to have to be considered as useful molecular descriptors. In a more recent study, Milne[10] analyzed some aspects concerned to the applications of graph theoretical molecular descriptors according to the publications in the *Journal of Chemical Information and Computer Sciences*. This author shown that 70% of the graph theory papers published in this journal are devoted to hydrocarbon molecules, which represent only 1% of the real organic chemistry. We consider that this is one of the main facts contributing to the misunderstanding of the role of these descriptors in chemistry and drug research. Among the others, we would like to mention that most of the QSPR applications are concentrated on the so-called "bulky" molecular properties, giving the impression that these theoretical approaches cannot go to other regions of the hypothetical "physicochemical properties space" of organic compounds.

2. On the Nature of Chemical Interactions

Chemical interactions in which molecules can be involved are of very different natures. In order to use the concept of chemical reactivity in the most general way, we will use an "artificial" subdivision of it according to the nature of such interactions. We call *local chemical reactivity* to such processes in which two or more chemical species interact through a well-localized chemical center, i.e., an atom or a chemical bond, as in the cases of reactions of addition, elimination, substitution, and so forth. On the other hand, *global chemical reactivity* is referred to the case in which the chemical species interact as a whole, such as in the cases of solvation and partition between two different phases. Topological, geometrical and electronic changes are currently involved in local chemical reactivity as consequences of bonds that are broken and new ones that are made, conformational changes produced by the action of heat or radiation on a localized center, and so forth. On the contrary, the global chemical reactivity does not influence over the topological structure of the molecules involved, modifying only the geometrical and electronic features of such molecules as a whole.

Global chemical reactivity is well described by the so-called topological descriptors, which are mainly derived from the graph-theoretic representation of molecules. Topological molecular descriptors are considered in many occasions as useless for the description of local chemical reactivity because, in general, they are designed to describe the molecule as a whole and they are unable of describing a chemical process occurring in a well-localized center of the molecule. The local chemical reactivity has been traditionally described well enough by using quantum chemical molecular descriptors and approaches. The use of electronic and steric constants of substituents at different positions of a defined framework is also an important alternative in such cases. These facts have conducted to believe that topological (more correctly graph theoretic) descriptors are of limited value in modeling chemical reactivity. For instance, Mekenyan and Basak[11] have recently concluded that "Topological indices have a predominant role in determining molecular reactivity where metric and electronic aspects of molecular architecture plays a very minor role in the reaction process." Here we will try to prove that the manipulation of chemical graphs in order to generate appropriate molecular descriptors open novel possibilities to solve the problems of modeling local chemical reactivity. By this way we are interested in showing some of the potentials that graph-theoretic molecular descriptors have in QSPR/QSAR studies beyond this frontiers previously (and sometime arbitrarily) established for these molecular descriptors.

3. Topological, Topographic and Quantum Chemical Descriptors

The topological indices are those structure molecular descriptors derived from a graph theoretical representation of molecules.[12] These molecular descriptors should fulfil most of the desired attributes for topological indices proposed by Randić.[9] On the other hand, the topographic molecular descriptors are those derived from a graph theoretical representation of molecules but including some three-dimensional features of the molecules so represented.[13-17] The inclusion of these three-dimensional effects can be carried out by using different weights for the vertices and/or edges of the molecular graph. It is clear that the topographic molecular descriptors always have a topological analogous because it is always possible to apply the same graph invariant to the graph without any weight. Finally, the quantum chemical molecular descriptors are those derived from the application of quantum chemical approaches to the molecular structure.[18] These descriptors can be generated from *ab initio* or semiempirical quantum chemical approaches.

The topological indices that we will use in the present study include only two classes of such molecular descriptors. The first, is the very well known series of molecular connectivity indices, which we will refer here as vertex connectivity indices.[19-21] These indices, firstly defined by Randić in 1975[22] and then extended to a series of descriptors and widely applied to QSPR and QSAR studies by Kier and Hall,[19, 20] are recognized as the most successful and applied series of topological indices in QSPR/QSAR studies. The second series of topological indices corresponds to the so-called edge connectivity indices. These descriptors were firstly introduced by Estrada in 1995[23, 24] and then extended by Estrada et al.[25] to a series of topological indices analogous of the vertex connectivity indices. Recent reports by several authors suggest that these indices are very promising in QSPR/QSAR studies.[26-31]

The topographic descriptors that we will employ here are divided in four groups. The first corresponds to the bond order weighted vertex connectivity indices proposed by Estrada and Montero in 1993.[32, 33] These indices are computed from molecular graphs with the edges weighted by the bond orders computed by semiempirical quantum chemical calculations. The graph-theoretical invariant of Randić[22] and the extensions of Kier and Hall[19] are applied to the definition of these indices. The second series is composed by the electron density weighted vertex connectivity indices introduced by Estrada in 1995.[33, 34] These indices are computed as the previous ones but using molecular graphs with vertices weighted by the atomic electron densities calculated from quantum chemical methods. A correction to these indices proposed by this author to include the effect of hydrogen atoms form the third group of descriptors.[33, 34] The last group of topographic indices is the so-called bond order weighted edge connectivity indices proposed by Estrada in 1996.[33, 35] These indices are the edge analogous of the bond order weighted vertex connectivity indices. The list of these topological and topographic molecular descriptors is given in Table 1.

The list of quantum chemical molecular descriptors used here is mainly that proposed by Kikuchi[36] and includes superdeslocalizability indices (electrophilic and nucleophilic) computed for σ or π electrons as well as the sum of both, charges, energies of the HOMO (highest occupied molecular orbital) and LUMO (lowest unoccupied molecular orbital) and so forth.

Finally, two other series of graph theoretical invariants are used here. The first is the vector of the first 15 spectral moments of the edge adjacency matrix of the molecular graph.[37-41] These moments have been successfully applied to a series of QSPR/QSAR studies including the design of novel bioactive molecules. These descriptors conform the basis of our approach to drug design called TOSS-MODE (*TO*pological *S*ub-*S*tructural *MO*lecular *DE*sign).[42] In order to account for the local topological effects of molecules we propose the use of the local spectral moments of the edge adjacency of the molecular graphs.[43] These descriptors are defined as the entries of the different powers of the edge adjacency matrix. For instance, the *k*th local spectral moment of the bond i in the molecular graph G is the corresponding entry e_{ii} of the kth power of the edge adjacency matrix of G.

Table 1. Symbols for topological, topographic and quantum chemical descriptors and their definitions.

${}^{h}\chi_{p}$	Path connectivity index of order h = 0 – 6
${}^{h}\chi_{C}$	Cluster connectivity index of order h = 3 – 6
${}^{h}\chi_{pC}$	Path-cluster connectivity index of order h = 4 – 6
${}^{h}\chi^{v}_{p}$	Valence path connectivity index of order h = 0 – 6
${}^{h}\chi^{v}_{C}$	Valence cluster connectivity index of order h = 3 – 6
${}^{h}\chi^{v}_{pC}$	Valence path-cluster connectivity index of order h = 4 – 6
${}^{h}\varepsilon_{p}$	Path bond connectivity index of order h = 1 – 6
${}^{h}\varepsilon_{C}$	Cluster bond connectivity index of order h = 3 – 6
${}^{h}\varepsilon_{pC}$	Path-cluster bond connectivity index of order h = 4 – 6
${}^{h}\Omega_{p}$	Path bond-order-based topographic connectivity index of order h = 0 – 6
${}^{h}\Omega_{C}$	Cluster bond-order-based topographic connectivity index of order h = 3 – 6
${}^{h}\Omega_{pC}$	Path-cluster bond-order-based topographic connectivity index of order h = 4 - 6
${}^{h}\Omega_{p}(q)$	Path charge-based topographic connectivity index of order h = 0 – 6
${}^{h}\Omega_{C}(q)$	Cluster charge-based topographic connectivity index of order h = 3 – 6
${}^{h}\Omega_{pC}(q)$	Path-cluster charge-based topographic connectivity index of order h = 4 – 6
${}^{h}\Omega^{c}_{p}(q)$	Path hydrogen-corrected charge-based topographic connectivity index of order h = 0 – 6
${}^{h}\Omega^{c}_{C}(q)$	Cluster hydrogen-corrected charge-based topographic connectivity index of order h = 3 – 6
${}^{h}\Omega^{c}_{pC}(q)$	Path-cluster hydrogen-corrected charge-based topographic connectivity index of order h = 4 – 6

$Q(i)$	Electronic charge on atom *i* of the furylethylene framework
$ES_{\sigma}(i)$	σ electrophilic superdeslocalizability on atom *i*
$ES_{\pi}(i)$	π electrophilic superdeslocalizability on atom *i*
$ES_{T}(i)$	Total electrophilic superdeslocalizability on atom *i*
$NS_{\sigma}(i)$	σ nucleophilic superdeslocalizability on atom *i*
$NS_{\pi}(i)$	π nucleophilic superdeslocalizability on atom *i*
$NS_{T}(i)$	Total nucleophilic superdeslocalizability on atom *i*
E_{HOMO}	Energy of the highest occupied molecular orbirtal
E_{LUMO}	Energy of the lowest unoccupied molecular orbirtal
μ_i	Total spectral moment of order *i*
$\mu_i(p-q)$	Local spectral moment of order *i* for the bond *p-q*
HB1	Hydrogen bonding potential of molecule

4. The MODEST/TOSS-MODE Computer Systems

An important question for the development of QSPR/QSAR models is the availability of computer softwares that permits the computation of the molecular descriptors to be used in such models. We have developed during the last five years two computer systems for personal computers. These systems are called MODEST[44] (*MO*lecular *DES*ign *T*ools) and TOSS-MODE[45] (*TO*pological *S*ub *S*tructural-*MO*lecular *DE*sign) both for Windows. These user-friendly computational systems permit the calculation of several topological, topographic and quantum chemical molecular descriptors. They were programmed by using object-oriented methodologies in Pascal.

The MODEST system uses the MOPAC[46] output files as inputs for the calculation of topographic and quantum chemical descriptors. The vertex and edges connectivity indices are also computed by this system, which also permits several other formats of input files. This system permits the calculation of these indices (see Table 1) for a single molecule or for a large number of them. In the last case a file with the name of the molecules and all the indices computed tabulated in columns are given as output. These files are ready to be manipulated by statistical packages in order to find the QSPR/QSAR models. In Fig. 1 we illustrate the desktop of the MODEST system.

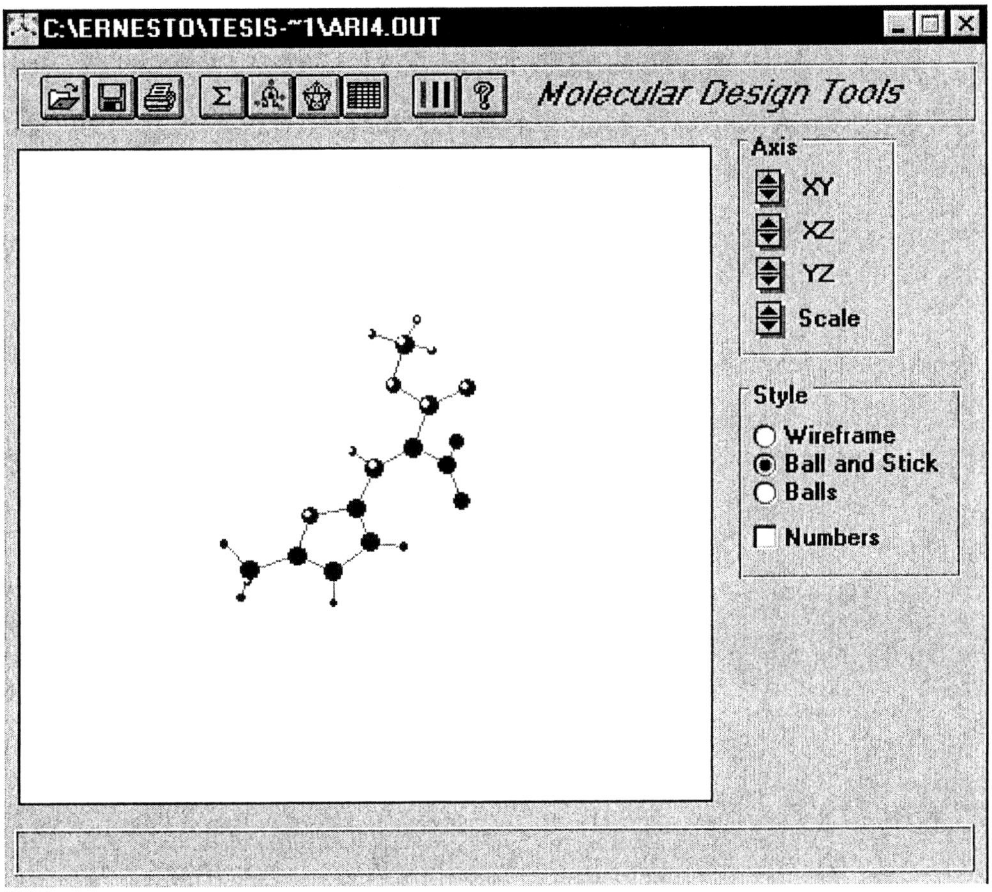

Fig. 1. Desktop of the MODEST system used to calculate topological, topographic and quantum chemical molecular descriptors.

The TOSS-MODE software is used to compute the spectral moments of the edge adjacency matrix of molecules. The molecules are drawn in an easy way on the desktop of the software including the different atoms selected from a periodic table. The global spectral moments can be computed by selecting any weight for the different bonds in the molecule, such as bond distances, bond dipole moments, bond polarizabilities, and so forth. The local moments, for single bonds or for a defined fragment in the molecule, can be computed on the same way after the selection of the bond/fragment. The outputs of this software are also given as a file ready to be manipulated by statistical packages. The desktop and the window for spectral moments calculations of the TOSS-MODEST system are shown in Fig. 2.

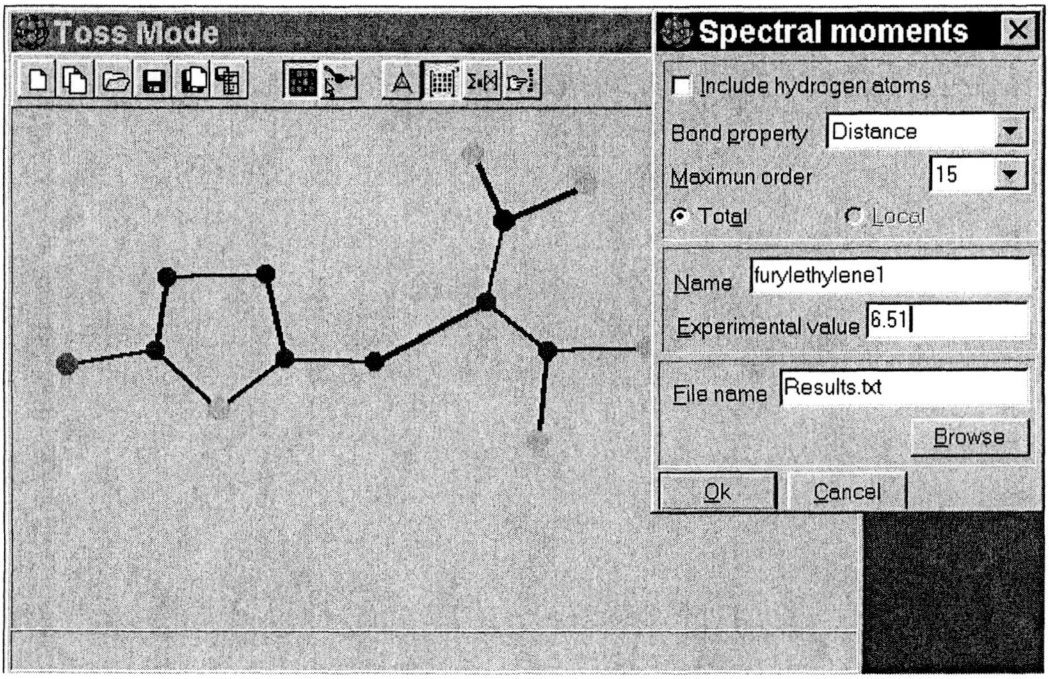

Fig. 2. Desktop and window for the calculation of the spectral moments of molecular graphs with the system TOSS-MODE.

5. Applications to QSPR/QSAR Studies

Here we will be concentrated in the study of two very important properties of 2-furylethylene compounds. These properties are the partition coefficient n-octanol/water, which is a measurement of the lipophilicity of such compounds and the rate constant of reaction for the nucleophilic addition of thiols to the exocyclic double bond of these chemicals. It is clear that the first of these properties can be considered as a "global" chemical reactivity property and the second as a "local" chemical reactivity one.

The 2-furylethylene compounds have been well known as antimicrobials, antitumoral and cytotoxic during many years.[47,48] The recent interest in such chemicals emerged from the strong antibacterial/antifungal activity of some derivatives with applications in the industry as well as in veterinary and human medicine.[49, 50] It has been clear from structure-activity relationship studies that the lipophilicity and the nucleophilic addition of thiols groups of some enzymes to the exocyclic double bond of such compounds are critical for the development of their antibacterial activity.[51] The role of the different substituents in the mutagenic activity observed in some derivatives of 2-furylethylenes has also been studied and we have found the main electronic structural features responsible for the development of such undesired effects.[52] From these studies it is clear the important role that the partition coefficient n-octanol/water (log P) and the specific constant of reaction for the nucleophilic addition to the double bond (log k) have for the understanding of the biological behavior of these chemicals. These quantities have been experimentally determined for a series of 34 2-furylethylene compounds and they are reported in the literature.[51] Here, we will use the topological/topographic/quantum chemical molecular descriptors in order to describe these two important reactivity indices (global and local).

The chemical structures and enumeration of the different atoms of the furylethylene framework are given in Table 2.

Table 2. Chemical structures and enumeration of atoms in the furylethyle compounds used in this study.

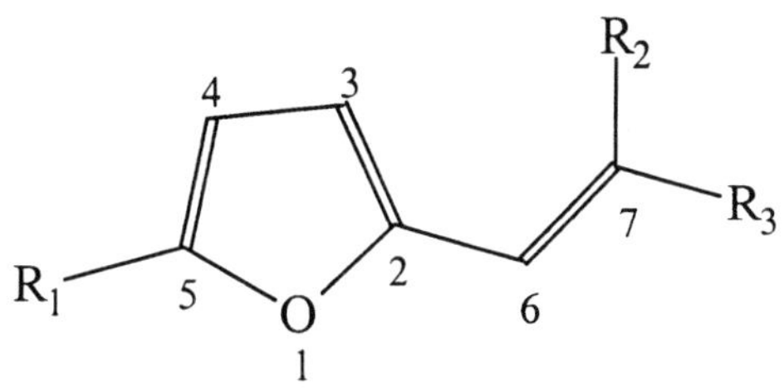

No.	R_1	R_2	R_3	No.	R_1	R_2	R_3
1	H	NO_2	$COOCH_3$	18	NO_2	H	$CONHCH(CH_3)C_2H_5$
2	CH_3	NO_2	$COOCH_3$	19	NO_2	H	$CONHC(CH_3)_3$
3	Br	NO_2	$COOCH_3$	20	NO_2	H	$CONHCH_2C(CH_3)_3$
4	I	NO_2	$COOCH_3$	21	NO_2	H	$COOCH_3$
5	$COOCH_3$	NO_2	$COOCH_3$	22	NO_2	H	$COOC_2H_5$
6	NO_2	NO_2	$COOCH_3$	23	NO_2	H	$COO(CH_2)_2CH_3$
7	NO_2	$COOC_2H_5$	$COOC_2H_5$	24	NO_2	H	$COOCH(CH_3)_2$
8	NO_2	H	NO_2	25	NO_2	H	$COO(CH_2)_3CH_3$
9	H	H	NO_2	26	NO_2	H	$COOCH_2CH(CH_3)_2$
10	NO_2	H	$CONH_2$	27	NO_2	H	$COOCH(CH_3)C_2H_5$
11	NO_2	H	$CONHCH_3$	28	NO_2	H	$COOC(CH_3)_3$
12	NO_2	H	$CON(CH_3)_2$	29	NO_2	H	$COO(CH_2)_4CH_3$
13	NO_2	H	$CONHC_2H_5$	30	NO_2	H	Br
14	NO_2	H	$CONH(CH_2)_2CH_3$	31	NO_2	H	CN
15	NO_2	H	$CONHCH(CH_3)_2$	32	NO_2	H	OCH_3
16	NO_2	H	$CONH(CH_2)_3CH_3$	33	NO_2	H	H
17	NO_2	H	$CONHCH_2CH(CH_3)_2$	34	NO_2	CN	$COOCH_3$

The computational strategy followed consisted in carrying out a full geometry optimization of the molecular structures of the furylethylene compounds by using the semiempirical quantum chemical method AM1.[53] This method was selected because we previously demonstrated that it reproduces the molecular geometry and conformational features of these compounds in an appropriated way.[54] After these calculations the output files were used as input for the system MODEST[44] in order to compute the topological, topographical and quantum chemical descriptors. The global and local spectral moments were computed by using the TOSS-MODE system.[45]

Our objective here is not to find the best QSPR models for describing log P and log k of this data set of compounds but to compare the possibilities of topological, topographic and quantum chemical descriptors in describing them. By this reason, we will obtain models that include only one of such kind of descriptors, for instance one model with topological indices, other with topographic indices, and so forth.

In describing the global chemical reactivity studied, i.e., the partition coefficient n-octanol/water, we found the following model by using the topological indices studied (vertex and edge connectivity indices):

$$\log P = 0.223 - 1.087\,{}^{4}\varepsilon_{p} + 0.763\,{}^{6}\chi_{pC} + 1.735\,{}^{1}\chi_{p}^{v} + 2.538\,{}^{5}\chi_{p}^{v} - 11.626\,{}^{6}\chi_{p}^{v}$$
$$- 3.250\,{}^{5}\chi_{pC}^{v} - 0.447HB1$$
$$N = 34 \quad R = 0.969 \quad s = 0.199 \quad s_{CV} = 0.247 \quad F(7.26) = 56.9$$

where N is the number of compounds, R is the correlation coefficient, s is the standard deviation of the regression, s_{CV} is the standard error of estimates of the leave-one-out cross validation and F is the Fisher ratio. As can be seen this model explains almost 94 % of the variance in the log P for this data set of compounds. An improvement is obtained by using topographic descriptors that are able to explain more than 96 % of the variance in this property. It is also clear from the cross validation experiment that the predictive ability of the topographic model represents an improvement of 29 % respect to that obtained with topological descriptors. The model obtained with this kind of molecular descriptors is given below:

$$\log P = 0.125 + 0.708\,{}^{1}\Omega_{p}(q) - 0.549\,{}^{4}\varepsilon_{p}(\rho) - 33.331\,{}^{5}\varepsilon_{C}(\rho) - 3.250\,{}^{5}\varepsilon_{C}(\rho)$$
$$+ 44.730\,{}^{5}\Omega_{C}^{c}(q) + 0.730\,{}^{2}\varepsilon_{p}(\rho) - 0{,}825\,{}^{3}\Omega_{C} - 0.590HB1$$
$$N = 34 \quad R = 0.982 \quad s = 0.155 \quad F(7.26) = 84.6 \quad s_{CV} = 0.176$$

When quantum chemical molecular descriptors were applied to describe this global reactivity property no one model significant from the statistical point of view could be obtained. By this reason, we used the Klopman approach[55] for describing the partition coefficient by using quantum chemical indices. In this approach the log *P* is expressed as a function of two variables, one is the sum of the atomic charges in the molecule and the other is the sum of the electrophilic superdelocalizabilities of all atoms in the molecule. We also included here the term *HB*1 in order to improve the quality of the model so developed. This model is given below:

$$\log P = 0.192 + 2.507\sum_i ES_i + 0.393\sum_i Q_i - 0.752HB1$$

$$N = 34 \quad R = 0.906 \quad s = 0.319 \quad s_{CV} = 0.37 \quad F(3,26) = 45.5$$

This model, however, is able to explain only 82 % of the variance in the log *P* for the data set of furylethylenes studied. This result can be considered as poor but no improvement could be obtained by using other of the quantum chemical descriptors studied.

The application of the global spectral moments of the edge adjacency matrix using bond distances as diagonal entries in the matrix does not produce any improvement respect to the topological indices. This model explains only 89 % of the variance in the log *P*:

$$\log P = 0.192 + 0.995\mu_1 + 0.431\mu_2 - 0.704\mu_3 + 0.157\mu_5 - 0.034\mu_6 + 3.25 \cdot 10^{-6}\mu_{12} - 0.698HB1$$

$$N = 34 \quad R = 0.942 \quad s = 0.283 \quad s_{CV} = 0.348 \quad F(7,26) = 26.8$$

As can be seen the inclusion of some electronic features (bond orders and electron charge densities) in the framework of the connectivity indices (vertex and edge) produces the best results for describing the partition coefficients n-octanol/water for the 34 furylethylenes studied. It has also been clear that the global chemical reactivity is well described by graph theoretical molecular descriptors in general and that the use of quantum chemical indices is not recommended in this case. The experimental values of log *P* as well as those calculated from the different models obtained here are given in Table 3.

Table 3. Experimental and calculated values of the partition coefficeint n-octanol/water (log *P*) for the furylethylenes studied.

	log *P*				
No.	**Exp.**	**Topol.**	**Topog.**	**QC**	**SM**
1	1.879	1.894	1.955	1.836	2.034
2	2.439	2.482	2.398	2.239	2.320
3	2.739	2.753	2.748	2.405	2.689
4	2.999	2.905	2.898	2.510	2.623
5	1.869	1.763	1.930	1.976	2.013
6	1.599	1.619	1.550	1.679	1.719
7	2.504	2.703	2.640	2.706	2.584
8	1.303	1.191	1.338	1.456	1.538
9	1.583	1.453	1.783	1.583	1.852
10	0.649	0.433	0.300	0.180	0.166
11	0.984	0.999	1.091	1.076	1.054
12	0.819	1.160	0.870	2.149	1.455
13	1.386	1.583	1.423	1.482	1.385
14	1.860	2.311	1.941	1.858	1.859
15	1.803	1.966	2.084	1.906	1.909
16	2.356	2.168	2.332	2.240	2.042
17	2.225	2.493	2.526	2.241	2.245
18	2.284	2.384	2.383	2.277	2.677
19	2.333	2.316	2.316	2.346	2.349
20	2.605	2.382	2.575	2.618	2.727
21	1.652	1.347	1.585	1.830	1.616
22	2.098	1.984	1.947	2.126	1.960
23	2.673	2.733	2.459	2.504	2.667
24	2.641	2.484	2.666	2.592	2.543
25	2.827	2.726	2.837	2.902	2.873
26	3.135	3.052	3.034	2.902	3.086
27	3.091	3.018	2.952	2.943	3.367
28	3.060	2.994	3.002	3.029	2.672
29	3.404	3.227	3.252	3.266	3.035

30	2.447	2.510	2.469	2.132	2.078
31	1.050	1.365	1.258	1.344	1.232
32	1.591	1.510	1.500	1.711	1.754
33	1.611	1.738	1.515	1.590	1.527
34	1.488	1.309	1.424	1.504	1.333

A very different picture is obtained when local chemical reactivity is to be studied by using topological and topographic molecular descriptors. As previously stated this kind of graph theoretical descriptors produce poor correlations with this important property. The best QSPR models obtained by using these molecular descriptors are given below:

$$\log k = 0.544 + 2.937\,{}^{6}\chi_{pC} - 5.647\,{}^{6}\chi_{p} - 3.954\,{}^{3}\chi_{C}^{v} + 2.778\,{}^{2}\chi_{p} - 9.742\,{}^{4}\chi_{p} + 7.996\,{}^{4}\varepsilon_{p} - 4.753\,{}^{5}\varepsilon_{p}$$

$$N = 34 \quad R = 0.906 \quad s = 0.681 \quad s_{CV} = 0.737 \quad F(7,26) = 17.1$$

and

$$\log k = 0.164 + 233.91\,{}^{5}\Omega_{C}^{c}(q) - 127.76\,{}^{5}\varepsilon_{p}(\rho) - 8.439\,{}^{6}\varepsilon_{p}(\rho) + 0.751\,{}^{1}\Omega_{p}(q) - 7.094\,{}^{5}\Omega_{pC}^{C}(q) + 2.114\,{}^{2}\Omega_{p}^{C}(q) - 6.513\,{}^{5}\Omega_{p}^{C}(q)$$

$$N = 34 \quad R = 0.915 \quad s = 0.513 \quad s_{CV} = 0.569 \quad F(7,26) = 13.8$$

As can be seen less than 84 % of the variance in the log k is explained by both kind of descriptors and no improvement is observed by using topographic instead topological indices. These results are expected from the consideration of the global nature of these descriptors that are unable for describing a local property such as log k for the nucleophilic addition of thiols to the exocyclic double bond of furylethylenes.

The use of the global spectral moments also produces similar results to that obtained by using topological and topographic descriptors, illustrating that the question is not concerned with the graph invariant used in the definition of the molecular descriptors but with the global nature of them. The QSPR model with the global spectral moments is given below:

$$\log k = -0.478 + 1.278\mu_1 + 0.085\mu_7 - 4.30\cdot10^{-6}\mu_{13} - 0.421\mu_5 + 0.583\mu_3 - 3.40\cdot10^{-3}\mu_{10} + 3.28\cdot10^{-4}\mu_{12}$$

$$N = 34 \quad R = 0.918 \quad s = 0.655 \quad s_{CV} = 0.711 \quad F(7,26) = 18.8$$

A dramatic improvement in the quality of the QSPR model is obtained by using the quantum chemical molecular descriptors. This model not only represents an improvement from the statistical point of view but also give clear insights about the chemical nature of the interaction. The model obtained is as follows:

$$\log k = 20.878208.914ES_{\sigma}(6) + 66.122ES_{\pi}(6) + 235.54ES_{T}(5) + 0.540NS_{\sigma}(5) - 0.938NS_{\pi}(2) - 0.284NS_{\pi}(7) + 3.256Q(7)$$

$$N = 34 \qquad R = 0.984 \qquad s = 0.288 \qquad s_{CV} = 0.305 \qquad F(7{,}26) = 112.2$$

As can be seen this model explain more than 96 % of the variance in the log k with a standard deviation that is less than a half of that obtained with the graph theoretical molecular descriptors. The molecular descriptors included in this equation clearly pointed to the identification of the reaction centers involved in the chemical interaction studied. The atoms 6 and 7 are those conforming the exocyclic double bond of the furylethylene that is attacked by the thiol group. Consequently, this QSPR model has a good quality from both statistical and chemical points of view.

At this point of our study it is clear that the real challenge for the design of novel graph theoretical indices consists in the development of molecular descriptors that are able of "capturing" the local molecular features of chemicals. There are some examples in the literature in this direction, such as the electrotopological state index which is a locally defined topological descriptor.[56] However, the graph theory is a very flexible mathematical tool that permits the generation of novel invariants[57] of interest in chemistry maintaining the chemical interpretability of the results. In this sense we will use here the local spectral moments of the edge adjacency matrix of molecular graphs as a sort of local graph theoretical descriptors to be applied in describing the log k under study. By this way we have computed the first 15 local moments for each of the bonds that conform the skeleton of the furylethylene framework. Consequently, 105 (15 x 7) local moments are obtained and the best QSPR model was obtained by using them as for the previously studied descriptors. This model is given below together with the statistical parameters:

$$\log k = 4.698 + 0.143\mu_6(6-7) + 0.0054\mu_{13}(6-7) - 0.504\mu_6(2-6) - 0..069\mu_{11}(6-7) - 0.044\mu_7(6-7) + 3.10\cdot 10^{-4}\mu_9(2-6) + 4.729\mu_3(6-7)$$

$$N = 34 \qquad R = 0.982 \qquad s = 0.320 \qquad s_{CV} = 0.339 \qquad F(7{,}26) = 70.4$$

This model explains more than 96 % of the variance in log k, similarly to that obtained by using quantum chemical descriptors, and also permits to interpret the results from the chemical point of view. As can be seen most of the local spectral moments included in this model are related to the bond 6-7, which is the bond directly implicated in the nucleophilic attack of the thiol groups. The other bond represented by the local moments included in this model is also involved in the chemical reaction under study because it represent the interaction of the carbon atom 6, the center attacked by the thiol group, with the carbon 2 which is in the furan ring. The experimental values of log k as well as those calculated by the different models developed here are given in Table 4.

Table 4. Experimental and calculated values of the specific constant for the reaction of nucleophilic addition of thiols (log *k*) to the exocyclic double bond of the furylethylenes studied.

	log *k*					
No.	**Exp.**	**Topol.**	**Topog.**	**QC**	**SM**	**LSM**
1	6.591	7.532	6.607	6.780	6.281	6.679
2	6.518	6.983	6.184	6.646	5.583	6.563
3	6.914	6.352	6.702	7.021	6.893	6.979
4	6.982	6.997	6.773	6.935	6.554	7.069
5	7.176	6.750	6.828	7.137	7.390	7.291
6	7.602	6.685	6.820	7.466	7.410	7.572
7	5.255	5.533	5.793	5.212	5.002	4.934
8	6.763	4.965	6.007	6.737	5.962	6.662
9	5.623	4.997	4.683	5.454	4.839	5.599
10	3.813	4.831	4.474	3.695	4.455	4.318
11	3.840	3.636	4.307	3.616	4.876	4.034
12	3.874	4.162	3.598	3.537	2.911	3.448
13	3.825	3.916	3.039	3.562	4.255	3.875
14	3.623	3.798	3.389	3.550	4.032	3.841
15	3.751	3.528	3.859	3.522	3.255	3.721
16	3.784	3.114	3.849	3.566	3.437	3.842
17	3.697	4.175	3.950	3.570	3.468	3.826
18	3.705	3.934	3.950	3.541	3.157	3.711
19	3.697	3.264	3.762	3.482	3.686	3.798
20	3.650	3.526	4.272	3.581	4.269	3.851
21	4.000	3.693	4.380	3.985	5.184	3.735
22	3.920	3.974	3.887	3.920	4.202	3.617
23	3.790	3.856	3.144	3.926	4.409	3.596
24	3.763	3.869	3.671	3.849	3.438	3.552
25	3.623	3.172	2.633	3.921	3.893	3.600
26	3.650	4.233	3.587	3.917	4.178	3.610
27	3.592	4.193	3.649	3.873	3.613	3.566
28	3.584	4.0586	3.531	3.819	3.569	3.881

29	3.590	3.478	3.555	3.918	3.204	3.600
30	2.987	3.463	2.842	3.281	3.534	2.785
31	3.273	3.070	3.881	4.089	3.779	3.651
32	2.140	3.070	2.378	2.287	2.794	2.751
33	3.553	3.780	3.918	3.338	2.716	3.485
34	5.557	5.114	5.346	4.969	5.474	5.524

We have previously demonstrated that the spectral moments of the edge adjacency matrix can be expressed as linear combinations of the different structural fragments of the molecular graphs.[37-40] By this way, we can find the contribution that any structural fragment makes to the property studied. The extension of this approach to the locally defined spectral moments of the edge matrix is straightforward. Consequently, the contribution of the different fragments containing the corresponding bond for which the local moment is defined can be obtained permitting a direct interpretation of the results in terms of the molecular structure. By using this approach we have found the contribution of the different fragments that contains bonds 6-7 and 2-6, which are those included in the spectral moments of the QSPR model found. In Fig. 3 we show some of these fragments in order to investigate the influence of the different substituents at position 5 of the furan ring. We show only a few fragments containing six, seven and eight bonds and using CH_3, F, Cl, Br, I, COOH and NO_2 as substituents at position 5 of the heterocyclic ring.

A very large number of fragments can be generated and their contributions can be computed by using the system TOSS-MODE.[45] As can be seen from the Fig. 3 the presence of the group CH_3 always produces a negative contribution to log *k*, while the greatest contribution are always made by the groups COOH and NO_2. This can be interpreted in terms of the electronic effects of these substituents and they are in complete agreement with the experimental results. For instances, compound number 2 having a methyl group at position 5 of the furan ring (see Table 2) has a value of log *k* lower than that of the unsubstituted compound (no. 1 in Table 2). The reactivity then increase in the order Br < I < $COOCH_3$ < NO_2. This is exactly the same order of the contributions of the different fragments illustrated in Fig. 3 (the fragment COO depicted in this figure also appears in the group $COOCH_3$).

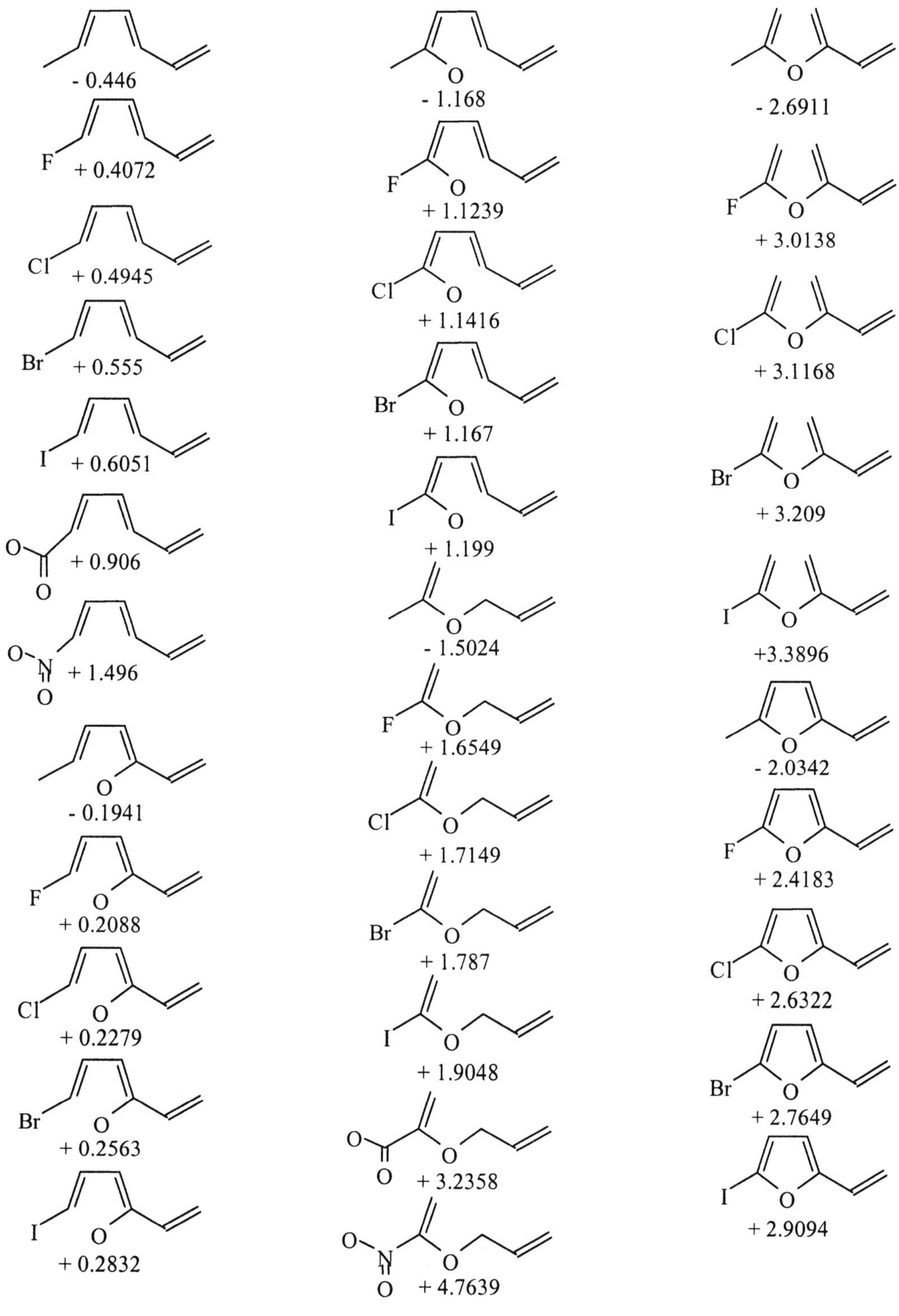

Fig. 3. Contribution of different structural fragments containing the exocyclic double bond of the furylethylene framework to the rate constant for the addition reaction of thiols.

By summing all the contributions of the different fragments containing a specific substructure or group we will obtain the contribution of this group to the property studied. By using this procedure we have computed the contributions of several groups that can be used as substituents at the position 5 of the heterocycle. We have computed these contributions by considering the groups NO_2 and $COOCH_3$ bounded at the β-position of the exocyclic double bond (carbon 7). In a similar way we also computed these group contributions considering NO_2 and Br as substituents in the before mentioned position. The groups considered here not only included those for which experimental values of log *k* exist but several others that can be interesting to investigate their influence over the reactivity of these chemicals. In Table 5 we give the values of these group contributions for the different substituents considered. In this Table we can observe that there are some differences in the absolute values of the group contributions calculated depending on the type of substituents in the exocyclic double bond. However, when these calculated quantities are correlated with the Hammett constant σ_p [58, 59] excellent correlations (R = 0.98) are observed for both series of group contributions. In Fig. 4 we illustrate these linear correlations.

Table 5. Values of the group contributions calculated from local moments for different substituents in the position 5 of the furan ring of the furylethylene compounds.

group	GC(1)[a]	GC(2)[b]	Group	GC(1)[a]	GC(2)[b]
H	0.00	0.00	c-C_3H_7	-0.32	-0.33
CH_3	-0.12	-0.28	i-C_3H_7	-0.12	-0.27
F	0.11	0.21	C_2H_5	-0.13	-0.27
Cl	0.25	0.25	C_6H_5	0.039	-0.10
Br	0.30	0.26	COOH	0.59	0.63
I	0.39	0.43	$COCH_3$	0.63	0.68
$COOCH_3$	0.61	0.61	CF_3	0.70	0.76
NO_2	0.89	1.10	CN	0.74	0.82
$N(CH_3)_2$	-0.62	-0.77	OH	-0.49	-0.41
NH_2	-0.54	-0.62	OCH_3	-0.38	-0.35
$C(CH_3)_3$	-0.12	-0.29			

[a] Group contribution when substituents in the exocyclic double bond are NO_2 and $COOCH_3$.
[b]Group contributions when the substituents in the exocyclic double bond are NO_2 and Br.

(A)

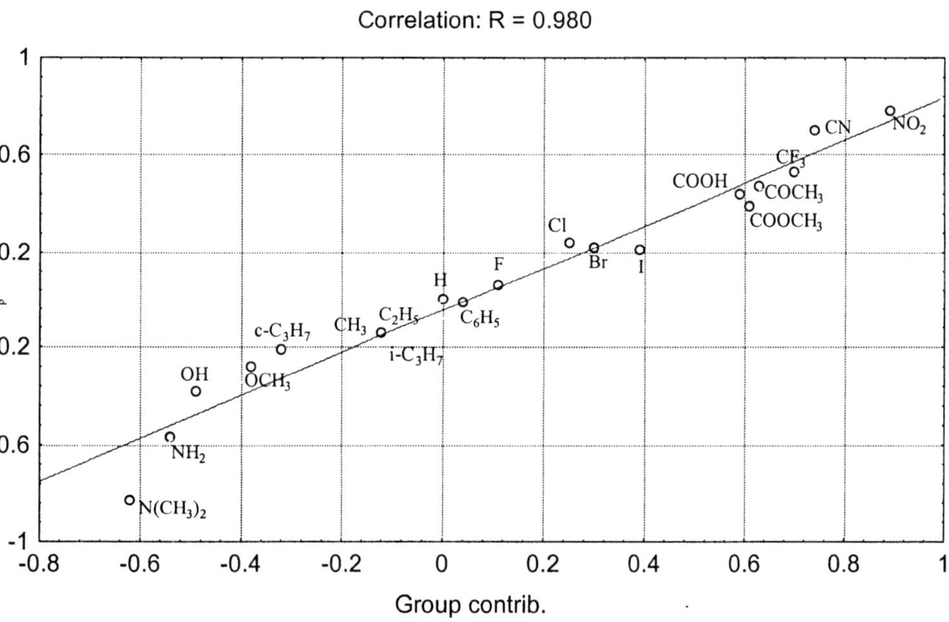

(B)

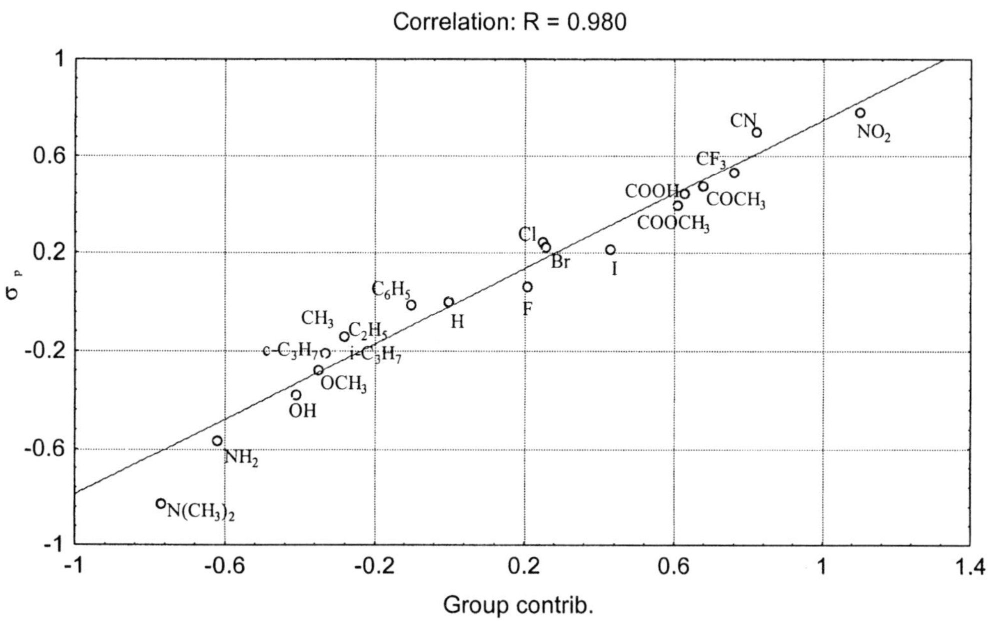

Fig. 4. Correlations between the group contribution of substituents at position 5 of the furan ring to log k and the Hammett σ_p constants when NO_2 and $COOCH_3$ are at position β of the double bond (A), and when NO_2 and Br are at this position (B).

With this example we have shown how the manipulation of (molecular) graphs permits the generation of molecular descriptors that are able to describe the local chemical reactivity of organic compounds. By this way we demonstrate that the use of this kind of molecular descriptors is not limited to the study of the global reactivity of chemicals. The statistically and chemically meaningful QSPR model obtained with the use of quantum chemical descriptors for the nucleophilic addition of thiols to furylethylenes obtained here prove that the electronic aspects of these molecules play a very important role in the explanation of this chemical process. By this way, we have proved that the chemical reactivity (global or local) can be studied with the use of appropriate graph theoretical descriptors even in the case where metric and electronic aspects of molecular architecture play an important role in the reaction process.

6. Conclusions and Future Outlook

The present study is only an example of the many possibilities that the application of graph theoretical concepts and ideas offers to the QSPR/QSAR studies. There has been severe criticism to the use of topological indices in QSAR, specially to the applications of the molecular connectivity indices. For instance, one of these critics formulated by Taylor[60] has been considered by Kubinyi in a recent text on QSAR[8]: "there has been some tendency, therefore, to use molecular connectivity in contexts for which it is unsuitable" and "regards molecular connectivity as an irrelevance witch has had the unfortunate effect of diverting attention from the real work that needs doing". In spite of the affirmation of Kubinyi that[8] "Nothing can be added to this criticism. To whom it may concern", we want to make some comments about the use and perspectives of this kind of descriptors in QSPR/QSAR studies. The use of molecular descriptors in contexts for which they are not suitable is not exclusive for molecular connectivity indices or for graph theoretical descriptors. Many examples are given in the literature where other approaches are used to solve problems completely outside the scope for which they were originally designed. As we stated in the introduction of this chapter there are some approaches that are considered as a "new fashion" and an explosion in their uses is immediately produced even in contexts for which it is unsuitable. However, the second critic is really discouraging and we only will give some examples that show its lack of precision. The molecular connectivity indices and other topological indices have been successfully applied to the design and discovery of novel analgesic compounds with greater therapeutic indices than that of the acetyl salicylic acid.[61, 62] Novel compounds with different biological activities were also discovered with these descriptors, such as antineoplasic,[63] β-blockers,[64] bronchodilators,[65] antifungal,[66] antiviral and others.[67] Other graph theoretical approaches have also been successfully applied in the design of novel compounds with biological activity. The TOSS-MODE approach has permitted the discovering of sedative/hypnotic activities of several classes of lead compounds.[42] This approach permitted the design and synthesis of several carbonucleosides with antineoplasic activity,[68] new compounds with antifungal activity,[69] novel antidepressant compounds,[70] and several series of anticonvulsants.[71] These are only some examples representing facts that can not be considered as "effect of diverting attention from the real work that needs doing".

The further development of the graph theoretical descriptors in QSPR/QSAR needs more applications of these descriptors to the real discovering of novel compounds with applications in the industry and in pharmaceutical sciences. In this sense, the use of the big arsenal of graph theoretical descriptors in a rational way for searching in data bases of chemical structures open novel possibilities for the topological indices in QSPR/QSAR studies. By this way, the 70 % of papers published with the use of graph theoretical ideas, which now is devoted to hydrocarbon molecules, should be dedicated to 99 % of organic chemicals that are not hydrocarbons. In doing so, the definition of novel descriptors that consider the different heteroatoms in the molecule is an urgent necessity for graph theoretical chemists.

Consequently, it is clear that the development of novel descriptors based on chemical graph theoretical concepts needs to receive an important attention of molecular descriptor designers. However, these novel graph theoretical descriptors need to solve some of the problems that the previous descriptors not solved. The mere exercise of using new graph invariants for producing novel descriptors that in general are similar to the "classic" topological indices only produce more criticism to the use of this kind of descriptors.

On the other hand, we believe that the development of user-friendly computer softwares is another point that should receive more attention in order to reach a wide application of these molecular descriptors in QSPR/QSAR studies. These computational systems should be designed for a wider spectrum of users in the same way that computational chemistry and molecular modeling programs are. They should also permits the manipulation of large data sets of compounds in a short time to be applied to the large data bases of chemical structures that are available for chemists today. Finally, it is hardly to believe the scarce use that the developers and users of graph theoretical molecular descriptors make on Internet as a source of information, experience and software interchange at the begin of the 21 century.

7. ACKNOWLEDGEMENT

E.E. thanks all his colleagues in Santa Clara, Cuba for the long continued support and collaboration during several years. The kindly hospitality of the members of Organic Chemistry Department, Faculty of Pharmacy, University of Santiago de Compostela, Spain is also acknowledged.

8. References

1. For instance, in the period 1993-spetember of 1997 the number of CoMFA papers was 383, see Kim, K. H. List of CoMFA References, 1993-1997. In *Persepective in Drug Discovery and Design*, **1998**, 12/13/14, 317-333.
2. Sablij, A.; Trinajstić, N. Quantitative structure-activity relationships: the role of topological indices. *Acta Pharm. Jugosl.* **1981**, 31, 189-194.
3. Mihalić, Z. and Trinajstić, N. A graph-theoretical approach to structure-property relationships. *J. Chem. Educ.* **1992**, 69, 701-712.
4. Trinajstić, N. *Chemical Graph Theory*; CRC Press: Boca Raton, Fl, 1992.
5. Devillers, J. and Balaban, A. T. (eds.) *Topological Indices and Related Descriptors in QSAR and QSPR.*, Gordon and Breach, Reading, UK, 1999.
6. Bonchev, D. *Information Theoretic Indices for Characterization of Chemical Structure*; Research Studies Press-Wiley: Chichester, 1993.
7. Albert, A. *Selective Toxicity. The Physico-Chemical Basis of Therapy*; Chapman and Hall: London, 1984.
8. Kubinyi, H. *QSAR: Hansch Analysis and Related Approaches*; VCH, Weinheim, 1993, p. 53, and references given therein.
9. Randić, M. Generalized molecular descriptors. *J. Math. Chem.* **1991**, 7, 155-168.
10. Milne, G. W. A. Mathematics as a basis for chemistry. *J. Chem. Inf. Comput. Sci.* **1997**, 37, 639-644.
11. Mekenyan, O. and Basak, S. C. Topological indices and chemical reactivity. In Bonchev, D. and Mekenyan, O. (eds.), *Graph Theoretical Approaches to Chemical Reactivity*; Kluwer Academic Pub., Amsterdam, 1994, pp. 221-239.
12. Randić, M. Topological indices. In *Encyclopedia of Computational Chemistry* (P. v. R. Schleyer, Ed.-in-Chief), 1997, J. Wiley and Sons, London.
13. Randić, M. On characterization of three-dimensional structures. *Int. J. Quantum Chem.: Quantum Biol. Symp.* **1988**, 15, 201-208.
14. Randić, M.; Jerman-Blazic, B.; Trinajstić, N. Development of 3-dimensional molecular descriptors. *Comput. Chem.* **1990**, 14, 237-246.
15. Bogdanov, B., Nikolić, S. and Trinajstić, N. On the three-dimensional Wiener number. *J. Math. Chem.* **1989**, 3, 299-309.
16. Randić, M.; Razinger, M. On characterization of three-dimensional molecular structure. In *From Chemical Topology to Three-Dimensional Geometry*; Balaban, A. T. (ed.); Plenum Press: New York, 1997, pp 159-236.
17. Diudea, M. V., Horvath, D. and Graovac, A. Molecular topology. 15. 3D distance matrices and related topological indices. *J. Chem. Inf. Comput. Sci.* **1995**, 35, 129-135.
18. *Computational Advances in Organic Chemistry: Molecular Structure and Reactivity.* C. Ögnetir, and I. G. Csizmadia, (eds.), Kluwer Academic, Dordrecht, 1991.
19. Kier, L. B.; Hall, L. H. *Molecular Connectivity in Chemistry and Drug Research*; Academic Press: New York, 1976.

20. Kier, L. B.; Hall, L. H. *Molecular Connectivity in Structure-Activity Analysis*; Research Studies Press: Letchworth, 1986.
21. Hall, L. H. Computational aspects of molecular connectivity and its role in structure-property modeling. In *Computational Chemical Graph Theory*; Rouvray, D. H. (ed.); Nova Science: New York, 1990; pp 202-233.
22. Randić, M. On characterization of molecular branching. *J. Am. Chem. Soc.* **1975**, 97, 6609-6615.
23. Estrada, E. Edge adjacency relationships and a novel topological index related to molecular volume. *J. Chem. Inf. Comput. Sci.* **1995**, 35, 31-33.
24. Estrada, E. Edge adjacency relationships in molecular graphs containing heteroatoms: a new topological index related to molar volume. *J. Chem. Inf. Comput. Sci.* **1995**, 35, 701-707.
25. Estrada, E.; Guevara, N.; Gutman, I. Extension of the edge connectivity index. Relationships to line graph indices and QSPR applications. *J. Chem. Inf. Comput. Sci.* **1998**, 38, 428-431.
26. Casch, G. G. Correlation of physicochemical properties of alkylphenols with their graph-theoretical ε parameter. *Chemosphere* **1995**, 31, 4307-4315.
27. Lekishvili, T.; Lekishvili, G.; Aleksidze, N. Mathematical investigation of the cancerogenic activity of some hormones. *Bull. Georgian Acad. Sci.* **1997**, 155, 441-443.
28. Nikolić, S.; Trinajstić, N. Comparison between the vertex- and edge-connectivity indices for benzenoid hydrocarbons. *J. Chem. Inf. Comput. Sci.* **1998**, 38, 42-46.
29. Plavšić, D.; Trinajstić, N.; Amić, D.; Solskic, M. Comparison between the structure-boiling points relationships with different descriptors for condensed benzenoids. *New J. Chem.* **1998**, 22, 1075-1078.
30. Nikolić, S.; Trinajstić, N. Modeling the aqueous solubility of aliphatic alcohols. *SAR QSAR Environ. Res.* **1998**, 9, 117-126.
31. Estrada, E.; Molina, E. 3D Connectivity Indices in **QSPR/QSAR** Studies. *J. Chem. Inf. Comput. Sci.* **2000**, submitted for publication.
32. Estrada, E.; Montero, L. A. Bond order weighted graphs in molecules as structure-property indices. *Mol. Eng.* **1993**, 2, 363-373.
33. Estrada, E. Novel graph theoretical concepts for molecular modeling in organic chemistry. Ph. Thesis. La Habana, 1997.
34. Estrada, E. Three-dimensional molecular descriptors based on electron charge density weighted graphs. *J. Chem. Inf. Comput. Sci.* **1995**, 35, 708-713.
35. Estrada, E.; Ramírez, A. Edge adjacency relationships and molecular topographic descriptors. Definition and QSAR applications. *J. Chem. Inf. Comput. Sci.* **1996**, 36, 837-843.
36. Kikuchi, O. Systematic QSAR procedures with quantum chemical descriptors. *Quant. Struct.-Act. Relat.* **1987**, 6, 179-184.
37. Estrada, E. Spectral moments of the edge adjacency matrix in molecular graphs. 1. Definition and applications to the prediction of physical properties of alkanes. *J. Chem. Inf. Comput. Sci.* **1996**, 36, 844-849.

38. Estrada, E. Spectral moments of the edge adjacency matrix in molecular graphs. 2. Molecules containing heteroatoms and QSAR applications. *J. Chem. Inf. Comput. Sci.* **1997**, 37, 320-328.
39. Estrada, E. Spectral moments of the edge adjacency matrix in molecular graphs.3. Molecules containing cycles. *J. Chem. Inf. Comput. Sci.* **1998**, 38, 23-27.
40. Estrada, E. Modelling the diamagnetic susceptibility of organic compounds by a sub-structural graph-theoretical approach. *J. Chem. Soc. Faraday Trans.* **1998**, 94, 1407-1410.
41. Estrada, E. Generalized spectral moments of the iterated line graph sequence. A novel approach to QSPR studies. *J. Chem. Inf. Comput. Sci.* **1999**, 39, 90-95.
42. Estrada, E.; Peña, A.; García-Domenech, R. Designing sedative/hypnotic compounds from a novel substructural graph-theoretical approach. *J. Comput.-Aided Mol. Des.* **1998**, 12, 583-595.
43. Estrada, E.; Molina, E. Novel Local (Fragment-based) Topological Molecular Descriptors for QSPR/QSAR and Molecular Design. *J. Mol. Graph. Modell.* **2000**, submitted for publication.
44. Rodríguez, L.; Estrada, E. MODEST ver. 3.0 for Windows. Central University of Las Villas, Santa Clara, Cuba, 1995.
45. Gutiérrez, Y.; Estrada, E.; Rodríguez, L.; Muñoz, I. TOSS-MODE ver. 2.5 for Windows. Central University of Las Villas, Santa Clara, Cuba, 1995.
46. Steward, J. J. P. MOPAC 6.0. Quantum Chemical Program Exchange No. 455, Bloomington, IN, 1990 .
47. Miyaji, T. Nitrofurans compounds as food additives. In *Mechanism of Toxicity and Metabolism, Vol. 6.* Karki, N. T. (ed.), Pergamon, Oxford, 1976, pp 127-136.
48. Dore, J. Ch.; Viel, C. Antitumoral chemotherapy: X. Cytotoxic and antitumoral activity of β-nitrostyrenes and nitrovinyl derivatives. *Farmaco*, **1975**, 30, 81-109.
49. (a) F. R. Gerns, L. D. Timberlake, U.S. Patent 5,138,076, Aug. 11 (1992). (b) W. K. Whitekettle, D. K Donofrio, U.S. Patent 5,158,972, Oct. 27 (1992). (c)W. F. McCoy and S. Thornburgh, U.S. Patent 5,090,990, Feb. 25 (1992).
50. N. Castañedo, R. Goizueta, J. Pérez, J. González, E. Silveira, M. Cuesta, A. Martínez, E. Lugo, E. Estrada, A. C. Carta, O. Navia and M. S. Delgado Cuban Patent 22446 (1994).
51. Balaz, S.; Sturdik, E.; Rosenberg, M.; Augustín, J.; Skada, B. Kinetics of srug activities as influences by their physico-chemical properties: Antibacterial effects of alkylating 2-furylethylenes. *J. Theor. Biol.* **1988**, 131, 115-134.
52. Estrada, E. Structure-mutagenicity relationships in 2-furylethylene derivatives. A molecular orbital study of the role of nitro groups. *Mutation Res.* **1998**, 420, 67-75
53. Deward, M. J. S.; Zoebish, E. G.; Healy, E. F.; Steward, J. J. P. AM1: a new general purpose quantum chemical molecular model. *J. Am. Chem. Soc.* **1985**, 107, 3902-3909.
54. Estrada, E.; Gómez, M.; Castañedo, N.; Pérez, C. Theoretical and experimental study on the structure of 1-(5-X-fur-2-yl)-2-nitro-2-Y-ethylenes. *J. Mol. Struct.* (THEOCHEM), 468,193-200.

55. Cited in: Franke, R. *Theoretical Drug Design Methods*. Elsevier, Amsterdam, 1984.
56. Kier, L. B.; Hall. L. H. *Molecular Structure Description: The Electrotopological State*. Academic Press, New York, 1999.
57. Randić, M. In search of structural invariants. *J. Math. Chem.* **1992**, 9, 97-146.
58. Hammett, L. P. *Physical Organic Chemistry*. McGraw-Hill, New York, 1940.
59. Perrin, D. D.; Dempsey, B.; Serjeant, E. P. *PKa Prediction for Organic Acids and Bases*. Chapman and hall, London, 1981.
60. Cited in ref. 8.
61. Gálvez, J.; García, R.; Moliner, R.; García, F. *Spanish patent* No. P9101034, 1991.
62. Gálvez, J.; García-Domenech, R.; De Julián-Ortíz, V.; Soler, R. Topological approach to analgesia. *J. Chem. Inf. Comput. Sci.* **1994**, 34, 1198-1203.
63. Gálvez, J.; Gómez-Lechón, M. J.; García-Domenech, R.; Castell, J. V. New cytostatic agents obtained by molecular topology. *Bioorg. Med. Chem. Lett.* **1996**, 6, 2301-2306.
64. García-Domenech, R.; de Gregorio-Alapont, C.; de Julián-Ortíz, J. V.; Gálvez, J. *Bioorg. Med. Chem. Lett.* **1997**, 7, 567-572.
65. Ríos-Santamaría, I.; García-Domenech, R.; Gálvez, J. New bronchodilators selected by molecular topology. *Bioorg. Med. Chem. Lett.* **1998**, 8, 477-482.
66. Pastor, L.; García-Domenech, R.; Gálvez, J. New antifungal selected by molecular topology. *Bioorg. Med. Chem. Lett.* **1998**, 8, 2577-2582.
67. Gálvez, J., García-Domenech, R., de Julian-Ortiz, J. V. and Soler, R. Topological approach to drug design. *J. Chem. Inf. Comput. Sci.* **1995**, 35, 272-284, and references cited therein.
68. Estrada, E.; Uriarte, E.; Montero, A.; Teijeira, M; Santana, L.;. De Clercq, E. A novel approach for the virtual screening and and rational design of anticancer compounds. *J. Med. Chem.* **2000**, 43, 1975-1985.
69. Arias-Cedeño, Q. Synthesis of Potentially Bioactive Compounds Derived from γ-Nitroketones. Ph.D. Thesis, Central University of Las Villas, Santa Clara, Cuba.
70. Estrada, E.; Peña, A. Unpublished results.
71. Estrada, E.; Peña, A. In-silico studies for the rational discovery of anticonvulsant compounds. *Bioorg. Med. Chem.* **2000**, 8, 2755-2770.

Chapter 6

THE CONCEPT OF GRAPH MASS IN MOLECULAR GRAPH THEORY. A CASE IN DATA REDUCTION ANALYSIS

Lionello Pogliani

Dipartimento di Chimica, Universita' della Calabria,
87030 Rende (CS), Italy

1. INTRODUCTION

A great deal of quantitative structure-property relationship (QSPR) studies are based on graph theoretical indices derived from hydrogen-suppressed chemical graphs and pseudo-graphs [1,2] the molecular connectivity χ indices, defined more than twenty years ago [3-7] and further refined over the last twenty-two years by several authors [8-58] into a self-consistent theoretical frame known as molecular connectivity, MC, theory (or RKH theory from Randić, Kier and Hall). It is a theory, which allows to model properties and activities of compounds with simple computational methods, once the basic mathematical tools needed to grasp the entire theory are mastered. Further, due to the introduction of an orthogonalization procedure, which allows to construct highly stable and useful relations [21-23] and of a procedure, which allows to revert from the molecular connectivity indices to the corresponding molecular graphs [34-35], this theory shows the characteristic of completeness. It is, in fact, possible to describe known properties or activities of molecules, and, also, from desired properties or activities revert back to the corresponding molecule.

Recently, with the methodical utilization of linear combinations of molecular connectivity indices (LCCI) [42-44,48-52] it has been possible to model many physicochemical properties of classes of substituted compounds, to detect association phenomena in solution, and even to model properties of inorganic compounds, and it has been possible, with specially designed molecular connectivity indices, to model properties of cis-trans isomers [41]. Use of linear combinations of molecular connectivity indices (LCCI) has lately been superseded by the introduction of linear combinations of second-level descriptors, like, squared, reciprocal and supramolecular connectivity indices [36,49,50] as well as higher-level molecular connectivity terms, $X = f(\chi)$, derived by the aid of a trial-and-error procedure based on a medium- or small-sized set of molecular connectivity χ indices [1,2,51,52,56,57]. Finally, to model different properties of highly heterogeneous classes of compounds have, quite recently, been introduced the semiempirical molecular connectivity terms [57], that is, terms that include empirical parameters. Molecular connectivity X terms, either normal or semiempirical, show the interesting property to be dominant descriptors, allowing to consistently reduce the combinatorial problem, as in many cases the total combinatorial technique for searching the best LCXCT (Linear Combination of X Molecular Connectivity Terms) can be replaced by the abridged forward selection technique [49,50]. The discovery of molecular connectivity terms has widened the possibility to design new and powerful connectivity descriptors, which can quite often be used as single descriptors but sometimes also in combination with other terms or χ indices. Further, the possibility to apply to the X terms of a LCXCT Randić's orthogonalization procedure [21-23], offers the chance to give rise to highly stable relations with enhanced utility.

All along preceding QSPR modeling the possibility to model the molar masses of compounds has never been considered quite seriously. That is, many times have molar masses been modeled with molecular connectivity, or different, indices but never with the aim to detect which molecular connectivity descriptor could be considered the exact counterpart of molar masses, both theoretically and experimentally. Now, the molecular connectivity version of chemical graph theory offers the possibility to define both an 'a priori' and an 'a posteriori' counterpart of the molar mass. In reality, we have to do with two theoretical graph mass descriptors because for every compound it is possible to draw two kinds of chemical graphs, the well-known graph and the less known pseudograph. Clearly, the problem cannot be solved at a purely theoretical level, the concept of molar mass should be compared with its experimental counterpart, the molar mass, and should be tested to check its descriptive power of physicochemical properties.

Aim of the present paper is to outline, without leaving the borders of molecular connectivity theory, the concept of graph mass, whose indices had already been defined not so long ago[31], to check the kind of relations they have with the molar mass, and further check which molecular connectivity indices are the best descriptors of the molar mass, and, finally to find out how far both theoretical and experimental graph mass descriptors are able to model the properties of different classes of compounds. Modeled properties are : the solubility, the side-chain molecular volume, the crystal densities, and the specific rotations of L-amino acids, the average <pk> values, and the solubility of purines and pyrimidines, five different properties of DNA-RNA bases, the melting points and motor octane number of alkanes, the lattice enthalpies of metal halides, the unfrozen water content of a heterogeneous class of amino acids and inorganic salts, the molar refractivities, the retention index, the refractivity, and the density of organic phosphoderivatives, and, finally, the boiling and melting points, the density, the refractive index, and the dielectric constant of a wide heterogeneous class of organic solvents.

2. METHOD

In graph theory the handshaking theorem occupies an important place, and it can be used to define two new kind of indices which can be regarded upon as graph mass indices. This theorem says : let G = (V, E) be a graph with E edges and V vertices, then, $2e = \Sigma_i\delta_i$, where e is the number of edges, and where δ_i is the vertex degree in a graph [1,2,58]. A similar definition can be derived for pseudographs, i.e., $2e^v = \Sigma_i\delta^v_i$, where apex v stands for valence, and δ^v_i is the vertex degree in a pseudograph. Since an edge (inclusive loops in pseudographs which contribute twice to the degree of a vertex) is incident with exactly two vertices, it contributes twice to the sum of the degree of the vertices. Handshaking because of the analogy between an edge having two end points and a handshake involving two hands. Clearly, for stereoisomers like amino acids L and D the vertex degree does not change, thus their sum is invariant for both L and D forms, just as the molar mass. Before, going into details let us have a look on chemical graphs and pseudographs. Cardinal numbers δ and valence δ^v are directly related to the degree of a vertex in a graph or pseudograph respectively, and indirectly they are related to the type of bond in a compound, that is, in the corresponding hydrogen-suppressed chemical graph or pseudograph. This last kind of graph allows, in fact, multiple edges and loops, which mimic multiple bonds and lone-pair electrons. In Figure 1 and 2 are shown the chemical graphs (left) and pseudographs (right) of an amino acid, Alanine, and of a pyrimidine base, Cytosine, respectively. Delta values can easily be derived counting the number of connections incident to a point, with loops counting twice. Now, reminding what has been said with the handshaking theorem, we can define the following graph or pseudograph mass indices, which are nonetheless than the sum-delta and valence sum-delta indices introduced six years ago into molecular connectivity theory [32]

$$D = 2e = \Sigma_i\delta_i \quad (1)$$

$$D^v = 2e^v = \Sigma_i\delta^v \quad (2)$$

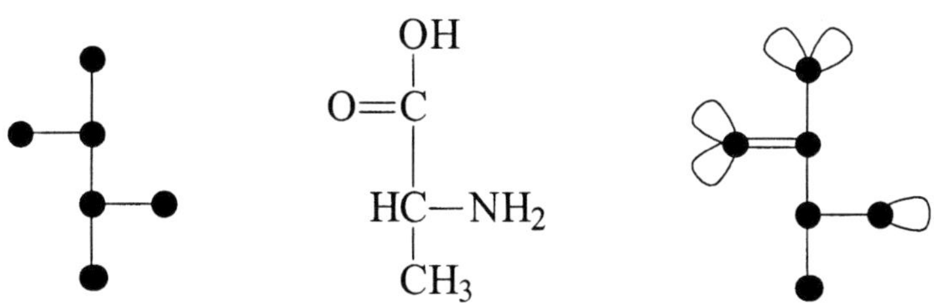

Figure 1. Graph (left) and pseudograph (right) of the amino acid Alanine.

Many of our preceding QSPR studies are based on the medium-sized set of molecular connectivity indices given by eq. 3. Now, it will be interesting to check if one of these indices has the right to be defined, on a purely experimental level, as graph mass index,

$$\{D, D^v, {}^0\chi, {}^0\chi^v, {}^1\chi, {}^1\chi^v, \chi_t, \chi_t^v\} \tag{3}$$

where the zeroth-, first-[12] and total [19]-order molecular connectivity indices are

$$ {}^0\chi = \Sigma(\delta_i)^{-0.5} \tag{4}$$

$$ {}^1\chi = \Sigma(\delta_i\delta_j)^{-0.5} \tag{5}$$

$$ \chi_t = (\delta_1\delta_2 \ldots\ldots \delta_N)^{-0.5} \tag{6}$$

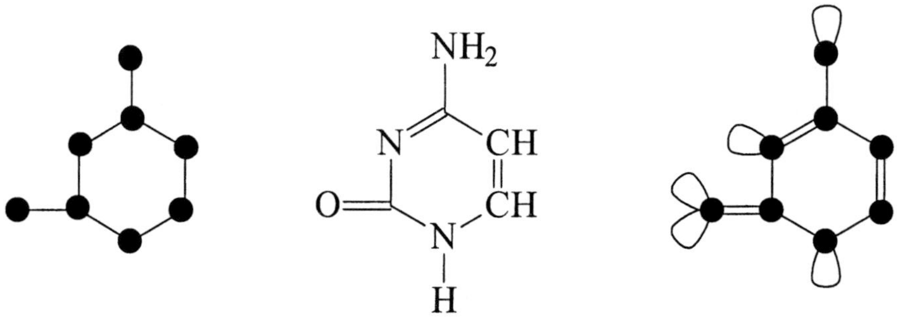

Figure 2. Graph (left) and pseudograph (right) of the pyrimidine base Cytosine.

Sums in eq. 4, and 5 run over the total number of N vertices (eqs. 4) and edges (eq. 5) of the hydrogen-suppressed molecular graph respectively, which correspond to heteroatoms and hetero-σ bonds, respectively (for atoms other than hydrogen). Replacing in eqs. 4-6 δ with valence δ^v, which represent the degree of a vertex in the corresponding pseudograph the corresponding χ^v indices are obtained. The δ^v(S) values in amino acids Cys and Met (0.56 and 0.67 respectively), as well as $\delta^v = Z^v / (Z - Z^v - 1)$, for the inorganic salts (here, metal chlorides) have been taken from Kier and Hall [12], where Z^v is the number of valence electrons and Z is the atomic number of the corresponding atom. From these eight structure-invariant parameters it is possible to build a whole hierarchy of higher-level indices, each level with its own family of indices [1,2,49,50,55-57].

The linear estimation problem of a physicochemical property P with χ indices or X terms is the estimation of the experimental property P_{exp} in terms of a linear function of χ, or X, which in matrix notation is given by the following dot product

$$P = |\mathbf{C} \cdot \chi| \tag{7}$$

where P is the calculated property of a compound. Row vector **C** (a 1·m vector) is the vector of coefficients c_k which are determined by the linear least-squares procedure and column (m·1) vector **χ** (or vector X) is the vector of the best molecular connectivity indices, derived by the aid of a combinatorial search procedure. The descriptor corresponding to the constant c_0 term is the unitary index $\chi^0 \equiv 1$. If χ is a m·n matrix, with n = number of compounds, then P becomes a column (1·n) vector **P** of the properties of the entire class of compounds. Bars in equation 5 stand for absolute value to get rid of negative P values with no physical meaning and simultaneously enhance the description of the property [46,48]. When properties with negative and antithetical values are modeled, as it has been the case for the specific SR rotations of L- and D-amino acids, eq. 7 has to be recast into the following form : $P_{L\cup D} = \mathbf{C}_{L\cup D}\cdot\mathbf{X}$, with, $\mathbf{C}_D = -\mathbf{C}_L$ (where sign $\cup$ stands for the logical sign '*or*').

For every coefficient c_k of the best χ_k index, including the constant coefficient of the unitary $\chi^0 \equiv 1$ index, the index utility, $u_k = |c_k/s_k|$, as well as the average index utility $<u> = \Sigma u_k/m$ will be estimated [1,2,38,50,55-57]. This statistics will be considered only if Q = r / s (the quality parameter), $F = fr^2/[(1-r^2)v]$ (the F ratio, f = degrees of freedom, v = number of χ parameters), r (correlation coefficient), and s (standard deviation of the estimate) statistics will show promising results.

3. Results and Discussion

In tables 1-15 are collected the statistical scores of the best single descriptor (1st row), of the molar mass, *M*, of the two best descriptors of *M* (that, from now on will be regarded upon as experimental graph mass descriptors), and of the theoretical graph, and pseudograph mass descriptors, as well as the simplest best linear combination of connectivity indices (LCCI) for a given property, and the same LCCI but with *M* replacing either the experimental or the theoretical graph mass descriptors. The molecular connectivity index values as well as the molar mass values for the different classes of compounds and the experimental data for the different properties have already been published elsewhere [43,46,48-50], but, for the sake of clarity, are here collected in tables 1A-11A.

Clearly, the validity of a descriptor resides in its capacity to model as many as possible properties of different classes of compounds. We will then check if the theoretical and the experimental graph mass descriptor can stand a comparison with the best molecular connectivity descriptor for the different properties of many classes of compounds, i.e., amino acids [n°(properties) = n(p) = 4], purines and pyrimidines [n(p) = 2], DNA-RNA bases [n(p) = 5], alkanes [n(p) = 2], metal halides [n(p) = 1], metal halides plus amino acids [n(p) = 1], organophosporous derivatives [n(p) = 4], and a wide heterogeneous set of organic compounds [n(p) = 5].

Table 1A. The molecular connectivity indices for 21 amino acids and their molar (MM) masses.

AA(*M*)	D	D^v	$^0\chi$	$^0\chi^v$	$^1\chi$	$^1\chi^v$	χ_t	χ_t^v
Gly (75)	8	20	4.28446	2.63992	2.27006	1.18953	0.40825	0.03727
Ala (89)	10	22	5.15470	3.51016	2.64273	1.62709	0.33333	0.03043
Cys (121)	12	23.56	5.86181	4.55358	3.18074	2.40290	0.23570	0.02875
Ser (105)	12	28	5.86181	3.66448	3.18074	1.77422	0.23570	0.00962
Val (117)	14	26	6.73205	5.08751	3.55342	2.53777	0.19245	0.01757
Thr (119)	14	30	6.73205	4.53473	3.55342	2.21862	0.19245	0.00786
Met (149)	16	26.67	7.27602	6.14607	4.18074	4.04355	0.11785	0.01859
Pro (115)	16	28	5.98313	4.55413	3.80453	2.76688	0.08333	0.00932
Leu (131)	16	28	7.43916	5.79462	4.03658	3.02094	0.13608	0.01242
Ile (131)	16	28	7.43916	5.79462	4.09142	3.07578	0.13608	0.01242
Asn (132)	16	36	7.43916	4.70278	4.03658	2.30434	0.13608	0.00254
Asp (133)	16	38	7.43916	4.57273	4.03658	2.23927	0.13608	0.00196
Lys (146)	18	32	7.98313	5.91594	4.68074	3.36624	0.08333	0.00439
Hyp (132)	18	34	6.85337	4.87159	4.19838	2.84158	0.06804	0.00340
Gln (146)	18	38	8.14627	5.40997	4.53658	2.80434	0.09623	0.00179
Glu (147)	18	40	8.14627	5.27984	4.53658	2.73927	0.09623	0.00139
His (155)	22	42	8.26758	5.81918	5.19838	3.15529	0.03402	0.00080
Arg (174)	22	42	9.56048	6.70883	5.53658	3.60022	0.04811	0.00078
Phe (165)	24	42	8.97469	6.60402	5.69838	3.72222	0.02406	0.00069
Tyr (181)	26	48	9.84493	6.97388	6.09222	3.85651	0.01964	0.00027
Trp (204)	32	54	10.83650	8.10402	7.18154	4.71624	0.00567	0.00009

The modeling of the molar *M* masses of 21 amino acids (AA, Hyp inclusive, see Table 1A) with the set of 8 molecular connectivity indices gives the following results for the four best descriptors:

$^0\chi$: Q = 0.156, F = 441, r = 0.979, s = 6.27, <u> = 10.7, **u** = (21, 0.34)

$^1\chi$: Q = 0.149, F = 401, r = 0.977, s = 0.56, <u> = 12.5, **u** = (20, 5.0)

$^0\chi^v$: Q = 0.107, F = 206, r = 0.957, s = 9.0, <u> = 8.1, **u** = (14, 1.9)

D : Q = 0.106, F = 203, r = 0.956, s = 9.0, <u> = 10.6, **u** = (14, 7.0)

The results for ${}^0\chi$ and ${}^1\chi$ are contradictory. While ${}^0\chi$ shows a better Q and F statistics, ${}^1\chi$ shows a much better utility, especially for what concerns the utility of the unitary term, which for the first index is completely unreliable. The low score of D index seems rather striking and even more striking the much worse score of D^v (Q = 0.07, F = 81). The theoretically defined graph mass, D, and pseudo-graph mass, D^v, do not correspond to the experimentally found graph mass descriptors. Such a finding will be confirmed with many other classes of compounds. It seems, thus, that theoretically defined graph mass indices have their own 'domain' which do not overlaps with the *M* 'domain'.

In the following analysis of 4 experimental properties of different sets of amino acids (n = 19, 18, 16, and 10, see Table 2A) the attention will be centered on the scores of D and D^v as well on the scores of the two best experimental, ${}^0\chi$ and ${}^1\chi$ graph mass descriptors. All along these sets of different numbers of amino acids, with the exception of the set n =10 amino acids, the 4 best descriptors for *M* (in decreasing Q and F order) are ${}^0\chi$, ${}^1\chi$, D and D^v, while for the class with 10 AA this ordering is : ${}^1\chi$, ${}^0\chi$, D, and D^v.

The different scores of descriptors, *M*, ${}^0\chi$, ${}^1\chi$, D, and D^v for the solubility, *S*, of 19 natural amino acids (Cys excluded) are collected in Table 1. The best descriptor is ${}^0\chi$, which is also the best descriptor for the activity [43,48]. The description of this property by *M*, ${}^0\chi$, ${}^1\chi$, D, and D^v is quite deceiving (in fact, only higher-level X terms will achieve a satisfactory modeling [2,50-51,56] for *S*), nevertheless interesting is the fact that the 'best' descriptor, together with *M*, is the found experimental ${}^0\chi$ graph mass index, it seems, thus, that we are on the right track for this index. Of the theoretical graph mass indices index D^v is the most similar to *M*. One of the best LCCI (linear combination of connectivity indices) for this property is the one shown in the 6th row of Table 1. Now, if we alternatively substitute each index of this combination with *M* we obtain the results shown in the 7th and 8th rows. These last results show that at the level of a linear combination, ${}^0\chi$ and ${}^1\chi$ are much better descriptor than *M*. To this it should added that for LCCI with growing number of χ parameters the descriptive capability between the given experimental graph mass indices and *M* diverges. Thus, results obtained at the level of a single index cannot be extrapolated to the level of a LCCI, as it seems that different components of the same index are activated at every level.

Table 2A. Calculated χ values for 23 Purine and Pyrimidine bases [a] and their molar masses.

PP (*M*)	D	D^v	$^0\chi$	$^0\chi^v$	$^1\chi$	$^1\chi^v$	χ_t	χ_t^v
7I8MTp (250.3)	38	62	13.61036	11.38981	8.34111	5.97071	0.003564	8.51E-05
7B8MTp (250.3)	38	62	13.44723	11.22667	8.48527	6.11486	0.003086	7.37E-05
7Itp (236.3)	36	60	12.74012	10.46716	7.93043	5.53989	0.004365	9.82E-05
7BTp (236.3)	36	60	12.57699	10.30402	8.07459	5.68405	0.00378	8.51E-05
1BTb (236.3)	36	60	12.57699	10.30402	8.07459	5.68405	0.00378	8.51E-05
7PTp (222.2)	34	58	11.86988	9.59691	7.57459	5.18405	0.005346	0.00012
1PTb (222.2)	34	58	11.86988	9.59692	7.57459	5.18405	0.005346	0.00012
7ETp (208.2)	32	56	11.16277	8.88981	7.07459	4.68405	0.00756	0.00017
1ETb (208.2)	32	56	11.16277	8.88981	7.07459	4.68405	0.00756	0.00017
Cf (194.2)	30	54	10.45567	8.1827	6.53658	4.10793	0.01069	0.00024
Tp (180.2)	28	52	9.58542	7.23549	6.1259	3.71758	0.013095	0.000269
Tb (180.2)	28	52	9.58542	7.23549	6.10906	3.7135	0.013095	0.000269
UA (168.1)	26	54	8.71518	5.72474	5.6647	3.11237	0.01604	0.00013
OA (156.1)	22	50	8.43072	5.24931	5.09222	2.66333	0.03928	0.00027
X (152.1)	24	48	7.84493	5.34106	5.27086	2.92873	0.01964	0.00034
IsoG (151.1)	24	46	7.84493	5.45738	5.27086	2.96049	0.01964	0.00043
G (151.1)	24	46	7.84493	5.45738	5.27086	2.96049	0.01964	0.00043
HypoX (136.1)	22	42	6.97469	4.95738	4.87701	2.74509	0.02406	0.00085
A (135.1)	22	40	6.97469	5.07369	4.87701	2.77277	0.02406	0.00108
T (126.1)	18	36	6.85337	4.89385	4.19838	2.4856	0.06804	0.00301
5MC (125.1)	18	34	6.85337	5.01016	4.19838	2.51736	0.06804	0.0038
U (112.1)	16	34	5.98313	3.9712	3.78769	2.06893	0.08333	0.00347
C (111.1)	16	32	5.98313	4.08751	3.78769	2.1007	0.08333	0.00439

[a] A = Adenine, G = Guanine, U = Uracil, T = Thymine, C = Cytosine, OA = orotic acid, UA = uric acid, X = Xanthine, M = methyl, P= propyl, B = butyl, I = isobutyl, Cf = Caffein =137MMMX = 7MTp, Tb = Theobromine = 37MMX, Tp = theophylline = 13MMX.

Table 1. Molar and graph mass descriptors for the solubility, *S*, 19 of natural amino acids.

Descriptor	Q	F	r	S
${}^0\chi$	0.001	3.0	0.386	350
M	0.0009	2	0.323	360
D^v	0.0008	1.5	0.286	364
${}^1\chi$	0.0007	1.2	0.256	367
D	0.0006	0.8	0.211	371
$\{{}^0\chi, {}^1\chi\}$	0.002	5.9	0.652	297
$\{{}^0\chi, M\}$	0.0016	3.0	0.520	334
$\{M, {}^1\chi\}$	0.0013	2.1	0.457	348

Table 2 shows that the best descriptor (1st row) for side-chain molecular volume, *V*, of 18 amino acids is ${}^0\chi^v$ [50], and the achieved description is quite remarkable. The description achieved by *M* is worse and is similar and midway the description offered by ${}^0\chi$ and ${}^1\chi$, the two experimental graph mass indices. Indices D and D^v do not at all mimic the behavior of *M*. But, indices ${}^0\chi$, ${}^1\chi$ and even D, which is a better descriptor of *V* than the pseudograph mass D^v index, play only minor roles in linear combinations of connectivity indices (LCCI) which are dominated by ${}^0\chi^v$, and ${}^1\chi^v$ valence indices. In fact, the 7th row of this table tells us that the best LCCI for this property is given by the set $\{D, {}^0\chi^v, {}^1\chi^v\}$, while the last row shows that when D is replaced by *M* a worse result is obtained. Thus, D, in a linear combination enhances the description more than *M*, even if as single descriptor is worse than *M*. A rapid check of the utilities of these two LCCI shows how, even at the level of *u* statistics, things get worse with *M*, in fact, $\langle u(D, {}^0\chi^v, {}^1\chi^v, \chi^0)\rangle = 4.8$, and $\mathbf{u} = (5.7, 6.9, 2.9, 3.9)$, while $\langle u(M, {}^0\chi^v, {}^1\chi^v, \chi^0)\rangle = 3.2$, and $\mathbf{u} = (4.0, 6.5, 0.4, 1.8)$, i.e., introduction of *M* strongly invalidates the utility of ${}^1\chi^v$, and, in a minor way, of the unitary index, $\chi^0 \equiv 1$. The molecular connectivity ${}^0\chi^v$ index together with D^v, is the basis index of the molecular connectivity X_V term, which in a linear combination with ${}^0\chi^v$, i.e., $\{X_v, {}^0\chi^v\}$ achieves a first-rate description for this property [50] with $Q = 0.424$ and $F = 989$. These results bring us to conclude that this property is not consistently dependent on the molar mass, and that pseudo-ramification, that is, ramification in pseudographs, plays a major role in modeling *V*, in fact the combination $\{X_V, {}^0\chi^v\}$ consists of valence indices alone.

Table 2. Molar and graph mass descriptors for the side-chain molecular volume, *V*, of 18 natural amino acids.

Descriptor	Q	F	R	s
$^0\chi^v$	0.250	691	0.989	3.9
M	0.087	83	0.916	10.5
$^0\chi$	0.090	89	0.920	10.3
$^1\chi$	0.085	79	0.912	10.7
D	0.076	64	0.894	11.7
D^v	0.043	20	0.749	17.4
$\{D, {}^0\chi^v, {}^1\chi^v\}$	0.433	688	0.997	2.3
$\{M, {}^0\chi^v, {}^1\chi^v\}$	0.349	447	0.995	2.9

The 'best' but deceiving modeling of specific rotations, SR_L, of 16 L-amino acids, shown in Table 3, is accomplished by index χ_t, the total molecular connectivity index, and the worse modeling by *M*. The optimal description for this property is only achieved by a combination of a molecular connectivity term and a normal connectivity index, that is, by $\{X_{SR}, {}^1\chi\}$ [2,56]. Theoretical graph mass and pseudograph mass indices score better than *M*, with D nearly mimicking χ_t, while the experimental graph mass index, $^0\chi$, roughly mimics *M*, a trend already detected with the preceding properties A close analysis of the best combination (3rd row from the bottom of Table 3) shows that sequential replacement of $^0\chi$ and D with *M* worsens the modeling consistently, especially when D is replaced by *M*. This fact again underlines again the differences between *M* and the theoretical graph mass indices, and between this last and the experimental graph mass index. Index D is here able to encode graph-molecular characteristics, not encoded by $^0\chi$, characteristics which are more apt to model this property than the bulk property *M*, a behavior already detected with the modeling of *V* by the best LCCI.

The single- (1st row) and multi-index modeling of the crystal densities, *CD*, of 10 amino acids [37,42], together with the modeling achieved by *M*, and by the four graph mass indices (2 experimental and 2 theoretical) is shown in Table 4. The best single index modeling is in reality achieved by a recently detected exponential molecular connectivity term, X_{CD} [56]. From this table we can again notice a trend already detected with the other properties (especially with the side-chain molecular volume *V*), that is, molar mass *M* and experimental graph mass indices, especially the zeroth-order molecular connectivity index, show similar modeling power, while the modeling power of D, and especially of D^v, theoretical graph mass indices are quite different from *M*. The third best experimental graph mass index, $^0\chi^v$, shows the characteristics of best single descriptor, but not as good as for the modeling of *V*. It becomes, thus, clear that at least for amino acids, the two theoretical graph mass indices encode molecular characteristics not encoded by *M*, while $^0\chi$, at least for amino acids, encode characteristics similar to the ones encoded by *M*, but, only at the level of single descriptor. In fact, this similarity between $^0\chi$ and M drastically disappears as soon as $^0\chi$ is replaced by M in the best multi-index description (3rd and 2nd row from bottom in Table 4). This 'drasticity' which is somewhat softened by replacing D^v with M. The lesson to be drawn here is that at the level of a LCCI the 'cards' are reshuffled again. It seems, thus, impossible to detect a graph mass index, both theoretical and experimental, that exactly mimics, at every level, the molar mass as descriptor. The individual character of each molecular connectivity index, grounded on graph structural characteristics, is at the origin of their particular modeling power, which is hardly mimicked by M. Let us now look if also with other classes of compounds the same trend can be found.

Table 3. Molar and graph mass descriptors for the specific rotations, SR_L, of 16 L-amino acids.

Descriptor	Q	F	r	s
χ_t	0.014	3.2	0.43	30
M	0.0003	0.12	0.091	34
D	0.009	1.3	0.293	32
$^1\chi$	0.006	0.58	0.200	33
D^v	0.005	0.41	0.169	33
$^0\chi$	0.0008	0.01	0.027	34
$\{D, {}^0\chi, \chi_t\}$	0.088	41	0.955	11.8
$\{D, M, \chi_t\}$	0.042	9.5	0.839	19.8
$\{M, {}^0\chi, \chi_t\}$	0.034	6.2	0.779	22.8

Table 4. Molar and graph mass descriptors for the crystal densities, CD, of 10 L-amino acids.

Descriptor	Q	F	R	s
$^0\chi^v$	3.43	3.9	0.570	0.17
M	1.87	1.14	0.354	0.19
$^0\chi$	1.96	1.26	0.368	0.19
$^1\chi$	1.71	0.95	0.326	0.19
D	1.58	0.80	0.302	0.19
D^v	0.039	0.0005	0.008	0.202
$\{D^v, {}^0\chi, {}^1\chi^v\}$	15.8	27.2	0.965	0.06
$\{D^v, M, {}^1\chi^v\}$	5.88	3.76	0.808	0.14
$\{M, {}^0\chi, {}^1\chi^v\}$	7.05	5.41	0.855	0.12

Modeling the molar masses of n = 25 purines and pyrimidines (see annex A, table 3) with the given set of molecular connectivity indices gives the following results

$^{0}\chi$: Q = 0.379, F = 7002, r = 0.998, s = 2.6, <u> = 43, **u** = (84, 2.2)

$^{1}\chi$: Q = 0.301, F = 4430, r = 0.997, s = 3.3, <u> = 34, **u** = (67, 1.0)

D : Q = 0.179, F = 1557, r = 0.993, s = 5.5, <u> = 20, **u** = (39, 1.4)

$^{1}\chi^{v}$: Q = 0.146, F = 1045, r = 0.989, s = 6.8, <u> = 22, **u** = (32, 12)

Statistical scores of $^{1}\chi^{v}$ and $^{0}\chi^{v}$ are quite similar ($^{1}\chi^{v}$ scoring a bit better), and D^{v} scores again rather badly with Q = 0.074, and F = 266. Comparison with the corresponding results in amino acids we notice that i) D, now, is the 3rd best descriptor, ii) $^{1}\chi^{v}$ replaces $^{0}\chi^{v}$ but in the 4th position, that iii) D^{v} is again in no way an optimal descriptor of *M*, that iv) index $^{0}\chi$ is again the best experimental graph mass descriptor, and that v) the only descriptor having good utilities on both first and 2nd parameter is the last one, $^{1}\chi^{v}$. Now, two properties of purine and pyrimidine (PP) bases will be analyzed, the solubility, *S*, of a set of n = 23 PP and the average <*pk*> values of n = 13 PP, whose values are given in Table 3A. The shrinking in the number of compounds with <*pk*> produces changes in the simulation of *M*. Here D^{v} becomes the 3rd best descriptor, with Q = 0.188, and F = 147, while D becomes the 4th best descriptor with Q = 0.188, and F = 104.

The modeling of 23 solubility values, *S*, of purines and pyrimidines can only be accomplished by the aid of higher-order molecular connectivity indices [44,49,50], thus, a valuable and direct comparison with molar masses is hardly possible. The modeling of *S* with normal indices (here not shown) is so poor that practically every given index, $^{0}\chi$, $^{1}\chi$, $^{1}\chi^{v}$, D and D^{v}, mimics the bad predictive power of *M*. Even if a satisfactory modeling of <*pk*> is not possible neither at the single- nor at the multi-index level description [49], nevertheless it is possible to detect the different modeling behaviors of $^{0}\chi$, $^{1}\chi$, D^{v}, and D indices (here, best descriptors of *M*) and draw a comparison with the modeling behavior of *M*. In Table 5 are collected the modeling results for <*pk*>, that offers some interesting clues. Best descriptor is a total connectivity descriptor, *M* shows a quite bad statistical score that is surpassed (negatively) by the statistical score of $^{0}\chi$ only. This last result and the fact that indices D and D^{v} are the farthest away (in the positive direction of the descriptive power) from *M*, with $^{1}\chi$ in between, mimics a general trend already detected with amino acids. Substitution of $^{1}\chi^{v}$ with *M* in the best two-index LCCI shows how even this index is only partially mimicked by *M*.

Table 3A. Experimental Solubilty, *S* (at 25°C in units of grams per kg of water), experimental side-chain molecular volume, *V* (in $Å^3$), experimental crystal *CD* densities for 10 amino acids (AA), experimental specific rotations in angular degrees, SR_L for L-AA in water (in parenthesis, ±1°C, when T≠20 °C), experimental unfrozen water content *UWC* (g H_2O/g AA) for 8 AA, experimental <*pk*> values [49], and experimental solubility, *S* (at the indicated T °C, in units of grams per 100 ml of water) for purines and pyrimidines (PP).

AA	S	V	CD	SR_L	UWC	PP	<pk>	S (T°C)
Gly	251	36.3	1.601			7I8MTp		0.63 (20)
Ala	167	52.6	1.401	2.7 (22)		7B8MTp		0.45 (20)
Cys	-					7ITp		2.7 (20)
Ser	422	54.9	1.537	-6.83	0.48	7BTp		0.37 (30)
Val	58	85.1	1.230	6.42		1BTb		0.56 (30)
Thr	97	71.2		28.4 (26)	0.72	7PTp		23.11 (30)
Met	56		1.340	-8.11 (25)		1PTb		1.38 (30)
Pro	1622	73.6		-85 (23)	1.07	7ETp		3.66 (30)
Leu	23	102	1.165	-10.8 (25)		1ETb		3.98 (30)
Ile	34	102		11.29		Cf		2.58 (30)
Asn	25	72.4				Tp		0.81 (30)
Asp	5	68.4	1.660	4.7 (18)		Tb		0.054 (30)
Lys	6	105.1		14.6	0.93	UA	8.35	0.002 (20)
Hyp	361			-75.2 (23)	0.70	OA	5.95	0.18 (18)
Gln	42	92.7				X	4.1	0.05 (20)
Glu	8.6	84.7	1.538	11.5 (18)	0.97	IsoG	6.75	0.006 (25)
His	43	91.1		-39.01 (25)	0.66	G	6.25	0.004 (40)
Arg	181	109.1	1.100	12.5	0.46	HypoX	5.45	0.07 (19)
Phe	29	113.9		-35.14		A	2.5	0.09 (25)
Tyr	0.5	116.2	1.456			T	12	0.40 (25)
Trp	12	135.4		-31.5 (23)		5MC	8.5	0.45 (25)
						U	5	0.36 (25)
						C	8.35	0.77 (25)
						7MG	6.7	
						5hyMC	8.65	

Table 5. Molar and graph mass descriptors for the average <*pk*> values of 13 purines and pyrimidines.

Descriptor	Q	F	r	s
χ_t	0.184	2.4	0.421	2.3
M	0.056	0.22	0.141	2.5
D	0.125	1.09	0.301	2.4
$^1\chi$	0.109	0.84	0.266	2.4
D^v	0.098	0.67	0.240	2.5
$^0\chi$	0.017	0.02	0.044	2.5
$\{^1\chi^v, \chi_t\}$	0.394	5.43	0.722	1.8
$\{M, \chi_t\}$	0.304	3.24	0.627	2.06

Now, we will try to check the behavior of graph mass indices and molar mass with 5 properties of the small set of nucleic acid bases, U, T, A, G, and C (see Table 4A). The following experimental properties of U, T, A, G, and C will, now, be simulated : first and second singlet excitation energy, ΔE_1 and ΔE_2, first and second oscillator strength of the first singlet excitation energies, f_1 and f_2, and molar absorption coefficient at 260 nm and pH=7, ε_{260} [49]. Even if the best descriptors for this properties are higher-level molecular connectivity terms [1,2,53,56] normal connectivity indices are, nevertheless, able of a valuable description. Table 6 tells us that, concerning the single index modeling, for the first singlet energy, the first oscillator strength, and the molar absorption coefficient, *M* and D^v behave similarly, while for the second singlet energy and for the second oscillator strength a similarity can be detected between *M* and $^0\chi$. Considering that $^0\chi$ also for ΔE_1, f_2 and ε_{260} show a behavior that is not too far away from *M*, we can conclude that even here the detected trend, i.e., similar behavior between M and $^0\chi$ at the single-index level, is confirmed. Not shown in this table are the similar behavior of $^1\chi^v$ and D for ΔE_1, ΔE_2, and for f_1, and the similar behavior of $^1\chi^v$ and $^1\chi$ for f_2 and ε_{260}. The best descriptor for f_1 and ε_{260} is a total molecular connectivity index (see first row) followed by D, a trend that mimics the trend already detected with the modeling of <*pk*>, and with the modeling of SR_L of amino acids. The theoretical graph mass index seems, sometimes, to have a strange predilection with the total χ_t index at the single-index level.

Table 4A. Experimental (exp) Molar Absorption Coefficient $\varepsilon_{260,exp}$ at 260 nm and pH=7.0, first ΔE_1 and second ΔE_2 singlet excitation energies in eV and first f_1 and second f_2 oscillator strength values (of the first singlet excitation energies) of the nucleotide DNA-RNA bases [a].

Bases	ε_{260}/1000	ΔE_1	ΔE_2	f_1	f_2
A	15.4	4.75	5.99	0.28	0.54
G	11.7	4.49	5.03	0.20	0.27
U	9.9	4.81	6.11	0.18	0.30
T	9.2	4.67	5.94	0.18	0.37
C	7.5	4.61	6.26	0.13	0.72

[a] A = Adenine, G = Guanine, U = Uracil, T = Thymine, C = Cytosine.

Table 6. Molar and graph mass descriptors for ΔE_1, ΔE_2, f_1, f_2 and ε_{260} of U, T, A, G, and C. Only Q/F values are given.

Descriptor	ΔE_1	ΔE_2	f_1	f_2	ε_{260}
χ_t			18.8 / 4.22*		0.42 / 6.47*
M	4.93 / 1.51	3.67 / 12.6	11.4 / 1.44	2.27 / 0.73	0.23 / 1.94
$^0\chi$	5.50 / 1.88*	3.88 / 14.1	9.03 / 0.97	2.47 / 0.87	0.18 / 1.23
$^1\chi$	4.09 / 1.03	2.71 / 6.87	14.2 / 2.39	1.68 / 0.40	0.31 / 3.46
D	3.97 / 0.98	2.62 / 6.40	14.5 / 2.52	1.60 / 0.36	0.32 /3.73
D^v	4.45 / 1.2	4.37 / 17.8 *	10.9 / 1.43	2.74 / 1.07 *	0.24 / 2.10

* this is the best index for this property.

Up to now we have analyzed the modeling power of graph mass descriptors for compounds for which valence and non valence molecular connectivity indices were different, that is, for compounds whose graph and pseudographs did not superpose. In alkanes, C_nH_{2n+2}, graphs and pseudographs coincide (graphs can be regarded upon as a special case of pseudographs), and the given set of indices of eq. 3 can be restricted to :{D, $^0\chi$, $^1\chi$, χ_t}. The modeling of the molar masses, *M*, of 56 alkanes of Table 5A with the new set of 4 molecular connectivity indices shows the following results

D : Q = 0.469, F = 6742, r = 0.996, s = 2.13, <u> = 48, **u** = (82, 14)

$^0\chi$: Q = 0.252, F = 1953, r = 0.986, s = 3.91, <u> = 23, **u** = (44, 1.0)

$^1\chi$: Q = 0.174, F = 934, r = 0.972, s = 5.57, <u> = 16, **u** = (30, 1.8)

Table 5A. Experimental melting point (*MP* in °K), motor octane numbers (*MON*) and calculated molecular connectivity indices for 56 alkanes and their molar masses *M*.

Names	**M**	**MP**	MON	D	$^0\chi$	$^1\chi$	χ_t
3	44.10	85.46		4	2.70710	1.41421	0.7071
4	58.12	89.80	90.1	6	3.41421	1.91421	0.5000
2	30.07	89.88		2	2.00000	1.00000	1.00000
2M4	72.15	113.25	97.6	8	4.28445	2.27005	0.4082
2M3	58.12	113.55	90.3	6	3.57735	1.73205	0.5774
2M5	86.18	119.48	73.5	10	4.99156	2.77005	0.2887
24MM6	114.23	113.65	69.9	14	6.56981	3.66390	0.1667
33MM5	100.21	138.69	86.6	12	5.91421	3.12132	0.2500
5	72.15	143.43	61.9	8	4.12132	2.41421	0.3536
23MM4	86.18	144.61	94.4	10	5.15470	2.64273	0.3333
235MMM6	128.26	145.35		16	7.43915	4.03658	0.1361
33MM6	114.23	147.05	83.4	14	6.62132	3.62132	0.1768
22MM5	100.21	149.34	95.6	12	5.91421	3.06066	0.2500
234MEM5	128.26	150.95		16	7.43915	4.09142	0.1361
22MM6	114.23	151.97	77.4	14	6.62132	3.56066	0.1768
2234(M)5	128.26	152.06		16	7.65470	3.85405	0.1667
4M7	114.23	152.20	39	14	6.40577	3.80806	0.1443
3M7	114.23	152.65	35	14	6.40577	3.80806	0.1443
224MMM6	128.26	153.15		16	7.49156	3.95450	0.1443
3M6	100.21	153.75	55.0	12	5.69867	3.30806	0.2041
24MM5	100.21	153.91	83.5	12	5.86180	3.12589	0.2357
23MM5	100.21	154.05	88.5	12	5.86180	3.18073	0.2357
3E5	100.21	154.55	65.0	12	6.69867	3.34606	0.2041
2M6	100.21	154.87	46.4	12	5.69867	3.27005	0.2041
3M5	86.18	155.15	74.3	10	4.99156	2.80806	0.2887
233MMM6	128.26	156.35		16	7.49156	4.00403	0.1443
23MM7	128.26	157.15		16	7.27602	4.18073	0.1179
23ME5	114.23	158.19	88.1	14	6.56891	3.71874	0.1667
3E7	114.23	158.25		16	7.11288	4.34606	0.1021

Table 5A continued.

244MMM6	128.26	159.77		16	7.49156	3.97716	0.1443
4M8	128.26	159.95		16	7.11288	4.30806	0.1021
22MM7	128.26	160.15		16	7.32842	4.06066	0.1250
223MMM5	114.23	160.88	99.9	14	6.78445	3.48138	0.2041
234MMM5	114.23	163.94	95.9	14	6.73205	3.55341	0.1925
2M7	114.23	164.11	23.8	14	6.40577	3.77005	0.1443
3M8	128.26	165.55		15	7.11288	4.30806	0.1021
224MMM5	114.23	165.77	100.0	14	6.78445	3.41650	0.2041
225MMM6	128.26	176.37		16	7.49156	3.91650	0.1443
26MM7	128.26	170.25		16	7.27602	4.12589	0.1179
2334(M)5	128.26	171.03		16	7.65470	3.88675	0.1667
334MMM6	128.26	171.95		16	7.49156	4.04204	0.1443
233MMM5	114.23	172.45	99.4	14	6.78445	3.50403	0.2041
22MM4	86.18	173.28	93.4	10	5.20710	2.56066	0.3536
223MME5	128.26	173.95		16	7.49156	4.01938	0.1443
6	86.18	177.80	26.0	10	4.82842	2.91421	0.2500
25MM6	114.23	181.95	55.7	14	6.56981	3.62589	0.1667
33ME5	114.23	182.28		14	6.62132	3.68198	0.1768
7	100.21	182.54	0.0	12	5.53553	3.41421	0.1768
2M8	128.26	192.75		16	7.11288	4.27005	0.1021
2244(M)5	128.26	206.61		16	7.70710	3.70710	0.1768
8	114.23	216.36		14	6.24264	3.91421	0.1250
9	128.26	219.63		16	6.94974	4.41421	0.0884
33EE5	128.26	240.04		16	7.32842	4.24264	0.1250
223MMM4	100.21	248.24		12	6.07735	2.94337	0.2887
22MM3	72.15	256.60	80.2	8	5.50000	2.00000	0.5000
2233(M)5	128.26	263.25		16	7.70710	3.81066	0.1768

Abbreviations as in ref. 60 : 2 = ethane, 3 = propane, etc.: M = methyl, E = Ethyl; e.g., 34ME6 = 3-methyl-4-ethylhexane.

The theoretical graph mass index , D, is here by far the best descriptor of *M*, and its excellent utility more than emphasizes his exceptional modeling power. The other two indices show a consistent worsening in every statistics, but especially in the utility of the unitary index. The total connectivity index, χ_t, is the worse descriptor for *M*. Two different properties of alkanes have recently been modeled, the melting points, *MP*, and the motor octane numbers, *MON* [44,56,2]. While a very good modeling for *MON* can be achieved only with a higher-level X_{MON} descriptors, a satisfactory modeling of the melting points of 56 alkanes can be achieved only after a segmentation of the set of 56 compounds into self-consistent subsets, that is, after what has recently been called a 'double sieve' procedure [57], where a set of compounds, after a first approximate modeling to detect patterned values is divided into subsets of more similar compounds. For the modeling of the melting points a subset of 14 {Mi + Ei} alkanes and a subset of 13 {MMMi + MEMi} alkanes will be chosen, while for the *MON* the full set of 30 alkanes will be chosen (see Table 5A). In Table 7 and 8 are collected the results of the modeling for these two properties. Table 7 tells us that for the modeling of *MP* of subset n = 14 (1st value before the slash) the molar mass *M* is the best descriptor, followed by the theoretical graph mass index, D, but with $^0\chi$ and $^1\chi$ showing a quite similar descriptive power. No better modeling can be achieved with a multi-index LCCI. For the subset of n = 13 alkanes (2nd value after the slash), things change consistently, best connectivity descriptor is χ_t (that is, the worse descriptor for *M* in alkanes), followed by $^1\chi$ and by D (thus, again in connection with χ_t), with *M* being the worse descriptor. This subset of alkanes shows a consistent improved description of *MP* with a 2-index LCCI (2nd row from bottom), in which D and χ_t are together. Now, modeling the first subset of n=14 alkanes with this LCCI and substituting D with *M*, things improve a bit (excluding the F statistics), while this substitution does not affect in any way the 2nd subset. This fact might be due to the somewhat better descriptive power of *M* for the first larger subset, but as a corresponding negative description cannot be detected for the 2nd subset with the same substitution (here M is a worse descriptor than D), such a conclusion should be excluded.

Table 7. Molar and graph mass descriptors for the melting points, *MP*, of two subsets of n=14 (1st descriptor), and n=13 of alkanes (2nd descriptor after the slash).

Descriptors	Q(14) / Q(13)	F(14) / F(13)	r(14) / r(13)	s(14) / s(13)
D / χ_t	0.069 / 0.053	29.5 / 22.1	0.843 / 0.817	12.2 / 15.4
M	0.073 / 0.034	33.1 / 10.3	0.857 / 0.771	11.7 / 22.6
D*	0.069 / 0.041	29.5 / 13.0	0.843 / 0.736	12.2 / 18.0
$^0\chi$	0.068 / 0.039	28.6 / 12.0	0.839 / 0.722	12.3 / 18.4
$^1\chi$	0.068 / 0.042	28.2 / 13.8	0.838 / 0.746	12.4 / 17.7
None[a] / {D, χ_t}	0.068 / 0.096	14.0 / 36.3	0.848 / 0.938	12.5 / 9.7
None[a] / {*M*, χ_t}	0.071 / 0.096	15.4 / 36.3	0.859 / 0.938	12.1 / 9.7

* This is the best connectivity descriptor for the n=14 subset (see 1st row).

[a] Statistical values are those from {D, χ_t} modeling (see text).

Table 8. Molar and graph mass descriptors for the motor octane number, *MON*, of 30 alkanes.

Descriptor	Q	F	r	s
χ_t	0.013	4.74	0.381	24.9
M	0.006	0.79	0.166	26.5
$^1\chi$	0.013	3.31	0.325	25.5
D	0.006	0.72	0.158	26.6
$^0\chi$	0.001	0.03	0.034	26.9
{D, $^0\chi$, $^1\chi$}	0.092	57.3	0.932	10.1
{*M*, $^0\chi$, $^1\chi$}	0.056	20.9	0.841	15.1
{D, $^0\chi$, *M*}	0.069	32.4	0.888	12.8
{D, *M*, $^1\chi$}	0.047	14.7	0.793	17.0

The modeling of *MON* of 30 alkanes by *M* is very bad and continues to be deceiving with the other connectivity indices. Here, like for the *MP* of the n=14 subset, index D mimics *M* in descriptive power, confirming, thus, the detected optimal description of *M* by D in alkanes. The theoretical graph mass index D achieves to be the best descriptor of the molar mass and parallels *M* in the description of two properties of alkanes. But, at the level of a LCCI things get reshuffled again: substituting D, in the best 3-index LCCI, with the apparently similar *M*, causes a consistent worsening of the modeling, while substitution of $^1\chi$, the worse descriptor of *M* and the best single descriptor of *MON*, causes only a moderate worsening. Again, the best 'companion' of *M* at the single-index level reveals to be the worse one at the multi-index level. That is, the portion of D which was similar to *M* in a single index description becomes irrelevant in a multi-index description.

If in alkanes normal and valence molecular connectivity indices coincide, metal halides do not have normal (non-valence) molecular connectivity indices, better said, these last have no use as every metal halide can be considered to be single connected (i.e., the gas molecule, see ref. 51). Thus, the set of χ values given by eq. 3 shrinks practically to {D^v, $^0\chi^v$, $^1\chi^v$}, where the total valence connectivity index equals $^1\chi^v$. The expression for the valence δ^v number used to derive the χ indices of metal halides, MeX, has been exposed in the method section. It should be underlined that the concept of pseudograph, as well of graph for these compounds becomes rather flurry as has already been noticed [51]. To these 3 indices a further index has been added based on the concept of valence δ^z number, i.e, $\delta^z = Z^v / n$, where n is the principal quantum number. From this number the following index can be defined : $D^z = \Sigma\delta^z_i$ [51]. In Table 6A are collected the values of the set of indices {D^v, $^0\chi^v$, $^1\chi^v$, D^z} for 20 MeX compounds as well their lattice enthalpies, $\Delta H_L^{\varnothing}$ in kJmol^{-1} at 298.15 K, and their molar mass *M*. The modeling of the molar mass M of the 20 metal halides by the given set of indices is summarized in the following set of statistical values

${}^{1}\chi^{v}$: Q = 0.030, F = 72.3, r = 0.895, s = 29.5, <u> = 6.7, **u** = (8.5, 4.5)

${}^{0}\chi^{v}$: Q = 0.027, F = 58.3, r = 0.874, s = 32.1, <u> = 4.3, **u** = (7.6, 0.9)

D^{z} : Q = 0.015, F = 18.0, r = 0.707, s = 46.7, <u> = 5.9, **u** = (4.3, 7.6)

D^{v} : Q = 0.009, F = 701, r = 0.530, s = 56.0, <u> = 6.0, **u** = (2.7, 9.3)

Table 6A. Lattice enthalpies $\Delta H_L^{\varnothing}$ at 298.15°K (kJ mol^{-1}) of 20 metal halides (MeX), their molar masses M, and their corresponding molecular connectivity values.

MeX	**M**	$\Delta H_L^{\varnothing}$	D^{v}	${}^{0}\chi^{v}$	${}^{1}\chi^{v}$	D^{Z}
LiF	25.94	1037	8	1.37796	0.37796	4
NaF	41.99	926	7.11111	3.37796	1.13389	3.83333
KF	50.10	821	7.05882	4.50107	1.55839	3.75000
RbF	104.47	789	7.02857	6.29404	2.23607	3.70000
CsF	151.90	750	7.01887	7.65807	2.75162	3.66667
LiCl	42.39	852	1.77778	2.13389	1.13389	2.83333
NaCl	58.44	786	0.88889	4.13389	3.40168	2.66667
KCl	74.55	717	0.83660	5.25700	4.67516	2.58333
RbCl	120.92	695	0.80635	7.04997	6.70820	2.53333
CsCl	168.36	678	0.79665	8.41400	8.25487	2.50000
LiBr	86.85	815	1.25926	2.96396	1.96396	2.25000
NaBr	102.89	752	0.37037	4.96396	5.89188	2.41667
KBr	119.00	689	0.31808	6.08707	7.09762	2.00000
RbBr	165.37	668	0.28783	7.88004	11.6190	1.95000
CsBr	212.81	654	0.27813	9.24407	14.2979	1.91667
LiI	133.85	761	1.15556	3.53546	2.53546	1.90000
NaI	149.89	705	0.26667	5.53546	7.60639	1.73333
KI	166.00	649	0.21438	6.65857	10.4540	1.65000
RbI	212.37	632	0.18413	8.45154	15.0000	1.60000
CsI	259.81	620	0.17442	9.81557	18.4585	1.56667

These values tell us that the best descriptor for M is $^1\chi^v$ at every statistical level, while D^z, and even more D^v, fail to achieve a satisfactory modeling for M. The modeling of the lattice enthalpies, instead, summarized in Table 9, offer an interesting insight about the different meanings of the connectivity indices relatively to M. Molar mass, M, and $^0\chi^v$ are the best (statistically identical) descriptors for $\Delta H_L^{\varnothing}$, but as soon as we look for a similar correspondence in the best 3-index LCCI things get mixed again. In fact, substitution of $^0\chi^v$ (the 2nd best descriptor of M) with M causes an abrupt worsening of the description, while substitution of the best descriptor of the molar mass, i.e., $^1\chi^v$ with M partially conserves the good quality of the modeling. Thus, again $^1\chi^v$ and especially $^0\chi^v$ have components, that at the multi-index level of a LCCI are not shared by M. Each descriptor uses different components at the single- and at the multi-index level.

Table 9. Molar and graph mass descriptors for the lattice enthalpies, $\Delta H_L^{\varnothing}$ at 298.15 K (kJ/mol) for 20 metal halides (MeX).

Descriptor	Q	F	r	s
M	0.015	45.4	0.846	57.3
$^0\chi^v$	0.015	45.4	0.846	57.3
$^1\chi^v$	0.013	35.9	0.816	62.2
D^z	0.010	21.7	0.739	72.5
$\{^0\chi^v, {}^1\chi^v, D^z\}$	0.043	130.5	0.980	22.6
$\{^0\chi^v, M, D^z\}$	0.038	98.0	0.974	25.9
$\{M, {}^1\chi^v, D^z\}$	0.017	20.3	0.890	52.1
$\{^0\chi^v, {}^1\chi^v, M\}$	0.016	18.2	0.879	67.7

Tables 1A, 3A, and 7A give us the possibility to check the best molar mass descriptor and their modeling power of the unfrozen water content, *UWC*, of a mixed set of 8 amino acids and 5 metal halides, MeX and MeX_2. The statistical ratings of the theoretical, D and D^v, molar mass descriptors and experimental molar mass descriptors, $^0\chi$ and $^1\chi$ reported in the following lines show that D, $^0\chi$, and $^1\chi$ have similar descriptive power and utility, while D^v has a worse descriptive power but a somewhat better utility.

$^0\chi$: Q = 0.038, F = 26.5, r = 0.841, s = 21.9, <u> = 5.3, **u** = (4.3, 6.4)

$^1\chi$: Q = 0.038, F = 26.3, r = 0.840, s = 21.9, <u> = 5.3, **u** = (4.2, 6.4)

D : Q = 0.037, F = 24.2, r = 0.829, s = 22.6, <u> = 5.5, **u** = (4.2, 6.7)

D^v : Q = 0.030, F = 16.4, r = 0.774, s = 25.6, <u> = 6.0, **u** = (4.6, 7.4)

Table 7A. Unfrozen water content *UWC* (g H_2O/g MeCl) for 5 metal chlorides, their molar masses *M*, and their corresponding molecular connectivity index values.

MeCl	M	UWC	D	$^0\chi$	$^1\chi$	D^v	$^0\chi^v$	$^1\chi^v$	χ_t^v
LiCl	42.39	6.5	2	2	1	1.7778	2.1339	1.1339	1.1339
NaCl	58.43	3.0	2	2	1	0.8889	4.1339	3.4016	3.4017
KCl	74.55	1.8	2	2	1	0.8366	5.2570	4.6752	4.6752
$CaCl_2$	110.98	4.0	4	2.7071	1.4142	1.6732	5.1832	6.6117	3.7485
$CuCl_2$	134.45	4.0	4	2.7071	1.4142	1.6325	5.8733	8.1777	4.6357

A satisfactory modeling of *UWC* can only be achieved by the aid of reciprocal molecular connectivity indices [51] or molecular connectivity terms [1,2,56] while LCCI of two indices improve the modeling only in a minor way. In Table 10 are collected the statistical scores for *M*, for the theoretical molar graph mass and for the experimental graph mass descriptors derived from the modeling of *UWC*. The best descriptor for this strange property being the pseudograph mass index, D^v, that is, the worse *M* descriptor. The worse descriptor of *UWC*, instead, is *M*, a seemingly expected result, confirmed by the substitution of D^v with *M* in the best 2-index LCCI, which is anyway a rather poor descriptor of *UWC*. The better score of index D, relatively to $^0\chi$, and $^1\chi$ seem to confirm this nearly reversed trend in the simulation of *UWC*. Thus, here again D and D^v indices, as for amino acids and purines and pyrimidines, are quite different from *M*, while $^0\chi$ index seems to confirm itself as the best candidate, at the single-index level, for the title of experimental graph mass index.

Table 10. Molar and graph mass descriptors for the unfrozen water content, *UWC*, of a set of 8 amino acids and 5 metal halides.

Descriptor	Q	F	r	s
M	0.438	8.09	0.651	1.5
D^v	0.705	20.9	0.810	1.1_5
$^0\chi$	0.655	18.1	0.788	1.2
D	0.654	18.0	0.788	1.2
$^1\chi$	0.644	17.4	0.783	1.2
$\{D^v, \chi_t^v\}$	0.818	14.1	0.859	1.0_5
$\{M, D^v\}$	0.675	9.58	0.811	1.2
$\{M, \chi_t^v\}$	0.506	5.41	0.721	1.4

Before starting to model the next group of compounds let us look if there is the possibility to model the molar mass of an heterogeneous group of compounds, composed of the classes of compounds studied up to now. The modeling of the molar mass for 43 amino acids plus purines and pyrimidines shows again that ${}^0\chi$ and ${}^1\chi$ indices are the best Q, F, and <u> experimental graph mass descriptors, even if the rather deceiving *u* value for the unitary index of ${}^0\chi$ constitutes a warning about the instability of this modeling equation [38]. Of the theoretical graph mass parameters, D scores quite satisfactorily with a quite good **u** vector, where both parameters, D and unitary $\chi^0=1$ index show a good utility,

${}^0\chi$: Q = 0.213, F = 3861, r = 0.995, s = 4.7, <u> = 32, **u** = (62, 1.1)

${}^1\chi$: Q = 0.156, F = 2070, r = 0.990, s = 6.3, <u> = 25, **u** = (46, 4.8)

D : Q = 0.095, F = 766, r = 0.974, s = 10.3, <u> = 18, **u** = (28, 7.9)

D^v : Q = 0.056, F = 266, r = 0.931, s = 16.6, <u> = 8.9, **u** = (16, 1.5)

Now, adding to these 43 [AA+PP] compounds the 56 alkanes (Alk), where it should be remembered that $\chi \equiv \chi^v$ for alkanes, the modeling of 96 molar masses of [AA+PP+Alk] show the following interesting results

${}^0\chi$: Q = 0.174, F = 5524, r = 0.991, s = 5.7, <u> = 48, **u** = (74, 6.2)

${}^1\chi$: Q = 0.165, F = 5017, r = 0.990, s = 6.0, <u> = 39, **u** = (71, 6.8)

D : Q = 0.125, F = 2875, r = 0.984, s = 7.9, <u> = 36, **u** = (54, 18)

D^v : Q = 0.044, F = 362, r = 0.888, s = 20, <u> = 19, **u** = (19, 20)

These results confirm preceding trend, here D has consistently improved his descriptive power, ${}^1\chi$ also has somewhat improved his score, ${}^0\chi$ and D^v have practically improved only their F and utility vector, and ${}^0\chi$ continues to be the best descriptor for *M*. Let us now add to these compounds the 20 metal halides, where it has to be remembered that now we have to add the following constant values for D, ${}^0\chi$, ${}^1\chi$, and χ_t : D = 2, ${}^0\chi$ = 2, ${}^1\chi = \chi_t = 1$, and to notice that : $\chi_t^v = {}^1\chi^v$. The modeling of *M* for these heterogeneous set of 119 compounds, even if quite unsatisfactory offers some interesting novelties, with ${}^0\chi^v$ as the best experimental graph mass descriptor, but with a poor utility vector at the level of the unitary index, resulting in an unstable predictive modeling equation,

${}^0\chi^v$: Q = 0.030, F = 238, r = 0.819, s = 27.2, <u> = 7.8, **u** = (15, 0.12)

D : Q = 0.019, F = 97.9, r = 0.675, s = 35.0, <u> = 11.2, **u** = (9.9, 13)

$^{1}\chi$: Q = 0.019, F = 93.4, r = 0.666, s = 35.4, <u> = 9.4, **u** = (9.7, 9.2)

D^{v} : Q = 0.018, F = 87.6, r = 0.654, s = 35.6, <u> = 13.4, **u** = (9.4, 18)

Theoretical graph mass descriptor D is the 2nd best but poor descriptor for *M*, his good utility is of no use with such a poor Q and F statistics. Well, if a search is started for the best LCCI descriptor for *M* for this group of compounds, index $^{1}\chi^{v}$, which alone rates, Q = 0.017, F = 73.5, and <u> = 10.6 (8.6, 12.6), becomes the turning point of a 2-, 3- and 4- index LCCI description, the best LCCI being

$\{D^{v}, {}^{0}\chi^{v}, {}^{1}\chi^{v}\}$: Q = 0.086, F = 647, r = 0.972, s = 11.3, <u> = 12.7, **u** = (22, 8.0, 17, 3.3)

where even the utility vector is quite satisfactory. The fact that in a LCCI an unexpected index becomes more important that other best single-indices, is not new in molecular connectivity, where the modeling power of each index plays different roles when used either in a single or in a multilinear modeling. This versatility of molecular connectivity indices can be better underlined with a LCOCI, i.e., with a linear combination of orthogonal molecular connectivity indices [21-23].

Tables 8A and 9A show a set of experimental properties of organophosphorous compounds : molar refractivities, MR_D, refractivity index, n_D^{20}, density, d_4^{20}, and retention index for paper chromatography, R_f, together with their molar mass values and molecular connectivity index values. For the first set of compounds of Table 8A a perfect collinearity between D and D^{v}, as well as between $^{0}\chi$ and $^{0}\chi^{v}$ but not between $^{1}\chi$ and $^{1}\chi^{v}$ reduces the set of meaningful indices to $\{D, {}^{0}\chi , {}^{1}\chi , {}^{1}\chi^{v} \}$, while for the second set of compounds of Table 9A total collinearity among D, D^{v}, and $^{0}\chi$ as well as between $^{1}\chi$ and $^{1}\chi^{v}$ reduces the set of meaningful indices to $\{{}^{0}\chi , {}^{1}\chi , {}^{1}\chi^{v}\}$. To derive χ^{v} values for the pseudographs of these phosphocompounds, a δ^{v}(P) value equal to 2.22 was assumed [12,44]. To notice that in a preceding works of ours (see Tables 6 and 7 in ref. 44) a $^{0}\chi^{v}$ instead of $^{1}\chi^{v}$ was erroneously reported. The simulation of the molar masses, *M*, of the entire class of 31 (i.e., 17 + 14) compounds with set $\{D, {}^{0}\chi , {}^{1}\chi , {}^{1}\chi^{v} \}$, gets the following result

$^{1}\chi^{v}$: Q = 0.200, F = 4490, r = 0.997, s = 5.0, <u> = 45, **u** = (71, 20)

$^{0}\chi$: Q = 0.198, F = 4886, r = 0.997, s = 5.0, <u> = 35, **u** = (70, 0.8)

$^{1}\chi$: Q = 0.183, F = 4160, r = 0.9966, s = 5.5, <u> = 38, **u** = (64, 12.2)

D : Q = 0.017, F = 34.0, r = 0.735, s = 44.5, <u> = 8.5, **u** = (5.8, 11.3)

Table 8A. Observed molar refractivities MR_D, refractivity index n_D^{20}, density d_4^{20}, calculated χ values, and molar masses, M, of 17 $MPO(OR')_2$ neutral organophosphorus compounds.

R'	M	MR_D	n_D^{20}	d_4^{20}	D	$^0\chi$	$^1\chi$	$^0\chi^v$
Butyl	208.24	54.42	1.4259	0.9638	24	10.15685	6.12132	5.48471
Isobu	208.24	54.86	1.4226	0.9653	24	10.48313	5.83300	5.19640
Secbu	208.24	54.81	1.4222	0.9657	24	10.48313	5.90901	5.34997
Terbu	208.24	54.46			24	10.91421	5.41421	4.90140
n-Pe	236.29	64.19			28	11.57107	7.12132	6.48471
IsoPe	236.29	63.61	1.5264	0.9529	28	11.89734	6.83300	6.19640
22MMP	236.29	64.27			28	12.32843	6.41421	5.77761
n-H	264.35	73.45	1.4353	0.9401	32	12.98528	8.12132	7.48471
c-H	260.32	69.23			36	12.13998	8.15660	7.59755
n-Hep	292.40	82.87	1.4401	0.9303	36	14.39949	9.12132	8.48471
Octyl	320.46	91.24	1.44	0.9257	40	15.81371	10.12132	9.48471
1Mhep	320.46	92.02	1.4381	0.9146	40	16.13998	9.90901	9.34997
2EH	320.46	91.18	1.4414	0.9289	40	16.13998	9.98502	9.34842
Nonyl	348.51	101.1	1.4445	0.9164	44	17.22792	11.12132	10.48471
Decyl	376.56	109.7	1.4427	0.9093	48	18.64213	12.12132	11.48471
Undec	404.62	119.8	1.4498	0.9077	52	20.05635	13.12132	12.48471
Dodec	432.67	129.3	1.4512	0.9012	56	21.47056	14.12132	13.48471

M = methyl, E = ethyl, P = prolyl, Bu = butyl, Pe = pentyl, H = hexyl, Hep = heptyl, Undec = undecyl, Dodec = dodecyl, c = cyclo.

From this simulation (up to now the best M simulation) it is evident the poor quality of the theoretical graph mass D index and the very good quality of $^1\chi^v$ which overrides $^0\chi$ index especially at the utility level of the unitary index. The fact that M can that well be described by a valence connectivity index could mean that i) these compounds are rather homogeneous in their structural and/or shape features, that ii) the $\delta^v(P)$ value plays an important role in stabilizing the predictive equation, and that iii) the different ratings of $^1\chi$ and $^1\chi^v$ underlines the fact that these two indices encode different portions of M. Thus, the two best experimental graph mass descriptors of M for this set of organophosphorus compounds are $^1\chi^v$ and $^0\chi$, while the theoretical graph mass descriptor D (or D^v, as they are collinear) with its poor descriptive power confirms its independent character from M. Let us now model 4 different properties of these organophosphorus : the molar refractivities, MR_D, the refractivity index, n_D^{20}, and the density, d_4^{20}, of a set of 17 and 14 (for the last two properties) MPO(OR')$_2$ compounds of Table 8A, and the retention index for paper chromatography, R_f, for 14 RPO(OR')$_2$ compounds of Table 9A.

Table 9A. Observed retention index, R_f, for paper chromatography, calculated connectivity χ values, and molar masses, M, for 14 RPO(OR')$_2$ neutral organophosphorus compounds.

R	R'	**M**	R_f	$^0\chi$	$^1\chi$	$^0\chi^v$
M	E	152.13	0.80	7.32843	4.12132	3.48471
M	P	180.19	0.71	8.74264	5.12132	4.48471
M	Bu	208.24	0.62	10.15685	6.12132	5.48471
E	Bu	222.27	0.59	10.86396	6.68198	5.99524
P	Bu	236.29	0.53	11.57107	7.18198	6.49524
M	Pe	236.29	0.48	11.57107	7.12132	6.48471
Bu	Bu	250.32	0.46	12.27817	7.68198	6.99524
M	H	264.35	0.38	12.98528	8.12132	7.48471
Pe	Bu	264.35	0.38	12.98528	8.18198	7.49524
H	Bu	278.37	0.34	13.69239	8.68198	7.99524
Hep	Bu	292.40	0.26	14.39949	9.18198	8.49524
M	Hep	292.40	0.24	14.39949	9.12132	8.48471
Oc	Bu	306.43	0.22	15.10660	9.68198	8.99524
M	Oc	320.46	0.15	15.81371	10.12132	9.48471

Abbreviations as in Table 6, Oc = octyl.

From Tables 10-13 we notice that M is the best single descriptor for MR_D, and R_f, (Tables 11 and 12) and that for the other two properties (Tables 13 and 14) it rates quite satisfactorily. Index $^1\chi$, which is not the best or 2nd best descriptor for M, becomes the best descriptor for n_D^{20}, and $^1\chi^v$ scores quite alike. The theoretical graph mass parameter D ($^0\chi$ in R_f plays also the role of D, see Table 12, bottom), a bad descriptor for M, is never the best descriptor for any of these properties, while the experimental graph mass parameters $^0\chi$ and $^1\chi^v$ are normally quite good descriptors for the 4 properties. It has been said [60,61] that MR_D and R_f are properties dependent more on the size of the molecule than on its shape, while n_D^{20} and d_4^{20} are more shape dependent. Such a difference can quite clearly be detected at the level of the exceptionally good ratings of M for MR_D and R_f, while for n_D^{20} and d_4^{20} a connectivity index accomplishes a better single-index description ($^1\chi$ and $^0\chi$, respectively). But, with the two-index description things change, M is no more a good descriptor, i.e., as good as $^0\chi$ and $^1\chi$, for MR_D while for R_f it maintains even at the level of the 2-index LCCI its good quality. For the two shape dependent properties, n_D^{20} and d_4^{20}, the 2-index LCCI, that show a worse F value, worsens with the introduction of M at the place of a connectivity index, a trend already detected in many other cases.

Table 11. Molar and graph mass descriptors for the molar refractivities, MR_D, for 17 organophosphorus, $MPO(OR')_2$, compounds.

Descriptor	Q	F	r	s
M	1.328	16299	0.9995	0.75
$^0\chi$	0.550	2831	0.997	1.8
$^1\chi^v$	0.413	1573	0.995	2.4
D	0.297	813	0.991	3.3
$\{^0\chi, {}^1\chi\}$	1.98	18116	0.9998	0.50
$\{^0\chi, M\}$	1.62	12093	0.9997	0.62
$\{M, {}^1\chi\}$	1.40	9008	0.9996	0.72

Table 12. Molar and graph mass descriptors for the retention index for paper chromatography, R_f, for 14 $RPO(OR')_2$, compounds.

Descriptor	Q	F	r	s
M *	44.5	970	0.994	0.022
$^0\chi$ *	44.5	970	0.994	0.022
$^1\chi^v$	43.6	935	0.994	0.023
$\{^1\chi, {}^1\chi^v\}$	57.5	809	0.997	0.017
$\{M, {}^1\chi^v\}$	"	"	"	"
$\{M, {}^1\chi\}$	"	"	"	"

* $^0\chi$ as well as D, D^v and *M* are collinear

Table 13. Molar and graph mass descriptors for the refractivity index, n_D^{20}, for 14 organophosphorus, $MPO(OR')_2$, compounds.

Descriptor	Q	F	r	S
$^1\chi$	404	195	0.971	0.002
M *	370	163	0.965	0.003
$^1\chi^v$	399	189	0.970	0.002
D *	370	163	0.965	0.003
$^0\chi$	340	138	0.959	0.003
$\{D, {}^0\chi\}$	461	127	0.979	0.002
$\{M, {}^0\chi\}$	412	102	0.974	0.002

* D as well as D^v and *M* are collinear

Table 14. Molar and graph mass descriptors for the density, d_4^{20}, for 14 organophosphorus, MPO(OR')$_2$, compounds.

Descriptor	Q	F	r	S
M *	140	148	0.962	0.007
$^0\chi$	143	155	0.963	0.007
D *	140	148	0.962	0.007
$^1\chi^v$	136	140	0.960	0.007
$\{^1\chi, ^1\chi^v\}$	141	75.1	0.965	0.007
$\{M, ^1\chi^v\}$	135	68.9	0.962	0.007
$\{M, ^1\chi\}$	137	71.2	0.963	0.007

* D as well as D^v and *M* are collinear

One of the main difficulties of molecular connectivity has been in the modeling of properties of random classes of organic compounds, i.e., classes build up by quite different type of compounds, i.e., saturated, unsaturated, non-substituted, slightly, and highly substituted compounds, whose properties are in many cases determined by non-covalent and/or hydrogen bond interaction. Quite recently semiempirical molecular connectivity terms have been introduced to describe different physicochemical properties of a random class of organic solvents [57] (ROS), and for many of these properties the description was quite satisfactory. In Tables 10A and 11A are collected five different properties, molar mass inclusive, of 63 random organic solvents and the corresponding molecular connectivity indices, respectively. We will try to check the modeling capabilities of molar mass, but before we will try to check the modeling power of the two theoretical graph mass indices, D and D^v, and derive the best experimental graph mass descriptors. The results of this last goal (n = 63) are

$^0\chi^v$: Q = 0.038, F = 104, r = 0.793, s = 21.1, $\langle u \rangle$ = 5.4, **u** = (10.2, 0.6)

$^1\chi^v$: Q = 0.027, F = 54.3, r = 0.686, s = 25.2, $\langle u \rangle$ = 5.7, **u** = (7.4, 4.1)

D : Q = 0.019, F = 25.9, r = 0.546, s = 29.0, $\langle u \rangle$ = 5.5, **u** = (5.1, 5.9)

D^v : Q = 0.010, F = 7.22, r = 0.325, s = 32.7, $\langle u \rangle$ = 5.0, **u** = (2.7, 7.2)

Table 10A. Physicochemical properties of 63 organic solvents : M = molar mass (g·mol^{-1}), T_m = melting points (°C), T_b = boiling points (°C), RI = refractive index (20°C), d = density (at 20°C±5°C relative to water at 4°C), ε=dielectric constant.

Solvent	**M**	T_m	T_b	**RI**	d	ε
Acetone	58.1	-94	56	1.3590	0.791	20.7
Acetonitrile	41.05	-48	82	1.3440	0.786	37.5
Benzene	78.1	5	80	1.5010	0.874	2.3
Benzonitrile	103.1	-13	188	1.528	1.010	25.2
1-Butanol	74.1	-90	117.7	1.3990	0.810	17.1
2-Butanone	72.1	-87	80	1.3790	0.805	18.5
Butyl Acetate	116.2	-78	125	1.3940	0.882	5.01
CS_2	76.1	-112	46	1.6270	1.266	2.6
CCl_4	153.8	-23	77	1.4595	1.594	2.2
Cl-Benzene	112.6	-45	132	1.5240	1.107	5.62
1Cl-Butane	92.6	-123	77.5	1.4024	0.886	7.39
$CHCl_3$	119.4	-63	61	1.4460	1.492	4.8
Cyclohexane	84.2	6.5	80.9	1.426	0.779	2.0
Cyclopentane	70.1	-94	50	1.4000	0.751	2.0
1,2-dCl-Benzene	147.0	-16.5	179.5	1.5510	1.306	9.9
1,2-dCl-Ethane	98.95	-35	83	1.4438	1.256	10.37
dCl-Methane	84.9	-97	39.9	1.4240	1.325	7.5
N,N-dM-Acetamd	87.1	-20	165.2	1.4380	0.937	37.8
N,N-dM-Formamd	73.1	-61	153	1.431	0.944	36.7
1,4-Dioxane	88.1	11.8	101	1.4220	1.034	2.2
Ether	74.1	-116	34.6	1.3530	0.708	4.3
Ethyl acetate	88.1	-84	77	1.3720	0.902	6.0
Ethyl alcohol	46.1	-130	78	1.3600	0.785	24.5
Heptane	100.2	-91	98	1.3870	0.684	1.92
Hexane	86.2	-95	69	1.3750	0.659	1.89
2-Methoxyethanol	76.1	-85	124.5	1.4020	0.965	16.0
Methyl alcohol	32.0	-98	64.6	1.3290	0.791	32.7
2-Methylbutane	72.15	-	30	1.3540	0.620	1.843
4-M-2-Pentanone	100.2	-80	117.5	1.3960	0.800	13.1
2-M-1-Propanol	74.1	-108	108	1.3960	0.803	17.7

2-M-2-Propanol	74.1	25	83	1.3870	0.786	10.9
DMSO	78.1	18.4	189	1.4790	1.101	46.7
Nitromethane	61.0	-29	100.9	1.3820	1.127	35.9
1-Octanol	130.2	-15	196	1.4290	0.827	10.34
Pentane	72.15	-130	35.5	1.3580	0.626	1.844
3-Pentanone	86.1	-40	102	1.3920	0.853	17.0
1-Propanol	60.1	-127	97	1.3840	0.804	20.1
2-Propanol	60.1	-89.5	82.4	1.3770	0.785	18.3
Pyridine	79.1	-42	115	1.5100	0.978	12.4
ttCl-Ethylene	165.8	-22	121	1.5056	1.623	2.3
tt-Hydrofuran	72.1	-108	67	1.4070	0.886	7.6
Toluene	92.1	-93	111	1.4960	0.867	2.4
1,1,2tCltFEthane	187.4	-35	47.5	1.3578	1.575	2.41
2,2,4-tM-Pentane	114.2	-107	98.5	1.3910	0.692	1.94
o-Xylene	106.2	-24	144	1.5050	0.870	2.568
p-Xylene	106.2	12.5	138	1.4950	0.866	2.374
Acetic acid	60.05	16.7	117.9	1.3719	1.049	6.1
Decaline	138.2	-43	191.7	1.4758	0.879	2.20
dBr-Methane	173.8	-52.6	97.0	2.4970	1.542	7.5
1,2-dCl-E-en(Z)	96.9	-80.0	60.6	1.4490	1.284	9.2
1,2-dCl-E-en(E)	96.9	-49.8	47.7	1.4462	1.255	2.1
1,1-dCl-E-en	96.9	-122.6	31.6	1.4247	1.213	4.6
Dmethoxymethane	76.1	-105.2	42.3	1.3563	0.866	2.6
DMethylether	46.1	-139	-24			5.02
E-enCarbonate	88.1	36.4	238	1.4250	1.321	89.6
Formamide	45.0	2.6	210.5	1.4475	1.133	109
Methyl chloride	50.5	-97.7	-24.1	1.3389	0.916	12.6
Morpholine	87.1	-3.1	128.9	1.4573	1.005	7.4
Quinoline	129.2	-14.9	237.1	1.6293	1.098	9.0
SO_2	64.1	-72.7	-10.0		1.434	17.6
2,2-ttCl-Ethane	167.8	-43.8	146.2	1.4868	1.578	8.2
ttM-Urea	116.2	-1.2	176.5	1.4493	0.969	23.1
tCl-E-en	131.4	-73	87.2	1.4800	1.476	3.4

Table 11A : Molecular connectivity indices for compounds of Table 10A.

Solvent	D	D^v	$^0\chi$	$^0\chi^v$	$^1\chi$	$^1\chi^v$	χ_t	χ_t^v
Acetone	6	12.0	3.57735	2.90825	1.73205	1.20412	0.57735	0.20412
Acetonitrile	4	10.0	2.70711	1.94721	1.41421	0.72361	0.70711	0.22361
Benzene	12	18	4.24264	3.46410	3	2	0.12500	0.03704
Benzonitrile	16	28	5.81999	4.33397	3.93185	2.38429	0.07217	0.00717
1-Butanol	8	12	4.12132	3.56853	2.41421	2.02333	0.35355	0.15811
2-Butanone	8	14	4.28446	3.61536	2.27006	1.76478	0.40825	0.14434
Butyl acetate	14	24	6.40578	5.43782	3.77006	2.90403	0.14434	0.02946
CS_2	4	5.33333	2.70711	2.94949	1.41421	1.22474	0.70711	0.75000
CCl_4	8	7.11112	4.50000	5.03557	2.00000	2.26778	0.50000	0.82653
Cl-Benzene	14	19.7778	5.11288	4.52064	3.39385	2.47763	0.10206	0.03637
1Cl-Butane	8	7.77778	4.12132	4.25521	2.41421	2.50889	0.35355	0.40089
$CHCl_3$	6	5.33334	3.57735	3.97903	1.73205	1.96396	0.57735	0.84169
Cyclohexane	12	12	4.24264	4.24264	3	3	0.12500	0.12500
Cyclopentane	10	10	3.53553	3.53553	2	2	0.17678	0.17678
1,2-dCl-Benzene	16	21.5556	5.98313	5.57718	3.80453	2.96124	0.08333	0.03571
1,2-dCl-Ethane	6	5.55556	3.41421	3.68200	1.91421	2.10357	0.50000	0.64286
dCl-Methane	4	3.55556	2.70711	2.97489	1.41421	1.60357	0.70711	0.90913
N,N-dM-Acetamd	10	18	5.15470	4.35546	2.64273	1.82216	0.33333	0.09129
N,N-dM-Formamd	8	16	4.28446	3.43281	2.27006	1.38833	0.40825	0.10541
1,4-Dioxane	12	20	4.24264	3.64492	3	2.15470	0.12500	0.04167
Ether	8	12	4.12132	3.82246	2.41421	1.99156	0.35355	0.20412
Ethyl acetate	10	20	4.99156	4.02360	2.77006	1.90403	0.28868	0.05893
Ethyl alcohol	4	8	2.70711	2.15432	1.41421	1.02333	0.70711	0.31623
Heptane	12	12	5.53553	5.53553	3.41421	3.41421	0.17678	0.17678
Hexane	10	10	4.82843	4.82843	2.91421	2.91421	0.25000	0.25000
2-Methoxyethanol	8	16	4.12132	3.26968	2.41421	1.51315	0.35355	0.09129
Methyl alcohol	2	6	2	1.44721	1	0.44721	1	0.44721
2-Methylbutane	8	8	4.28446	4.28446	2.27006	2.27006	0.40825	0.40825
4-M-2-Pentanone	12	18	5.86181	5.19271	3.12590	2.62063	0.23570	0.08333
2-M-1-Propanol	8	12	4.28446	3.73167	2.27006	1.87918	0.40825	0.18257
2-M-2-Propanol	8	12	4.5	3.94721	2	1.72361	0.5	0.22361

DMSO	6	8.66667	3.57735	3.63299	1.73205	2.94948	0.57735	0.5
Nitromethane	6	18	3.57735	2.26371	1.73205	0.81236	0.57735	0.07454
1-Octanol	16	20	6.94975	6.39696	4.41421	4.02333	0.08839	0.03953
Pentane	8	8	4.12132	4.12132	2.41421	2.41421	0.35355	0.35355
3-Pentanone	10	16	4.99156	4.32246	2.80806	2.32544	0.28868	0.10206
1-Propanol	6	10	3.41421	2.86143	1.91421	1.52333	0.5	0.22361
2-Propanol	6	10	3.57735	3.02456	1.73205	1.41290	0.57735	0.25820
Pyridine	12	20	4.24264	3.33397	3	1.84973	0.12500	0.02869
ttCl-Ethylene	10	11.1111	5.15470	5.53557	2.64273	2.51778	0.33333	0.41326
tt-Hydrofuran	10	14	3.53553	3.23668	2.5	2.07735	0.17678	0.10206
Toluene	14	20	5.11288	4.38675	3.39385	2.41068	0.10206	0.03208
1,1,2tCltFEthane	14	31.3333	7	5.53557	3.25	2.51778	0.25	0.01968
2,2,4-tM-Pentane	14	14	6.78446	6.78446	3.41650	3.41650	0.20412	0.20412
o-Xylene	16	22	5.98313	5.30940	3.80453	2.82735	0.08333	0.02778
p-Xylene	16	22	5.98313	5.30940	3.78769	2.82137	0.08333	0.02778
Acetic acid	6	16	3.57735	2.35546	1.73205	0.92773	0.57735	0.09129
Decaline	22	22	6.81155	6.81155	4.96633	4.96633	0.02083	0.02083
dBr-Methane	4	2.51852	2.70711	4.63502	1.41421	2.77746	0.70711	2.72740
1,2-dCl-E-enZ	6	7.55556	3.41421	3.42248	1.91421	1.64264	0.5	0.42857
1,2-dCl-E-enE	6	7.55556	3.41421	3.42248	1.91421	1.64264	0.5	0.42857
1,1-dCl-E-en	6	7.55556	3.57735	3.47489	1.73205	1.48745	0.57735	0.45457
DMethoxymethane	8	16	4.12132	3.52360	2.41421	1.39385	0.35355	0.11785
dMethyl ether	4	8	2.70711	2.40825	1.41421	0.81650	0.70711	0.40825
E-enCarbonate	10	26	4.99156	3.04817	2.77006	1.27581	0.28868	0.01521
Formamide	4	12	2.70711	1.56295	1.41421	0.56904	0.70711	0.13608
Methyl chloride	2	1.77778	2	2.13389	1	1.13389	1	1.3389
Morpholine	12	18	4.24264	3.73667	3	2.28446	0.125	0.05103
Quinoline	22	34	6.81155	5.48867	4.96633	3.26450	0.02083	0.00239
SO_2	4	13.6667	2.70711	1.59109	1.41421	0.63245	0.70711	0.12910
2,2-ttCl-Ethane	10	9.11112	5.15470	5.69027	2.64273	2.95194	0.33333	0.55102
ttM-Urea	14	24	6.73205	5.80268	3.55342	2.44019	0.19245	0.04082
tCl-E-en	8	9.33334	4.28446	4.47903	2.27006	2.07722	0.40825	0.42085

An acceptable modeling is achieved only by valence type indices, and, especially, by the $^{0}\chi^{v}$ index, which, nevertheless, fails in the utility of the unitary index, $^{1}\chi^{v}$ instead shows a more reliable utility, but a worse Q and F statistics. Thus, first index gives rise to quite unstable non optimal predictive equations (for a detailed discussion about stability and prediction see ref. 38), while the second gives rise to quite stable but even worse predictive equations. The modeling of the two theoretical graph mass descriptors are, again, quite unsatisfactory, with D index faring better than D^{v}. The only conclusion could be that even the molar mass (and not only its properties) of a random class of compounds is quite difficult to be modeled with normal molecular connectivity indices.

Well, even if a satisfactory modeling of the properties of these compounds can be achieved only by the aid of semiempirical molecular connectivity terms, it is nevertheless interesting to detect the best and second best molecular connectivity descriptors, together with *M*, for the given 5 properties of Table 10A. Results collected in Table 15 show that *M* is, by far, the best descriptor for the density and the refractive index, an expected result for *d*, as density depends on the mass of a compound, and the fact that here D is the 2nd best descriptor should not impress as the description is really quite poor. Index D is the best descriptor for T_b, followed by D^{v}, while for T_m this order is reversed, and *M* plays in both cases a quite marginal role. Thus, here again we detect the opposing trends between *M* and the graph and pseudograph mass descriptors. Only for the dielectric constant the experimental graph mass descriptors, $^{0}\chi^{v}$ and $^{1}\chi^{v}$ offer a better modeling than the theoretical graph mass descriptors. Interestingly enough, the semiempirical molecular connectivity terms for T_b and T_m have D as a constituent index, the semiempirical term for the density has *M* in its expression, and the semiempirical term for the dielectric constant has both $^{0}\chi^{v}$ and *M* in its expression [57].

Table 15. Molar Mass and 1st and 2nd best descriptors for the boiling and melting temperatures, T_b, and T_m, density, *d*, refractive index, *RI*, and dielectric constant, ε, for a random class of organic solvents.

Property	Descriptor	Q	F	r	S
T_b *(n = 63)*	**M**	0.006	7.81	0.337	54.5
	D	0.013	33.3	0.594	45.6
	D^{v}	0.012	29.9	0.574	47.4
T_m (n = 62)	**M**	0.006	5.14	0.281	45.4
	D^{v}	0.010	14.4	0.440	42.4
	D	0.009	10.2	0.381	43.7
ε (n = 63)	**M**	0.017	6.51	0.310	17.8
	$^{1}\chi^{v}$	0.028	16.6	0.462	16.6
	$^{0}\chi^{v}$	0.025	13.7	0.428	16.9
d (n = 62)	**M**	2.45	27.2	0.559	0.23
	D	0.485	1.07	0.132	0.27
RI (n = 61)	**M**	3.40	15.9	0.461	0.14
	$^{1}\chi^{v}$	1.56	3.35	0.232	0.15

4. CONCLUSION

All along this excursus centered on the concept of graph mass defined within the frame of graph theory it has been possible to detect that for the simulation of the molar mass of many classes of compounds (AA, PP, [MeX+AA], [PP+AA], [PP+AA+Alk]) $^0\chi$ is the best or nearly the best descriptor, followed by $^1\chi$, which can thus be considered kind of experimental graph mass descriptors, while the simulation of the molar mass of 'less obvious' classes of compounds (MeX, [PP+AA+Alk+MeX], ROS) requires, normally, a valence type of experimental graph mass descriptor, normally $^1\chi^v$ or $^0\chi^v$. For $MPO(OR')_2$, and RPO(OR') classes of compounds both type of indices, $^0\chi$ and $^1\chi$ as well as $^1\chi^v$ and $^0\chi^v$, are good descriptors. Theoretical graph, D, and pseudograph, D^v, mass descriptors, are normally quite poor descriptors of *M*. Only for alkanes, experimental and theoretical graph mass coincide : for these compounds D is the best descriptor (or D^v, as for alkanes graphs and pseudographs are coincident). This could mean that as soon as graph and pseudograph do not superpose anymore both D and D^v become parameters by their own, with no or only minimal superposition with *M*. Theoretical graph mass parameters cannot thus be exchanged with *M* or be considered redundant with it. Further, simulation of different properties of the given classes of compounds shows that it should clearly be differentiated between single-index and multi-index LCCI description, as the two kind of descriptions activate different components within a connectivity index, and an index which can mimic *M* at the level of a single-index description of a property, can become its 'opponent' at the level of just a two-index LCCI description. Experimental and theoretical graph mass descriptors can be compared with M only at the level of a single-index modeling.

Thus, while the experimental graph mass does not have a specific identity, as it is dependent on the class of compounds examined, and it can be any of the molecular connectivity indices, excluding the total connectivity indices, the theoretical graph mass descriptors are defined once for all and are an independent concept not related to the molar mass concept, and sometimes, but only sometimes, even sharing their fate with the total connectivity indices.

Let us end this special case of data reduction analysis with some interesting words of E. Mach, which nicely fit the general aim of QSAR/QSPR studies and which constitute an appropriate comment to the many tables of this work : '*Because our memory is limited, data must be reduced. If, for example, to every time of falling, we knew the corresponding space fallen through, we could be satisfied with that. Only, what a gigantic memory would be needed to contain the table of the correspondences of s and t. Instead of this we remember the formula* $s = gt^2/2$*, that is to say, the rule of derivation by means of which we find from a given t, the corresponding s, and this replaces the table just mentioned in a very complete, convenient and compendious manner*'.

5. ACKNOWLEDGEMENTS

I am indebted to Professor Mircea Diudea of the University of Cluj, Romania, for interesting suggestions. I would also like to thank Professors L.B. Kier (Virginia University) and S. Basak (University of Minnesota) for their continuous attention, support and help.

6. REFERENCES

1. L. Pogliani, Modeling properties of biochemical compounds with connectivity terms. *Amino Acids* 13 (1997) 237-255.
2. L. Pogliani, Properties of molecular connectivity terms and physicochemical properties. *J. Mol.Struct. (Theochem)* **1997**, *13*, 237-255.
3. Randić, M. On characterization of molecular branching. *J.Am.Chem.Soc.* **1998**, (in press).
4. Kier, L.B.; Hall, L.H.; Murray, W.J.; Randić, M. Molecular Connectivity I : relationship to nonsppecific local anesthesia. *J.Pharm.Sci.* **1975**, *64*, 1971-1974.
5. Hall, L.H.; Kier, L.B.; Murray, W.J. Molecular Connectivity II : relationship to water solubility and boilng point. *J.Pharm.Sci.* **1975**, *64*, 1974-1977.
6. Murray, J.M.; Hall, L.H.; Kier, L.B. Molecular Connectivity III : relationship to partition coefficients. *J.Pharm.Sci.* **1975**, *64*, 1978-1981.
7. Kier, L.B.; Hall. L.H. Molecular Connectivity VII : specific treatment of heteroatoms. *J.PharmSci.* **1976**, *65*, 1806-1809.
8. Balaban, A.T. (Ed.) *Chemical applications of Graph theory*. Academic Press : London, 1976.
9. Hall, L.H. ; Kier, L.B. A molecular connectivity study of electron density in alkanes. *Tetrahedron* **1977**, *33*, 1953-1957.
10. Kier, L.B. ; Hall, L.H. Derivation and significance oof valence molecular connectivity indices. *J.Pharm.Sci* **1981**, *70*, 583-589.
11. Trinajstić, N. *Chemical graph theory*, CRC Press : Boca Raton, Fl, 1983 (2nd ed. 1992).
12. Kier, L.B.; Hall, L.H. *Molecular connectivity in structure-activity analysis*. Wiley : New York, 1986, and references therein.
13. Turro, N.J. Geometric and topological thinking in organic chemistry. *Angew.Chem.Int.Edn. Engl.* **1986**, *25*, 882-901.
14. Seybold, P.G.; May, M.; Bagal, A.U. Molecular structure-property relationships. *J.Chem. Ed* **1987**, *64*, 575-581.
15. Randić, M. On characterization of three-dimensional structures. *Int.J.Quant.Chem: Quant. Biol.Symp.* **1988**, *15*, 201-208.
16. Randić, M.; Hansen, P.J.; Jurs, P.C. Search for useful graph theoretical invariants of molecular structure. *J. Chem.Inf.Comput.Sci.* **1988**, *28*, 60-68.

17. Basak, S.C.; Magnuson, V.R.; Niemi, G.J.; Regal, R.R. Determining structural similarity of chemicals using graph-theoretical indices. *Discr.Appl.Math.* **1988**, *19*, 17-44.
18. Hansen, P.J.; Jurs, P.C. Chemical applications of graph theory. *J.Chem.Ed.* **1988**, *65*, 574-580.
19. Needham, D.E.; Wei, I-C.; Seybold, P.G. Molecular modeling of the physical properties of the alkanes. *J.Am. Chem.Soc.* **1988**, *110*, 4186-4194.
20. Rouvray, D.H. The limits of applicability of topological indices. *J Mol Struct (Theochem)* **1989**, *185*, 187-201.
21. Randić, M. Orthogonal molecular descriptors. *N.J.Chem.* **1991**, *15*, 517-525.
22. Randić, M. Resolution of ambiguities in structure-property studies by use of orthogonal descriptors. *J.Chem. Inf.Comput.Sci.* **1991**, *31*, 311-320.
23. Randić, M. Search for optimal molecular descriptors. *Croat.Chim.Acta* **1991**, *64*, 43-54.
24. Basak, S.C.; Niemi, G.J.; Veith, G.D. Predicting properties of molecules using graph invariants. *J.Math.Chem* **1991**, *7* : 243-272.
25. Balaban, A.T. Using real numbers as vertex invariants for third-generation topological indices. *J.Chem.Inf. Comput.Sc.* **1992**, *32*, 23-28.
26. Maier, B.J. Wiener and Randić topological indices for graphs. *J.Chem.Inf.Comput.Sci.* **1992**, *32*, 87-90.
27. Mihalić, Z.; Trinajstić, N. A graph-theoretical approach to structure-property relationships. *J.Chem.Ed.* **1992**, *69*, 701-712.
28. Mihalić, Z.; Nikolić, S.; Trinajstić, N. Comparative study of molecular descriptors derived from the distance matrix. *J.Chem.Inf.Comput.Sci.* **1992**, *32*, 28-37.
29. A.T. Balaban, Using real numbers as vertex invariants for third-generation topological indexes. *J.Chem.Inf.Comput.Sci.* 32 (1992) 23-28.
30. Balaban, T.A. ; Kier, L.B. ; Joshi, N. Structure-Property analysis of octane numbers for hydrocarbons (Alkanes, Cycloalkanes, Alkenes). *match*, (*Comm.Math.Chem*) **1992**, *28*, 13-27.
31. Pogliani, L. Molecular connectivity model for determination of isoelectric points of amino acids. *J.Pharm. Sci.* **1992**, *81*, 334-336.
32. Pogliani, L. Molecular Connectivity : treatment of the electronic structure of amino acids. *J.Pharm.Sci.* **1992**, *81*, 967-969.
33. Stanton, D.T.; Jurs, P.C. Computer-assisted study of the relationship between molecular structure and surface tension of organic compounds. *J.Chem.Inf.Comput.Sci.* **1992**, *32*, 109-115.
34. Kier, L.B,; Hall, L.H.; Frazer, J.W. Design of molecules from quantitative structure-activity relationship models. 1. Information transfer between path and vertex degree counts. *J.Chem.Inf.Comput.Sci* **1993**, *33*, 143-147.
35. Hall, L.H.; Kier, L.B.; Frazer, J.W. Design of molecules from quantitative structure-activity realtionship models. 2. Derivation and proof of information transfer relating equations. *J.Chem.Inf.Comput.Sci.* **1993**, *33*, 148-152.

36. Pogliani, L. Molecular connectivity model for determination of T_1 relaxation times of α-carbons of amino acids and cyclic dipeptides. *Comput.Chem.* **1993**, *17*, 283-286.
37. Pogliani, L. Molecular connectivity model for determination of physicochemical properties of α-amino acids. *J.Phys.Chem.* **1993**, *97*, 6731-6736.
38. Randić, M. Curve-Fitting paradox. *Int.J.Quant.Chem. : Quant.Biol.Symp* **1994**, *21*, 215-225.
39. Balaban, A.T. ; Bertelsen, S. ; New centric topological indexes for acyclic molecules (trees) and substituents (rooted trees) and coding oofrooted trees. *match* **1994**, *30*, 55-72.
40. Basak, S.C.; Grunwald, G.D. Molecular similarity and risk assessment : analog selection and property estimation using graph invariants. *SAR & QSAR Environ.Res.* **1994**, *2*, 289-307.
41. Pogliani, L. On a graph theoretical characterization of cis/trans isomers. *J.Chem.Inf. Comput.Sci.* **1994**, *34*, 801-804.
42. Pogliani, L. Molecular connectivity descriptors of the physicochemical properties of the α-amino acids. *J. Phys.Chem.* **1994**, *98,* 1494-1499.
43. Pogliani, L. Modeling the solubility and activity of amino acids with the LCCI method. *Amino Acids* **1995**, *9*, 217-228.
44. Pogliani, L. Molecular modeling by linear combinations of connectivity indices. *J.Phys.Chem.* **1995**, *99*, 925-937.
45. Lucić, B.; Nikolić, S.; Trinajstić, N.; Juretić, D.; Jurić, A. A novel QSPR approach to physicochemical properties of the α-amino acids. *Croat.Chim. Acta* **1995**, *68*, 435-450.
46. Galvez, J. ; Garcia-Domenech, R. ; de Julian-Ortiz, J.V. ;Soler, R. Topological approach to drug design. *J.Chem.Inf.Comput.Sci.* **1995**, *35*, 272-284.
47. Galvez, J. ; Garcia-Domenech, R. ; de Gregorio Alapont C. ; de Julian-Ortiz, J.V. ;Popa, L. Pharmacological distribution diagrams : a tool for *de novo* drug design. *J.Mol.Graph.* **1996**, *14*, 272-276.
48. Pogliani, L. A strategy for molecular modeling of a physicochemical property using a linear combination of connectivity indices. *Croat.Chim.Acta* **1996**, *69*, 95-109.
49. Pogliani, L. Modeling purines and pyrimidines with the linear combination of connectivity indices - molecular connectivity "LCCI-MC" method. *J.Chem.Inf.Comput.Sci.* **1996**, *36*, 1082-1091.
50. Pogliani, L. Modeling with special descriptors derived from a medium-sized set of connectivity indices. *J.Phys.Chem.* **1996**, *100,*: 18065-18077.
51. Pogliani, L. Modeling enthalpy and hydration processes of inorganic compounds. *Croat.Chem.Acta* **1997**, *70*, 803-817.
52. Pogliani, L. Modeling biochemicals with leading molecular connectivity terms. *Med. Chem.Res.* **1997**, *7*, 180-393.
53. Garcia-Domenech, R. ; de Gregorio Alapont, C. ; de Julian-Ortiz, J.V. ; Galvez, J. Molecular connectivity to find β-blockers with low toxicity. *Bioorg.&Med.Chem.Letters* **1997**, *7*, 567-572.

54. Galvez, J. On a topological interpretation of electronic and vibrational molecular energies. *J.Mol.Struct.(THEOCHEM)* **1998**, *429*, 255-264.
55. Kuanar, M. ; Mishra, B.K. Optimization of a regression model for a quantitative structure mutagenicity relationship of some natural amino acids. *Bull.Chem.Soc.Jpn.* **1998**, *71*, 191-198.
56. L. Pogliani, Modeling properties with higher-level molecular connectivity descriptors. *J. Chem.Inf.Comput.Sci.* **1999**, *39*, 104-111.
57. L. Pogliani, Modeling with semiempirical molecular connectivity terms. *J.Phys.Chem.* **1999**, *103*, 1598-1610.
58. K. H: Rosen, Discrete mathematics and its Applications, McGraw-Hill, New York, 1995.
59. Kier, L.B.; Hall, L.H. *Molecular Connectivity in Chemistry and Drug Research*, Academic Press, New York, 1976.
60. Xu, L.; Yun, H.; Su, Q. A newly proposed molecular topological index for the discrimination of *cis/trans* isomers and for the studies of QSAR/QSPR. *Computers Chem.* **1992**, *16*, 187-194.
61. Xu, L.; Yun, H.; Su, Q. Correlation analysis in structure and chromatographic data of organophosphorus compounds by GAI. *Computers Chem.* **1992**, *16*, 195-199.

Chapter 7

EIGENVALUES AS MOLECULAR DESCRIPTORS

Milan Randić*, Marjan Vračko and Marjana Novič
National Institute of Chemistry
1001 Ljubljana, POB 3430 Slovenia

1. INTRODUCTION

Recent years have witnessed increasing expansion of the development of molecular descriptors for use in data reduction [1, 2]. Several computer programs [3] were developed over the years that generate molecular descriptors for use in multivariate regression analyses [4] as well as other statistical techniques: PCA, the Principal Component Analysis [5], the pattern recognition [6], the artificial neural networks [7], the cluster analysis [8], the sensitivity analysis [9], the similarity analysis [10], and such. Novel descriptors continue to be proposed, regardless whether such efforts are adequately justified or not. Apparently construction of novel descriptors is likely to continue for a while until sufficiently general, or sufficiently flexible, descriptors emerge.

In this chapter we will not consider arguments in favor or against construction of novel descriptors, except to mention that introduction of novel descriptors, in our view, should *always* be accompanied with an illustration of the use of such descriptor outlining their advantages. It may be that a novel descriptor has simple structural interpretation, leads to better quality statistical characterization of a regression, can be applied to diverse classes of compounds, or offers description of variety of molecular properties of a set of compounds investigated. Some time ago Read [11] suggested a dozen desirable requirements for the construction of molecular codes, which included some obvious features, and some less obvious. For example, the codes should be linear string of symbols, the codes should be unique, the codes should be simple, the codes should be easily understood, etc. In the same spirit a dozen requirements for satisfactory topological indices as molecular descriptors were also proposed [12, 13].

---

* On leave from Department of Mathematics & Computer Science, Drake University, Des Moines, IA 50311

In Table 1 we have reproduced the list of the desirable attributes for topological indices as outlined by Balaban [12] and Randić [13]. According to Balaban the first five requirements are to be considered mandatory, but one may somewhat relax some of the conditions. For example, the condition that descriptors have low degeneracy or no degeneracy is desirable, but since topological indices have limitations as a tool for graph isomorphism problem the presence of the degeneracy is not so critical. After all, molecules may have some properties equal or almost equal, hence descriptors that are degenerate or almost degenerate will not be at disadvantage in such applications. The first requirement of Randić is not listed among the requirements of Balaban: Molecular codes should have a direct structural interpretation. The second requirement of Randić agrees with that that Balaban (stated there as the first condition): The codes should show good correlation with some molecular property. Both these conditions deserve to remain as the leading conditions for introduction of novel descriptors. Unfortunately these two conditions appear often to have been overlooked by practitioners in the field. It suffice to point out that structural interpretation of Wiener index [14], one of the earliest graph theoretical molecular descriptors, despite that fifty years passed of Wiener's celebrated paper, still is somewhat obscure. The same can be said about linear combinations of descriptors that appear as the principal components in the PCA (the Principal Component Analysis) of Hotelling [5]. The situation is no better in the case of the multiple regression analysis, or the artificial neural networks, when the output is given as a combination of descriptors. While individual descriptors may have plausible structural interpretation, it is not clear at all what represents linear combination of such descriptors which are inter-correlated (often highly intercorrelated and sometimes almost collinear).

We will in this chapter re-examine some of the above mentioned objections, and hope to show how some of the difficulties can be resolved. But the focus of this chapter is on eigenvalues as molecular descriptors. Eigenvalues of a matrix are well defined mathematical quantities, nevertheless, use of eigenvalues as descriptors does not relieve us from the before mentioned obstacles: a need for clarification of their structural interpretation, and a need for resolution of ambiguities resulting from their interrelation with other descriptors. Eigenvalues of adjacency matrix have received considerable attention and will only briefly be considered here. Most of our review will concern eigenvalues of various graph matrices, and their use as molecular descriptors.

Browsing through the literature one will notice almost unlimited variety of molecular descriptors [15]. Even if one confines attention to hydrocarbons, the compound ideal for testing novel descriptors, because of lack of heteroatoms and the abundance of reported molecular properties, variations of the possibilities to define a descriptor appear unlimited. Conspicuous, however, is absence of eigenvalues as molecular descriptors. Yet eigenvalues of a matrix, including then also any matrix associated with a molecular graph or molecular structure, represent one of the most elementary structural invariant. Why is that the case? Is there a need for eigenvalues of graph matrices to be included as molecular descriptors in the arsenal of mathematical tool for the characterization of molecules?

Table 1

Balaban		Importance
1	Good correlational ability	xx
2	Low or no degeneracy	x
3	Easily computed	x
4	Increase with branching	
5	Adjustable to Unsaturation and heteroatoms	xxx
6	Complete non degeneracy	x

Randić		Importance
1	Direct structural interpretation	xxx
2	Correlation with at least one property	xx
3	Discrimination of isomers	x
4	Locally defined	xx
5	Generates higher analogues	xx
6	Linearly independent	xxx
7	Simple	x
8	Not based on properties	
9	Not trivially related to other descriptors	xxx
10	Efficiency of construction	x
11	Based on familiar structural concepts	xx
12	Show correct size dependence	
13	Gradual change on perturbation	xx

2. Adjacency Matrix and its Eigenvalues

One of the reasons why the eigenvalues of the adjacency matrix of a graph have not been considered seriously as molecular descriptors may be due to early recognition of the fact that the egenvalues of the adjacency matrix are not size-dependent. In Table 2 we have listed the leading eigenvalues of alkane graphs having from 2 to 7 carbon atoms. As we see regardless the size of a molecule the leading eigenvalues do not exceed 4, the maximal valence for saturated hydrocarbons. On the other hand most physico-chemical properties of molecules, alkanes in particular, such as the boiling points, the heats of formation, the molar refraction, the densities, the entropy, etc. are size-dependent. It is well known in linear algebra (Frobenius theorem) that the upper bound on the leading eigenvalue of a matrix is the maximal row (or column) sum. In the case of the adjacency matrix of molecular graphs each row sum equals to the valence of the vertex represented by the row. Hence, the leading eigenvalue for molecular graphs of most organic molecules will be at most equal to four. Similarly in the case of compounds having at each carbon atom pi-electron, such as polycyclic aromatic hydrocarbons, the leading eigenvalues will be at most equal to three. By being thus confined to a small interval for their magnitude eigenvalues offer rather limited variations for almost unlimited variations in molecular connectivity even when one considers molecules of the same size (isomers) only.

Table 2

ethane	1.000000
propane	1.414214
butane	1.618034
isobutane	1.732051
pentane	1.732051
isopentane	1.847759
neopentane	2.000000
n-hexane	1.847759
2-methylpentane	1.902113
3-methylpentane	1.931852
2,2-dimethylbutane	2.074313
2,3-dimethylbutane	2.000000
n-heptane	1.879385
2-methylhexane	1.931852
3-methylhexane	1.969616
3-ethylpentane	2.000000
2,2-dimethylpentane	2.101003
2,3-dimethylpentane	2.052881
2,4-dimethylpentane	2.000000
3,3-dimethylpentane	2.135779
2,2,3-trimethylbutane	2.175328

An additional reason for a lack of interest in eigenvalues of graphs as molecular descriptors may be due to the occurrence of isospectral graphs. Already during World War II Sinogowitz [16] noted that different trees may have all eigenvalues of adjacency matrix identical. In Fig. 1 we show the smallest known isospectral graphs: acyclic [16], cyclic [17], and acyclic having double bond [18]. In Fig. 2 we have illustrated molecular skeletons of isospectral nonanes, while in Fig. 3 we illustrate a selection of isospectral graphs from the chemical and the mathematical literature. Since the early studies of isospectral graphs many additional graphs were found or constructed that have identical spectra [19]. As the size of a graph become larger frequency of the occurrence of isospectral graphs increases so that isospectral graphs become a rule rather than an exception. Mathematician A. Schwenk [20] in an article entitled : "Almost all trees are isospectral" has proved that as the size of trees (acyclic graphs) increases the probability that a graph has an isospectral companion tends towards 1, the certainty.

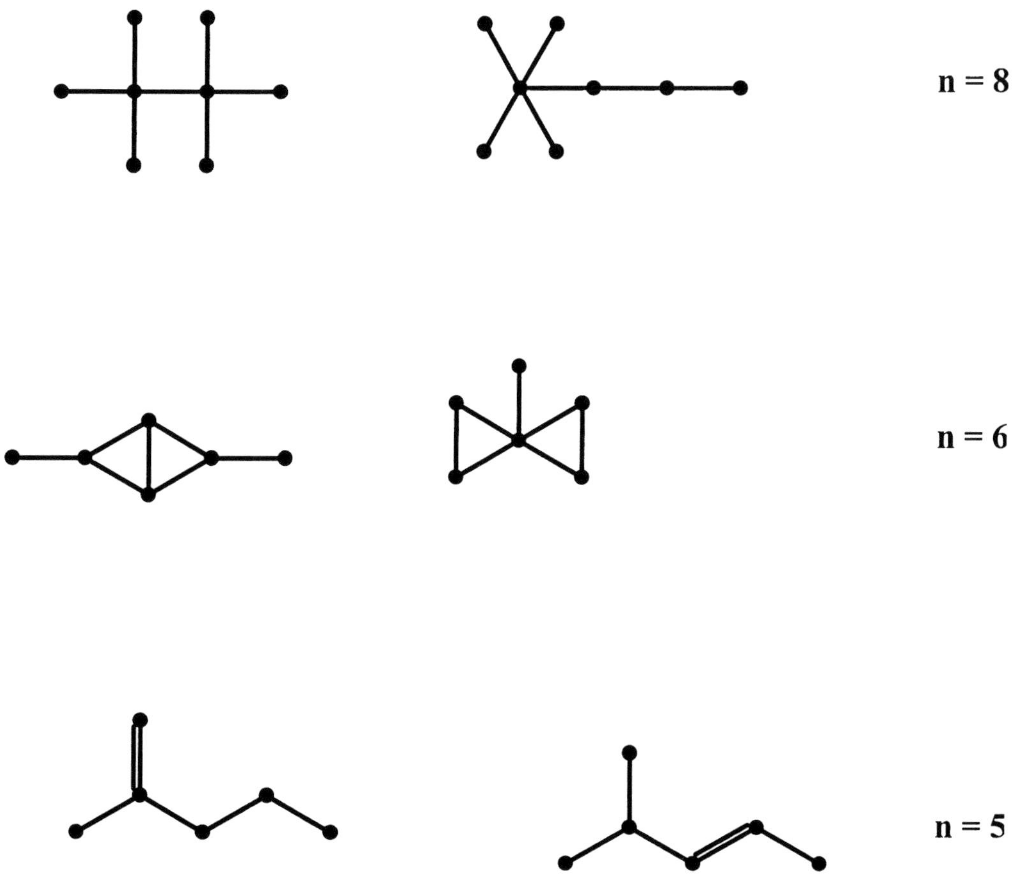

Figure 1

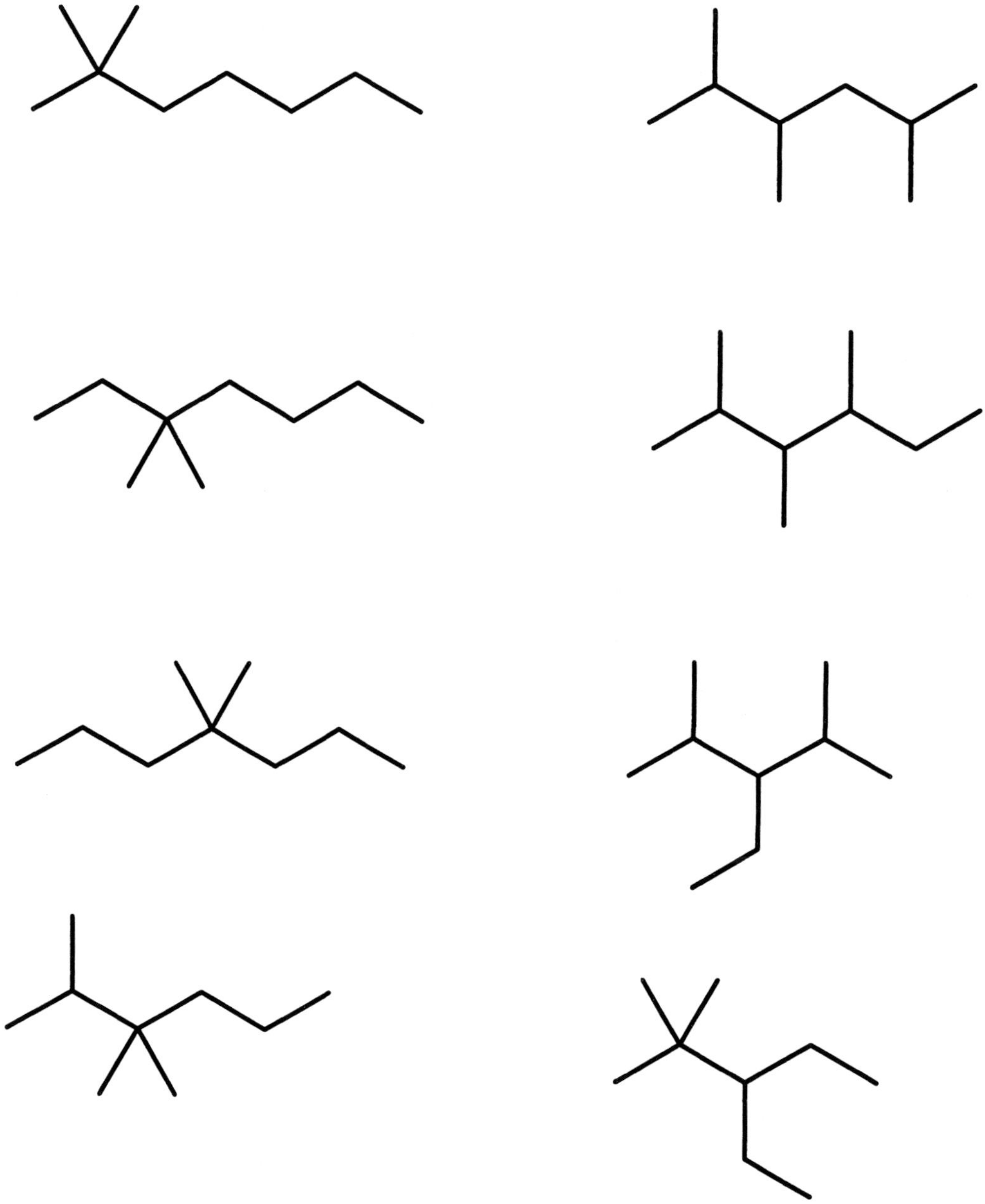

Figure 2

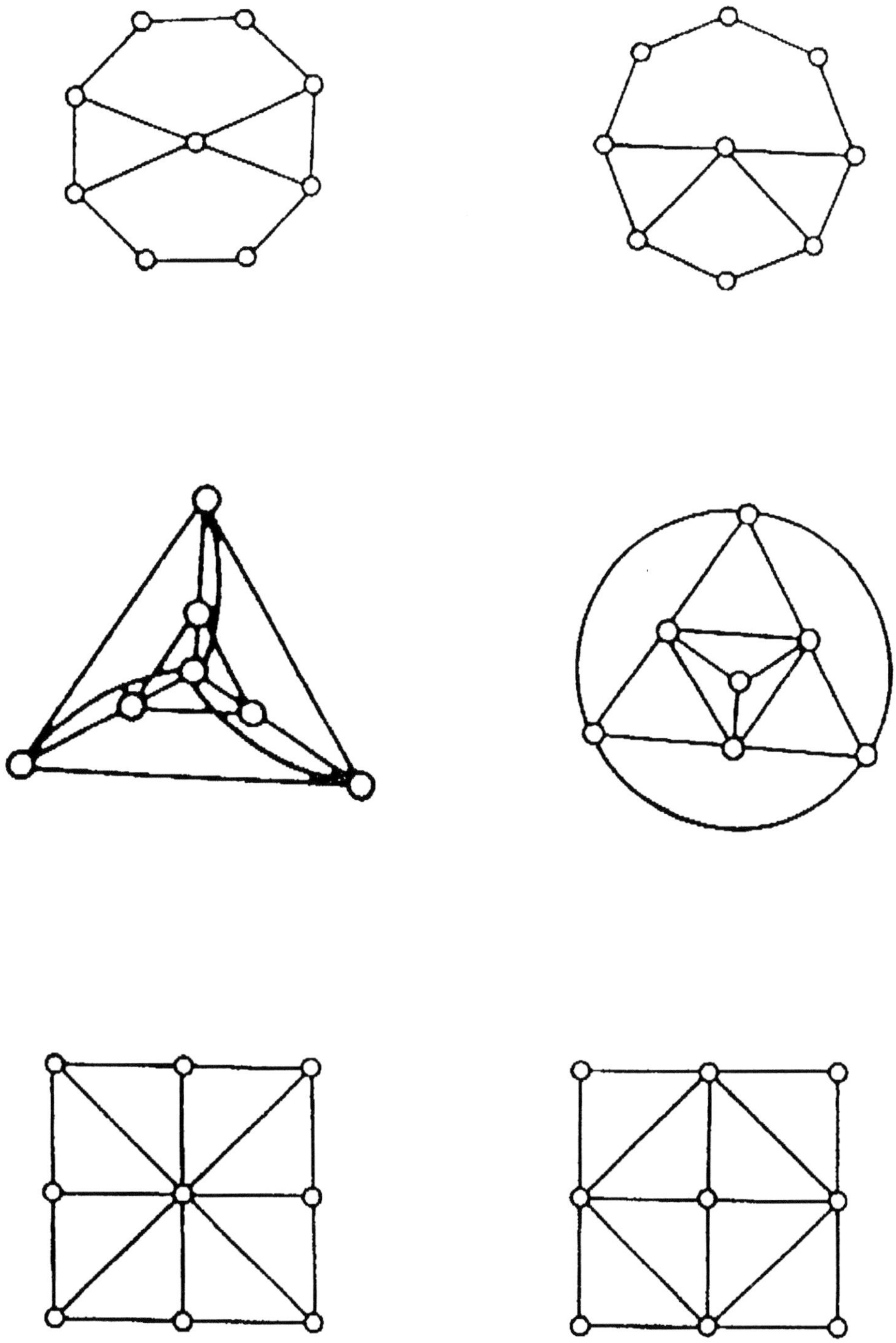

Figure 3

In the early 1940s - 1950s the eigenvalues of the adjacency matrix of graphs of benzenoid hydrocarbons and other polycyclic aromatic compounds played the central role in Hückel Molecular Orbital theory [21], HMO. Over the time the HMO, that was initially viewed as enlightening, as it offered insights into the nature of chemical bonding for various organic compounds, gradually was replaced by more sophisticated quantum chemical models [21a]. Subsequently HMO was viewed as simple, and finally as simplistic. The problem with HMO was not solely in the underlying simplifying assumptions (due to Felix Bloch [22]) of "either/or" interactions that lead to binary matrices for accompanying hamiltonians, but also in the limitation of assuming that eigenvalues of individual orbital energies, even with an independent particle model, well characterize orbital energies. To demonstrate limitations of HMO Heilbronner and Jones [23] reported photoelectron spectra of two benzene derivatives (shown in Fig. 4), 1,4-divinylbenzene and 2-phenylbutadiene, the structures that are within HMO isospectral. The actual spectra, and the computed spectra as the difference of the respective eigenvalues (that are in mathematical literature referred to as "spectra"), were distinctively different. This contribution may have been viewed by some as "the last nail in the coffin" of the HMO, but if the authors wanted to kill HMO, which was at the time for most practical purposed already dead, it would have sufficed to show photoelectron spectra of a *single* molecule, whether it is isospectral to another, or not!

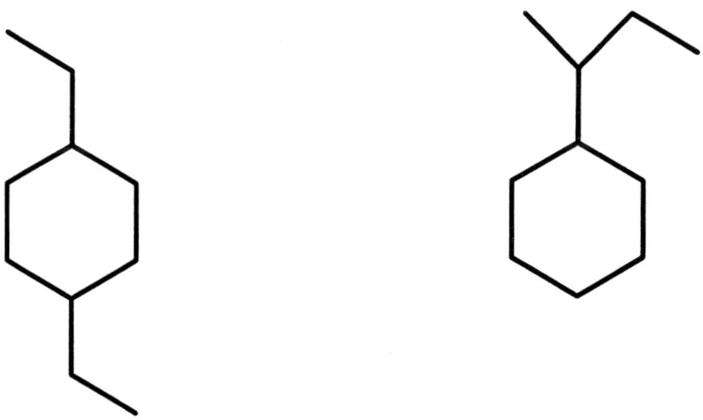

Figure 4

It is interesting to mention that during the "prosperous times of HMO" the presence of isospectral graphs, which would be of considerable interest them, has not been recognized at all at that time. Useful source of computed data on polycyclic aromatic compounds was the book of Coulson and Streitwieser [24], "The Dictionary of π-electron Calculations" which catalogued the eigenvalues, the eigenvectors, and additional construction of MO theory (the atom and the molecular polarizabilities) and it contained, among others, also 1,4-divynylbenzene and 2-phenylbutadiene (Fig. 4), two molecules that are isospectral. It was only in 1973 that Živković [25] noticed that these two molecules, separated by few pages, have all their eigenvalues identical!

On the other hand, we could add that with proper precautions and adequate modifications even today HMO offers some useful insight in large systems, or for large collection of structures, as demonstrated among others by Hoffmann when developing his "Extended Hückel Method" [26].

3. THE EARLY BRANCHING INDEX

By reviewing the spectra of trees Lovasz and Pelikan [27] suggested in 1973 the leading eigenvalue of adjacency matrix as an index of molecular branching. In Fig. 5 we show the molecular graphs of 18 isomers of n-octane together with the corresponding leading eigenvalues. Clearly, as the number of branches in a molecule increases so increases also the leading eigenvalue of the structure. However, there are some limitations of viewing the leading eigenvalue as an index of branching. For example, 4-methylheptane and 2,5-dimethylphexane, which clearly have distinct branching patterns, both have identical leading eigenvalue. Nevertheless, the proposal of Lovasz and Pelikan offers some quantitative characterization of branching, an important but elusive structural concept, that has hitherto remained qualitative. The paper by Lovasz and Pelikan has not been overlooked in the chemical literature, and one may say that it may have stimulated interest in characterization of molecular branching, which later lead to alternative characterizations of molecular branching.

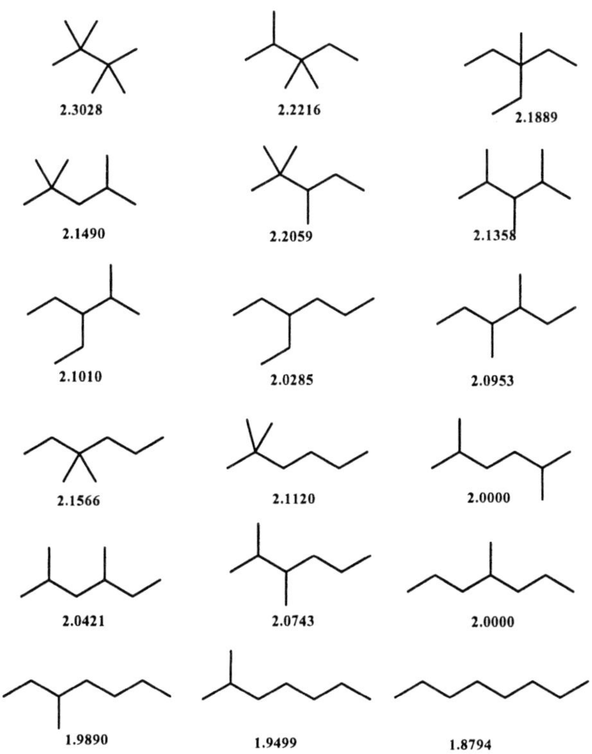

Figure 5

That the leading eigenvalues for octane isomers of Fig. 5 show structural regularity can be observed by using the so called (p_2, p_3) path diagram shown in Fig. 6 [28]. Here p_2 and p_3 are the number of paths of length two and the number of paths of length three of each isomer, respectively. For example, n-octane has six paths of length two and five paths of length three, hence it is placed on the coordinate (6, 5). As we see from Fig. 6, except in two cases, each point on the (p_2, p_3) grid belongs to a different isomer. If we now replace isomers by the corresponding value of their leading eigenvalue λ_1 we obtain diagram shown in Fig. 7. As we see there is a regular increase of λ_1 as both p_2 and p_3 increase, with a minor exception for 3,3-dimethulhexane and 2,3,4-trimethylpentane.

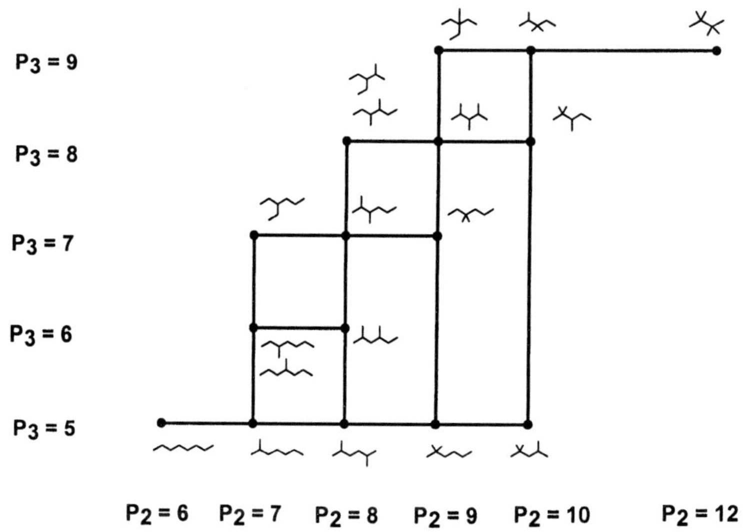

Figure 6

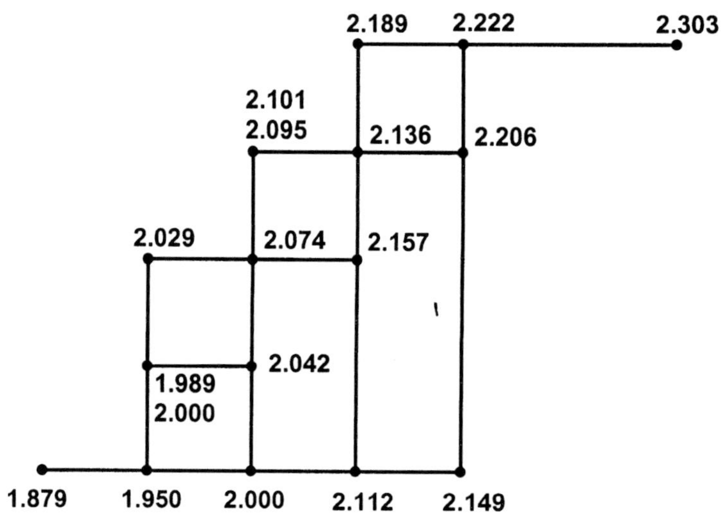

Figure 7

Molecular branching received considerable attention in the chemical literature [29]. One of the motivations for the interest in molecular branching is generally known fact that many physicochemical properties of molecules, such as the boiling points of alkanes, depend inherently on molecular branching. Wiener [14], in his pioneering work on use of mathematical descriptors in structure-property correlation when he introduced W, today known as Wiener index, was motivated by a statement that he found (as an undergraduate student) in standard chemistry textbooks that the boiling points of paraffins depend on branching. Yet, there were no further clarifications in these textbooks as to how boiling points depend on branching, or even how is branching defined.

In concluding this section we may observe that the leading eigenvalue of the adjacency matrix has been relatively early recognized as potentially useful molecular descriptor, but were later overlooked, probably deliberately, in view of the limited flexibility in its applications to the structure-property studies.

4. Graph Matrices

Before we continue to explore use of eigenvalues as molecular descriptors we ought to enlist matrices that one can associate with graphs. For quite a long time the only matrices that were "recognized" in chemical graph theory (and graph theory in general) were the adjacency matrix (which is probably almost as old as the graph theory) and the distance matrix, that has been introduced in graph theory by Frank Harary [30]. In Table 3 we show the adjacency and the distance matrix for graph of Fig. 8 (that belongs to 2-methylheptane, or the corresponding unsaturated hydrocarbon having identical connectivity). There is considerable literature on the distance matrix and its use in chemical graph theory [31]. In particular, it is worth mentioning that the sum of all entries above the main diagonal in the distance matrix, as demonstrated the first time by Hosoya [32], gives the Wiener number of a graph. This is the same W parameter that Wiener has introduced in 1947 in order to account for isomeric variations of molecular properties [14].

Another matrix that Harary introduced at the same time when distance matrix is the detour matrix. In contrast to the distance matrix it has been only in recent time that the detour matrix received attention in the chemical literature [33]. The verdict is still not out whether the detour matrix is sufficiently useful in the structure-property-activity studies. On the other hand it seems that the detour matrix has some potential for characterization of cyclic and polycyclic structures [34]. The detour matrix has been used for construction of several topological indices [35]. It is not surprising to see that several molecules have identical topological indices derived from detour matrix. However, it is interesting and unexpected to find that different graphs have identical detour matrix [36]. Such graphs will necessarily have identical all invariants derived from the detour matrix. Hitherto, the detour matrix is the only matrix of graphs that can be identical for non isomorphic graphs.

Table 3

Adjacency matrix

0	1	0	0	0	0	0	0
1	0	1	0	0	0	0	0
0	1	0	1	0	0	0	1
0	0	1	0	1	0	0	0
0	0	0	1	0	1	0	0
0	0	0	0	1	0	1	0
0	0	0	0	0	1	0	1
0	0	1	0	0	0	1	0

Distance matrix

0	1	2	3	4	5	6	3
1	0	1	2	3	4	5	2
2	1	0	1	2	3	4	1
3	2	1	0	1	2	3	2
4	3	2	1	0	1	2	3
5	4	3	2	1	0	1	4
6	5	4	3	2	1	0	5
3	2	1	2	3	4	5	0

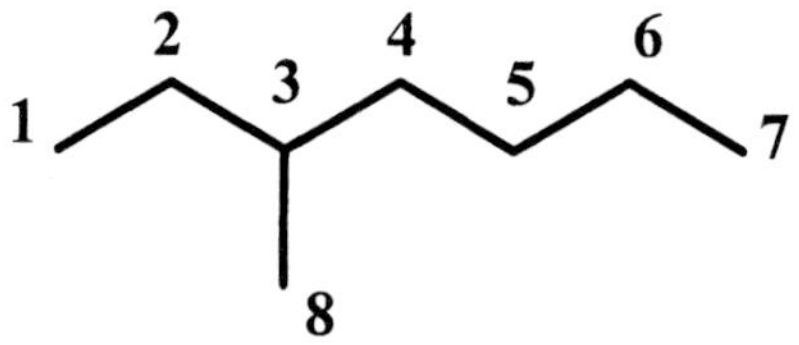

Figure 8

In Table 4 we list several matrices that one can construct for molecular graphs. They have all been illustrated on molecular graph of 3-methylheptane. As a historical fact one should mention: (1) the property matrices of Balandin constructed prior to 1940 [37] and (2) the alphanumerical matrices that Spialter introduced for chemical documentation in 1963 [38]. It passed almost about 50 years before novel matrices for molecular re-appeared in chemical graph theory. The list of these is given in Table 5 in more-less chronological order. Among the first were the matrices of Tratch, Stankevitch and Zefirov [39], Kier and Hall's matrix of "electrotopological" state [40], and Wiener and Hosoya matrices, introduced by Randić [41, 42 respectively], in which the Wiener number W and the Hosoya topological index Z have been generalized.

Table 4

Wiener matrix

0	7	6	4	3	2	1	1
	0	12	8	6	4	2	2
		0	16	12	8	4	7
			0	15	10	5	4
				0	12	6	3
					0	7	2
						0	1
							0

Reversed distance

0	7	6	5	4	3	2	5
	0	7	6	5	4	3	6
		0	7	6	5	4	7
			0	7	6	5	6
				0	7	6	5
					0	7	4
						0	3
							0

Hosoya matrix

0	13	5	3	2	1	1	5
	0	4	3	2	1	1	5
		0	6	4	2	2	10
			0	9	5	5	6
				0	7	7	4
					0	11	2
						0	2
							0

The generalized matrices include also the "restricted random walk" matrix [43] which is non symmetrical, and the distance/distance matrix [44], that will be considered in the next section, which is defined for a structure that is rigidly embedded in 2-dimensional or 3-dimensional space. It appears that just as the early topological indices, the Wiener number [14], the Hosoya Z index [32], the connectivity index [45], and the higher order connectivity indices [46], were followed by a proliferation of other topological indices the emergence of novel graph matrices, the extended connectivity matrix[39], the electrotopological matrix [40], the Wiener matrix [41], and Hosoya matrix [42], has been followed by construction of increasing number of novel graph matrices [47, 48].

Table 5. Chronological list of graph matrices

Year	Name	Authors	Reference
	Adjacency		
	Distance	Harary	30
	Detour	Harary	30
1990	Expanded distance	Trach, Stankevich Zefirov	39
	Electrotopological	Kier and Hall	40
1993	Wiener	Randić	41
1993	Resistance distance	Klein and Randić	
1994	Distance/distance	Randić Kleiner DeAlba	44
1994	Hosoya matrix	Randić	42
1995	Restricted random walk	Randić	43
	Path matrix	Randić Plavšić Razinger	49
	Szeged matrix	Gutman	47
1997	Cluj matrix	Diudea	47

Among novel matrices we want to draw attention of readers to one matrix in particular, the path matrix [49, 50], which is the subject of the following section. Before going to the new section let us just observe that very little has been reported on eigenvalues of all these novel matrices. Only in a study on Wiener matrix [31], however, attention was given to eigenvalues of the newly introduced matrix. Perhaps not surprisingly the leading eigenvalue of the Wiener matrix does show some structural regularities. In order to see the regularity of the leading eigenvalues of the Wiener matrix we plotted in Fig. 9 for octane isomers λ_1 on the (p_2, p_3) coordinate grid. As we see from Fig. 9 the first eigenvalue of the Wiener matrix vary regularly for the 18 isomers of octane over the (p_2, p_3) coordinate grid. However, in contrast to the behavior of the leading eigenvalue of the adjacency matrix, which increases with the increase of p_2 and p_3, the leading eigenvalue of Wiener matrix decreases as p_2 and p_3 increase.

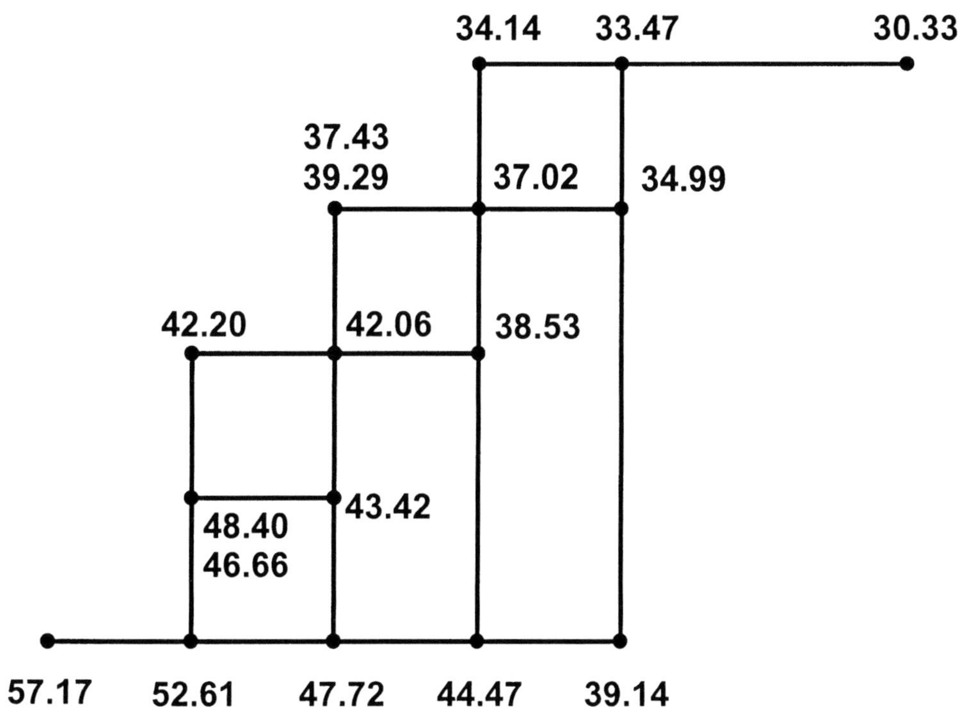

Figure 9

Because many physicochemical properties of octanes show a regular variation on the (p_2, p_3) grid the regular variation of λ_1 on the (p_2, p_3) grid suggests that the leading eigenvalue may serve as a descriptor in structure-property correlations. The Wiener matrix, which is defined so that its i, j element counts path subgraphs in a graph G that contain the path from vertex i to vertex j, is size dependent. For octane isomers its leading eigenvalue vary in the range between approximately 30 (for 2,2,3,3-tertramethylbutane) to about 60 (for n-octane). In contrast the smallest eigenvalue, the most negative eigenvalue, of the Wiener matrix for octane isomers is almost constant for all isomers (being close to between -17 and -18).

The leading eigenvalue of the Wiener matrix show strong correlation with the leading eigenvalue of the adjacency matrix [51]. Since, the leading eigenvalue of the adjacency matrix, according to Lovasz and Pelikan [27], is an index of branching in a graph the correlation between the first eigenvalue of the Wiener matrix and the first eigenvalue of the adjacency matrix (shown in Fig. 10) suggests the leading eigenvalue of the Wiener matrix as an alternative branching index for octane isomers. The coefficient of regression between the two leading eigenvalues was found to be r = 0.958, and the Fisher ratio is 176, which are quite a respectable values for correlations of properties of molecules of the same size.

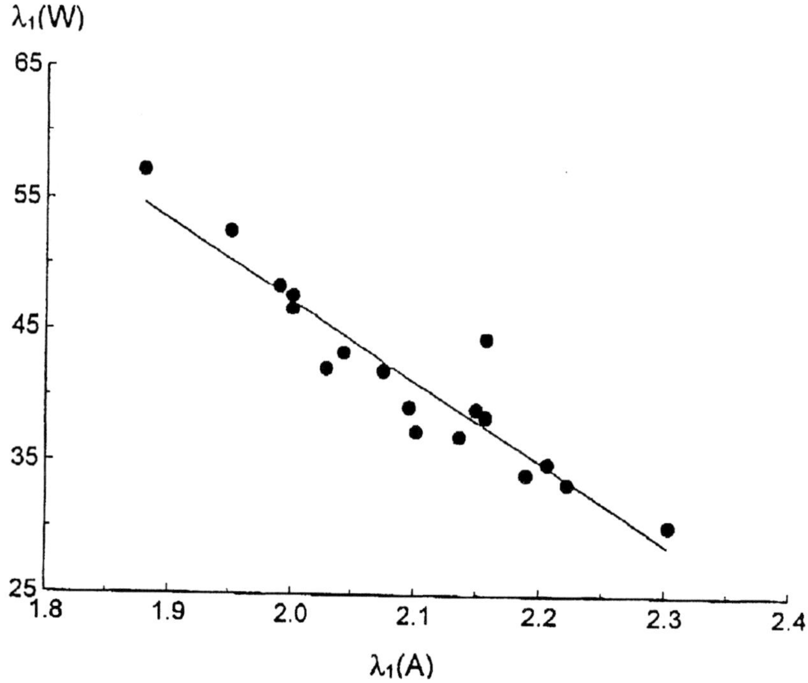

Figure 10

The leading eigenvalue of the Wiener matrix was tested as a descriptor for structure-property by considering variation of selected properties of octane isomers. In Table 6 we have collected the regression coefficients for regression using two descriptors, which among others include the leading eigenvalue of the Wiener matrix λ_1, and λ_2, the second largest eigenvalue. The other descriptors used are the Wiener number W, the hyper-Wiener number WW [52], and the JJ index [51], derived from row sums of the Wiener matrix in an analogy with Balaban's J index [53], the quotients of paths and walks of length two (q_2) and three (q_3), the sum of the positive eigenvalues (eig sum), and the multiplicity of the zero eigenvalue (μ_0). As we see from Table 6 several regression listed are characterized by the regression coefficient of over 0.900, which is not so easy to attain for the regression when all molecules are of the same size. Some of the better regressions are obtained when the leading eigenvalues of the Wiener matrix was one of the descriptors used.

Table 6. Two parameter regressions

	WW,W	WW, λ_1	WW, JJ	W, λ_1	W, JJ	λ_1, λ_2	q_2, q_3	eig sum μ_0
BP		0.902	0.775		0.763	0.810	0.914	0.890
S	0.874	0.857	0.854	0.874	0.881	0.904	0.950	0.864
ΔH							0.954	0.874
Ac							0.920	
R^2	0.858	0.932	0.916	0.941	0.944	0.923	0.854	
T_c							0.910	
P_c							0.987	
V_c		*		0.822	0.769	*	0.703	
MR							0.995	
ρ							0.991	

5. Path Matrices -- Branching Revisited

All hitherto mentioned matrices had as matrix elements numerical entries, except for the Spialter's alpha-numeric matrix [38] in which the diagonal entries are atomic labels, while off-diagonal entries indicate the connectivity. The path matrix can be viewed as a special case of even more general graph matrix built from subgraphs as its elements. In the case of path matrices all the subgraphs are the shortest paths between the corresponding vertices, hence its matrix elements are non numerical quantities. Such matrices were introduced by Randić, Plavšić and Razinger [49] in an effort to arrive at novel structural invariants for use in the structure-property regression analysis. Their article outlining the path matrices was entitled "Double Invariants," because they lead to two choices in construction of a novel invariant: (1) one has the liberty to select a particular invariant of the subgraphs when constructing numerical form for the matrix elements; (2) After arriving at a numerical matrix one can select a particular matrix invariants as a descriptor. Moreover, for the most general case one could add that one has a possibility even to select a kind of subgraphs that form the matrix elements of these generalized matrices; and then proceed with the choices listed above.

If we select as subgraphs the shortest paths between vertices i and j we obtain the "Path matrix" of a graph. In Table 7 we show the path matrix for 3-methylheptane, and in Fig. 11 we show graphically elements of path matrices of several cyclic graphs as reported in ref. [49]. To avoid possible confusion, let us mention that label "path matrix" has been used also by Diudea and collaborators for a non symmetrical matrix in which the elements above the main diagonal count the number of the shortest paths between two vertices while the corresponding entry below the main diagonal indicates the number of the longest paths between the same pair of vertices.

Table 7

Path matrix

0	p_1	p_2	p_3	p_4	p_5	p_6	p_3
p_1	0	p_1	p_2	p_3	p_4	p_5	p_2
p_2	p_1	0	p_1	p_2	p_3	p_4	p_1
p_3	p_2	p_1	0	p_1	p_2	p_3	p_2
p_4	p_3	p_2	p_1	0	p_1	p_2	p_3
p_5	p_4	p_3	p_2	p_1	0	p_1	p_4
p_6	p_5	p_4	p_3	p_2	p_1	0	p_5
p_3	p_2	p_1	p_2	p_3	p_4	p_5	0

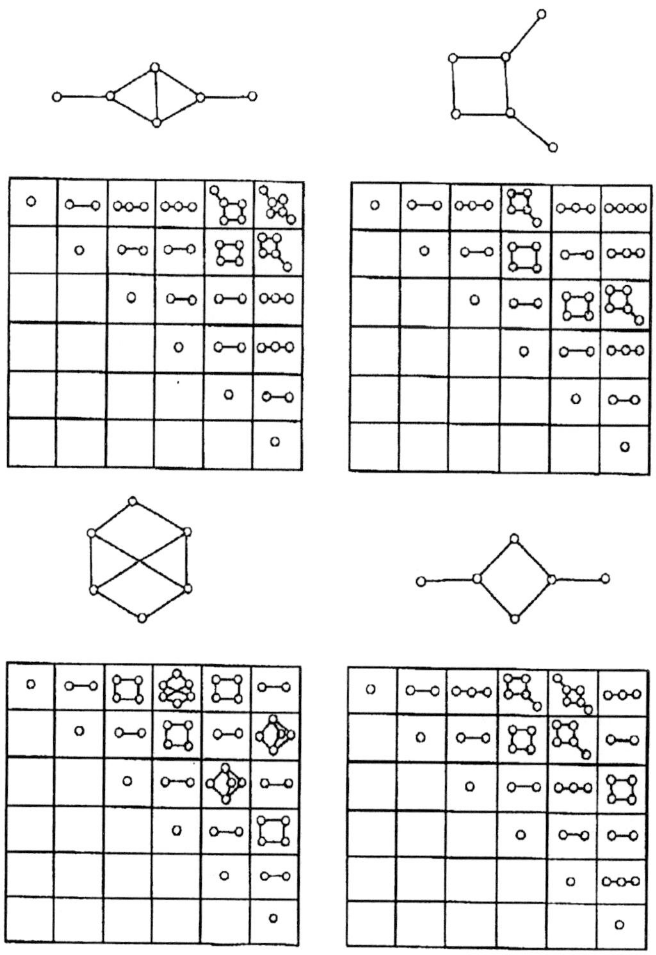

Figure 11

For trees there is only one path between any two vertices, hence, the elements of the path matrices are paths p_k or length k. If we select the leading eigenvalue of path p_k as the invariant of choice and replace each path subgraph by its leading eigenvalue we obtain the corresponding numerical matrix [49, 50, 54, 55]. In Table 8 we show the numerical matrix for 3-methylheptane derived by replacing p_k entries with the leading eigenvalues of the corresponding path (listed in Table 9). Thus entry p_1 is replaced by 1 because the leading eigenvalue of p_1 is 1. Similarly the entry p_2 is replaced by 2, the leading eigenvalue of path of length two. In Table 9 we listed the leading eigenvalues of longer paths that are needed when considering numerical path matrices of larger systems.

Table 8

0	1	1.41421	1.61803	1.73205	1.80194	1.84776	1.61803
	0	1	1.41421	1.61803	1.73205	1.80194	1.41421
		0	1	1.41421	1.61803	1.73205	1
			0	1	1.41421	1.61803	1.41421
				0	1	1.41421	1.61803
					0	1	1.73205
						0	1
							0

Table 9

path	eigenvalue
1	1
2	1.41421356
3	1.61803399
4	1.73205081
5	1.80193774
6	1.84775907
7	1.87938524
8	1.90211303
9	1.91898595
10	1.93185165
11	1.94188363
12	1.94985582
13	1.95629520
14	1.96157056
15	1.96594620

Let us label the leading eigenvalue of such path matrix as $\lambda\lambda_1$, to remind us that the elements of the matrix itself are the leading eigenvalues of paths occurring between pair of vertices. The leading eigenvalue of path matrices for 18 octane isomers are shown in

Fig. 12 on the (p_2, p_3) grid. First, observe that all the leading eigenvalues $\lambda\lambda_1$ are distinct, which was not the case with the leading eigenvalues of the adjacency matrix that Lovasz and Pelikan proposed as an index of branching. Neither is unique the Wiener number W, which Bonchev and Trinajstić [56] used as guide in their attempt to derived rules for characterization of molecular branching. Calculation of the leading eigenvalue for nonane and decane trees similarly has not revealed any pair of isomers having duplicate leading eigenvalue $\lambda\lambda_1$[55]. This in itself is of some significance because many common topological indices have degeneracy already for trees having eight or less carbon atoms. It remains to be seen whether lack of degeneracy so far observed will hold when larger trees are examined [57].

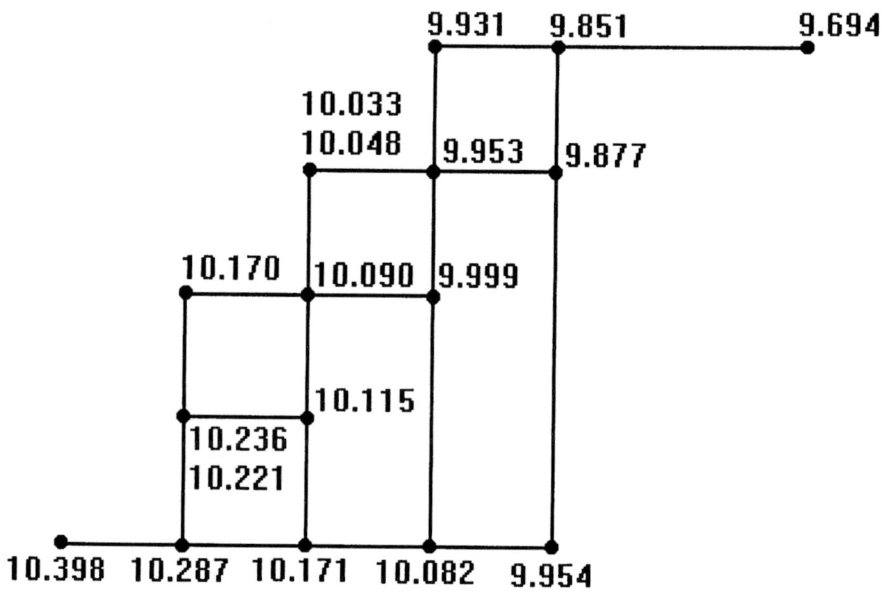

Figure 12

A correlation between $\lambda\lambda_1$ and λ_1, the leading eigenvalue of the path matrix and the leading eigenvalue of the adjacency matrix, shows considerable parallelism between the two invariants (Fig. 13). The regression coefficient is 0.9820 and the Fisher ratio is 377.5, which is a high value when one consider isomers of any structure. On the basis of this correlation we can indeed interpret $\lambda\lambda_1$ as a "novel" branching index. Advantage of $\lambda\lambda_1$ against λ_1 as a branching index is that now there are no degeneracies, hence there is no need to consider special rules to resolve ambiguities arising when two structures have the same leading eigenvalue λ_1 or the same Wiener index W.

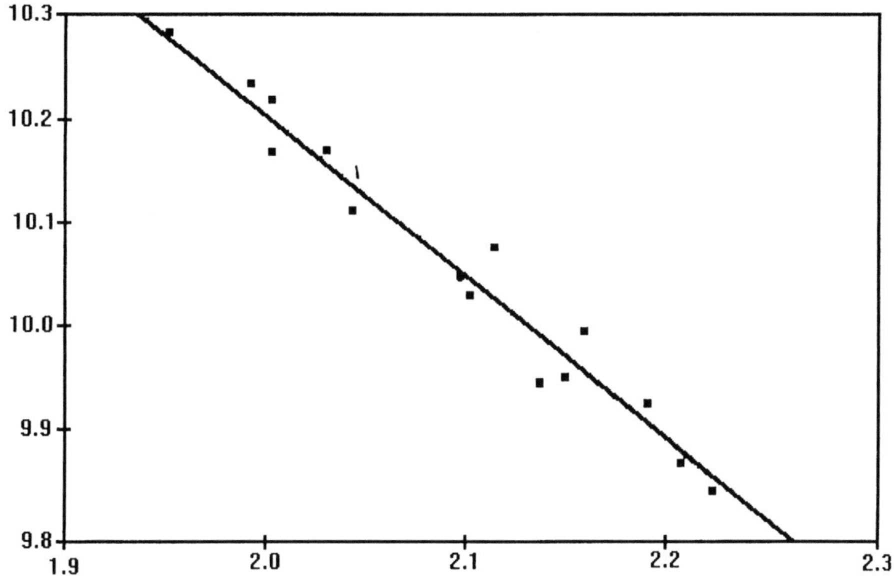

Figure 13

How well can the leading eigenvalue of path matrices serve as molecular descriptor in structure-property-activity correlations? Does the new descriptor, $\lambda\lambda_1$, lead to some good correlations? In Table 10, again for octane isomers, we have collected results of regressions for motor octane numbers (MON) based on several different descriptors. In the upper part of the table are the results based on linear regression model, while the lower part summarizes the results based on quadratic regression model. As we see from Table 10 the connectivity index as a single descriptor for octane motor numbers shows limited ability. The zero order connectivity index (that Kier introduced in extending the concept of the connectivity indices [58]) shows a somewhat better performance. The leading eigenvalue of the adjacency matrix λ_1, and the Balaban's J index, perform slightly better. However, the leading eigenvalue of the path matrix, $\lambda\lambda_1$, and the Wiener index, W, are still better, the Wiener index being the best. The coefficient of the regression is r = 0.957 and the standard error becomes s = 7.40.

By introducing some "corrective" steps, which effectively amounts to use of two descriptors rather then having a single descriptor, Kirby [59] reported for the same property of octanes regression with the regression coefficient above 0.977. One of Kirby's regression even has r = 0.994, but we could not reproduce this particular result from the given information. If we use two descriptors for correlation of motor octane numbers we also see improvement in the results. For example, by using the zero order and the first order connectivity indices, $^0\chi$ and $^1\chi$, respectively, one obtains for the correlation of the octane numbers r = 0.9591 and s = 7.5 [50].

Table 10. Correlations of MON

	r	s	F
Linear Model			
$^{1}\chi$	0.780	16.01	
$^{0}\chi$	0.913	10.40	
λ	0.925	9.07	
J	0.928	9.52	
$\lambda\lambda_1$	0.954	7.65	
W	0.957	7.40	
Quadratic Model			
λ	0.9648	6.98	87.4
I_D	0.9689	6.56	99.5
W	0.9711	6.33	107.5
$\lambda\lambda_1$	0.9891	3.91	292.1

By use of quadratic regression rather than linear regression one obtains much better statistical results, all listed in the lower part of Table 10. The best is the quadratic regression based on the leading eigenvalue $\lambda\lambda_1$, shown in Fig. 14. It is interesting to observe that while for linear model W is slightly better than $\lambda\lambda_1$ when we go to quadratic model the opposite is the case. Moreover, the regression based on quadratic $\lambda\lambda_1$ is visibly better than the corresponding quadratic regression based on the Wiener number.

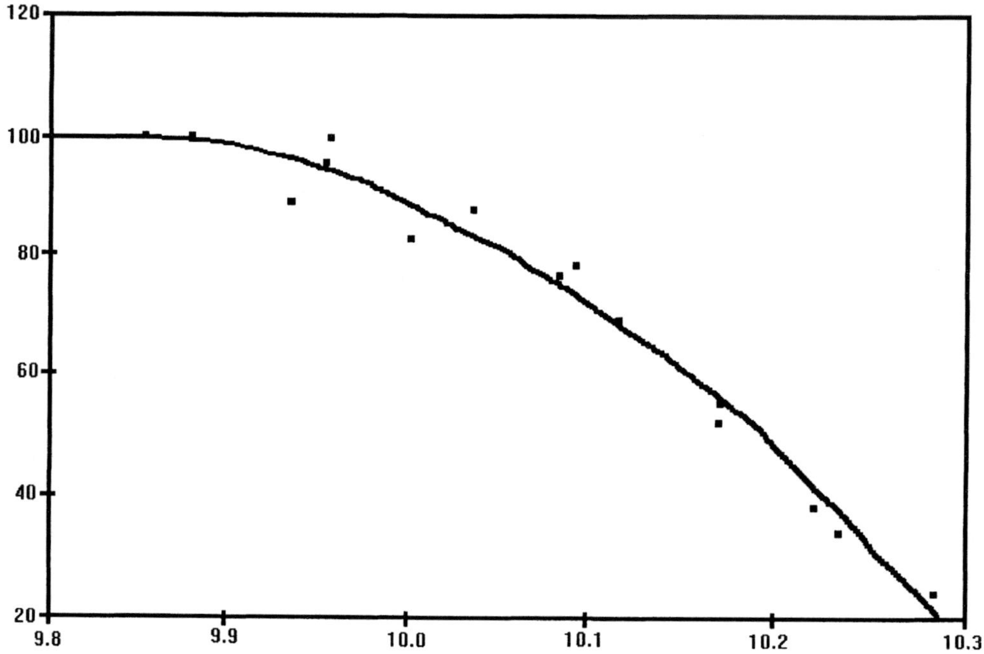

Figure 14

6. D/D MATRICES

Consider graphs of Fig. 15, all assumed to be embedded on a graphite lattice. For embedded graphs, which have rigid geometry, one can construct the geometric distance matrix, the matrix elements of which are defined so that element i, j represents the Euclidean distance between the vertices (atoms) i and j. In Table 11 (top part) we show the adjacency matrices for the three graphs of Fig. 15 by assuming that the length all edges is equal to 1. The last two graphs of Fig. 15 both represent a chain have necessarily identical adjacency matrix. In the middle part of Table 11 we give the graph theoretical distance matrix for the three graphs of Fig. 15. Again, the matrices of the last two graphs are the same, because the two graphs are acyclic and posses the same distance relationships. Finally, at the bottom of Table 11 we show the Euclidean distance matrices for all three structures. Now the first two graphs have identical matrix, because through space distance between any pair of vertices in the first structure (benzene ring) is precisely the same as through space (Euclidean) distance in the second graph (folded chain). The fact that the pair (1, 6) is in one structure adjacent and in the other at maximal through bond separation does not change the fact that they are at the same Euclidean distance.

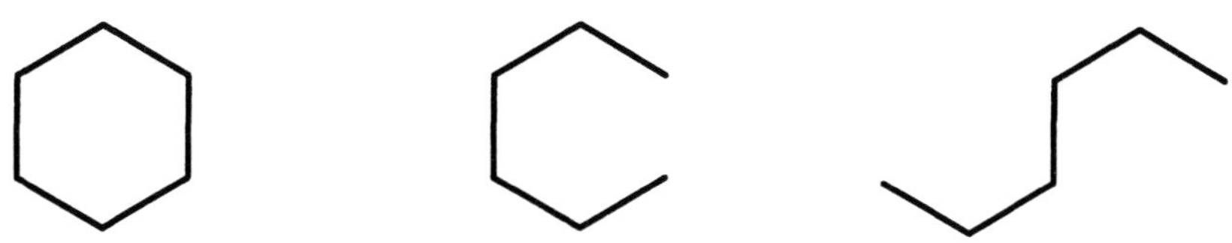

Figure 15

As we see from the illustration given neither the Euclidean distance matrix nor the graph theoretical distance matrix have preserved all the information of interest in molecular modeling. The former lacks the information on the connectivity, the later is devoid of the information on the 3-dimensional geometry. It would be useful to combine the information on the geometry with the information on the connectivity in a single matrix, and this is possible: The answer is D/D matrices [44].

The D/D matrix is constructed from the matrix elements of the Euclidean distance matrix and the matrix elements of the graph theoretical distance matrix by considering the quotients of the corresponding entries as an element of the new matrix. In Table 12 we show the D/D matrix for the three embedded graphs of Fig. 15. As we see all the three D/D matrices are different. Hence, D/D matrices can differentiate among distinct molecular geometries and at the same time they will discriminate structures of different connectivity. Clearly, because the Euclidean distance (or through-space distance) is always smaller, or at most equal to, the graph theoretical distance (or through-bond distance) for any two vertices all the entry of a D/D matrix are smaller than one, or at most equal to one.

Table 11

Adjacency matrix

0	1	0	0	0	1
1	0	1	0	0	0
0	1	0	1	0	0
0	0	1	0	1	0
0	0	0	1	0	1
1	0	0	0	1	0

0	1	0	0	0	0
1	0	1	0	0	0
0	1	0	1	0	0
0	0	1	0	1	0
0	0	0	1	0	1
0	0	0	0	1	0

0	1	0	0	0	0
1	0	1	0	0	0
0	1	0	1	0	0
0	0	1	0	1	0
0	0	0	1	0	1
0	0	0	0	1	0

Graph Theoretical Distance matrix

0	1	2	3	2	1
1	0	1	2	3	2
2	1	0	1	2	3
3	2	1	0	1	2
2	3	2	1	0	1
1	2	3	2	1	0

0	1	2	3	4	5
1	0	1	2	3	4
2	1	0	1	2	3
3	2	1	0	1	2
4	3	2	1	0	1
5	4	3	2	1	0

0	1	2	3	4	5
1	0	1	2	3	4
2	1	0	1	2	3
3	2	1	0	1	2
4	3	2	1	0	1
5	4	3	2	1	0

Euclidean Distance matrix

0	1	3	2	3	1
1	0	1	3	2	3
3	1	0	1	3	2
2	3	1	0	1	3
3	2	3	1	0	1
1	3	2	3	1	0

0	1	3	2	3	1
1	0	1	3	2	3
3	1	0	1	3	2
2	3	1	0	1	3
3	2	3	1	0	1
1	3	2	3	1	0

0	1	3	2	3	13
1	0	1	3	7	3
3	1	0	1	3	2
2	3	1	0	1	3
3	7	3	1	0	1
13	3	2	3	1	0

While, as we have seen, D/D matrices have desired properties concerning characterization of geometrical and topological molecular features this alone is not enough to qualify such entities as "of interest" for structure-property-activity studies. The final, and the only relevant, criterion of importance in QSAR is usefulness of such matrices in structure-property-activity regressions. This is and this remains also the ultimate criterion for justification of introducing of novel topological indices in molecular modeling and QSAR. However, there are two additional hurdles to cross before such innovations, as the new graph matrices, and the D/D matrices in particular, may become of interest in QSAR: (1) How to find and how to select structural invariants from such matrices that may be of interest in QSAR and (2) What is structural interpretation of the so introduced invariants, if any, that may be of interest in molecular model building.

Table 12

Benzene

0	1	3/2	2/3	3/2	1
	0	1	3/2	2/3	3/2
		0	1	3/2	2/3
			0	1	3/2
				0	1
					0

Hexatriene bent

0	1	3/2	2/3	3/4	1/5
	0	1	3/2	2/3	3/4
		0	1	3/2	2/3
			0	1	3/2
				0	1
					0

Hexatriene extended

0	1	3/2	2/3	3/4	13/5
	0	1	3/2	7/3	3/4
		0	1	3/2	2/3
			0	1	3/2
				0	1
					0

Because of the great importance of interpretation of the results of regression analysis, and other data reduction techniques, before we continue with an outline of use of D/D matrices in structure-property-activity studies we will address the issue of interpretation of molecular descriptors.

7. On the Interpetation of Molecular Descriptors

Strange as it may sound, while there is an explosion of novel molecular descriptors, and continued interest in developing additional ones, apparently, there has been little effort made during all this time in trying to illuminate their structural interpretation. Even the structural interpretation of one of the oldest topological index, the Wiener index, is far from accomplished. Platt [60] was first to recognize the importance of the Wiener number W (and was first to refer to W as the Wiener number), tried to propose an interpretation of W. He argued that W is a quantity that parallels or reflects to considerable extent molecular volume. Many publications and many applications were focused on the Wiener number over the past many years since the emergence of W and we are hardly closer to its interpretation then was Platt 50 years ago! A special issue of both, Discrete Applied Mathematics [61] and MATCH (Communication in Mathematical Chemistry) [62] were devoted to the Wiener number on the occasion of 50-th anniversary of the paper of Harry Wiener but no contribution concerning the meaning of Wiener numbers was considered.

The search for structural *interpretation* of a descriptor should not be confused with structural *definition* of a descriptor. All mathematical descriptors are, as a rule, *well defined,* otherwise they would not qualify as mathematical! They are constructed usually by manipulating selected structural elements, hence, their definition is clearly based on structural elements. But by combining elements one can create quantities , the immediate interpretation of which became obscured. Consider in parallel elementary algebra, which is based on simple mathematical operations -- yet their combination results in endless forms, the interpretation of which could become cumbersome! E. g., while the formula for the roots of the quadratic equation is simple, involving the discriminate as a useful descriptor, already the Cardano formula for the roots of the cubic equation is more involved and less ready for interpretation.

The Wiener number W can be defined as the sum of all through-bond or graph theoretical distance in a molecule, but that does not explain what this quantity represents in terms of structural concepts. The situation was similar with the leading eigenvalue of the adjacency matrix λ_1. Clearly, from the mathematical point of view there could be no simpler interpretation: diagonalization of a matrix represents a similarity transformation in which eigenvectors of a matrix serve as the basis vectors for the vector space considered, and consequently matrix adopts a diagonal form. But do the eigenvalues have some recognizable structural interpretation? As we have seen, according to Lovasz and Pelikan [27], in the case of trees they can be viewed as a branching index.

As one can infer from the above discussion we consider an "interpretation" as something expressed in the already *known* structural concepts. Suppose, for a moment, that we have an acceptable structural interpretation of the Wiener number. Then, if we succeed to "explain" another, more involved construction, such as for example, the hyper-Wiener number, in terms of the Wiener number we could say that we arrived at structural interpretation of the more complex invariant. Hence, (1) interpretation of topological indices and other mathematical descriptors require acceptance of some structural concept as *elementary*, and (2) interpretation may vary with time as the number of *elementary invariants* used as the basis for interpretation of others may also vary, if new structural concepts become recognized as elementary.

Randić and Zupan [63] have recently raised the question of interpretation of structural invariants and mathematical descriptors. They have selected as the most elementary structural concepts *paths* and *walks*, assumed as well understood and as the simplest components of a structure. By considering weights for paths and edges one immediately obtains powerful tool for characterization of many more involved structural components. Using such approach Randić and Zupan then continued with interpretation of the three well known and widely used molecular descriptors in terms of weighted paths or edges: the connectivity index $^1\chi$, the Wiener index W, and the Hosoya index Z.

An edge can be considered as a path of length one or a walk of length one. In Fig. 16 we show partitioning of the connectivity index, the Wiener number, and the Hosoya's index for 3-methylheptane in terms of weighted paths (edges). We can now arrived at structural interpretation of these three descriptors in terms of weighted paths. In the case of the connectivity index and the Hosoya's Z index, as can be seen from Fig. 16, the terminal edges (i. e., C-CH_3; C-CH_2; and C-CH) have greater weights than the internal edges (such as -CH_2-CH_2-). The situation is opposite with the Wiener number! This may be one of the reasons why interpretation of W remains elusive. It is not that W could not be partitioned, but that the contributions so arrived at appear counterintuitive. Perhaps this should not be surprising after all, since W is based on the topological distance matrix and the distance matrix itself is counterintuitive. It has large entries between vertices (atoms) at the large separations while the opposite is expected for realistic models of chemical structure. A distance matrix in which to elements corresponding to longer distances one assigns smaller numerical values would better reflect the actual interactions between atoms within a molecule. In fact, several authors considered invariants constructed from matrices in which the reciprocal distances were used for matrix elements [64]. An alternative that has a similar effect is to reverse the assignment of the weights for bonds when constructing graph distance matrix and give the largest weights to bonds at shorter distance [48].

We should mentioned that Lukovits [65] was among first to consider partitioning of Wiener number for various benzenoids into bond contributions. However, as we see from Fig. 16 we are no closer to a better understanding of the physical significance of the Wiener number now with W partitioned to bond contributions them we were when viewing W as a global molecular descriptor. On the other hand the connectivity index $^1\chi$ and the Hosoya index Z can be understood as bond-additive quantities in which the external bonds play more prominent role. This is consistent with our notion of molecular surface where also external bonds make larger contributions merely by being more exposed. Hence, one may expect that the connectivity index and the Z index will be useful descriptors for molecular properties that are characterized by surface, such as the boiling points.

Connectivity index χ
$\chi = 3.681$

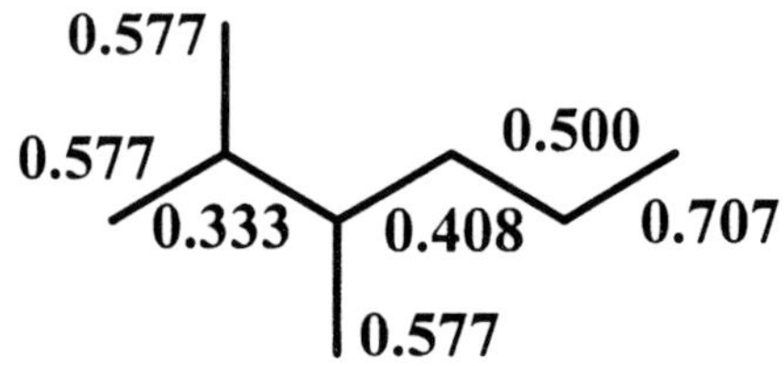

Wiener index W
W = 70

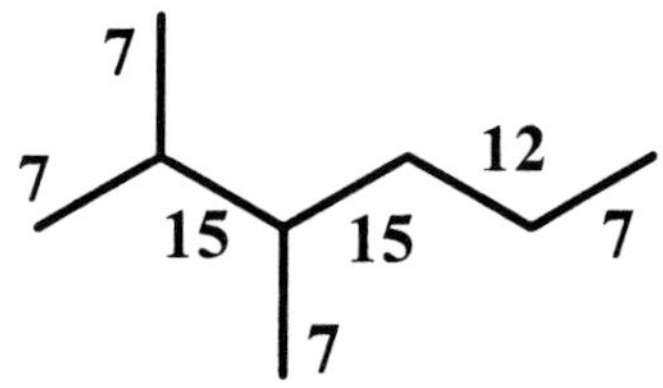

Hosoya Z index
Z = 26 + 1 = 27

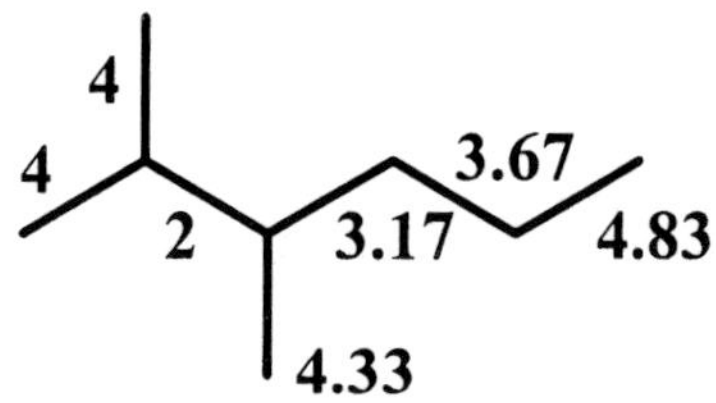

Figure 16

How and why W is also good descriptors for the same surface-dependent properties? The answer may lie in often overlooked aspect of regression analyses -- regression does not signify a cause/effect relationship, it merely points to a parallelism of the quantity considered. If, for all the molecules considered, W correlates well with another molecular descriptor, say M, then not only that structural interpretation of M can tell us something about W, but one can argue in reverse and claim that W is good descriptor precisely because it correlates with M (for which we will assume to have adequate structural interpretation in terms of elementary concepts, paths and walks). This is precisely what has been shown to be the case for octane isomers. Instead of considering W, which can be written as a sum of weighted paths:

$$W = 1 \cdot p_1 + 2 \cdot p_2 + 3 \cdot p_3 + 4 \cdot p_4 + 5 \cdot p_5 + 6 \cdot p_6 + 7 \cdot p_7$$

Randić [48] considered an alternative index M defined as:

$$W = 7 \cdot p_1 + 6 \cdot p_2 + 5 \cdot p_3 + 4 \cdot p_4 + 3 \cdot p_5 + 2 \cdot p_6 + 1 \cdot p_7$$

in which the magnitudes of the weights were reversed. Somewhat unexpectedly the two indices, W and M not only that correlate well, but they are strictly collinear! Hence, one can argue, W is good descriptor because M is good descriptor, and M assigns to vertices at larger distances smaller weight.

The concepts of paths and walks are among the first defined in any text on graph theory. A number of structural concepts are directly or indirectly defined using combinations of paths and walks. These include hamiltonian cycles, Kekulé valence structures, conjugated circuits, the characteristic polynomial and the matching polynomial, the complexity, etc. Considerable attention has been given to paths [66] and walks [67] in chemical literature.

8. Leading Eigenvalue of D/D Matrices -- Folding

We will examine use of the leading eigenvalue of the D/D matrices as molecular descriptor. In Fig. 17 we show all conformers of C_8H_{10} embedded on a graphite lattice. In Table 13 we have listed normalized leading eigenvalues of different conformers of C_8H_{10}. Visual inspection of the figure and the table shows that structures that are more folded have a smaller leading eigenvalue while those that are more extended have a larger leading eigenvalue. This kind of observation prompted Randić, Kleiner and DeAlba [44] to interpret the leading eigenvalue of the D/D matrix as an index of folding of a structure.

The leading eigenvalue of the D/D matrix can be correlated with the first moment for the structures considered. The first moment is defined by the sum of the distances of all atoms (vertices) from the center of molecule. Recall that the second moment is similarly defined by the sum of the squares of the distances of all atoms from the center of molecule, and represents for planar molecules the moment of inertia around the axis perpendicular to the molecular plane. For molecules with the center of symmetry the calculation of moments is not difficult, for more general cases one has, using an arbitrary Cartesian coordinate system first to find the center of molecule, and then to calculate using the coordinates of the center and the coordinates of all the vertices the corresponding moments. Because the moments depend only on the coordinates of points considered, and not on the connectivity, that is whether there is a bond between two points or not, we find that TTCCC and CTCCC conformations have exactly the same first (or any) moment, (printed in Table 13 as bold).

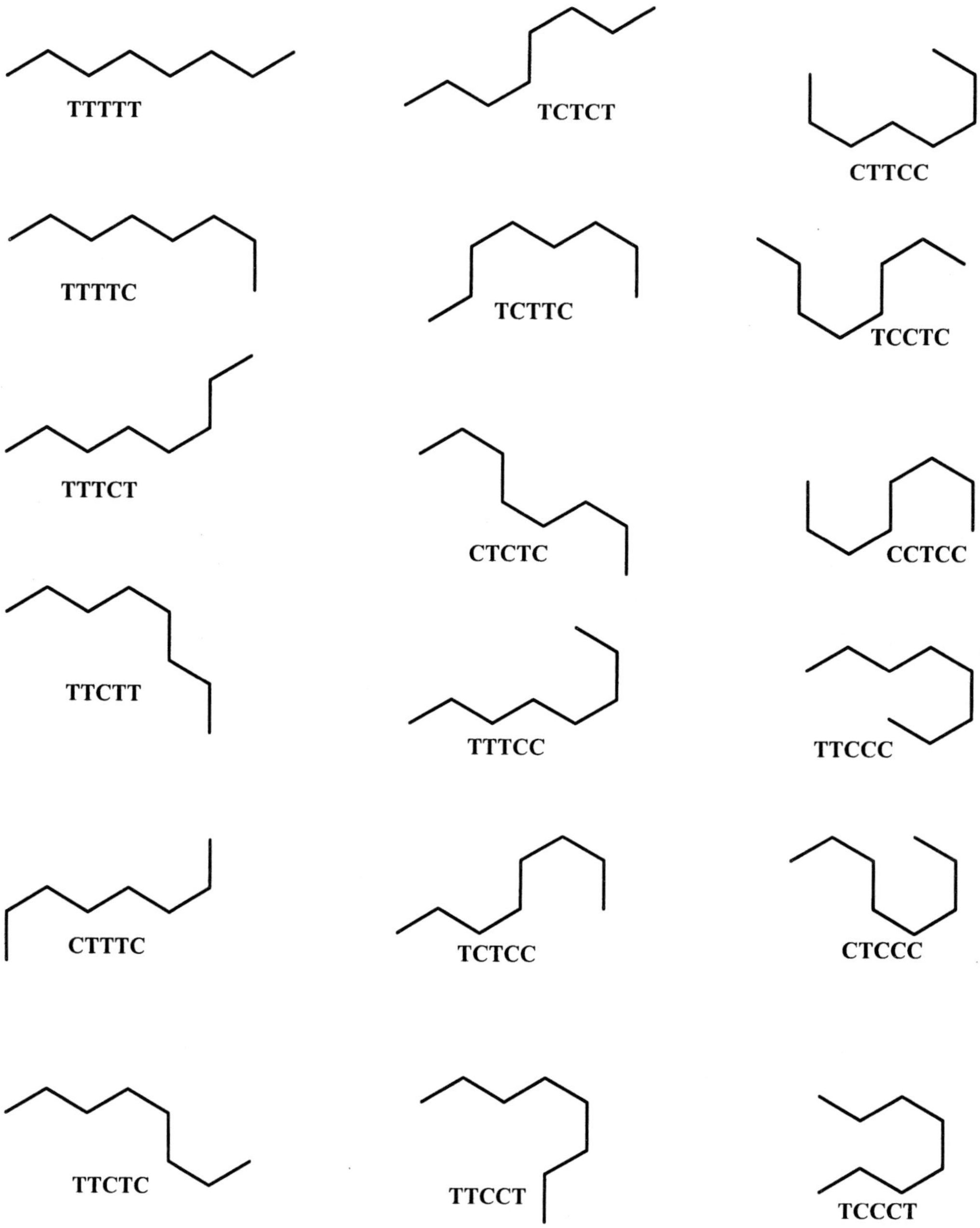
TTTTT
TCTCT
CTTCC
TTTTC
TCTTC
TCCTC
TTTCT
CTCTC
CCTCC
TTCTT
TTTCC
TTCCC
CTTTC
TCTCC
CTCCC
TTCTC
TTCCT
TCCCT

Figure 17

Table 13

Conformer	Normalized D/D matrix leading eigenvalue	Normalized Line Adjacency leading eigenvalue	First moment
TTTTT	0.7903	0.8571	14.08741
TTTTC	0.7695	0.7191	13.56574
TTTCT	0.7613	0.5916	13.25778
TTCTT	0.7541	0.5208	13.29150
CTTTC	0.7506	0.5858	13.00465
TTCTC	0.7451	0.4688	13.01638
TCTCT	0.7448	0.4019	12.81907
TCTTC	0.7365	0.4748	12.69023
CTCTC	0.7336	0.3836	12.66945
TTTCC	0.7250	0.5793	11.97183
TCTCC	0.7112	0.3773	11.77755
TTCCT	0.7021	0.4464	11.53252
CTTCC	0.6997	0.4533	11.36715
TCCTC	0.6966	0.3538	11.46839
CCTCC	0.6786	0.3375	10.85685
TTCCC	0.6654	0.4426	**10.02216**
CTCCC	0.6587	**0.3347**	**10.02216**
TCCCT	0.6472	**0.3347**	9.56493

Obviously more folded molecules will have smaller moments since then atoms are at shorter distances from the center of the molecule. Thus one anticipates that the first moment will correlate with the folding index derived from the first eigenvalue of D/D matrix. That this is indeed the case can be seen from Fig. 18 in which we have correlated for the 18 structures of Fig. 17 their first moment against the computed folding index. The correlation coefficient r = 0.9934, the standard error of estimate s = 0.15 and the Fisher ratio F = 1277.

In order to avoid "surprises" further testing is essential before the suggestion that normalized leading eigenvalue qualifies and should be accepted as the folding index of a structure. Several mathematical curves displaying different degrees of folding have therefore been examined [68]. In Fig. 19 we show a spiral embedded on Cartesian coordinate grid, Hilbert curve, Peano curve, and Knuth curve, all displaying different pattern of folding [69]. In addition one could add a zig-zag curve of Buckminster Fuller [70] (Fig. 20), which has a simple structure and for which one can derive upper and low bound for the leading eigenvalue for the limiting structure when size of curve increased to infinity. In Table 14 are listed for the above mentioned mathematical curves the normalized leading eigenvalues λ_1/n as a function of the size. Because λ_1 increases with the size of a matrix we have to scale down the size dependence, hence: λ_1/n is taken as the folding index.

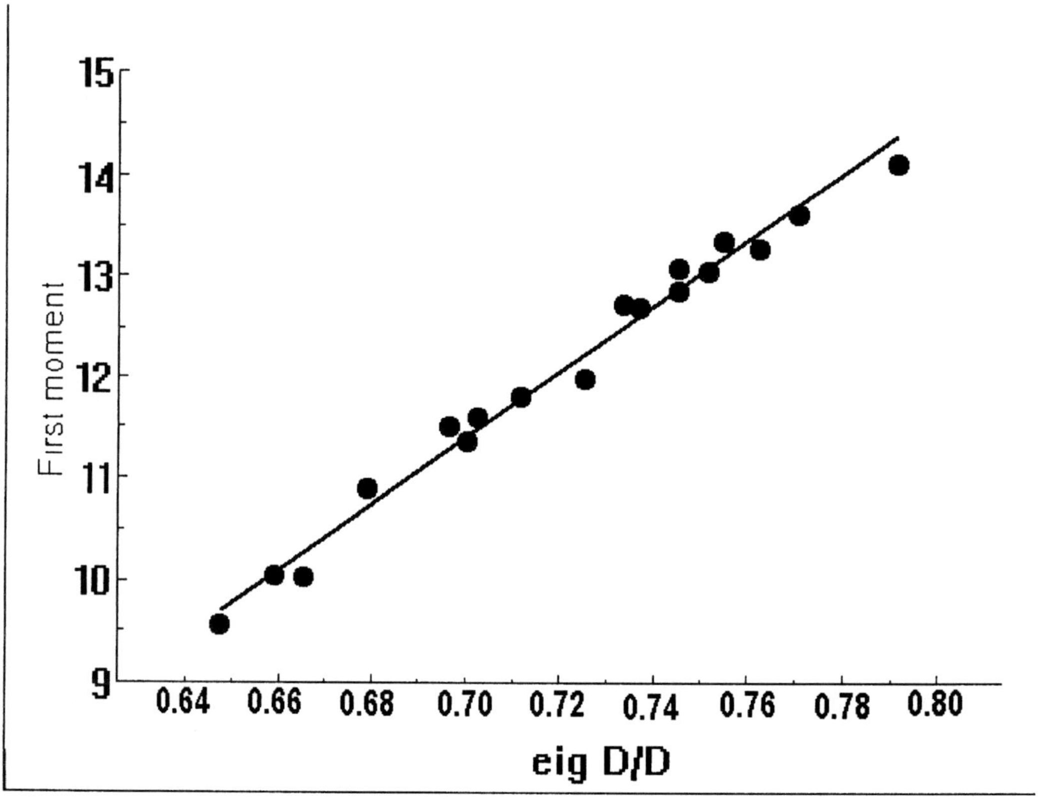

Figure 18

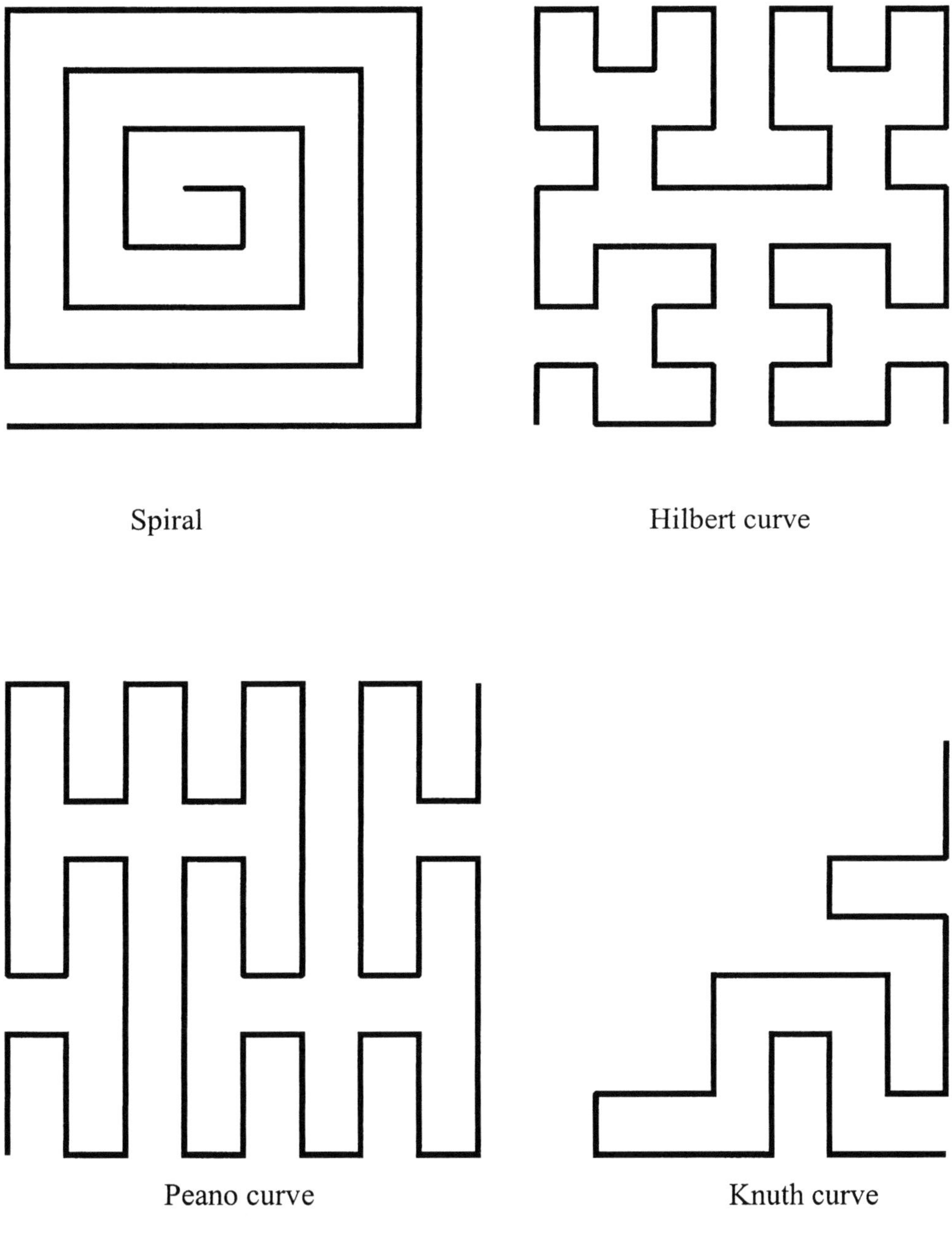

Figure 19

Table 14

Conformer	eigenvalue	Conformer	eigenvalue
TTTTT	0.8571	**TCTTC**	0.4748
TTTTC	0.7191	**TCTCT**	0.4018
		TCTCC	0.3773
TTTTC	0.7191	**TCCTC**	0.3538
TTTCT	0.5916	**TCCCT**	0.3347
TTCTT	0.5208	**CTTTC**	0.5858
TTCTC	0.4688	**CTTCC**	0.4533
TTCCT	0.4464	**CTCCC**	0.3347
TTCCC	0.4426		
		CCTTT	0.5793
		CCTTC	0.4533
		CCTCT	0.3773
		CCTCC	0.3375

The major conclusions to be extracted from the study of mathematical curves (like those of Fig. 19 and data of Table 14) is that our intuitive ideas of foldedness are confirmed by the numerical values of the leading eigenvalues of considered curves. That λ_1/n decreases as curves increase is to be expected because the row sums in the D/D matrices, which give an upper and the lower bound on the leading eigenvalue increase very slowly. The apparently most folded among the considered cases, the Hilbert curve, is indeed associated with the smallest leading eigenvalue for curves of the same length. The next smallest leading eigenvalue belongs to the Knuth curve, which again appears more folded than the simple spiral of the same length or the Peano curve. A comparison of the leading eigenvalues of the spiral and the Peano curve shows some alternation in the relative magnitudes indicating some limitations of characterization when considering truncated curves. Inspection of Fig. 19 suggests that eventually Peano curve will show larger folding as n increases. As we see, the longest stretch of linear segments in the Peano curve are of limited size, while as the spiral continue to grow the length of linear segments of the spiral will increases indefinitely, suggesting very slow decrease of its normalized leading eigenvalue λ_1/n.

It is not difficult to conclude that for fully extended "straight" chain structure the folding index λ_1/n tends to 1 as n increases indefinitely. In contrast, without a more detailed analysis it is not clear whether in all cases (i.e., for any folded curve) as n increases the normalized leading values λ_1/n has finite limit or the limit is zero. In the case of zig-zag curve of Buckminster Fuller (Fig. 20) one can show that the limiting value of λ_1/n is small, but not zero.

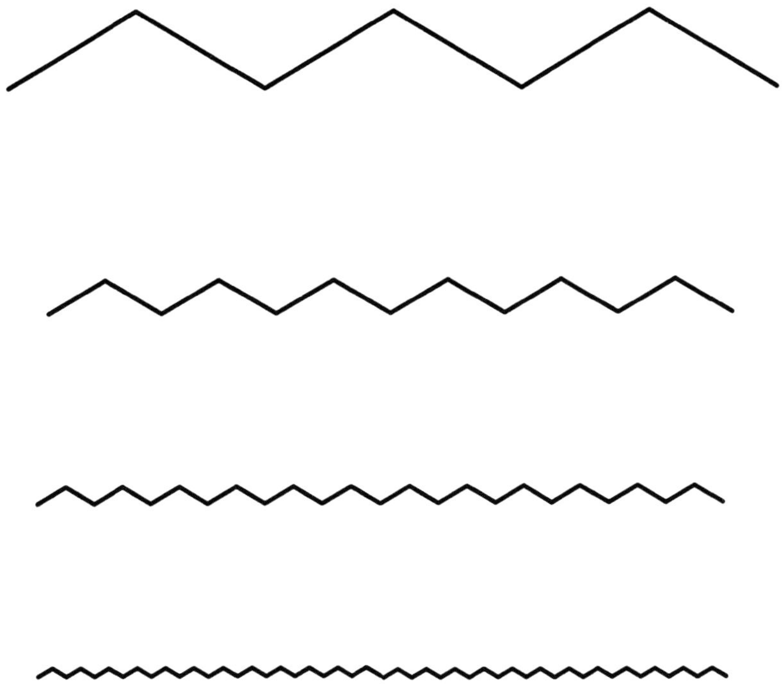

Figure 20

Table 15

	Spiral	Hilbert	Peano	Knuth
n=5	0.442864	0.369552	0.442864	0.512311
n=10	0.333861	0.237927	0.313206	0.278165
n=15	0.256300	0.159588	0.338181	0.224850
n=20	0.201004	0.123730	0.253739	0.176033
n=25	0.202867		0.203353	

9. Characterization of Folded Proteins

A single index, such as λ_1/n, can hardly be expected to offer sufficiently complete characterization of large, highly folded structures, such as DNA and proteins. Even already small folded structures, such as model proteins of Tang and coworkers [71] having only 27 units (amino acids), illustrated in Fig. 21, would be better characterized by a set of descriptors rather than by a single "folding" index. Visual inspection of Fig. 21, or even an inspection of the models made to correspond to the diagrams in the figure, would be of little help for quantitative considerations. However, recently Randić and Krilov [72] extended the considerations of the "folding" index and considered matrices $^kD/^kD$, derived from D/D matrices by raising each element of these matrices to k-th power. The approach is analogous to earlier extension of the topographic index of Randić and Razinger [71, 73] which has lead to sequence of descriptors, referred to as molecular profile [74], and shape profile [75], in which entries of a distance matrix were raised to increasing powers. In this way instead of a single descriptor one obtains a sequence, ^1D, ^2D, ^3D, ^4D, . . . which when suitably normalized offer better characterization of molecules. Initially only the distances between atoms were considered when constructing the ^3D distance matrices, but later the approach was extended by considering geometrical points along edges [72, 76], so that geometrical objects, such as cuboctahedron and twisted cuboctahedron could be differentiated [77]. Finally Randić and Krilov have extended the approach to molecular surfaces of arbitrary shape [78]. All these application have resulted in a sequence of structural invariants for the system considered, given by the average element of the corresponding ^kD matrix. This same approach can be extended to $^kD/^kD$ matrices. Instead of the average matrix element one can use the leading eigenvalue as the invariant of choice. As a result a single index, the leading eigenvalue λ_1/n is replaced by a sequence of indices $^1\lambda_1/n$, $^2\lambda_1/n$, $^3\lambda_1/n$, $^4\lambda_1/n$, . . . each successive number representing the normalized leading eigenvalue of the $^kD/^kD$ matrix obtained by increasing the exponent of the power k to which the elements are raised.

The infinite sequence $^1\lambda_1/n$, $^2\lambda_1/n$, $^3\lambda_1/n$, $^4\lambda_1/n$, . . . , where $^k\lambda_1/n$ signifies the leading eigenvalue of $^kD/^kD$ matrix, has introduced a conceptual, even if not computational, novelty in the characterization of (finite) structures: The question of convergence of such sequence. We have already seen one aspect of convergence when considering the spiral and Hilbert curve of ever increasing length. In other applications, including modeling of proteins, structures are not increasing in size indefinitely, but their mathematical characterization does. In practice, at least for molecules of intermediate size, it was observed that the first 15-20 powers of $^kD/^kD$ matrices suffice for characterization of a structure and that the sequence can be truncated after the leading 15-20 terms. Namely as the exponent k increases all the entries in a matrix steadily decrease except those having the value one. It is not difficult to see that as k tends to infinity all entries in $^kD/^kD$ matrices that are not equal to one will tend to zero. Hence, in the limit we obtain for $^kD/^kD$ a binary matrix with only zero and one as entries. The entry one will appear only next to the main diagonal and at adjacent places if the adjacent vertices are geometrically in line, because only then of Euclidean distance and graph theoretical distance are equal and their quotient equals 1. The limiting matrix has been referred to as the line adjacency matrix. If viewed as the adjacency matrix of a graph the matrix has been known in Graph Theory as Menger graph of a configuration [79).

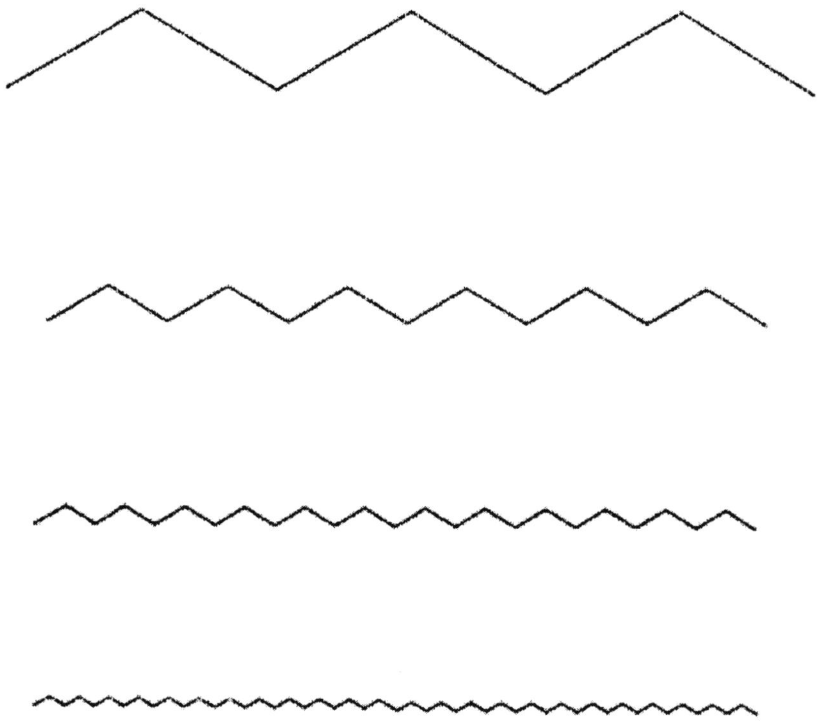

Figure 21

10. The Leading Eigenvalue of Line Adjacency Matrix -- Flexibility

In Table 13 under the heading "Normalized line adjacency leading eigenvalue" we listed the leading eigenvalues of the line adjacency matrix for the line graphs that one can associate with each of the conformer of Fig. 17. Line graph L(G) of graph G is defined as a graph in which edges in G become vertices of L(G), and the adjacency of new vertices is determined by incidence of the edges in G [30]. Two edges are said to be incident if they have a common vertex. Since the graphs of Fig. 17 are already embedded (on a graphite lattice) the constructed line graphs will also be embedded. In Fig. 22 we have depicted the embedded line graphs for the 18 conformers of Fig. 17 and above each diagram we indicated the length of the straight line segments present in the line graph. For example the last graph of Fig. 17, TCCCT, is associated with the line partitioning 2, 1, 1, 2, which signifies that it consists of two line segments of length two interrupted by two line segments of length one.

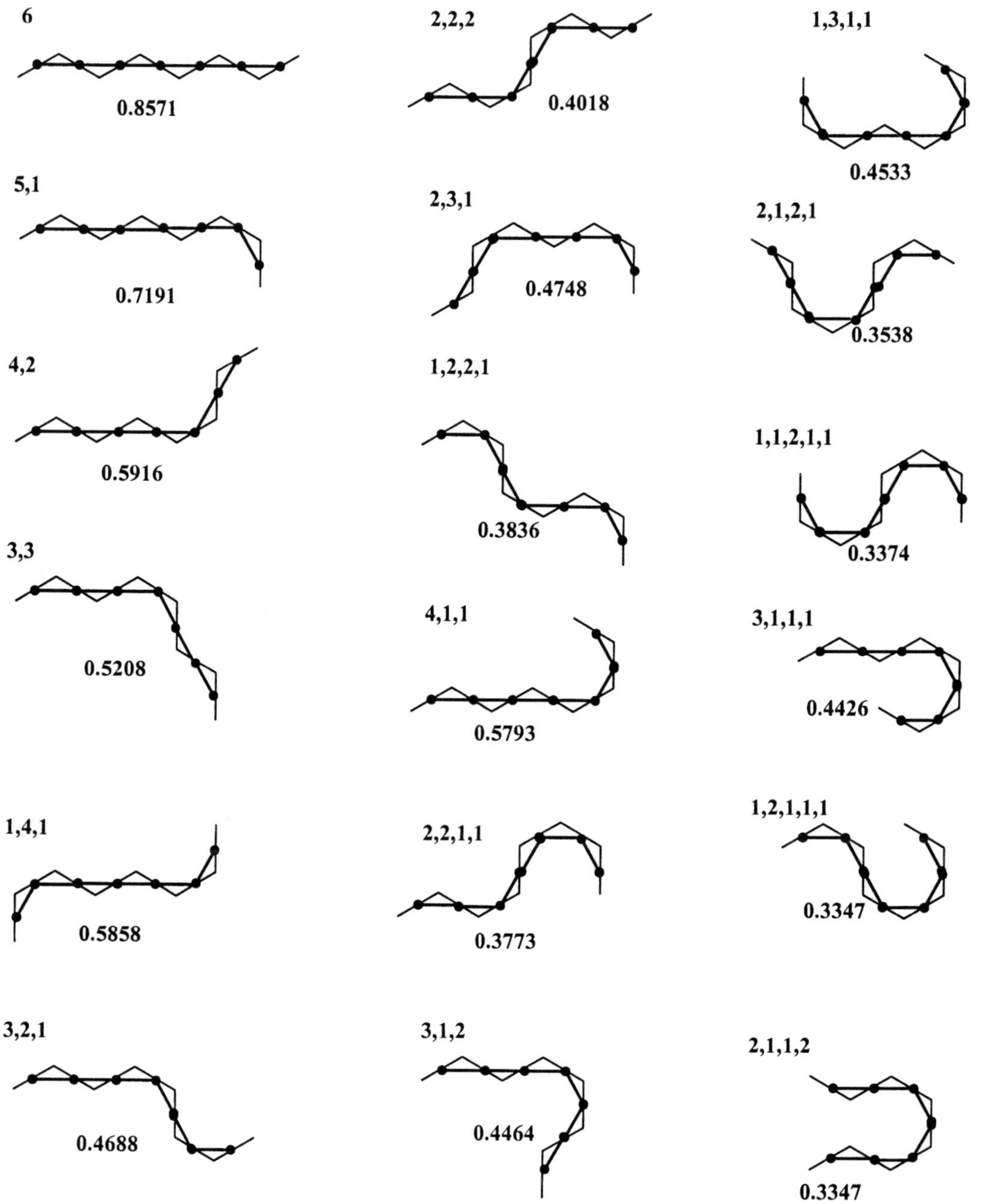

Figure 22

The line adjacency matrix is here defined for embedded graphs (i.e., graphs with rigid geometry). It appears as the augmented adjacency matrix in which besides the non zero entries for adjacent vertices also non zero entries appear whenever vertices are on the same geometrical line. Thus, for example, for TCCCT the line adjacency matrix is:

0	1	1	0	0	0
1	0	1	0	0	0
1	1	0	1	0	0
0	0	1	0	1	1
0	0	0	1	0	1
0	0	0	1	1	0

As we see the line adjacency matrix of (an embedded) graph is built from submatrices of the complete graphs K_n (n = 1, 2, 3 . . .) along the main diagonal.

It is interesting to observe from Fig. 22 that all 18 conformers of Fig. 17 have a different partitioning of the line segments in their line graphs. This is a consequence of the fact that graphs are embedded on a graphite lattice where a change of direction of a line segments necessarily involves change of *cis* and *trans* labels.

A comparison of the two columns of Table 13, listing the normalized leading eigenvalues of D/D matrix and the normalized leading eigenvalue of the Line Adjacency matrix L, shows some parallelism between them. However, the parallelism is not as strong as has been the case between the leading eigenvalue of D/D matrix and the first moment. In several places there is significant departure in the respective relative magnitudes. For example, TCTTC and TTTCC both have values much larger than the structures listed immediately above or below them. This apparent irregularity is not accidental. The two quantities, the leading eigenvalue of D/D matrix and the leading eigenvalue of the Line Adjacency matrix, (which in fact is the limiting matrix of D^k/D^k as k), represent different molecular properties. The first gives an index of folding of a system and the second gives an index of flexibility of a structure.

That the eigenvalues of the Line Adjacency matrix also show regularity of their own can be seen from Table 14 in which we have grouped the embedded line graphs so that they have the same initial T and C labels. Because the five letter codes consisting of labels T and C can be read from the left to the right and also from the right to the left, the observed regularity that always *trans* isomer precede *cis* (other parts of the structures being the same) holds in both cases, as illustrated by the last group of conformers obtained by reversing the codes. As we see T label dominates C label, the corresponding eigenvalue is larger, and the corresponding structure can be viewed as more "stiff," or less "flexible." The assumption here is that molecule can flex only around joints in which the line segments end, while central parts of the line segments do not allow flexibility. This need not be the case with alkanes, or alkenes, but this seems to be a good model regarding the flexibility of nitrogen chains in diazoazides, already discussed in the literature using simple molecular orbital theory by Roberts [80]. Incidentally, the degeneracy, the two identical eigenvalues that appear for line matrices of CTCCC and TCCCT (see Table 13) have no apparent structural explanation so far. One needs additional cases of similar "accidental" degeneracy before attempting to find underlying structural factors causing the degeneracy.

In Table 16 we show the line adjacency matrix for truncated spiral of Fig. 19, containing first 17 points. As we see the matrix is built from overlapping blocks of increasing size that correspond to the line segments of the spiral and represent the adjacency matrices of the complete graphs K_n. Clearly, in view of this simple structural characteristics one can easily construct the limiting matrix D^k/D^k as k , by simply searching for line segments in a structure.

Table 16

Spiral

0	1	0	0	0	0	0	0	0	0	0	0	0	0	0	0	0
	0	1	0	0	0	0	0	0	0	0	0	0	0	0	0	0
		0	1	1	0	0	0	0	0	0	0	0	0	0	0	0
			0	1	0	0	0	0	0	0	0	0	0	0	0	0
				0	1	1	0	0	0	0	0	0	0	0	0	0
					0	1	0	0	0	0	0	0	0	0	0	0
						0	1	1	1	0	0	0	0	0	0	0
							0	1	1	0	0	0	0	0	0	0
								0	1	0	0	0	0	0	0	0
									0	1	1	1	0	0	0	0
										0	1	1	0	0	0	0
											0	1	0	0	0	0
												0	1	1	1	1
													0	1	1	1
														0	1	1
															0	1
																0

From the limiting matrix D/ D matrices we can calculate their leading eigenvalue, which reflects the pattern of folding of a curve in a somewhat different manner then is given by the D/D matrix or any of the ${}^kD/{}^kD$ matrices. From the form of the limiting matrix (the line-adjacency matrix) we can immediately deduce for example that Hilbert curves represents a more folded case, because, regardless the size of the Hilbert curve, the linking of self similar fragments in Hilbert curve introduces at most three vertices on a line, while as the spiral grows so does the number of vertices on a line segments grows without limit.

We should maintain a distinction between the description given by the leading eigenvalue of D/D matrix and the characterization given by the leading eigenvalue of the line adjacency matrix, the limiting form of D^k/D^k as k . The former, as has been stated before, gives an index of folding of a chain (polymer). That is not the case for the leading eigenvalue of the limiting matrix. Consider, for example, the eight graphs of Fig. 23, which all consist of linkage of identical segments, two of length one and three of length two, embedded on the Cartesian x, y grid. Clearly they show different patterns of folding, yet they all have the same line adjacency matrix, and hence the same limiting leading eigenvalue of ${}^kD/{}^kD$ matrix. It appears that the leading eigenvalue of the line-adjacency represents an index of molecular flexibility. The smaller is the leading eigenvalue of the line adjacency matrix the chain has more sites at which it can show flexibility. Chains having smaller leading eigenvalue also have more conformers when compared to chains of the same length associated with a greater leading eigenvalue. This follows from the fact that chains having fewer line segments will have more submatrices belonging to adjacency matrices of K_n, complete subgraphs, and will consequently have larger row sums. Matrices with larger row sums, as a rule, have large leading eigenvalue.

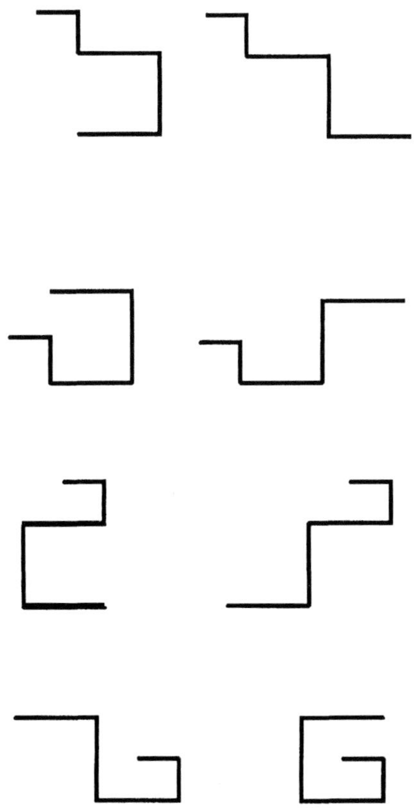

Figure 23

11. On Characterization of DNA

Table 17

Human beta globin (length 1424 bases)
ID HSHBB - Beta globin sequence extract
exons: **1-92**, **223-445**, **1296-1424**; introns: 93-222, 446-1295
SQ Hshbb.MK1 -- Segment from 62205 To 63628 of HSHBB

ATGGTGCACCTGACTCCTGAGGAGAAGTCTGCCGTTACTGCCCTGTG
GGGCAAGGTGAACGTGGATGAAGTTGGTGGTGAGGCCCTGGGCAGGTT
GGTATCAAGGTTACAAGACAGGTTTAAGGAGACCAATAGAAACTGGGCATG
TGGAGACAGAGAAGACTCTTGGGTTTCTGATAGGCACTGACTCTCTCTGCCTA
TTGGTCTATTTTCCCACCCTTAG**GCTGCTGGTGGTCTACCCTTGGACCCAG**
AGGTTCTTTGAGTCCTTTGGGGATCTGTCCACTCCTGATGCTGTTATGGG
CAACCCTAAGGTGAAGGCTCATGGCAAGAAAGTGCTCGGTGCCTTTAGT
GATGGCCTGGCTCACCTGGACAACCTCAAGGGCACCTTTGCCACACTGA
GTGAGCTGCACTGTGACAAGCTGCACGTGGATCCTGAGAACTTCAGGGT
GAGTCTATGGGACCCTTGATGTTTTCTTTCCCCTTCTTTTCTATGGTTAAGTTC
ATGTCATAGGAAGGGGAGAAGTAACAGGGTACAGTTTAGAATGGGAAACAG
ACGAATGATTGCATCAGTGTGGAAGTCTCAGGATCGTTTTAGTTTCTTTTATT
TGCTGTTCATAACAATTGTTTTCTTTTGTTTAATTCTTGCTTTCTTTTTTTTTCTT
CTCCGCAATTTTTACTATTATACTTAATGCCTTAACATTGTGTATAACAAAAG
GAAATATCTCTGAGATACATTAAGTAACTTAAAAAAAAACTTTACACAGTCT
GCCTAGTACATTACTATTTGGAATATATGTGTGCTTATTTGCATATTCATAATC
TCCCTACTTTATTTTCTTTTATTTTTAATTGATACATAATCATTATACATATTTA
TGGGTTAAAGTGTAATGTTTTAATATGTGTACACATATTGACCAAATCAGGGT
AATTTTGCATTTGTAATTTTAAAAAATGCTTTCTTCTTTTAATATACTTTTTTGT
TTATCTTATTTCTAATACTTTCCCTAATCTCTTTCTTTCAGGGCAATAATGATA
CAATGTATCATGCCTCTTTGCACCATTCTAAAGAATAACAGTGATAATTTCTG
GGTTAAGGCAATAGCAATATTTCTGCATATAAATATTTCTGCATATAAATTGT
AACTGATGTAAGAGGTTTCATATTGCTAATAGCAGCTACAATCCAGCTACCAT
TCTGCTTTTATTTTATGGTTGGGATAAGGCTGGATTATTCTGAGTCCAAGCTA
GGCCCTTTTGCTAATCATGTTCATACCTCTTATCTTCCTCCCACAG**CTCCTGG**
GCAACGTGCTGGTCTGTGTGCTGGCCCATCACTTTGGCAAAGAATTCAC
CCCACCAGTGCAGGCTGCCTATCAGAAAGTGGTGGCTGGTGTGGCTAAT
GCCCTGGCCCACAAGTATCACTAA

Some of the ideas for characterization of conformers, mathematical curves, and model proteins can be extended to characterization of DNA, though with an important distinction. In all the cases hitherto mentioned the characterization applied to the actual geometries and the actual 3-dimensional conformations of the structures. Such considerations, of course, can be similarly applied without difficulties directly to known folded DNA, such as to chains of length 80-85 of t-RNA, the folded clover-leaf. However, the geometry of most DNA is unknown. All that is known is the primary sequence of the four nucleic bases, adenine, guanine, cytosine and thymine, A, G, C, T briefly. Such sequences can be very long, having over 1000, 10,000 and even 100,000 nucleic bases. In Table 17 we show human beta globin of length 1424, as an illustration of the data available.

Is there an alternative representation and characterization of such data that offers more insights? With increasing accumulation of primary sequences a need for alternative characterization of such data became acute. In recent years, indeed, graphical representation of primary DNA sequences has been considered by several researches [81]. One of the pioneers of graphical representation of DNA, A. Nandy, suggested a "transform" of a primary sequence of a DNA to a graph by drawing a path on x, y coordinate grid, moving in the positive and the negative direction along x axis for A and G respectively and along the positive and the negative y axis for C and T respectively [82]. The first 92 bases of the beta globin of Table 17 are thus "translated" into the graph of Fig. 24. This graph, of course, has nothing to do with the actual geometrical form and the folding of DNA, but represent a projection of a "virtual" folding of DNA. Once the graphical representation of DNA is generated its D/D matrix can be constructed and the folding of such diagrams can be quantitatively characterized.

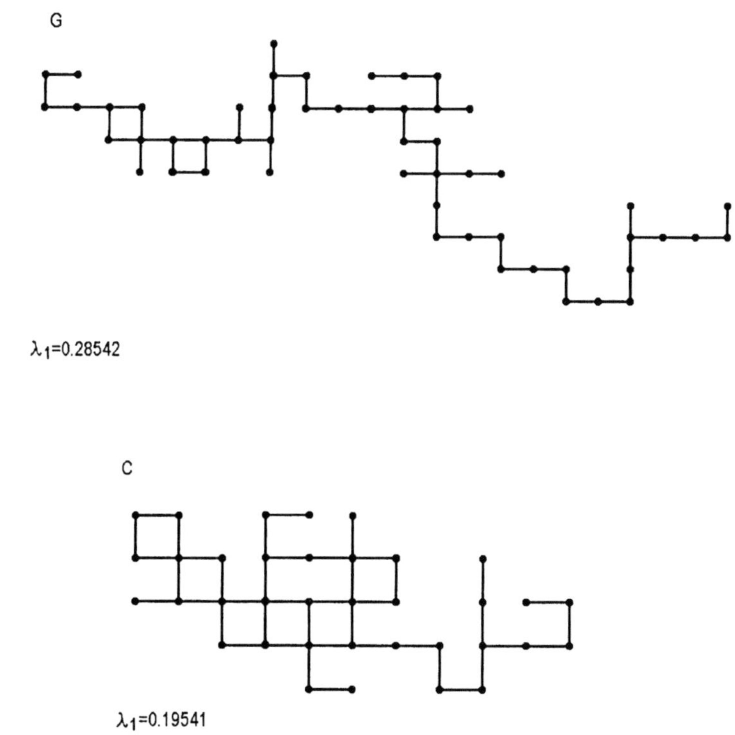

Figure 24

That the leading eigenvalue of D/D matrices of primary sequences of DNA reflects correctly the "virtual" folding of the graphical representations of DNA has been recently verified [83]. Randić and Vračko [84] considered graphical representation of DNA primary sequences for eight beta globins of different species using the approach developed by Nandy. In Table 18 we show the primary sequences of Exon 1 of beta globin DNA considered. The exons (belonging to a variety of animals, human included) had between 86 and 93 nucleic bases in their primary sequences, thus the corresponding D/D matrices have between 86 and 93 eigenvalues. In Fig. 25 we show graphical representations of the exons associated with the extreme values of the leading eigenvalues λ_1/n: 0.285242 (beta globin of rabbit) the largest value, and 0.195441 (beta globin of opossum), the smallest value. As we see, indeed, the two extreme values are associated with an apparently "extended" x, y path projection and a highly overlapping, condensed, or more folded, x, y path projection, respectively. This not only agrees with the suggested interpretation of the leading eigenvalue of D/D matrix as an index of folding of a chain but suggests also that the characterization based on D/D matrix can be extended meaningfully from chains also to branched curves.

Table 18

A **human** **92 bases**
ATGGTGCACCTGACTCCTGAGGAGAAGTCTGCCGTTACTGCCCTGTGGGGC
AAGGTGAACGTGGATTAAGTTGGTGGTGAGGCCCTGGGCAG

B **goat** **86 bases**
ATGCTGACTGCTGAGGAGAAGGCTGCCGTCACCGGCTTCTGGGGCAAGGT
GAAAGTGGATGAAGTTGGTGCTGAGGCCCTGGGCAG

C **opossum** **92 bases**
ATGGTGCACTTGACTTCTGAGGAGAAGAACTGCATCACTACCATCTGGTCT
AAGGTGCAGGTTGACCAGACTGGTGGTGAGGCCCTTGGC AG

D **gallus gallus** **92 bases**
ATGGTGCACTGGACTGCTGAGGAGAAGCAGCTCATCACCGGCCTCTGGGG
CAAGGTCAATGTGGCCGAATGTGGGGCCGAAGCCCTGGCCAG

E **lemur** **92 bases**
ATGACTTTGCTGAGTGCTGAGGAGAATGCTCATGTCACCTCTCTGTGGGGC
AAGGTGGATGTAGAGAAAGTTGGTGGCGAGGCCTTGGGCAG

F **mouse** **93 bases**
ATGGTTGCACCTGACTGATGCTGAGAAGTCTGCTGTCTCTTGCCTGTGGGC
AAAGGTGAACCCCGATGAAGTTGGTGGTGAGGCCCTGGGCAGG

G **rabbit** **90 bases**
ATGGTGCATCTGTCCAGTGAGGAGAAGTCTGCGGTCACTGCCCTGTGGGGC
AAGGTGAATGTGGAAGAAGTTGGTGGTGAGGCCCTGGGC

H **rat** **92 bases**
ATGGTGCACCTAACTGATGCTGAGAAGGCTACTGTTAGTGGCCTGTGGGGA
AAGGTGAACCCTGATAATGTTGGCGCTGAGGCCCTGGGCAG

G

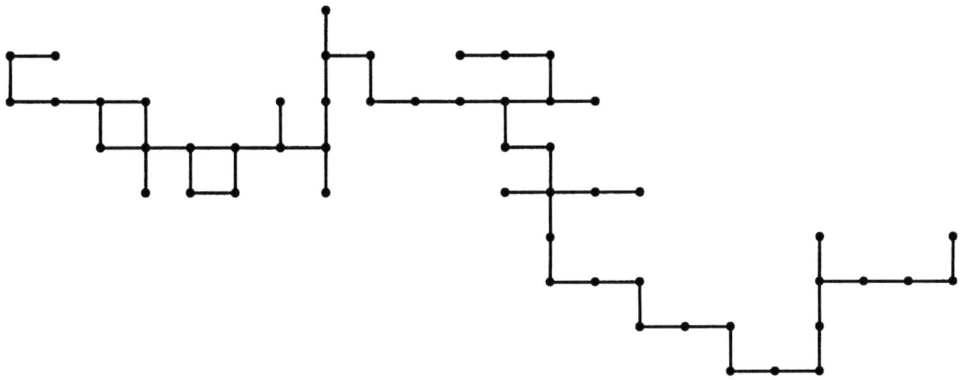

$\lambda_1 = 0.28542$

C

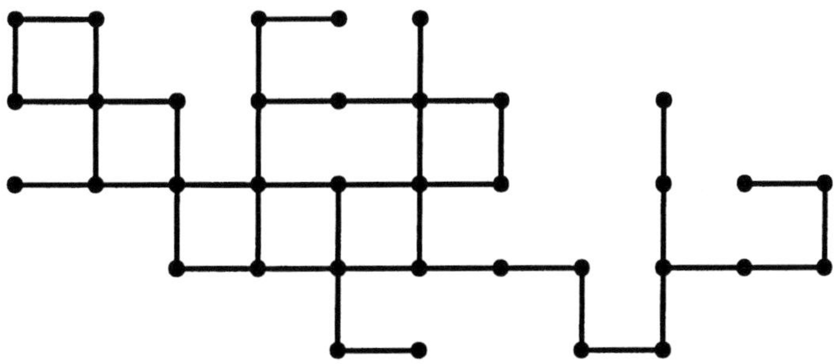

$\lambda_1 = 0.19541$

Figure 25

Numerical characterization of DNA, and eventually proteins, by using graphical invariants has only been initiated. One can expect further developments in this direction. For example, instead of using the four direction given by ±x and ±y axes one can select the four directions of tetrahedron to represent graphically primary sequences of DNA [85]. In this case DNA graph is embedded in 3D (on a diamond lattice characterized by tetrahedral angels). This 3D space curve can then be directly used for construction of D/D matrices. It is interesting to observe that projection of this spatial graph on x, y plane gives the very graphical curve for primary DNA sequences as outlined by Nandy. Now we have in addition two more planar projection, (x, z) and (y, z), which would allow more detailed characterization of DNA primary sequences. In Fig. 26 we show a part of a 3-D representation of human beta globin obtained by assigning to the four nucleic bases the four equivalent tetrahedral directions.

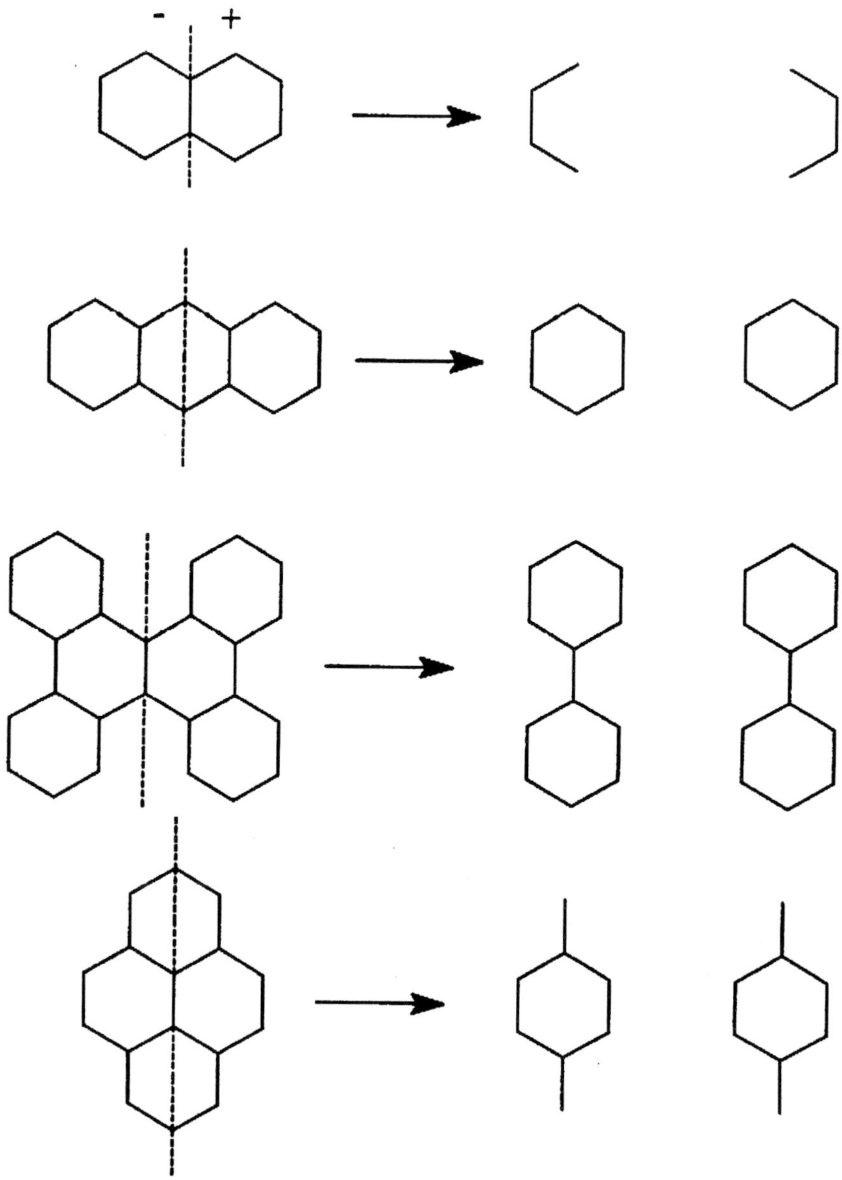

Figure 26

12. EIGENVALUES -- ALL

In previous sections we have mostly focused attention on the leading eigenvalue of graph matrices of graphs. What about other eigenvalues? In the study of isospectral graphs and subspectral graphs other eigenvalues also play important role, although mostly as one set to be compared with another set to check if they are the same. Do other eigenvalues have some application in chemistry?

It is our feeling that eigenvalues as invariants have not received sufficient attention, and have been mostly ignored despite their potential as molecular descriptors. Occasionally authors have mentioned other eigenvalues of graphs. For example, Fowler, Pisanski and collaborators [86] considered eigenvectors associated with the three leading eigenvalues of adjacency matrix. These are the eigenvectors with no nodal surface, with a single nodal surface, and with two nodal surfaces. For a number of cage structures, including fullerenes, they found that these eigenvectors when interpreted as coordinates offer an alternative graphical representation of such structures that displays "nice" geometry.

Recently Randić and Vračko [87] considered all positive eigenvalues of a graphical representation of DNA primary sequences and used them to arrive at partial ordering for exon 1 of beta globin DNA of different species. The exons considered (belonging to a variety of animals, human included) had between 86 and 93 nucleic bases in their primary sequences, thus the corresponding D/D matrices would have between 86 and 93 eigenvalues. Of these eigenvalues typically about 1/3 was positive. In Table 18 we have already shown the primary sequences for eight beta globins considered and to be compared later.

In order to restrict the overwhelming output of the data (list of all eigenvalues for all DNA considered) we will restrict attention to the positive eigenvalues alone. Under these conditions each DNA structure is represented by a sequence of between 25 - 30 entries. Now we will try to "digest" this, still relatively bulky, information. The process has been reduces from comparisons of the primary sequences to comparison of numerical sequences. Bur the latter have been subject of mathematical studies, initiates almost a hundred years ago by Muirhead, Scottish mathematician.

Instead directly comparing sequences of computed eigenvalues (belonging to different DNA), according to Muirhead [88, 89] one should compare entries of the sequences of the corresponding partial sums. That is, instead of listing: $\lambda_1, \lambda_2, \lambda_3, \lambda_4, \lambda_5, \ldots$, we have to consider the list: $\lambda_1, \lambda_1 + \lambda_2, \lambda_1 + \lambda_2 + \lambda_3, \lambda_1 + \lambda_2 + \lambda_3 + \lambda_4, \lambda_1 + \lambda_2 + \lambda_3 + \lambda_4 + \lambda_5, \ldots$ etc.

According to Muirhead two sequences A, B, defined by elements $\{a_1, a_2, a_3, a_4, \ldots\}$ and $\{b_1, b_2, b_3, b_4, \ldots\}$, respectively, are comparable if all the corresponding partial sums of one sequence dominate the partial sums of the other sequence. That is, for A to dominate B the following inequalities have to be satisfied:

$$
\begin{gathered}
a_1 > b_1 \\
a_1 + a_2 > b_1 + b_2 \\
a_1 + a_2 + a_3 > b_1 + b_2 + b_3 \\
a_1 + a_2 + a_3 + a_4 > b_1 + b_2 + b_3 + b_4 \\
\cdots
\end{gathered}
$$

If these inequalities are not satisfies then the two sequences A and B are said not to be comparable. Even though two sequences may be found not comparable they both can dominate another sequence, or be dominated by another sequence.

In Table 19 we show all the eigenvalues of D/D matrix for the exon 1 of human beta globin A of Table 18. In Table 20 we have listed partial sums obtained from the positive eigenvalues of D/D matrices for the eight DNA sequences of Table 18. The first column of Table 20 is obtained from the positive eigenvalues of Table 19. We will now outline the search for ordering of the sequences following the prescribed procedure proposed by Muirhead. More detailed description of the procedure can be found in ref. [87]. Consider first two sequences that have been labeled A, and B in Table 20. As we see from Table 20 while at the beginning the partial sums of A are larger than those of B by about half way down the sequences the opposite is the case, the partial sums of B are greater than those of A. Hence, the sequences A and B are not comparable. Sequence C, however, is dominated by both, the sequence A and the sequence B, because at each row in Table 20 the corresponding entry (partial sum) in column C is smaller than the corresponding entries in column A and B. When all comparisons are completed we arrive at the partial order illustrated in Fig. 27.

Table 19

All eigenvalues:

-0.01208	-0.01211	-0.01202	-0.01195	-0.01224	-0.01227	-0.01180
-0.01164	-0.01149	-0.01259	-0.01131	-0.01115	-0.01278	-0.01282
-0.01088	-0.01084	-0.01303	-0.01319	-0.01335	-0.01046	-0.01013
-0.01008	-0.01001	-0.01369	-0.00944	-0.00912	-0.00886	-0.01416
-0.00852	-0.00824	-0.00802	-0.00776	-0.01447	-0.01476	-0.00728
-0.00657	-0.00631	-0.00619	-0.00595	-0.01560	-0.01568	-0.01589
-0.00534	-0.00509	-0.01633	-0.00476	-0.01695	-0.00395	-0.01745
-0.00336	-0.00319	-0.00292	-0.00242	-0.00215	-0.01827	-0.01842
-0.00109	-0.00069	-0.01941	-0.00009	0.00071	0.00063	-0.02077
0.00196	-0.02149	0.00349	-0.02249	0.00451	-0.02367	0.00596
0.00650	0.00678	-0.02493	0.00931	0.00996	-0.02688	0.01070
0.01314	0.01438	0.01527	0.01565	0.01820	0.02071	0.02429
0.02563	0.02842	0.03236	0.03315	0.04361	0.06208	0.07010
0.27136						

Table 20

Partial sum of positive eigenvalues

A	B	C	D	E	F	G	H
0.27136	0.28493	0.19541	0.26262	0.25947	0.24354	0.28542	0.24036
0.34146	0.36659	0.29176	0.34453	0.34028	0.33812	0.35174	0.33949
0.40354	0.40749	0.35302	0.40490	0.40738	0.39572	0.41231	0.40971
0.44715	0.44888	0.40870	0.45212	0.44820	0.45056	0.45503	0.45861
0.48030	0.48590	0.44423	0.48600	0.48410	0.48537	0.49361	0.49641
0.51266	0.52292	0.47572	0.51788	0.51367	0.51609	0.53150	0.53030
0.54108	0.54959	0.50414	0.54852	0.54117	0.54262	0.55911	0.55825
0.56671	0.57539	0.53046	0.57504	0.56331	0.56821	0.58478	0.58331
0.59100	0.59924	0.55621	0.59912	0.58382	0.58885	0.60614	0.60648
0.61171	0.61768	0.57813	0.62079	0.60263	0.60818	0.62554	0.62684
0.62991	0.63416	0.59879	0.63675	0.61845	0.62734	0.64399	0.64428
0.64556	0.64916	0.61885	0.65127	0.63335	0.64249	0.65921	0.66019
0.66083	0.66308	0.63481	0.66529	0.64744	0.65671	0.67641	0.67522
0.67521	0.67443	0.64948	0.67862	0.66109	0.67008	0.69051	0.68916
0.68835	0.68542	0.66261	0.68966	0.67088	0.68206	0.70304	0.70001
0.69905	0.69501	0.67498	0.70000	0.67972	0.69240	0.71349	0.71050
0.70901	0.70398	0.68505	0.70822	0.68772	0.70206	0.72153	0.72056
0.71897	0.71195	0.69437	0.71516	0.69518	0.71111	0.72957	0.72855
0.72575	0.71887	0.70206	0.72115	0.70233	0.71846	0.73062	0.73552
0.73225	0.72513	0.70966	0.72687	0.70859	0.72506	0.74208	0.74089
0.73821	0.73006	0.71601	0.73191	0.71349	0.73082	0.74682	0.74514
0.74272	0.73455	0.72076	0.73561	0.71775	0.73634	0.74925	0.74848
0.74621	0.73767	0.72450	0.73900	0.72158	0.73993	0.75039	0.75043
0.74817	0.74032	0.72799	0.74174	0.72495	0.74264	0.75138	0.75202
0.74888	0.74193	0.73049	0.74344	0.72749	0.74506		0.75216
0.74951	0.74327	0.73265	0.74486	0.72927	0.74623		
	0.74352	0.73387	0.74538	0.73008			
		0.73439	0.74554	0.73160			
				0.73220			

There are different ways how can one graphically represent the same partial order. It is important that any such graphical visualization of a partial order preserves the relative positioning of the elements of the partial order (DNA sequences) as dictated by the dominance relationships. As we see the structures A and B, that are not comparable, are located in different branches of the partial order diagram. The partial ordering of the eight sequences of Table 20 illustrated in Fig. 27. The diagram allows one to visualize the relationships and possible similarities among DNA primary sequences considered, which although contain all the necessary information in their primary sequences do not offer easy comparisons.

Information content of the partial order is different then that obtained from the regression analysis, the similarity analysis, the sensitivity analysis, etc. Two elements (DNA sequence) may be similar, as is the case with sequences F (mouse) and H (rat), yet this need not be reflected in the partial order. Partial orders (Hesse diagrams and lattices as objects of mathematics) have some relation to tabular representation of data, such as is given by the Periodic Table of Elements, by the (p_2, p_3) path diagrams for study of isomeric variations of physicochemical properties in alkanes [28,90], by ordering of biologically active compounds in searching for common pharmacophore [91], or ordering of benzenoids according to the empirical formulas [92].

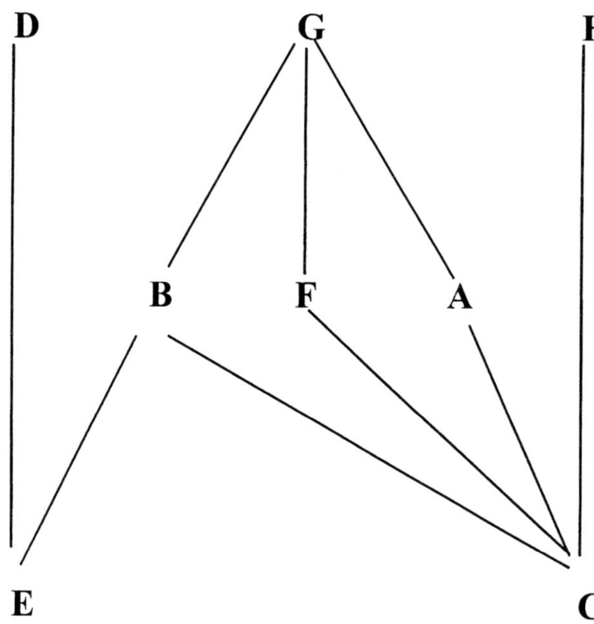

Figure 27

To illustrate use of the partial order of Fig. 27 we have reproduced (twice) the partial order in Fig. 28. We will examine now two mathematical quantities, the leading eigenvalue λ_1, and the total sum of all positive eigenvalues $\Sigma\, \lambda_i$, as the "properties" of DNA. Instead of using labels A, B, C, . . . in the diagrams of the partial order in Fig. 28 we have replaced them with the respective values of the leading eigenvalue (top) and the positive eigenvalue sum (bottom). As we see from Fig. 28 in both cases the partial order with labeled magnitudes does not show contradictions, that is, the numerical values follow the dominance relationship of the sequences characterized by the partial order.

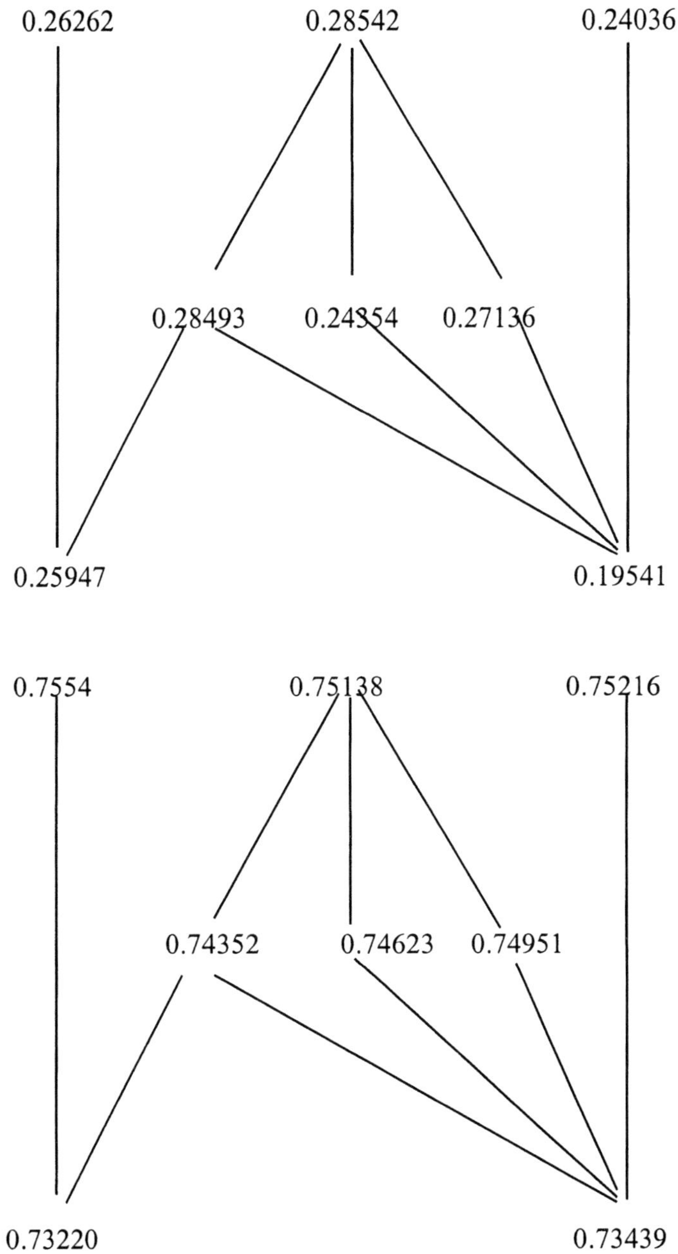

Figure 28

13. Eigenvalue Sums

In the previous section we have introduced as a mathematical property of a structure the positive eigenvalue sum. Construction of novel invariants by "synthesis" *(composition)* of local or partial structural features is not so common, neither in the mathematical analyses nor in the chemical applications. The opposite is apparently more common: *decomposition* of a global property into local components, partitioning of a molecular (global) property to local properties. It suffice to mention various bond additivities, including celebrated introduction of bond dipoles, non observable quantities, as components of total molecular dipole (observable quantity). Each partitioning formally decomposes property into local contributions, whether we identify such contributions as local or not. For example, we often speak of bond energy (derived from decomposition of the total energy to bond contributions), but almost never we speak of bond boiling point, even though both are equally virtual (except when considering diatomic molecules).

Here, however, we are interested in the opposite process -- the *synthesis* of local properties of molecular fragments to global molecular property. Among few quantities so constructed (derived from experimental measurements of suitable property) we may mention the chemical shift sum, the sum of all C^{13} chemical shifts in a hydrocarbon [93]. By adding all carbon-13 chemical shifts in a molecule one obtains a single numerical quantity that belongs to a molecule, rather than individual atoms. Hence, while carbon-13 chemical shifts is an atom property the chemical shift sum is a molecular property. Any similar construction using local characteristics thus lead to a "molecular property." Besides local atomic attributes one can consider selected bond properties, or properties of other constitutional fragments. However, for such constructions to be of interest in chemistry they must have some relevance to molecular modeling, be of interest in structure-property study, or show some regularity in the data reduction procedures. When chemical shifts sums of octanes are displayed on the p_2, p_3 coordinate grid, indeed, a very regular isomeric variation in magnitudes for different isomers is observed, not dissimilar to similar regularities typifying isomeric variations of the traditional physico-chemical properties of alkanes [28, 941], boiling points, heats of formation, entropy, density, molar magnetic susceptibilities, critical pressure, molar volumes, heat of combustion, surface tension, critical temperatures, etc.

One can view as another such composite property molecular resonance energy (RE) when obtained from resonance energies associated with individual Kekulé valence structures, or from conjugated circuits [95]. In such an approach one consider conjugated circuits as the most elementary contributions to RE and then by decomposition of each Kekulé valence structure into contributions from R_1, R_2 and R_3 conjugated circuits (corresponding to 6, 10 and 14 member conjugated circuits) by summation obtains molecular RE as a molecular property.

Positive eigenvalues have been selected because they result in a numerical magnitude for a sum, while if one is to add all the eigenvalues of a matrix one obtains zero, (an invariant of no particular interest here). By adding all positive eigenvalues one obtains a well defined, at least mathematically well defined, quantity. That alone, however, is not enough reason for investigating such invariant in the applied mathematics. The distinction between the mathematics and the applied mathematics is that in the latter we have no luxury of investigating interesting and intriguing relations, unless they offer some results of potential interest in applications. In the early days of HMO by adding all the positive eigenvalues of the adjacency matrix one would obtain molecular energy, one of the central concepts of quantum chemistry of those days. Today, this is primarily (but not exclusively) of historic and educational value. Nevertheless, the example clearly shows that eigenvalue sum (as we will continue to refer to the sum of the positive eigenvalues of a matrix) could be not only an interesting but also an important structural invariant. Already Fig. 28 has shown that eigenvalue sum, at least among structurally similar systems, does follow some structural features of systems considered. A random distributions of the eigenvalue sums for the eight DNA species is more than likely to introduce contradictions within the Hesse diagram shown.

In order to investigate the structural regularities for the eigenvalue sum we have collected in Table 21 data for 18 isomers of octane. Fig. 29 shows that indeed eigenvalue sum displays regular variation along the p_2, p_3 coordinate grid of octanes. This finding is significant, as it suggests that the eigenvalue sum could be useful molecular descriptor for selected physico-chemical properties, because most of those properties show also a regular variation along the p_2, p_3 path axes. We may say, in other words, that the eigenvalue sum satisfy the necessary conditions to qualify as a molecular descriptor, but that alone is not sufficient. As the saying goes: The proof is in eating the cake! A descriptor, any descriptor, is not useful unless shown to be useful in at least a single structure-property correlation, or some other statistical data reduction procedure.

Table 21

Eigenvalue sums and zero eigenvalue multiplicities (μ_0) for octane isomers

	eig sum	μ_0		eig sum	μ_0
n-octane	4.7588	0	3,3-MM	4.2596	1
2-M	4.3814	1	3,4-MM	4.6659	0
3-M	4.7046	0	2M,3E	4.3603	1
4-M	4.3814	1	3M,3E	4.6458	0
3-E	4.7229	0	2,2,3-MMM	4.1305	1
2,2-MM	4.1565	1	2,2,4-MMM	3.6924	2
2,3-MM	4.3235	1	2,3,3-MMM	4.1876	1
24-MM	4.2826	1	2,3,4-MMM	4.2122	1
2,5-MM	4.2360	1	2,2,3,3-MMMM	3.6050	2

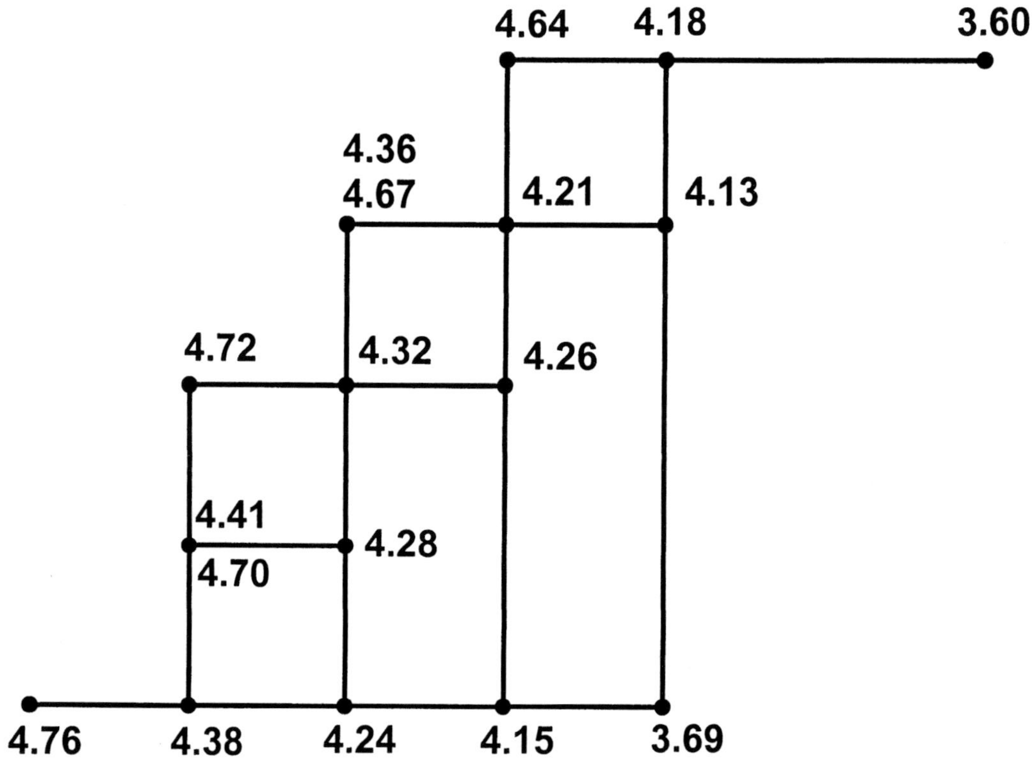

Figure 29

By examining correlations of several physico-chemical properties of octane isomers with the eigenvalue sum we did observe promising results. The best single descriptor regressions had the correlations coefficient of r = 0.881 for the boiling points of octanes, which is only slightly below the best single correlation for the boiling points based on the Hosoya Z topological index (r=0.888). The correlation coefficients below 0.900 may not appear impressive, however, one should keep in mind that for the regressions restricted to octane isomers, molecules of the same size, it is generally difficult to obtain regression coefficient above 0.900, particularly when using a single descriptor. In Table 22 we have collected the regression coefficient and the standard error for several properties of octanes and several well-known molecular descriptors for the sake of comparison.

Table 22

Linear regressions

	$^1\chi$	$^3\chi$	ID	J	P'/P	WW	Z	W
BP	0.821						0.888	
S	0.906		0.926	0.896	0.888	0.821		
ΔH	0.958		0.951	0.797	0.842	0.798	0.971	0.820
σ		0.765						
N	0.778		0.921	0.932	0.942	0.957		0.957
Ac	0.855		0.983	0.970	0.945	0.933	0.791	0.964
R^2	0.770		0.814	0.858	0.873	0.903	0.747	0.890
T_c								
P_c								
V_c			0.760	0.793	0.798	0.785		0.780
MV		0.978						
MR		0.970						
Σ δ			0.921					

Linear and quadratic regressions

	W/Z	p_2/w_2	p_3/w_3	WW/W	x_1	x_2	JJ	eig sum
BP	0.872	0.701				0.786		0.881
S				0.853	0.826	0.856	0.849	0.726
ΔH	0.840	0.735						0.823
σ	0.916							
N								
Ac		0.917						
R^2		0.840						0.892
T_c	0.836		0.865					
P_c		0.731	0.872	0.886	0.908		0.937	
V_c	0.752							
MV								
MR			0.990					
ρ			0.990*					
Σ δ	0.929							

An examination of the correlation of the eigenvalue sum against the connectivity index (Fig. 30) shows clustering of the 18 octane isomers in three groups. The first group consisted of only 2,2,4-trimethylpentane and 2,2,3,3-tetramethylbutane. The second group involved: n-octane, 3-methylheptane, 3-ethylheptane, 3,4-dimethylhexane and 3-ethyl-3-methylpentane. The remaining 11 isomers comprised the third group. Immediately a question can be raised how and why these particular grouping of isomers and not some other combinations? What have, for example, n-octane, 3-methylheptane, 3-ethylheptane, 3,4-dimethylhexane and 3-ethyl-3-methylpentane in common to form a single cluster? A close look at the eigenvalues of the 18 octane isomers gave the answer: The first group has zero as the eigenvalue with the multiplicity two, the second group has zero as the eigenvalue of multiplicity one, and the third group has no zero as its eigenvalue. This immediately suggested that the eigenvalue sum and the zero eigenvalue multiplicity should be combined as descriptors.

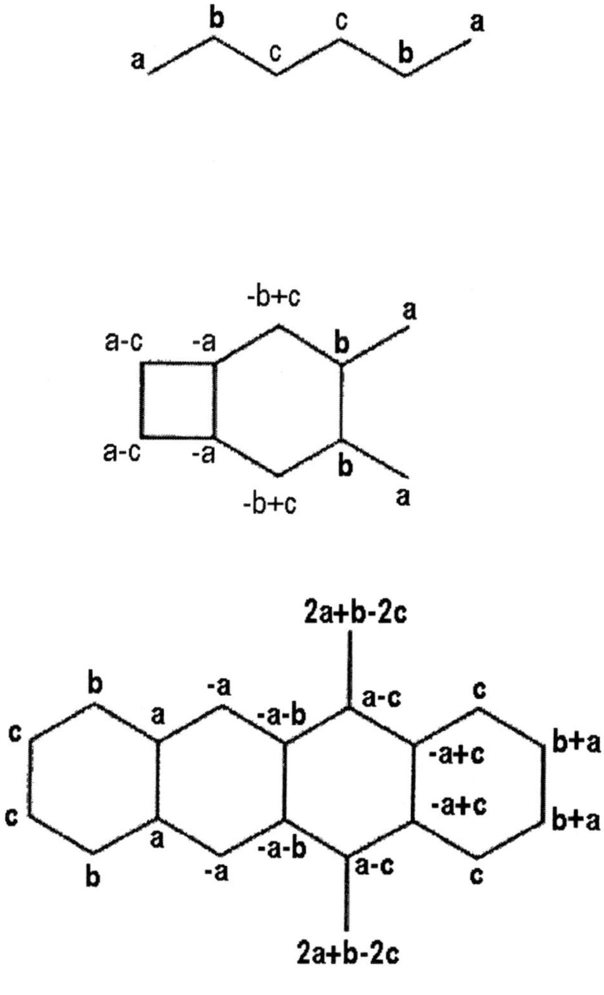

Figure 30

Using as descriptors p_2, p_3 and zero multiplicity we obtain for regression of the eigenvalue sum very good statistical parameters r = 0.9972, and F = 819. This suggests that p_2, p_3 diagram of Fig. 29 could lead to quantitative description of high quality if the eigenvalue sum is "corrected" when a jump in the zero eigenvalue multiplicity for an isomer occurs. A two parameter regression of the connectivity index against the eigenvalue sum and the zero multiplicity resulted in regression coefficient r = 0.9957 and the Fisher ratio of 866, which are statistical parameters almost impossible to achieve when sample of compounds is limited to octane isomers (molecules of the same size, differing only in shape).

Hence, even though the eigenvalues themselves have not lead to high quality regressions, the eigenvalue sum combined with the zero eigenvalue multiplicity as second descriptor appear promising molecular descriptor for structure-property-activity studies.

14. REFERENCES

1. M. Randić, Topological indices, The Encyclopedia of Computational Chemistry, Schleyer, P. v. R.; Allinger, N. L., Clark, T., Gasteiger, J., Kollman, P. A., F. Schaefer, III, H. F., Schreiner, P. R. (Eds.); John & Sons, Chichester, 1998, pp. 3018-3032.
2. M. Randić, M,. Novic and M. Vracko, Topological Indices, New and Old, Lecture Notes in Chemistry (submitted)
   R. Todeschini and V. Consonni, Handbook of Molecular Descriptors, Wiley – VCH
   M. I. Stankevitch, I. V. Stankevitch, and N. S. Zefirov, Topological indexes in organic chemistry, Usp. Khim., **1988**, *57,* 337-366.
3. CODESSA: A. R. Katritzky, V. S. Lobanov, M. Karelson, QSPR: The correlation and quantitative prediction of chemical and physical properties from structure, Chem. Soc. Rev., **1995**, *24,* 279-287.
   POLLY MOLCONN, Molconn=Z software Package: Hall Associates Consulting: 2 Davis Street, Quincy, MA 02170, USA.
4. Malinowski, Factor Analysis in Chemistry, Wiley-Interscience, New York, (1990)
5. H. Hotelling, Analysis of a complex of statistical variables into principal components, J. Educ. Psych., **1933**, *24,* 417-441 and 489-520.
6. K. Varmuza, Chemometrics: Multivariate view on chemical problems, The Encyclopedia of Computational Chemistry, Schleyer, P. v. R.; Allinger, N. L., Clark, T., Gasteiger, J., Kollman, P. A., F. Schaefer, III, H. F., Schreiner, P. R. (Eds.); John & Sons, Chichester, 1998, pp. 346-366.
7. J. Zupan and J. Gasteiger, Neural Networks for Chemists, VCH, Weinheim (1993)
8. P. Willet, Similarity and Clustering in Chemical Information Systems, Research Studies Press, Letchworth, 1987.
9. M. S. Okino and M. L. Mavrovouniotis, Chemical reaction systems model reduction, The Encyclopedia of Computational Chemistry, Schleyer, P. v. R.; Allinger, N. L.,

Clark, T., Gasteiger, J., Kollman, P. A., F. Schaefer, III, H. F., Schreiner, P. R. (Eds.); John & Sons, Chichester, 1998, pp. 329-334.

10. Concept and Applications of Molecular Similarity; M. A. Johnson and G. M Maggiora, Eds, John Wiley & Sons, New York 1990.
M. Randić, Similarity methods of interest in chemistry, in: Mathematical Methods in Contemporary Chemistry, (S. I. Kuchanov, Ed.), Gordon & Breech, Amsterdam, (1996), pp. 1-100.
11. R. C. Read, A new system for the designation of chemical compounds. 1. Theoretical preliminaries and coding of acyclcic compounds, J. Chem. Inf. Comput. Sci., **1983**, *23,* 135.
12. A. T. Balaban, Topological indices and their uses: A new approach for coding of alkanes, J. Mol. Structure (Theochem), **1988**, *165,* 243-253.
13. M. Randić, Generalized molecular descriptors, J. Math. Chem, **1991**, *7,* 155-168.
14. H. Wiener, Structural determination of paraffin boiling points, J. Am. Chem. Soc., **1947**, *69,* 17-20.
15. I. Motoc, A. T. Balaban, Ov. Mekenyan and D. Bonchev, Topological indices: Inter-relations and composition, MATCH, **1982**, *13,* 369-404.
A. T. Balaban, A. Chiriac, I. Motoc, and Z. Simon, Steric Fit in Quantitative Structure-Activity Relations, (Chapter 3), Lecture Notes in Chemistry, Springer, Berlin, 1980.
16. L. Collatz and U. Sinogowitz, Spectra of finite graphs, Abhandl. Math. Sem. Univ. Hamburg, **1957**, *21,* 64-77.
17. A. T. Balaban and F. Harary, The characteristic polynomial does not uniquely determines the topology of a molecule, J. Chem. Docum., **1971**, *11,* 258-259.
18. 18 . M. Randić and B. Baker, Isospectral multigraphs, J. Math. Chem., **1988**, *2,* 249-265.
19. G. A. Baker, Jr., Drum shapes and isospectral graphs, J. Math. Phys., **1966**, *7,* 2238-2242.
M. Fisher, J. Combinatorial Theory, **1966**, *7,* 2238.
W. C. Herndon, Isospectral molecules, Tetrahedron Lett., **1974**, 671-674.
T. Živković, N. Trinajstić and M. Randić, On conjugated molecules with identical topological spectra, Mol. Phys., **1975**, *30,* 517-532.
W. C. Herndon and M. L. Ellzey, Jr., Isospectral graphs and molecules, Tetrahedron, **1975**, *31,* 99-107.
M. Randić, N. Trinajstić and T. Živković, Molecular graphs having identical spectra, J. Chem. Soc. Faraday Trans. II, **1976**, *72,* 244-256.
T. Živković, N. Trinajstić and M. Randić, On the topological spectra of composite molecular systems, Croat. Chem. Acta, **1977**, *49,* 89-100.
E. Heilbronner, Some comments on cospectral graphs, MATCH, **1979**, *5,* 105-133.
J. P. Lowe and M. R. Soto, Isospectral graphs, symmetry, and perturbation theory, MATCH, **1986**, *20,* 21-51.
J. P. Lowe and M. W. Davis, Isospectral points and edges in graph theory, J. Math. Chem., **1990**, *5,* 275-285.
Y. Jiang, Problems on isospectral molecules, Sci. Sin., **1984**, *27,* 236.

J. V. Knop, W. R. Müller, K. Szymanski, N. Trinajstić, A. F. Kleiner and M. Randić, On irreducible endospectral graphs, J. Math. Phys., **1986**, *27,* 2601-2612.
W. C. Herndon and M. L. Ellzey, Jr., The construction of cospectral graphs, MATCH, **1986**, *20,* 53-79.
M. Randić and A. F. Kleiner, On the construction of endospectral graphs, Ann. New York Acad. Sci. **1989**, *555,* 320-331.
M. Randić, M. Barysz, J. Nowakowski, S. Nikolić and N. Trinajstić, Isospectral graphs revisited, J. Mol. Struct. (Theochem), **1989**, *185,* 95-121.
20. A. J. Schwenk, in: New Directions in Theory of Graphs, (F. Harary, ed.), Academic press, New York, (1973), p. 275
21. E. Hückel, Quantentheoretische Beitrage zum Benzolproblem, I. Die Elektronenkonfiguration des Benzols und verwandter Verbindungen, Zeit. fur Physik, **1931**, *70,* 204
E. Hückel, Quantentheoretische Beitrage zum Problem der aromatischen und ungesattigten Verbindungen III, Zeit. fur Physik, **1932**, *76,* 628-648
E. Hückel, Grundzuge der Theorie ungesattiger und aromatischer Verbindungen, Verlag Chemie, Berlin, 1938.
21a J. M. Andre, D. H. Mosley, M.-C. Andre, B. Champagne, E. Clementi, J. G. Fripiat, L. Leherte, L. Pisani, D. Vercauteren, M. Vracko. Exploring Aspects of Computational Chemistry: Concepts and Exercises, Presses Universitaires de Namur, Belgium, 1997.
22. F. Bloch, Uber die Quantenmechanik der Elektronen in Kristallgittern, Zeit. fur Physik, **1929**, *52,* 555-600.
F. Bloch, Zeit. fur Physik, **1930**, *61,* 206
23. E. Heilbronner and T. B. Jones, Spectral differences between "isospectral" molecules, J. Am. Chem. Soc., **1978**, *100,* 6506
24. C. A. Coulson and A. Streitweiser, Jr., Dictionary of π-electron Calculations, Freeman, San Francisco (1965).
25. T. Živković, reported at the Quantum Chemistry School of USSR Academy of Science, Repino, USSR (December 1973)
26. R. Hoffmann, An extended Hueckel Theory. I. Hydrocarbons, J. Chem. Phys., **1963**, *39,* 1397-1412.
R. Hoffmann, Extended Hueckel theory. II. Compounds of boron and nitrogen, J. Chem. Phys., **1964**, *40,* 2474-2480.
27. L. Lovasz and J. Pelikan, I. On the eigenvalues of trees, Period. Math. Hung., **1973**, *3,* 175-182.
28. M. Randić and C. L. Wilkins, On a graph theoretical basis for ordering of structures, Chem. Phys. Lett., **1979**, *63,* 332-336.
M. Randić and C. L. Wilkins, Graph theoretical ordering of structures as a basis for systematic searches for regularities in molecular data, J. Phys. Chem., **1979**, *83,* 1525-1540.
29. 29. I. Gutman, B. Ruščič, N. Trinajstić and C. F. Wilcox, Jr., Graph theory and molecular orbitals, XII. Acyclic polyenes, J. Chem. Phys., **1975**, *62,* 3399

D. Bonchev and N. Trinajstić, Information theory, distance matrix and molecular branching, J. Chem. Phys., **1977**, *67,* 4517-4533.
D. Cvetković and I. Gutman, Note on branching, Croat. Chem. Acta, **1977**, *49,* 115
D. Bonchev, J. V. Knop and N. Trinajstić, Mathematical models for branching, MATCH, **1979**, *6,* 21-47.
W. Hasselbarth, Die Verzweighheit von Graphen, MATCH, **1984**, *16,* 3
M. Barysz, J. V. Knop, S. Pejakovic, and N. Trinajstić, Characterization of branching, Polish J. Chem., **1985**, *59,* 405-432.
S. H. Bertz, Branching in graphs and molecules, Disc. Appl. Math., **1988**, *19,* 65-83.
D. Bonchev, V. Kamenska and O. Mekenyan, Comparability graphs and molecular properties: IV. Generalizations and applications, J. Math. Chem., **1990**, *5,* 43072.
D. Bonchev, Topological order in molecules, 1. Molecular branching revisited, J. Mol. Struct. (Theochem), **1995**, *336,* 137-156.

30. F. Harary, Graph Theory, Addison-Wesley, Reading, MA (1969)
31. F. Buckley and F. Harary, Distance in Graphs, Addison-Wesley, Reading, MA, 1989
D. Bonchev and N. Trinajstić, Information theory, distance matrix, and molecular branching, J. Chem. Phys., **1977**, *67,* 4517-4533.
D. J. Klein, Graph geometry, graph metrics, & Wiener, MATCH, **1997**, *35,* 7-27.
D. J. Klein and H.-Y. Zhu, Distances and volumina for graphs, J. Math. Chem., **1998**, 1-17.
32. H. Hosoya, Topological index. A newly proposed quantity characterizing the topological nature of structural isomers of saturated hydrocarbons, Bull. Chem. Soc. Japan, **1971**, *44,* 2332-2339.
33. N. Trinajstić, S. Nikolić, B. Lučić, D. Amić and Z. Mihalić, The detour matrix in chemistry, J. Chem. Inf. Comput. Sci., **1997**, *37,* 631-6381.
34. M. Randić, On characterization of cyclic structures, J. Chem. Inf. Comput. Sci., **1997**, *37,* 1063-1071.
T. Pisanski, D. Plavšić and M. Randić, On numerical characterization of cyclicity, J. Chem. Inf. Comput. Sci., (in press)
35. D. Amić and N. Trinajstić, On the detour matrix, Croat. Chem. Acta, **1995**, *68,* 53-62.
I. Lukovits, The detour index, Croat. Chem. Acta, **1996**, *69,* 873-882.
S. Nikolić, N. Trinajstić, A. Jurić, and Z. Mihalić, The detour matrix and the detour index of weighted graphs, Croat. Chem. Acta, **1996**, *9,* 1557-1591.
I. Lukovits and M. Razinger, On calculation of the detour index, J. Chem. Inf. Comput. Sci., **1997**, *37,* 283-286.
36. M. Randić, L. M. DeAlba and F. E. Harris, Graphs with identical detour matrix, Croat. Chem. Acta, **1998**, *71,* 53-68.
37. A. A. Balandin, Structurnaya algebra v khimii, Uspekhi Khimii, **1940**, *9,* 390
38. L. Spialter, The atom connectivity matrix (ACM) and its characteristic polynomial (ACMP): A new computer oriented chemical nomenclature, J. Amer. Chem. Soc., **1963**, *85,* 2012-2013.
L. Spialter, The atom connectivity matrix (ACM) and its characteristic polynomial, J. Chem. Docum., **1964**, *4,* 261-269.

L. Spialter, The atom connectivity matrix characteristic polynomail (ACMCP) and its physico-geometrical (topological) significance, J. Chem. Docum., **1964**, *4,* 269-274.
39. S. S. Tratch, M. I. Stankevitch, N. S. Zeforov, Combinatorial models and algorithms in chemistry. The expanded Wiener number - A novel topological index, J. Chem. Inf. Comput. Sci., **1990**, *11,* 899-908.
40. L. B. Kier and L. H. Hall, Molecular Structure Description: Their Electrotopological State, Academic Press (in press).
41. M. Randić, Novel molecular descriptor for structure-property studies. Chem. Phys. Lett., **1993**, *211,* 478-43.
42. M. Randić, Hosoya matrix - a source of new molecular descriptors, Croat. Chem. Acta, **1994**, *67,* 415-429.
A. Hermann and P. Zinn, List operations on chemical graphs. 6. Comparative study of combinatorial topological indexes of the Hosoya type, J. Chem. Inf. Comput. Sci., **1995**, *35,* 551-560.
43. M. Randić, Restricted random walk on a graph as a source of novel molecular descriptors, Theor. Chem. Acta, **1995**, *92*, 97-106.
44. M. Randić, A. F. Kleiner and L. M. DeAlba, Distance/distance matrices, J. Chem. Inf. Comput. Sci., **1994**, *34,* 277-286.
45. M. Randić, On characterization of molecular branching, J. Amer. Chem. Soc., **1975**, *97,* 6609-6615.
46. L. B. Kier, W. J. Murray, M. Randić and L. H. Hall, Molecular connectivity V: Connectivity series applied to density, J. Pharm. Sci., **1976**, *65,* 1226-1230.
47. M. V. Diudea, Cluj matrix *CJu*: Source of various graph descriptors, MATCH, **1997**, *35,* 169-183.
M. V. Diudea, Cluj matrix invariants, J. Chem. Inf. Comput. Sci., **1997**, *35,* 300-305.
M. V. Diudea, O. M. Minailiuc, G. Katona and I. Gutman, Szeged matrices and related numbers, , MATCH, **1997**, *35,* 129-143.
M. V. Diudea, O. M. Minailiuc, S. Nikolić and N. Trinajstić, Matrices of reciprocal distance , MATCH, **1997**, *35,* 243-259.
M. V. Diudea , Wiener and hyper-Wiener numbers in a single matrix, J. Chem. Inf. Comput. Sci., **1996**, *36,* 833-836.
I. Gutman and M. V. Diudea, Correcting the definition of Cluj matrices, MATCH **1998**, *37,* 195-201.
48. M. Randić, Linear combinations of path numbers as molecular descriptors, New J. Chem., **1997**, *21,* 945-951.
49. M. Randić, D. Plavšić and M. Razinger, Double invariants, MATCH, **1997**, *35,* 243-259.
50. M. Randić, On molecular branching, Acta Chim. Slovenica, **1997**, *44,* 57-77.
51. M. Randić, X. Guo, T. Oxley, H. Krishnapriyan and L. Naylor, Wiener matrix invariants, J. Chem. Inf. Comput. Sci., **1994**, *34,* 361-367.
52. M. Randić, X. Guo, T. Oxley, and H. Krishnapriyan, Wiener matrix: Source of novel graph invariants, J. Chem. Inf. Comput. Sci., **1993**, *33,* 709-716.
53. A. T. Balaban, Highly discriminating distance-based topological index, Chem. Phys. Lett., **1982**, *89,* 399-404.

54. M. Randić, On structural ordering and branching of acyclic saturated hydrocarbons, J. Math. Chem, **1998**, *24,* 345-358.
55. M. Randić, X. Guo and S. Bobst, Use of path matrices for characterization of molecular structures, DIMACS Series in Discrete Math. and Theor. Comput. Sci. (in press).
56. D. Bonchev and N. Trinajstić, On topological characterization of molecular branching, Int. J. Quant. Chem: Quant. Chem. Symp., **1978**, *12,* 293-303.
57. W. R. Müller, J. V. Knop and M. Randić (work in progress)
58. L. B. Kier and L. H. Hall, Molecular Connectivity in Chemistry and Drug Research, Academic Press, New York, (1976).
59. E. C. Kirby, Sensitivity of topological indices to methyl group branching in octanes and azulenes, or what does topological index index?, J. Chem. Inf. Comput. Sci., **1994**, *34,* 1030-1035.
60. J. R. Platt, Prediction of isomeric differences in paraffin properties, J Phys. Chem., **1952**, *56,* 328-336.
61. Special issue of Discrete and Appl. Math., (I. Gutman, S. Klavzar and B. Mohar, eds).
62. Special issue of MATCH (Communication in Mathematical and Computer Chemistry), vol. 35 (I. Gutman, S. Klavzar and B. Mohar, eds).
63. M. Randić and J. Zupan, On the interpretation of well known topological indices, J. Chem. Inf. Comp. Sci. (in press).
64. D. Plavšić, S. Nikolić, N. Trinajstić and Z. Mihalić, On the Harary index for the characterization of chemical graphs, J. Math. Chem., **1993**, *12,* 235-250.
O. Ivanciuc, T. S. Balaban and A. T. Balaban, Design of topological indices. Part 4. Reciprocal distance matrix, related local vertex invariants and topological indices, J. Math. Chem., **1993**, *12,* 309-318.
M. V. Diudea, O. M. Minailiuc, S. Nikolić and N. Trinajstić, Matrices of reciprocal distance, MATCH, **1997**
65. I. Lukovits, An algorithm for computation of the Wiener index, Croat. Chem. Acta, **1995**, *68,* 99-103.
I. Lukovits and I. Gutman, Edge-decomposition of the Wiener number, MATCH, **1994**, *31,* 133-144.
M. Juvan and B. Mohar, Bond contribution to the Wiener number, J. Chem. Inf. Comput. Sci., **1995**, *35,* 217-219.
66. J. R. Platt, Influence of neighbor bonds on additive bond properties in paraffins, J. Chem. Phys., **1947**, *15,* 419-420.
M. Randić, Characterization of atoms, molecules, and classes of molecules based on path enumeration, MATCH, **1979**, *7,* 3-60.
M. Randić, Representation of molecular graphs by basic graphs, J. Chem. Inf. Comput. Sci., **1992**, *32,* 57-69.
67. M. Randić, Random walks and their diagnostic value for characte4ization of atomic environment, J. Comput. Chem., **1980**, *1,* 386-399.

J. V. Knop, W. R. Müller, K. Szymanski, M. Randić and N. Trinajstić, Note on acyclic structures and their self-returning walks, Croat, Chem. Acta, **1983**, *56,* 405-409.
M. Razinger, Discrimination and ordering of chemical structures by the number of walks, Theor. Chim. Acta, **1986**, *70,* 365-378.
G. Rücker and C. Rücker, Counts of all walks as atomic and molecular descriptors, J. Chem. Inf. Comput. Sci., **1993**, *33,* 683-695.
O. Ivanciuc and A. T. Balaban, The characterization of chemical structures by the atomic counts of self-returning walks: on the construction of isocodal graphs, Croat. Chem. Acta, **1996**, *69,* 66-74.
M. V. Diudea, Walk numbers $^{e}W_{M}$: Wiener-type numbers of higher rank, J. Chem. Inf. Comput. Sci., **19962**, *36,* 535-540.
G. Rücker and C. Rücker, Walk counts, labyrinthicity, and complexity of acyclic and cyclic graphs ands molecules, J. Chem. Inf. Comput. Sci., 2000, 40, 99-106.

68. M. Randić and M. Razinger, On characterization of 3D molecular structure, in: *From Chemical Topology to Three-Dimensional Geometry,* (A. T. Balaban, ed.), Plenum Press, New York, (1997).
69. D. Hilbert, Math. Ann., **1891**, *38,* 459.
G. Peano, Math. Ann., **1890**, *36,* 157.
D.E. Knuth (see V. Batagelj)
V. Batagelj, Drawing space-filling curves in Logo, Univ. of Ljubljana, Slovenia (preprint)
70. A.C. Edmondson, "A Fuller Explanation: The Synergetic geometry of R. Buckminster Fuller" (1987).
71. H. Li, R. Helling, C. Tang, N. Wingreen, Emergence of preferred structures in a simple model of protein folding, Science, **1996**, *273,* 666-669..
72. M. Randić and G. Krilov, On a characterization of the folding of proteins, Int. J. Quant. Chem. 1999, (in print).
73. M. Randić and M. Razinger, Molecular topological indices, J. Chem. Inf. Comput. Sci., **1995**, *35,* 140-147.
74. M. Randić, Molecular profiles -- novel geometry0dependent molecular descriptors, New J. Chem., **1995**, *19,* 781-791.
75. M. Randić and M. Razinger, On characterization of molecular shapes, J. Chem. Inf. Comput. Sci., **1995**, *35,* 594-606.
M. Randić, Molecular shape profiles, J. Chem. Inf. Comput. Sci., **1995**, *35,* 373-382.
76. M. Randić, Molecular bonding profiles, J. Math. Chem., **1996**, *19,* 375-392.
77. M. Randić and G. Krilov, Bond profiles for cuboctahedron and twist cuboctahedron, Int. J. Quantum Chem: Quantum Biol. Symp., **1996**, *23,* 127-139.
78. M. Randić and G. Krilov, On characterization of molecular surfaces, Int. J. Quantum Chem., **1997**, *65,* 10657-1076.
79. H. S. M. Coxeter, Self dual configurations and regular graphs, Bull. Amer. Math. Soc., **1950**, *56,* 413-455.
T. Pisanski and M. Randić, Hexagonal systems and their Menger and Levi graphs (to be published)

80. J. D. Roberts, Notes on Molecular Orbital Calculations, Benjamin, New York, (1962) pp. 131 - 139.
81. C. Raychaudhury, A. Nandy, Indexing scheme and similarity measures for macromolecular sequences, J. Chem. Inf. Comput. Sci., **1999**, *39,* 243-247.
82. A. Nandy, A new graphical representation and analysis of DNA sequence structure. I. Methodology and application to globin genes, Current Science, **1994**, *66,* 309-313.
A. Nandy, Graphical analysis of DNA sequence structure: III. Indications of evolutionary distinctions and characteristics of introns and exons, Current Science, **1996**, *70,* 661-668.
A. Roy, C. Raychaudhury, A. Nandy, J. Biosci., **1998**, *23,* 55.
83. M. Randić, A. Nandy and S. C. Basak, On numerical characterization of DNA primary sequences, J. Math Chem. (in press).
84. M. Randić and M. Vraćko, Novel Numerical characterization of DNA primary sequences based on sequential indices of nucleic acids (to be published).
85. M. Randić, M. Vraćko, A. Nandy and S. C. Basak, On 3D graphical representation of DNA primary sequences and their numerical characterization. J. Chem. Inf. Comp. Sci. 2000, 40, 1235-1244.
86. D. E. Manolopoulus and P. W. Fowler, J. Chem. Phys., **1992**, *96,* 7603.
P. W. Folwer, T. Pisanski, and J. Shave-Taylor, in: Graph Drawing, Lecture Notes in Computer Science, Springer Verlag, Berlin (R. Tamassia and I. G. Tollis, Eds.), **1995**, *894*, 282.
T. Pisanski, B. Plestenjak, and A. Graovac, NiceGraph program and its applications in chemistry, Croat. Chem. Acta, **1995**, *68,* 283-292.
87. M. Randić and M. Vraćko, On similarity of DNA primary sequences J. Chem. Inf. Comp. Sci. 2000, 40, 599-606.
88. R. F. Muirhead, Proc. Edinburgh Math. Soc., **1903**, *21,* 144-
89. O. J. Heilmann and E. H. Lieb, Theory of monomer-dimer systems, Commun. Math. Phys., **1972**, *25,* 190-232.
E. Ruch, Acc. Chem. Res., **1972**, *5,* 49-
E. Ruch, Theor. Chim. Acta. 1975, 38, 167.
M. Randić, On comparability of structures, Chem. Phys. Lett., **1978**, *55,* 547-551.
90. M. Randić and N. Trinajstić, Isomeric variations in alkanes: Boiling points in nonanes, New J. Chem., **1994**, *18,* 179-189.
91. M. Randić, B. Jerman-Blažić, S. C. Grossman and D. H. Rouvray, A Rational approach to the optimal drug design, Math. Modelling, **1986**, *8,* 571-582.
M. Randić, B. Jerman-Blažić, D. H. Rouvray, P. G. Seybold, and S. C. Grossman, The search for active substructure in structure-activity studies, Int. J. Quant. Chem. Quant. Biol. Symp., **1987**, *14,* 245-260.
92. J. R. Dias, A periodic table for aromatic hydrocarbons. Isomer enumeration of fused polycyclic aromatic hydrocarbons, J. Chem. Inf. Comput. Sci., **1982**, *22,* 15-22.
J. R. Dias, A formula periodic table for benzenoid hydrocarbons and the aufbau and excised internal structure concept in benzenoid enumerations, Zeit. Naturforsch., **1989**, *44a,* 765-771.
J. R. Dias, A periodic table for polycyclic aromatic hydrocarbons, Acc. chem. Res.,

1985, *18,* 241-248.
J. R. Dias, the formula periodic table set for benzenoid hydrocarbons and the unifying theory of a periodic table set, Polycyclic Aromatic Compounds, **1994**, *4,* 87-106.
J. R. Dias, Setting benzenoids to order, Chem. Brit., **1994**, 384-386.
J. R. Dias, Formula periodic tables - their construction and related symmetries, J. Chem. Inf. Comput. Sci., **1996**, *36,* 361-366.
93. M. Randić, Chemical shift sums, J. Magn. Res., **1980**, *39,* 431-436.
M. Randić and N. Trinajstić, Composition as a method for data reduction. Application to carbon-13 NMR chemical shifts, Theor. Chim. Acta, **19882**, *73,* 233-246.
Y. Miyashita, H. Ohsako, T. Okuyama, S. Sasaki and M. Randić, Computer assisted studies of structure-property relationship, Magn. Res. Chem.., **1991**, *29,* 362-365.
94. M. Randić, On characterization of chemical structure, J. Chem. Inf. Comput. Sci., **1997**, *37,* 672-687.
95. M. Randić and N. Trinajstić, Critical test for resonance energies, J. Am. Chem. Soc., **1987**, *109,* 6923-6926.
M. Randić, S. Nikolić, and N. Trinajstić, The conjugated circuit model. On selection of the parameters for computing the resonance energies, in: Graph Theory and Topology in Chemistry (R. B. King and D. H. Rouvray, eds.), Studies Phys. Theor. Chem., **1987**, *51,* 429-447.
S. Nikolić, M. Randić, D. J. Klein, D. Plavšić, and N. Trinajstić, The conjugated circuit model: Application to benzenoid hydrocarbons, J. Mol. Struct. (Theochem), **1989**, *198,* 223-237.
D. J. Klein, M. Randić, D. Babić and N. Trinajstić, On conjugated circuit polynomials, Int. J. Quant. Chem, **1994**, *50,* 369-384.
M. Randić, Resonance in very large benzenoids, Acta Chim. Slovenica, **1996**, *43,* 255-267.
M. Randić, Resonance in catacondensed benzenoid hydrocarbons, Int. J. Quant. Chem., 1997, 63, 585-600.
M. Randić, D. J. Klein, S. El-Basil and P. Calkins, Resonance in large benzenoid hydrocarbons, Croat. Chem. Acta, **1996**, *69,* 1639-1660.

Chapter 8

NEW NEURAL NETWORKS FOR STRUCTURE-PROPERTY MODELS

Ovidiu Ivanciuc
University "Politehnica" of Bucharest,
Department of Organic Chemistry
Faculty of Industrial Chemistry,
Oficiul 12 CP 243, 78100
Bucharest, Romania
E-mail: ivanciuc@netscape.net

1. INTRODUCTION

The growing interest in the application of Artificial Neural Networks (ANN)[1-4] in chemistry,[5-8] in chemical engineering,[9] and in biochemistry[10] is a result of their demonstrated superiority over the traditional models. Neural networks were used in quantitative structure-property relationships (QSPR) and quantitative structure-activity relationships (QSAR) studies to predict various physical, chemical, and biological properties of organic compounds. Conventional QSPR and QSAR require the user to specify the mathematical function of the model. If these functions are highly nonlinear then considerable mathematical and numerical expertise is needed to obtain significant models. In recent years this problem was solved with ANN that generate highly non-linear models between input and output variables; an important advantage of ANN is the fact that the mathematical form of the relationship between the input and output variables is not specified by the user. An ANN may be represented as an assembly of units (artificial neurons) that performs some basic mathematic operations and that receive and send signals through connections. Each connection between two neurons has an adjustable weight that modifies the signal send through that connection. The artificial neuron is a simplified model of a neuron having four basic functions: receives input signals from the environment or from the neurons in the previous layer; makes a summation of the inputs signals; the result of summation is passed to the activation function and transformed with a mathematical function; the result of the activation function is used by a transfer function to produce an output value that is send to the neurons in the next layer. The most important activation functions are: linear, $Act(x) = x$; sigmoid, $Act(x) = 1/(1 + e^{-x})$; hyperbolic tangent, $Act(x) = tanh(x)$; symmetric logarithmoid, $Act(x) = \text{sign}(x) \ln(1+|x|)$; bell, $Act(x) = 1/(1 + x^2)$.[11-15]

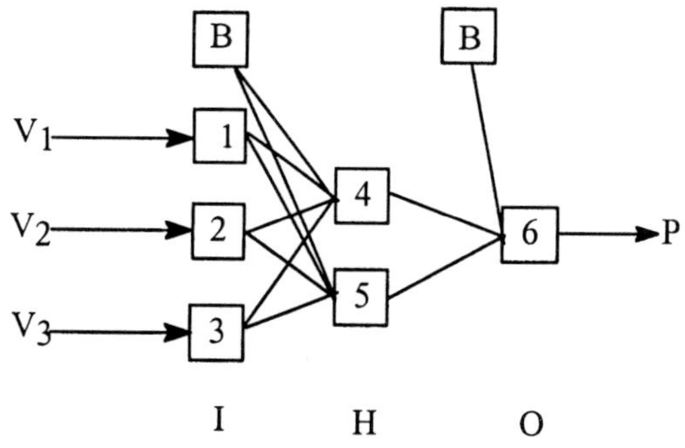

Figure 1. The topology of a multilayer feed-forward neural network with three layers

In multi-layer feedforward (MLF) networks, usually used in QSPR and QSAR studies, the neurons are arranged in distinct layers, with connections between the neurons in different layers; the structure of a simple MLF network with three layers is presented in Figure 1. The input layer I receives the input signals from the environment and sends them to the next layer. The middle layer H is called the hidden layer because it is not connected directly to the environment, but receives signals from the input layer, transforms them, and sends information to the output layer or to the next hidden layer. The output layer O receives signals from the hidden layer, processes them, and sends to the environment the result computed by the network. Each neuron in the hidden and output layers is connected to a bias neuron B. An MLF contains a number of input neurons equal to the number of descriptors that describe the structure of each chemical compound, and a number of output neurons equal to the number of physical, chemical, or biological properties modeled by the ANN. The network in Figure 1 has three input neurons, meaning that the chemical structure is represented with three descriptors, denoted here V_1, V_2, and V_3. When a pattern representing in numerical form the structure of a certain molecule is presented to the network, descriptor V_1 goes to input neuron 1, V_2 goes to input neuron 2, and V_3 goes to input neuron 3. In this way the information regarding the chemical structure of a molecule is entered into the ANN. The hidden layer is formed by neurons 4 and 5, and the output layer contains neuron 6. The output neuron 6 offers the computed value of the property P for the compound whose structure was encoded in descriptors V_1, V_2, and V_3. We have to note here that the multilinear regression model, widely used in QSPR and QSAR, is equivalent with a multi-layer feedforward network without hidden layer and with one output neuron provided with linear activation function.

An important problem for the QSPR and QSAR applications of ANN remains the numerical representation of the chemical structure used as input by the ANN; a recent review presents the molecular graph descriptors used as input data for ANN models.[16] The molecular graph descriptors[17-21] represent an important class of structural descriptors for QSPR and QSAR studies; these descriptors present important advantages when compared with other classes of descriptors because they can be easily computed from the molecular graph and they do not require the computation of the molecular geometry. For example, simple graph descriptors (the number of carbon atoms and the number of pairs of methyl groups separated by 3 up to 8 carbon-carbon single bonds) were used to obtain an ANN model for six physical properties of alkanes.[22]

The usual structure of an MLF network is not dependent on the chemical structure of the molecules from the calibration and prediction sets. Three new neural networks were defined in order to encode into their topology the chemical structure of each compound presented to the network: the Baskin-Palyulin-Zefirov neural device,[23] ChemNet defined by Kireev,[24] and MolNet introduced by Ivanciuc.[25,26] All the above neural networks change their topology (the number of neurons in the input and hidden layers, together with the number and type of connections) according to the molecular structure of the chemical compound presented to the network. The structure of each molecule is represented as a molecular graph that is used to set the ANN topology. In this review we present the rules that define the three neural models together with examples of network generation from the molecular graph.

2. THE BASKIN, PALYULIN, ZEFIROV NEURAL DEVICE

The Baskin, Palyulin, Zefirov (BPZ)[23] neural device is a special MLF neural network that generates nonlinear QSPR and QSAR correlations using as input data local invariants describing the atomic environment or bonding relationships. The structure of the BPZ neural device, presented in Figure 2, is constructed by analogy with a biological vision system and contains a sensor field, a set of eyes, and a brain. A chemical structure modeled by the BPZ neural device is represented as a molecular matrix that is superimposed over a sensor field. The sensor field receives the network input from the numerical representation of the chemical structure. The information received by the sensor field is transmitted to a set of eyes that transform it in several MLF networks, and sends signals to the next block, the brain. All output signals from the eyes are processes in the brain with the aid of an MLF ANN that offers at its output the computed values of the investigated properties. According to a set of rules the structure of the sensor field and of the eyes depends on the chemical nature of the atoms and their bonding relationships for each molecule presented to the neural device.

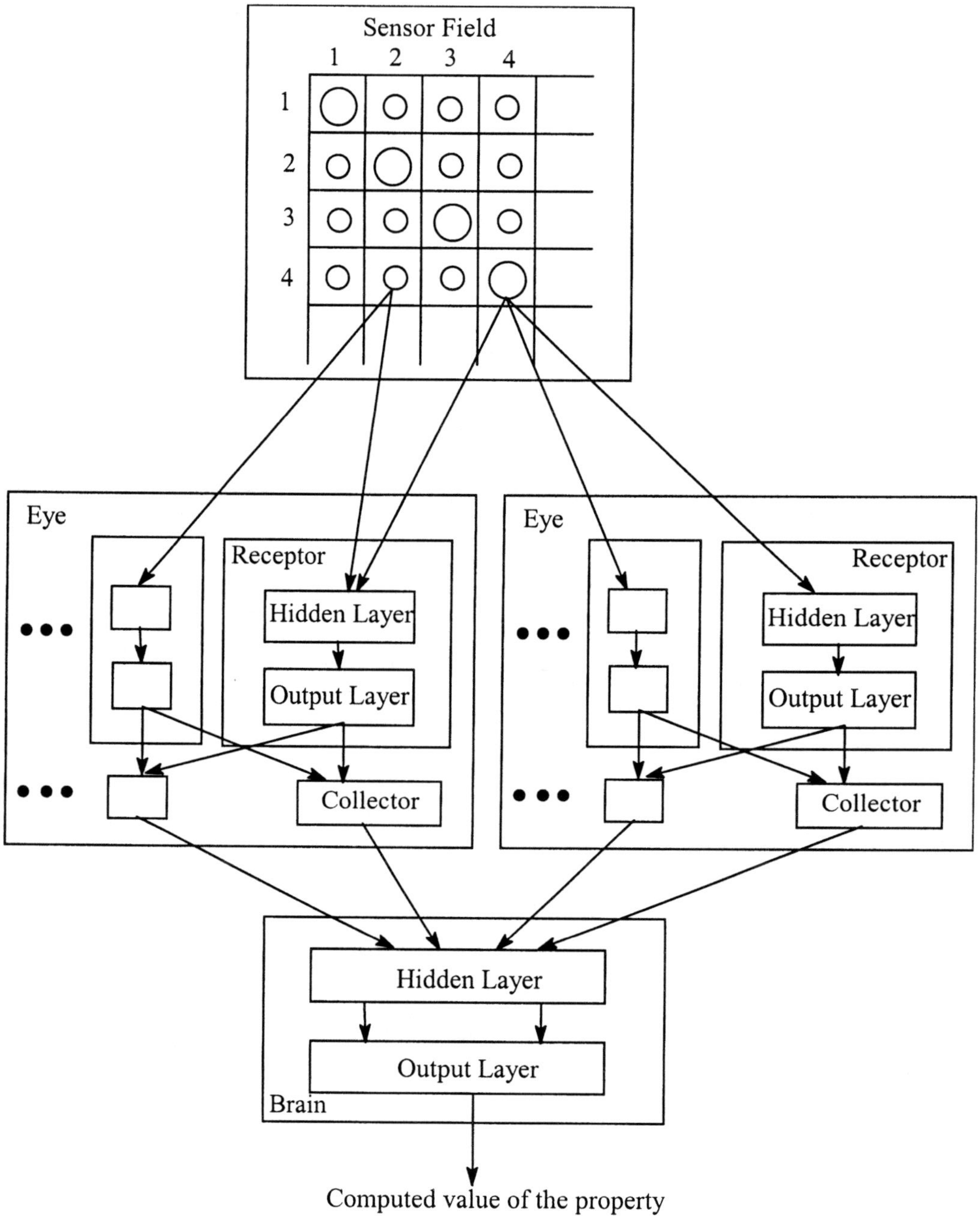

Figure 2. The structure of the Baskin, Palyulin, Zefirov neural device.

All input neurons in the sensor field receive specific structural elements from a chemical compound and send this information to the neural networks situated in the eyes. The neurons that form the eyes and the brain receive signals, sum them, transform the sum, and send output signals. These neurons are connected to a bias neuron; in the mathematical equations that describe their function the connection from the bias neuron is represented as a threshold. The three building blocks that form the BPZ neural device are presented in detail below.

Using a matrix representation, the chemical structure of each organic compound presented to the BPZ neural device is encoded into the sensor field. The atoms are labeled from 1 to N, where N is the number of non-hydrogen atoms from the current molecule. The molecular structure is represented by an $N \times N$ matrix in which the ii-th element (situated on i-th position of the diagonal) corresponds to a certain property of the ith atom in the current molecule, and the ij-th element (situated at the intersection of the ith row with the j-th column) is a numerical value representing some relationship between atoms i and j from the current molecule. This molecular matrix is symmetric, i.e. the ij-th element is identical with the ji-th element. The atomic properties that can be used on the main diagonal of this matrix are the principal quantum number, the electronegativity, the atomic charge, the number of valence electrons, the number of hydrogen atoms attached to the atom. The nondiagonal matrix elements represent various interatomic relationships, such as connectivity information, the interatomic distance or the bond order. The sensor field is formed by input neurons arranged in a square $N \times N$ matrix. Each neuron corresponds to an element in the molecular matrix from the current molecule. A sensor neuron receives the value of the corresponding molecular matrix element and sends the structural information through weighted connections to the eyes.

The BPZ neural device contains two or more eyes, each one receiving specific information about the chemical structure of the current molecule. An eye contains a set of identical receptors and one or more collectors. All receptors situated in an eye are identical, containing the same number of neurons, the same weights for connections between identical pairs of neurons, and equal thresholds for identical neurons situated in different receptors. A receptor is an MLF network that receives signals from the sensor field, processes them in a hidden layer, and from the output layer sends signals to the collector(s). The hidden layer can have any number of neurons, but the output layer always contains one neuron that sends signals to the collectors from the same eye. Each eye receptor is connected to a specific field from the sensor field that contains a part of the information related to the chemical structure. For each receptor there is an ordered vector $\{v_1, v_2, ..., v_i, ... v_n\}$, where n is the number of atoms sending signals to the receptor and v_i is the label of the corresponding atom in a molecule. This specific vector is called a receptor identifier and represents the molecular substructure perceived by a specific receptor. The number of receptors situated in an eye is equal to the number of different receptor identifiers that can be generated, i.e. $N!/(N-n)!$, where N is the number of non-hydrogen atoms in the molecule encoded in the sensor field, and n is the number of atoms in a receptive field. A receptor identifier containing n atoms is called n-atomic. A molecule that contains three non-hydrogen atoms can be analyzed by the BPZ neural device in three ways: with three receptors receiving signals from the one-atomic receptor identifiers {1}, {2}, and {3}; with six receptors receiving signals from the two-atomic receptor identifiers {1, 2}, {1, 3}, {2, 1}, {2, 3}, {3, 1}, and {3 ,2}; with six receptors receiving signals from the three-atomic receptor identifiers {1, 2, 3}, {1, 3, 2}, {2, 1, 3}, {2, 3, 1}, {3, 1, 2}, and {3, 2, 1}.

The signals processed in each receptor from an eye are send to one or more collectors from the same eye. Each collector contains a neuron that receives signals, sums them, transforms the sum, and sends a signal to the brain of the BPZ neural device. The brain is a feed-forward neural network that receives signals from every collector, processes them in a hidden layer, and from the output layer sends signals that represent the computed value of the investigated molecular property. The hidden layer can contain any number of neurons, but the output layer always contains a number of neurons equal to the number of molecular properties modeled with the BPZ neural device. Each output neuron corresponds to one and only one molecular property.

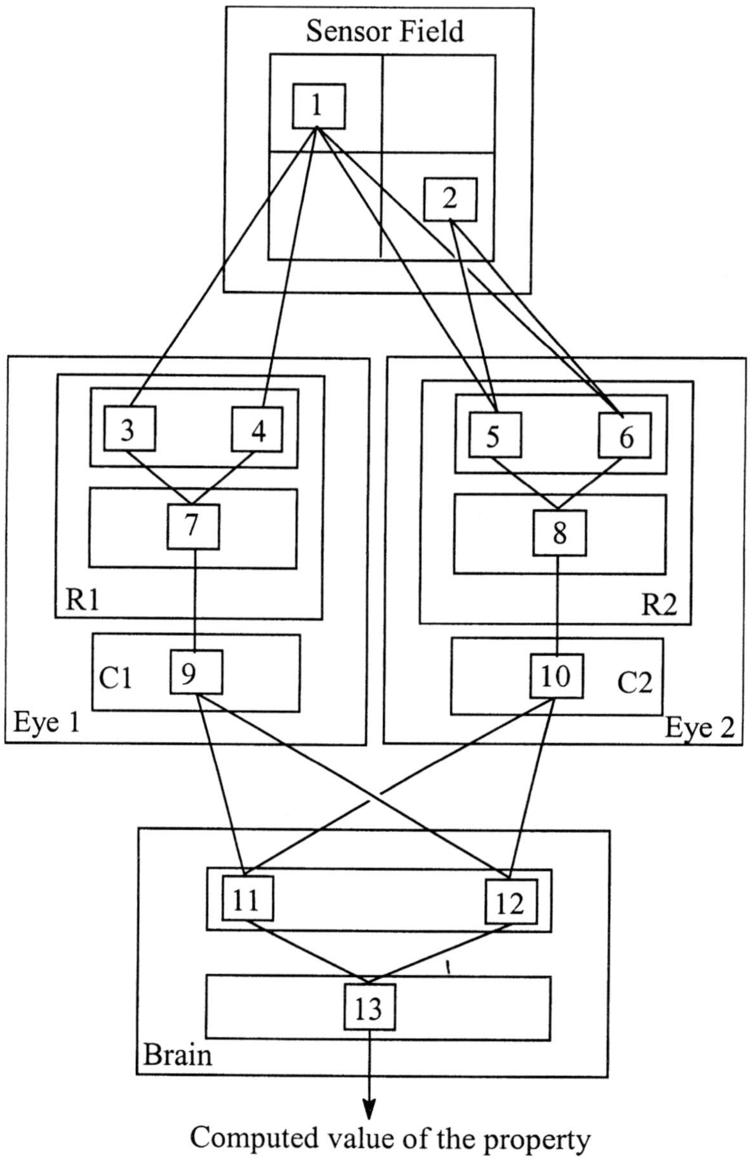

Figure 3. A minimal configuration of the Baskin, Palyulin, Zefirov neural device.

The BPZ neural device that contains all receptors needed for the perception of a molecule represents the configuration for that molecule. A BPZ neural device with a minimal configuration, presented in Figure 3, has one receptor in each eye and contains only mutually independent adjustable parameters. A minimal configuration can be used as a template for the construction of the BPZ neural device for any molecule presented to the neural device and encoded in the sensor field. In this case, the sensor field is a square matrix containing only atomic sensors situated on the diagonal of the matrix. The minimal configuration has two eyes with different functions: eye 1 receive signals from individual atoms, while eye 2 receives from the sensor field signals corresponding to pairs of bonded atoms. The signals from the sensor neuron 1 go to neurons 3 and 4 that represent the hidden layer of the receptor R1 from Eye 1. The processed signals are send to the output neuron 7. The collector C1 has one neuron, 9, that gets the signal from the eye receptor and sends it to the brain. From the neurons in the sensor field Eye 2 receives signals from pairs of bonded atoms: neurons 1 and 2 send two signals to receptor neuron 5, and another pair of signals to receptor neuron 6. The signal flow in Eye 2 is similar with that from Eye 1: from the input neurons 5 and 6 to the output neuron 8 and then to the collector neuron 10. The brain has an input layer that contains neurons 11 and 12, and an output layer containing the neuron 13. The brain input neurons 11 and 12 receive signals from the two eyes collector neurons 9 and 10, respectively. Brain output neuron 13 offers the computed molecular property of the molecule encoded in the sensor field.

The structure of the BPZ neural device for ethane is presented in Figure 4. Ethane is considered here as its hydrogen-depleted molecular graph. The threshold of a neuron i is denoted with θ_i and the weight of the connection between neurons i and j is denoted with w_{ij}. According to the rules for generating a BPZ neural device, certain connections weights and neuron thresholds have identical values. In this way, the number of adjustable parameters is much lower than the number of connections between neurons. For ethane, the receptor field is a square 2×2 matrix, containing only atomic sensors (neurons 1 and 2) situated on the diagonal of the matrix, corresponding to the two carbon atoms in ethane. The input value for the sensor neurons can be any property of the corresponding atom; if this property is the atomic number Z, both sensor neurons in ethane receive the value 6. The neural device presented in Figure 4 consists of two eyes, Eye 1 and Eye 2, with different functions: each receptor situated in Eye 1 receives signals from only one sensor neuron representing an atom, while each receptor from Eye 2 receives signals from two-atomic receptive fields corresponding to atoms that have a bond between them in the molecule encoded in the sensor field. Each eye has two receptors and one collector. The ethane BPZ neural device is generated from the minimal configuration neural device presented in Figure 3, and as one can see from Figure 4, each receptor has two hidden and one output neuron. From the BPZ neural device generation algorithm it results that the following eye neurons thresholds are identical: $\theta_3 = \theta_5$, $\theta_4 = \theta_6$, $\theta_7 = \theta_9$, $\theta_8 = \theta_{10}$, $\theta_{11} = \theta_{12}$, and $\theta_{13} = \theta_{14}$. Some connections between neurons in the sensor field and neurons in the receptors input layers have identical weights: $w_{1,3} = w_{2,5}$, $w_{1,4} = w_{2,6}$, $w_{1,7} = w_{2,9}$, $w_{1,9} = w_{2,7}$, $w_{1,8} = w_{2,10}$, and $w_{1,10} = w_{2,8}$. One finds also identical weights for certain connections between neurons in the receptor input and output layers:

$w_{3,11} = w_{5,12}$, $w_{4,11} = w_{6,12}$, $w_{7,13} = w_{9,14}$, and $w_{8,13} = w_{10,14}$. Finally, the following connections between receptors and collectors have identical weights: $w_{11,15} = w_{12,15}$, and $w_{13,16} = w_{14,16}$. Each eye contains a single collector containing one neuron, namely neurons 15 and 16, and each eye sends signals to the brain. The BPZ neural device was successfully used in the prediction of alkanes boiling points, hydrocarbons viscosity, heat of evaporation, and density, cyclohexane heat of solvation, organic compounds polarizability, and gases anesthetic pressure.

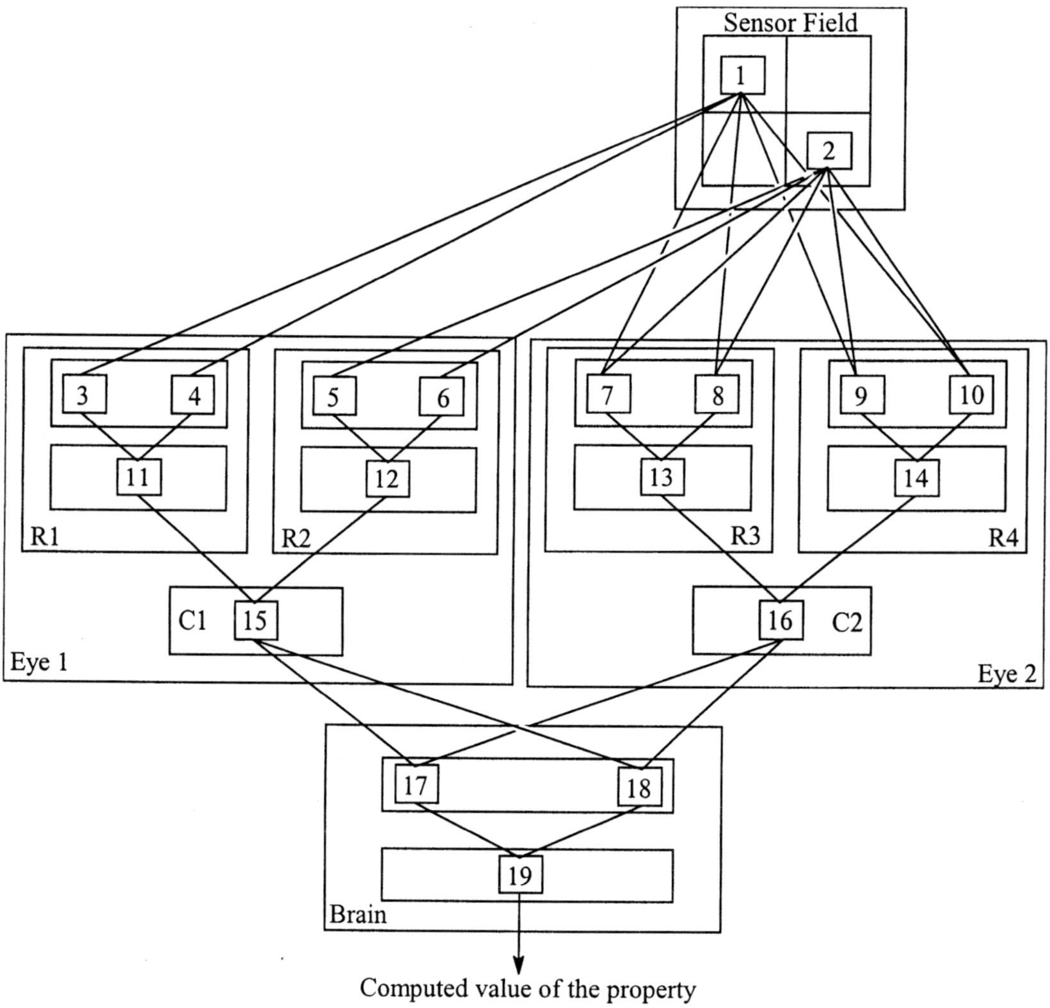

Figure 4. The structure of the Baskin, Palyulin, Zefirov neural device for ethane.

3. ChemNet

ChemNet is an MLF neural network that encodes in its topology the structure of each molecule presented to the network, and computes an atomic property, such as the atomic charge.[24] Each molecule is represented by its labeled hydrogen-depleted molecular graph. For each atom *i* from the molecular graph ChemNet has two corresponding neurons with the same label *i*, one in the input layer and the second one in the hidden layer. The output layer has only one neuron, representing the atom from the molecular graph whose property is computed with ChemNet. The network contains also a bias neuron, connected to the hidden and output neurons. ChemNet changes the number and significance of the neurons with each molecule presented to the network. The connections between the input and hidden layers correspond to the bonding relationships between pairs of atoms, i.e. two pairs of atoms separated by the same number of bonds have identical connection weights.

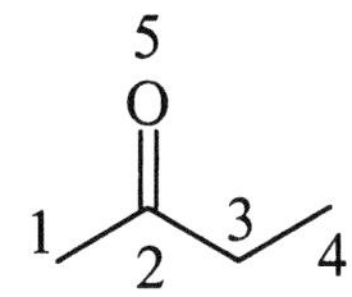

1

As an example of ChemNet structure we present the network generation for butanone **1**. In ChemNet the bonding relationship that determines the type of the connections between input and hidden layers considers only the number of bonds separating a pair of atoms. These relationships can be determined from the distance matrix of the molecular graph computed by considering that all atoms are carbons and all bonds are single. The distance matrix of the molecular graph **1**, **D(1)**, is:

D(1)

	1	2	3	4	5
1	0	1	2	3	2
2	1	0	1	2	1
3	2	1	0	1	2
4	3	2	1	0	3
5	2	1	2	3	0

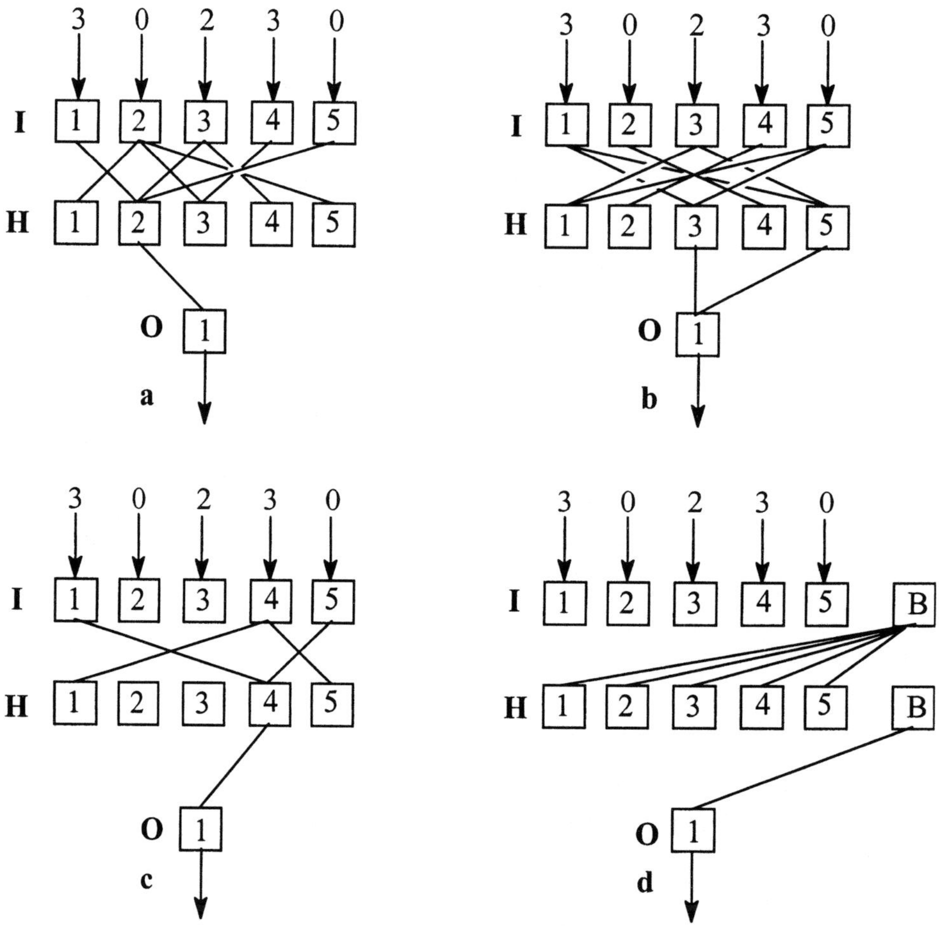

Figure 5. The ChemNet topology for butanone **1** that computes a property of atom 1. Each neuron in the input (**I**) and hidden (**H**) layers corresponds to the atom with the same label from the molecular graph **1**. The connections between atoms situated at distances 1, 2, and 3 are presented in **a**, **b**, and **c**, respectively, while the connections from the bias neuron B are presented in **d**. Input values represent the number of hydrogen atoms attached to each atom in the molecular graph **1**.

The molecular graph of butanone has 5 atoms and the corresponding ChemNet has 5 input and 5 hidden neurons. Each neuron from the input and hidden layers of ChemNet corresponds to the atom with the same label in the molecular graph **1**, as presented in Figure 5a-d; for example, the oxygen atom is represented by the input and hidden neurons labeled with 5. All pairs of atoms in **1** that are separated by the same number of bonds are characterized by input-hidden connections with identical weights. A bonding relationship between two atoms i and j corresponds to two identical input-hidden connections: the first from input neuron i to hidden neuron j, and the second from input neuron j to hidden neuron i. In **1** there are 4 pairs of atoms separated by one bond, as can be seen also from the distance matrix **D(1)**. In Figure 5a we present the ChemNet connections corresponding to pairs of atoms separated by one bond, giving the following equalities between the corresponding weights: $w_{1,2} = w_{2,1} = w_{2,3} = w_{3,2} = w_{3,4} = w_{4,3} = w_{2,5}$

$= w_{5,2}$. The ChemNet connections corresponding to pairs of atoms separated by two bonds are presented in Figure 5b. From the molecular graph of **1** and its corresponding distance matrix it follows that $w_{1,3} = w_{3,1} = w_{1,5} = w_{5,1} = w_{2,4} = w_{4,2} = w_{3,5} = w_{5,3}$. The 4 input-hidden connections corresponding to pairs of atoms separated by three bonds are presented in Figure 5c; they give the following equalities between the corresponding weights: $w_{1,4} = w_{4,1} = w_{4,5} = w_{5,4}$. All connections from the bias neuron to the 5 hidden neurons, presented in Figure 5d, have the same weight: $w_{B,1} = w_{B,2} = w_{B,3} = w_{B,4} = w_{B,5}$.

In Figure 5 we present the ChemNet structure for butanone when atom 1 is the output atom, i.e. the network computes an atomic property of the atom 1. In this case, the output layer contains one neuron representing the atom 1 from butanone. The type of a hidden-output connection joining a hidden neuron *i* with an output neuron *j*, denoted v_{ij}, is determined by the number of bonds between atoms *i* and *j*. There is one hidden-output connection corresponding to atoms one bond away from atom 1, representing the bond between atoms 2 and 1, as presented in Figure 5a. The ChemNet hidden-output connections corresponding to atoms two bonds away from atom 1 are presented in Figure 5b. From the molecular graph of **1** and its corresponding distance matrix it follows that two hidden-output connections have identical weights, namely $v_{3,1} = v_{5,1}$. The connection between atoms 4 and 1, separated by three bonds, is depicted in Figure 5c.

The ChemNet topology that computes an atomic property for atom 2 in butanone is given in Figure 6. The input and hidden layers, together with the connections between them, are identical with those from the ChemNet network generated for the output atom 1, as can be seen by comparing Figures 5 and 6. Therefore, we will explain in detail only the connections between the hidden and output layers. The ChemNet hidden-output connections corresponding to atoms one bond away from atom 2 are presented in Figure 6a, and correspond to three hidden-output connections with identical weights: $v_{1,2} = v_{3,2} = v_{5,2}$. There is one hidden-output connection corresponding to atoms two bonds away from atom 2, representing the path between atoms 4 and 2, as presented in Figure 6b, and there is no atom three bonds away from atom 2, as can be seen from Figure 6c. The connections from the bias neuron to the 5 hidden neurons, and to the output neuron representing atom 2 are depicted in Figure 6d. ChemNet was applied for the computation of AM1 atomic charges.

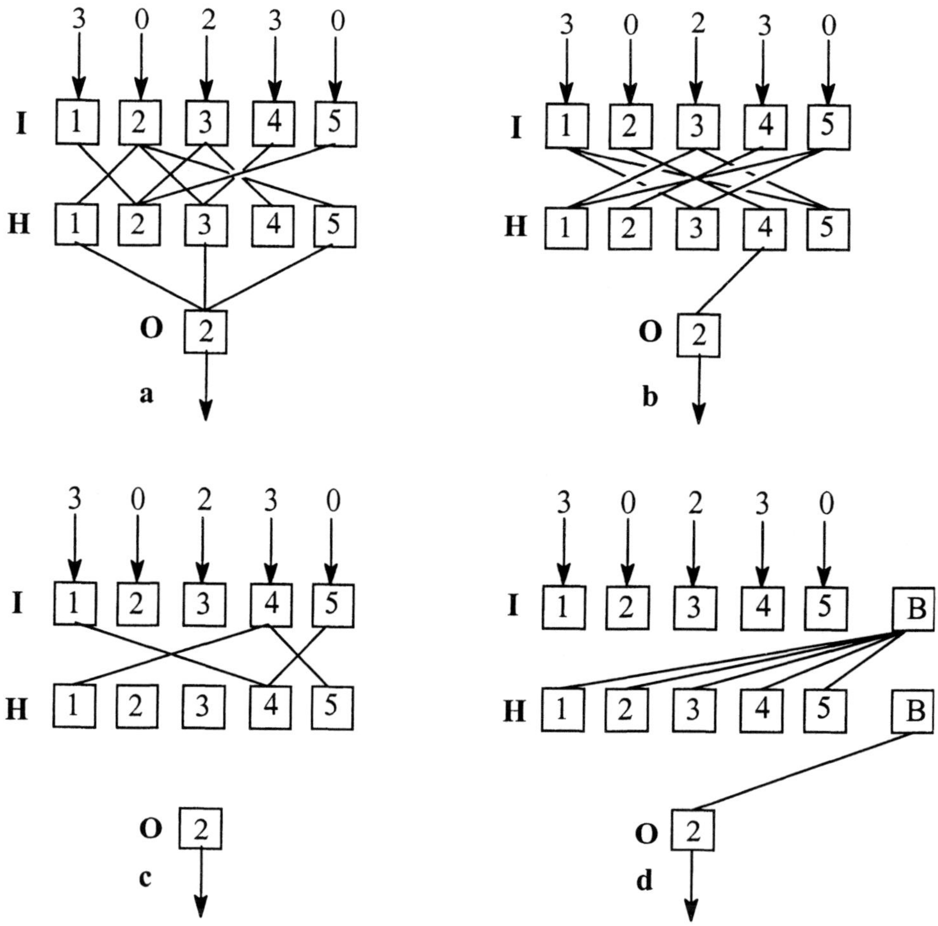

Figure 6. The ChemNet topology for butanone **1** that computes a property of atom 2. Each neuron in the input (**I**) and hidden (**H**) layers corresponds to the atom with the same label from the molecular graph **1**. The connections between atoms situated at distances 1, 2, and 3 are presented in **a**, **b**, and **c**, respectively, while the connections from the bias neuron B are presented in **d**. Input values represent the number of hydrogen atoms attached to each atom in the molecular graph **1**.

4. MolNet

MolNet is a multi-layer feedforward neural network that can be used to compute molecular properties on the basis of chemical structure descriptors.[25,26] A specific feature of MolNet is that the number of neurons and the connections between them depend on the chemical structure of each molecule presented to the network. Molecules are represented by the corresponding hydrogen-suppressed molecular graph. Each non-hydrogen atom in a molecule has a corresponding neuron in the input and hidden layers. The number of neurons in the input and hidden layers is equal to the number of atoms from the molecular graph. The output layer has only one neuron, providing the calculated value of the molecular property under investigation. The network has a bias neuron, connected to all hidden and output neurons.

The connection between an input and a hidden neuron characterizes the bonding relationship between the corresponding atoms. Input-hidden connections corresponding to the same bonding relationship between two atoms, either in the same molecule or in different molecules, belong to the same connection class and they have identical weights. In MolNet the bonding relationship considers the shortest path between a pair of atoms. Two identical paths contain the same ordered sequence of atoms and bonds; such paths belong to the same connection class. A neuron that corresponds to an atom *i* in the input layer is connected to the neuron corresponding to the same atom *i* in the hidden layer by a connection; these connections are classified according to the chemical nature of the atoms.

The topology of the connections between the hidden and output layers is determined by the partitioning in classes of the atoms from the molecule presented to MolNet. The atoms are partitioned according to the atomic number *Z*, the hybridization state and the degree. All atoms from a class, either in the same molecule or in different molecules, correspond to the same type of hidden neurons. We have to point here that even for neurons in the same class their contribution to the molecular property depends also on the signal received from the input layer, signal that can be different for neurons in the same class. Each neuron in the hidden layer is connected to the bias neuron by connections partitioned in the same way with the connections between the hidden and output layers, i.e. according to the atom types as defined above. Also, the bias neuron is connected with the output neuron.

For a molecule with N non-hydrogen atoms, there are N^2 connections between the input and hidden layers, N connections between the hidden and output layers, N connections from the bias neuron to the hidden neurons, and one connection from the bias neuron to the output neuron. Some connections may have identical weights according to the partitioning schemes described above. This implies that for MolNet the number of adjustable parameters is much smaller than the number of connections. When a molecule is presented to MolNet input neuron *i* receives a signal representing an atomic property computed for the atom *i* of the respective molecular graph. Any vertex invariant computed from the structure of the molecular graph can be used as input for MolNet.

As an example of MolNet generation we consider *t*-butylcyclopropane **2** whose molecular graph is presented below:

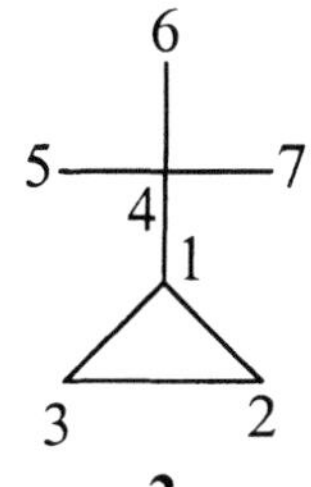

2

In the molecular graph of an alkane, the topological distance between two vertices *i* and *j*, d_{ij}, is equal to the number of edges (corresponding to carbon-carbon single bonds) on the shortest path between the vertices *i* and *j*. Distances d_{ij} are elements of the distance matrix of a molecular graph *G*, **D** = **D**(*G*). The distance matrix of the molecular graph of **2**, **D**(**2**), is:

D(2)

	1	2	3	4	5	6	7
1	0	1	1	1	2	2	2
2	1	0	1	2	3	3	3
3	1	1	0	2	3	3	3
4	1	2	2	0	1	1	1
5	2	3	3	1	0	2	2
6	2	3	3	1	2	0	2
7	2	3	3	1	2	2	0

Molecule **2** contains 7 carbon atoms. Each carbon atom from the molecular graph **2** has a corresponding neuron with the same label in the input and hidden layers of MolNet, as presented in Figure 7a-d. The distance matrix of *t*-butylcyclopropane has 4 classes of topological distances: 7 distances 0; 7 distances 1; 8 distances 2; 6 distances 3. The 4 types of graph distances correspond to four IH (input-hidden) connection types or parameters that are adjusted during the calibration phase. A bonding relationship between two atoms *i* and *j* corresponds to 2 identical IH connections: the first from input neuron *i* to hidden neuron *j*, and the second from input neuron *j* to hidden neuron *i*. As an example of identical IH connections, consider the 6 pairs of atoms: 2 and 5; 2 and 6; 2 and 7; 3 and 5; 3 and 6; 3 and 7. The graph distance between the atoms in the above pairs is 3. Therefore, for molecule **2** there are 12 IH connections with identical weights between the above 6 pairs of atoms, as depicted in Figure 7d. These 12 connections have an identical weight and correspond to the parameter for two carbon atoms situated at distance 3.

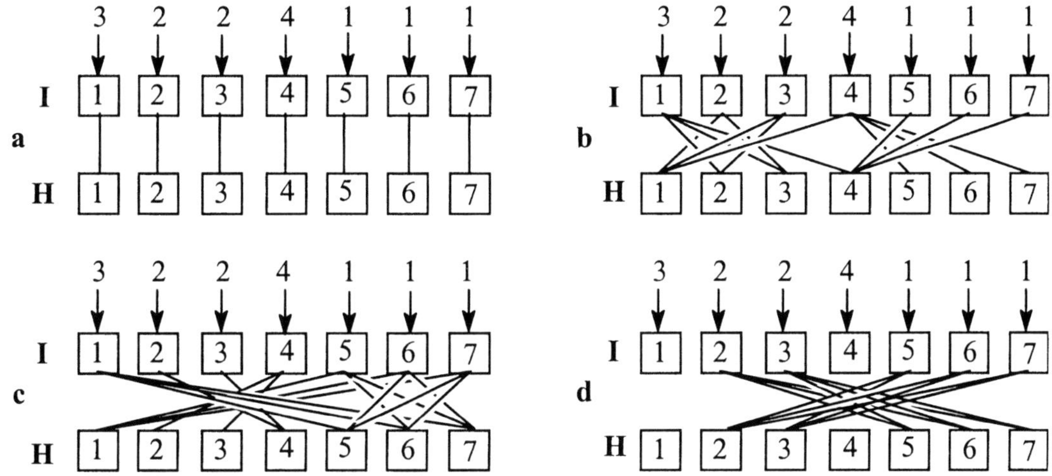

Figure 7. The structure of the MolNet IH connections between the input (**I**) and hidden (**H**) layers for *t*-butylcyclopropane **2**; each neuron corresponds to the carbon atom with the same label from the molecular graph **2**. The connections between atoms with the same label are presented in **a**, while the connections between atoms situated at distances 1, 2, and 3 are presented in **b**, **c**, and **d**, respectively. Input values represent vertex degrees.

In Figure 7a-d we present the structure of IH connections according to the classes of identical weights: there are 7 connections corresponding to distance 0 (Figure 7a), which in our case have identical weights because all non-hydrogen atoms are carbon atoms: $w_{1,1} = w_{2,2} = w_{3,3} = w_{4,4} = w_{5,5} = w_{6,6} = w_{7,7}$; the 7 pairs of atoms situated at distance 1 correspond to the 14 connections with identical weights in Figure 7b: $w_{1,2} = w_{2,1} = w_{1,3} = w_{3,1} = w_{1,4} = w_{4,1} = w_{2,3} = w_{3,2} = w_{4,5} = w_{5,4} = w_{4,6} = w_{6,4} = w_{4,7} = w_{7,4}$; Figure 7c presents the 16 connections between the 8 pairs of atoms situated at distance 2, with the following equalities between connection weights: $w_{1,5} = w_{5,1} = w_{1,6} = w_{6,1} = w_{1,7} = w_{7,1} = w_{2,4} = w_{4,2} = w_{3,4} = w_{4,3} = w_{5,6} = w_{6,5} = w_{5,7} = w_{7,5} = w_{6,7} = w_{7,6}$; the 12 connections corresponding to the 6 pairs of atoms situated at distance 3 are presented in Figure 7d: $w_{2,5} = w_{5,2} = w_{2,6} = w_{6,2} = w_{2,7} = w_{7,2} = w_{3,5} = w_{5,3} = w_{3,6} = w_{6,3} = w_{3,7} = w_{7,3}$.

The connections between the hidden and output layers (the HO connections) are determined by the structure of the molecule presented to MolNet. In alkanes the HO connections are classified according to the degree of the carbon atoms: hidden neurons representing atoms with identical degrees are linked to the output neuron with connections having identical weights. Because the molecular graph of *t*-butylcyclopropane contains three atoms with degree 1, two atoms with degree 2, one atom with degree 3, and one atom with degree 4, the 7 HO connections belong to four classes (i.e. adjustable parameters). The connections between the bias neuron and the neurons in the hidden layer (the BH connections) are classified according to the same rules used for the HO connections, giving in the case of molecule **2** four adjustable weights. For example, there are 3 atoms with degrees 1 in *t*-butylcyclopropane, namely 5, 6, and 7. Figure 8a presents their connections from the bias neuron and to the output neuron. From the rule used to generate the MolNet connections it follows that the 3 atoms with degrees 1 have HO connections with identical weights. If we denote with $v_{i,o}$ the weight of the connection between hidden neuron *i* and output neuron *o*, and with $v_{b,i}$ the weight of the connection between the bias neuron *b* and the hidden neuron *i*, we have the following equalities: $v_{5,o} = v_{6,o} = v_{7,o}$ and $v_{b,5} = v_{b,6} = v_{b,7}$. Because the 3 atoms are also topologically equivalent, the signal send to the output neuron is identical. The same Figure 8a depicts the 3 identical BH connections to the 3 atoms with degrees 1. As a consequence, the signal received from the bias by the neurons 5, 6, and 7 is identical.

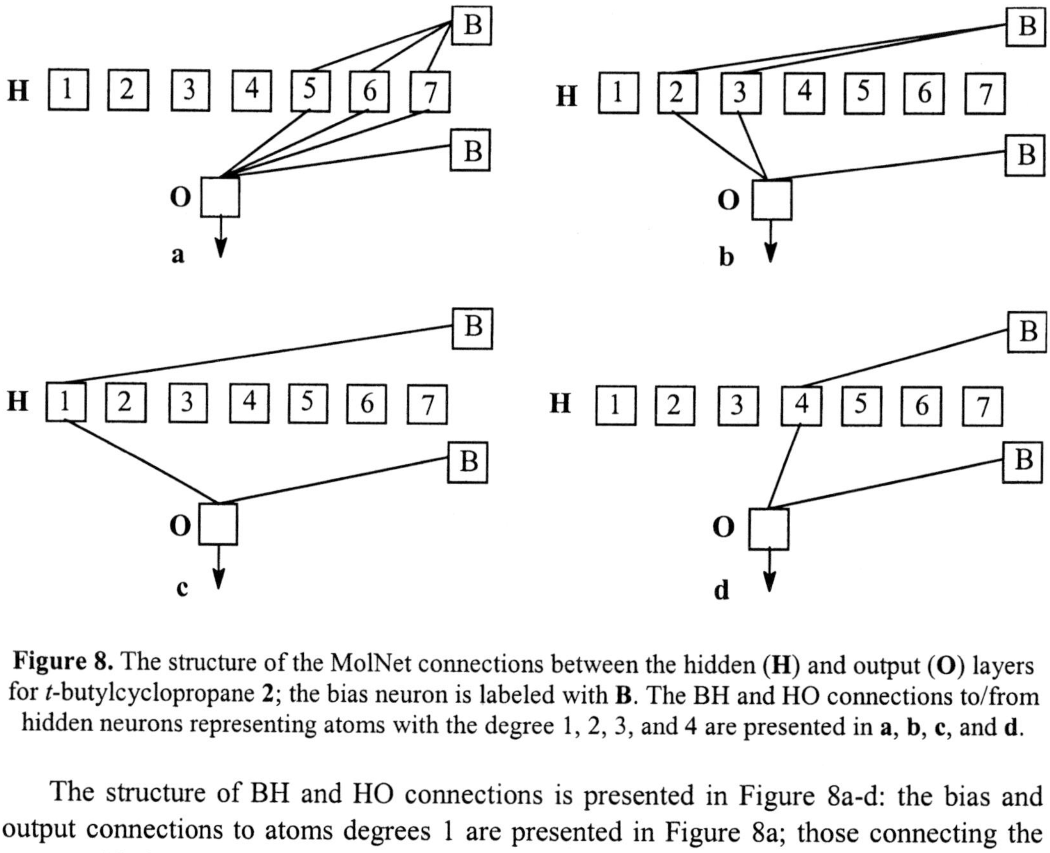

Figure 8. The structure of the MolNet connections between the hidden (**H**) and output (**O**) layers for *t*-butylcyclopropane **2**; the bias neuron is labeled with **B**. The BH and HO connections to/from hidden neurons representing atoms with the degree 1, 2, 3, and 4 are presented in **a**, **b**, **c**, and **d**.

The structure of BH and HO connections is presented in Figure 8a-d: the bias and output connections to atoms degrees 1 are presented in Figure 8a; those connecting the atoms with degrees 2, 3, and 4 are depicted in Figure 8b-d, respectively. The bias neuron has also a connection to the output neuron (BO connection).

Considering all connection types present in the case of *t*-butylcyclopropane the total number of adjustable weights is: 4 (IH connections) + 4 (BH connections) + 4 (HO connections) + 1 (BO connection) = 13. MolNet can contain more parameters, corresponding to bonding relationships that are not present in this example, but are found in one or more molecules from the calibration set. A certain connection type has the same weight in all molecules that contain it.

MolNet is an MLF network and its use involves two phases: a calibration (learning) and a prediction phase, respectively. The target of the calibration phase is to compute an optimal set of IH, HO, BH and BO connection types (adjustable parameters) that minimizes the error in computing the investigated molecular property for the calibration set of molecules. Any optimization algorithm can be used to determine an optimal set of connection types. In the prediction phase MolNet uses the weights determined in calibration to compute the investigated molecular property for molecules that were not present in the calibration set. If the set of molecules used in the prediction phase contains bonding relationships that are absent in the molecules used in the calibration phase these bonding relationships are neglected in predicting the molecular property.

Using a vector of input data computed from the molecular graph, we present the signal flow through MolNet. The degree of an atom i from a molecular graph G, $\mathbf{DEG}_i = \mathbf{DEG}_i(G)$, is computed with the formula:

$$\mathbf{DEG}_i = \sum_{j=1}^{N} \mathbf{A}_{ij} \tag{1}$$

where $\mathbf{A} = \mathbf{A}(G)$ is the adjacency matrix. The degree vector of *t*-butylcyclopropane **2** is **DEG(2)** = {3, 2, 2, 4, 1, 1, 1}. After the generation of MolNet as presented in Figures 7 and 8, the vector of atomic descriptors is entered into the network through the neurons in the input layer. As is usual with neural networks, the input and output values are scaled. Each input neuron receives a numerical value representing the degree of the atom with the same label from the molecular graph. In the case of *t*-butylcyclopropane, input neuron 1 receives the value 3, neuron 2 receives the value 2, neuron 3 receives the value 2, neuron 4 receives the value 4, and neurons 5, 6, and 7 all receive the same value 1. In this way the **DEG** vector is entered into MolNet and is then propagated through the network following the rules of MLF ANN. The signal that is offered by the output neuron represents the computed value of the investigated property for *t*-butylcyclopropane.

5. Conclusions

Usually, a multi-layer feedforward neural network has a topology that does not depend on the structure of the chemical compounds used in calibration or prediction. The network receives information about the structure of the compounds only from the atomic or molecular descriptors received by the neurons in the input layer. In this review we have presented three new MLF neural models that encode the molecular structure into the topology of the neural network: ChemNet defined by Kireev, the neural device introduced by Baskin, Palyulin and Zefirov, and MolNet introduced by Ivanciuc. These neural models are developed specifically for chemical applications; using a set of rules each network encodes into its topology the structure of the molecule examined by the ANN. Depending on the structure of each molecule, the network changes the number of neurons in the input and hidden layers, together with the number and type of connections. Such neural models that use information on the chemical structure to generate the network were applied with success to QSPR studies.

6. References

1. Hopfield, J.J. Neural Networks and Physical Systems with Emergent Collective Computational Abilities. *Proc. Natl. Acad. Sci. U.S.A.* **1982**, *79*, 2554-2558.
2. Rumelhart, D.E.; Hinton, G.E.; Williams, R.J. Learning Representations by Back-Propagating Errors. *Nature* **1986**, *323*, 533-536.
3. Rumelhart, D.E.; McClelland, J.L. *Parallel Distributed Processing*; MIT Press: Cambridge, MA, USA, 1986.
4. Wasserman, P.D. *Neural Computing*; Van Nostrand Reinhold: New York, 1989.
5. Zupan, J.; Gasteiger, J. Neural Networks: A New Method for Solving Chemical Problems or Just a Passing Phase? *Anal. Chim. Acta* **1991**, *248*, 1-30.
6. Gasteiger, J.; Zupan, J. Neural Networks in Chemistry. *Angew. Chem. Int. Ed. Engl.* **1993**, *32*, 503-527.
7. Burns, J.A.; Whitesides, G.M. Feed-Forward Neural Networks in Chemistry: Mathematical Systems for Classification and Pattern Recognition. *Chem. Rev.* **1993**, *93*, 2583-2601.
8. Zupan, J.; Gasteiger, J. *Neural Networks for Chemists*; VCH: Weinheim, 1993.
9. Bulsari, A.B. *Neural Networks for Chemical Engineers*; Elsevier: Amsterdam, 1995.
10. Devillers, J. *Neural Networks in QSAR and Drug Design*. Academic Press, London, 1996.
11. Ivanciuc, O. Artificial Neural Networks Applications. Part 5. Prediction of the Solubility of C_{60} in Organic Solvents. *Rev. Roum. Chim.* **1998**, *43*, 775-783.
12. Ivanciuc, O. Artificial Neural Networks Applications. Part 6. Use of Non-Bonded van der Waals and Electrostatic Intramolecular Energies in the Estimation of ^{13}C-NMR Chemical Shifts in Saturated Hydrocarbons. *Rev. Roum. Chim.*, **1995**, *40*, 1093-1101.
13. Ivanciuc, O. Artificial Neural Networks Applications. Part 8. The Influence of the Activation Function in the Estimation of the Sensorial Scores of Red Wine Color. *Rev. Roum. Chim.* **1998**, *43*, 545-551.
14. Ivanciuc, O.; Rabine, J.-P.; Cabrol-Bass, D.; Panaye, A.; Doucet, J.P. ^{13}C NMR Chemical Shift Prediction of sp^2 Carbon Atoms in Acyclic Alkenes using Neural Networks. *J. Chem. Inf. Comput. Sci.* **1996**, *36*, 644-653.
15. Ivanciuc, O.; Rabine, J.-P.; Cabrol-Bass, D.; Panaye, A.; Doucet, J.P. ^{13}C NMR Chemical Shift Prediction of the sp^3 Carbon Atoms in the α Position Relative to the Double Bond in Acyclic Alkenes. *J. Chem. Inf. Comput. Sci.* **1997**, *37*, 587-598.
16. Ivanciuc, O. Molecular Graph Descriptors Used in Neural Network Models. In: *Topological Indices and Related Descriptors in QSAR and QSPR*; Devillers, J., Balaban, A.T., Eds.; Gordon and Breach Science Publishers: The Netherlands, 1999, pp. 697-777.
17. Ivanciuc, O.; Balaban, A.T. Graph Theory in Chemistry. In: *The Encyclopedia of Computational Chemistry*; Schleyer, P. v. R., Allinger, N. L., Clark, T., Gasteiger, J., Kollman, P. A., Schaefer III, H. F., Schreiner, P. R., Eds.; John Wiley & Sons: Chichester, 1998, pp. 1169-1190.

18. Ivanciuc, O.; Balaban, A.T. The Graph Description of Chemical Structures. In: *Topological Indices and Related Descriptors in QSAR and QSPR*; Devillers, J., Balaban, A.T., Eds.; Gordon and Breach Science Publishers: The Netherlands, 1999, pp. 59-167.
19. Ivanciuc, O.; Ivanciuc, T.; Balaban, A.T. Vertex- and Edge-Weighted Molecular Graphs and Derived Structural Descriptors. In: *Topological Indices and Related Descriptors in QSAR and QSPR*; Devillers, J., Balaban, A.T., Eds.; Gordon and Breach Science Publishers: The Netherlands, 1999, pp. 169-220.
20. Ivanciuc, O.; Ivanciuc, T.; Diudea, M.V. Molecular Graph Matrices and Derived Structural Descriptors. *SAR QSAR Environ. Res.* **1997**, *7*, 63-87.
21. Diudea, M.V.; Gutman, I. Wiener-Type Topological Indices. *Croat. Chem. Acta* **1998**, *71*, 21-51.
22. Gakh, A.A.; Gakh, E.G.; Sumpter, B.G.; Noid, D.W. Neural Network-Graph Theory Approach to the Prediction of the Physical Properties of Organic Compounds. *J. Chem. Inf. Comput. Sci.* **1994**, *34*, 832-839.
23. Baskin, I.I.; Palyulin V.A.; Zefirov, N.S. A Neural Device for Searching Direct Correlations between Structures and Properties of Chemical Compounds. *J. Chem. Inf. Comput. Sci.* **1997**, *37*, 715-721.
24. Kireev, D.B. ChemNet: A Novel Neural Network Based Method for Graph/Property Mapping. *J. Chem. Inf. Comput. Sci.* **1995**, *35*, 175-180.
25. Ivanciuc, O. Artificial Neural Networks Applications. Part 9. MolNet Prediction of Alkane Boiling Points. *Rev. Roum. Chim.* **1998**, *43*, 885-894.
26. Ivanciuc, O. The Neural Network MolNet Prediction of Alkane Enthalpies. *Anal. Chim. Acta* **1999**, *384*, 271-284.

Chapter 9

3D QSAR MODELS

Ovidiu Ivanciuc
Department of Organic Chemistry, Faculty of Chemical Technology
University "Politehnica" of Bucharest, Oficiul 12 CP 243,
78100 Bucharest, Romania
E-mail: ivanciuc@netscape.net

1. INTRODUCTION

Drug discovery was mainly the result of chance discovery and massive screening of large corporate libraries of synthesized or naturally-occurring compounds. Computer-aided drug design is an approach to rational drug design made possible by the recent advances in computational chemistry in various fields of chemistry, such as molecular graphics, molecular mechanics, quantum chemistry, molecular dynamics, library searching, prediction of physical, chemical, and biological properties.

An important step in drug design is to find a lead, a compound that binds to the target receptor. Leads can be generated using techniques of *de novo* drug design or can be discovered by *in vitro* screening of large corporate libraries. We have to mention that the lead identification is only the beginning of a long and expensive process that eventually yields a commercial drug. A lead may have a low affinity for the target receptor, may be too unstable in solution, too toxic, too rapidly eliminated, too quickly metabolized, too difficult or too expensive to synthesize in large quantities. Because the screening procedures generally give leads that are not suitable as commercial drugs, these compounds have to be optimized using various techniques of computer-aided drug design. The availability of three-dimensional (3D) structural information of biological receptors and their complexes with various ligands can be extremely useful in suggesting ways to improve the affinity of the lead to the target. Because in many cases such detailed structural information is still unavailable, the drug design process must rely upon a more indirect approach, the quantitative structure-activity relationships (QSAR) approach.

In the absence of detailed structural data upon biological receptors, a QSAR model establishes a statistical relationship between the biological activity exerted by a series of compounds and a set of parameters determined from the structures of the compounds. The central assumption of a QSAR model is that the numerical value of a specified biological activity measured for a set of molecules depends on the structure of these molecules. In order to correlate with a QSAR model the biological activity and the molecular structure, the structure must be adequately described in a numerical form with a large variety of structural descriptors: empirical (Hammett and Taft substituent constants), physical properties (octanol-water partition coefficient, dipole moment, aqueous solubility), constitutional (counts of various molecular subgraphs), topological indices, geometrical descriptors (molecular surface and volume), quantum (atomic charges, HOMO and LUMO energies), molecular fields (steric, electrostatic, and hydrophobic).

The first studies that use QSAR notions to explain the biological activity of sets of compounds were published by Kopp,[1] Crum-Brown and Frazer,[2] Meyer,[3] and Overton.[4] However, the background for a quantitative understanding of relationships between chemical structure and reactivity was performed by Hammett who introduced the linear free energy relationship (LFER) model in physical organic chemistry. In a study published in 1962,[5] Hansch extended these ideas and developed the most widely and effectively used QSAR model for congeneric series of compounds, expressed by a multilinear regression equation:[5-7]

$$\log(1/C) = a_0 + a_1\,\pi + a_2\,\pi^2 + a_3\,\sigma + a_4\,E_S \qquad (1)$$

Here, C is the concentration (or dose) of congeneric members that gives a standard response such as EC_{50}, LD_{50}, etc., on a molar basis; π is the hydrophobic substituent parameter defined from 1-octanol/water partition coefficients P as:[8]

$$\pi = \log P_{RX} - \log P_{RH} \qquad (2)$$

where subscripts RX and RH denote substituted and unsubstituted compounds, respectively; σ is the Hammett constant for the electronic property of substituents derived from dissociation constants of benzoic acids; E_S is the Taft constant that measures the steric effect of the substituent. Depending on the situation, the hydrophobicity parameter of the whole molecule, log P, can sometimes be used in place of π; also, the term π^2 can be ignored if it lacks statistical significance. Depending on the chemical structure of the molecules, the electronic parameters for aliphatic substituents such as σ_I and σ_R replace the Hammett constant, and the steric effect can be measured by modified E_S substituent constants, the volume of the substituent, or the STERIMOL parameters.

The Hansch model from Eq. (1) was developed from the assumption that the biological activity of a certain molecule depends on the transport from the site of application to its site of action and on the ligand-receptor interaction. The transport depends in a nonlinear (parabolic) manner on the lipophylicity of the molecule, while the binding affinity to the receptor depends on the lipophylicity, electronic properties, steric effect, or other properties of the ligand. Because the effect of structural modification is separated into components, and significant physicochemical factors are indicated quantitatively, the Hansch model may reveal molecular mechanisms involved in the transport and ligand-receptor interaction of drugs.

The Hansch model was applied with success in hundreds of QSAR studies; however, the empirical parameters employed in this equation are not available for all substituents. Moreover, the use of substituent parameters limits the applicability of this model to series of congeneric compounds. To overcome this problem, computational chemistry techniques were employed to obtain various structural descriptors from the three-dimensional molecular structure. Such geometric, electrostatic, or quantum descriptors, used in a Hansch-like multilinear regression equation, represent a first type of 3D QSAR models.[9,10] In recent years the availability of detailed, three-dimensional structural information of biological receptors and their complexes with various ligands has revolutionized the drug-design process. However, in most instances such information is still unavailable. Therefore, when the structure of the biological target is not known the drug design process must rely upon a more indirect 3D QSAR approach that uses molecular alignment of atoms, pharmacophores, volume, or fields to generate a virtual receptor. Whenever the receptor structure is known, it is possible to investigate the ligand-receptor interactions and to derive 3D QSAR models from the corresponding parameters. The precise definition of 3D QSAR is still lacking, but we can identify two components that are essential for this type of models. The first component in the definition of a 3D QSAR model is the computation of the structural descriptors from the three-dimensional molecular structure; various geometrical, quantum, or molecular field descriptors were proposed in recent years to substitute the Hansch substituent constants. The second component in a 3D QSAR model is an explicit mathematical structure-activity relationship established between a dependent variable (biological activity) and a set of independent variables (3D structural descriptors); the mathematical 3D QSAR equations can be computed with the help of a large number of statistical models, such as multilinear regression, partial least squares (PLS), or neural networks. Some 3D QSAR models contain also a third component, a graphical representation of the three-dimensional information relative to the ligand-receptor interactions encoded into the structure-activity equation. Some representative 3D QSAR descriptors and ligand-receptor models will be presented in this review.

2. Mass Distribution Descriptors

The van der Waals atomic radius is a successful concept for the computation of molecular size and shape descriptors, even if in a quantum chemical description the electron cloud has no well-defined boundary surface. In this theory, each atom of the molecule is represented as a sphere centered at the equilibrium position of the atomic nucleus having a radius equal to the van der Waals radius of the corresponding atom. The exterior surface of all atomic spheres defines the van der Waals surface, which delimits the van der Waals volume of the molecule.

In the QSAR program CODESSA[11] Katritzky defined two geometric descriptors that compute the mass distribution in a molecule. Gravitation indexes for all pairs of atoms G_1 and for all bonded pairs of atoms G_2 are defined as follows:

$$G_1 = \sum_{\text{all pairs}} \frac{m_i m_j}{r_{ij}^2} \tag{3}$$

$$G_2 = \sum_{\text{all bonds}} \frac{m_i m_j}{r_{ij}^2} \tag{4}$$

where m_i and m_j are the atomic weights of atoms i and j, and r_{ij} is the interatomic distance.

3. Geometric Descriptors from Information-Theory Operators

Numerous attempts have been made in theoretical chemistry to develop molecular graph descriptors that express in a numerical form the chemical structure. Such structural descriptors are widely used in modeling physical, chemical, or biological properties, in similarity and diversity assessment, drug design, database mining, and in the screening of virtual combinatorial libraries. Recently, the mathematical equations used to define molecular graph descriptors were extended to molecular matrices derived from the three-dimensional molecular geometry.[12-18] These numerical measures of the chemical structure, called topographic indices, offer a simple and efficient way for the computation of structural descriptors.

The information on distance topological indices U, V, X, and Y[19] were extended to three-dimensional molecular matrices, giving the information-theory operators **U(3M)**, **V(3M)**, **X(3M)**, and **Y(3M)**.[20] These operators are computed from atomic invariants that measure the information content of the matrix elements associated with the respective atom. Three-dimensional descriptors can be computed for the hydrogen-depleted molecular structure, i.e. the heavy-atom molecular structure, denoted with G, or for the whole molecule, denoted with H. These four operators can be computed from any molecular matrix **3M** derived from three-dimensional molecular geometry, such as the geometric distance matrix or the reciprocal geometric distance matrix.

The three-dimensional distance matrix, **3D** = **3D**(G), of a molecular structure G with N atoms is a real symmetric $N \times N$ matrix with the element $[\mathbf{3D}]_{ij} = [\mathbf{3D}]_{ji}$ representing the shortest Cartesian distance between atoms i and j in G; all geometric distances from the examples presented below are in Å. The reciprocal geometrical distance matrix of a molecular structure G with N atoms, **3RD** = **3RD**(G), is the square $N \times N$ symmetric matrix whose entries $[\mathbf{3RD}]_{ij}$ are equal to the reciprocal of the geometric distance between atoms i and j, i.e. $1/[\mathbf{3D}]_{ij}$, for non-diagonal elements, and is equal to zero for the diagonal elements:

$$[\mathbf{3RD}]_{ij} = \begin{cases} 1/[\mathbf{3D}]_{ij} & \text{if } i \neq j \\ 0 & \text{if } i = j \end{cases} \tag{5}$$

As mentioned above, these molecular matrices can be computed both for the hydrogen-depleted molecular structure G, or for the whole molecule H.

The graph vertex operators **VUinf(3M,**G**)**, **VVinf(3M,**G**)**, **VXinf(3M,**G**)**, and **VYinf(3M,**G**)** apply the information theory equations to the non-zero elements of the molecular matrix **3M** that correspond to an atom i:

$$\mathbf{VUinf(3M)}_i = -\sum_{\substack{j=1 \\ j\neq i}}^{N} \frac{[\mathbf{3M}]_{ij}}{\mathbf{AS(3M)}_i} \log_2 \frac{[\mathbf{3M}]_{ij}}{\mathbf{AS(3M)}_i} \tag{6}$$

$$\mathbf{VVinf(3M)}_i = \mathbf{AS(3M)}_i \log_2 \mathbf{AS(3M)}_i - \mathbf{VUinf(3M)}_i \tag{7}$$

$$\mathbf{VXinf(3M)}_i = \mathbf{AS(3M)}_i \log_2 \mathbf{AS(3M)}_i - \mathbf{VYinf(3M)}_i \tag{8}$$

$$\mathbf{VYinf(3M)}_i = \sum_{\substack{j=1 \\ j\neq i}}^{N} [\mathbf{3M}]_{ij} \log_2 [\mathbf{3M}]_{ij} \tag{9}$$

where $\mathbf{AS(M)}_i$ represents the atom sum of the atom i, and the summations in equations (6) and (9) are done for the non-zero elements of the molecular matrix **3M**, $[\mathbf{3M}]_{ij} \neq 0$. The atom sum operator of the atom i, $\mathbf{AS(3M)}_i$, of a molecular structure G or H with N atoms, is defined as the sum of the elements in the column i, or row i, of the molecular matrix **3M**:

$$\mathbf{AS(3M)}_i = \sum_{j=1}^{N} [\mathbf{3M}]_{ij} = \sum_{j=1}^{N} [\mathbf{3M}]_{ji} \tag{10}$$

For a general molecular matrix **3M** derived from three-dimensional molecular geometry, the matrix elements $[\mathbf{3M}]_{ij}$ may have values lower than 1, giving negative terms for certain vertex structural descriptors computed with the graph vertex operators **VUinf(3M)**, **VVinf(3M)**, **VXinf(3M)**, and **VYinf(3M)**. The Randić-like formula used in the case of the indices U, V, X, and Y is therefore replaced by the following equation:

$$f(x,y) = \begin{cases} (xy)^{-1/2} & \text{if } xy > 0 \\ -(|xy|)^{-1/2} & \text{if } xy < 0 \end{cases} \quad (11)$$

The operators **U(3M)**, **V(3M)**, **X(3M)**, and **Y(3M)**, representing information on matrix elements, are computed with the equations:

$$\mathbf{U(3M)} = \frac{M}{\mu+1}\sum_{\text{bonds}} f\left(\mathbf{VUinf(3M)}_i, \mathbf{VUinf(3M)}_j\right) \quad (12)$$

$$\mathbf{V(3M)} = \frac{M}{\mu+1}\sum_{\text{bonds}} f\left(\mathbf{VVinf(3M)}_i, \mathbf{VVinf(3M)}_j\right) \quad (13)$$

$$\mathbf{X(3M)} = \frac{M}{\mu+1}\sum_{\text{bonds}} f\left(\mathbf{VXinf(3M)}_i, \mathbf{VXinf(3M)}_j\right) \quad (14)$$

$$\mathbf{Y(3M)} = \frac{M}{\mu+1}\sum_{\text{bonds}} f\left(\mathbf{VYinf(3M)}_i, \mathbf{VYinf(3M)}_j\right) \quad (15)$$

where M is the number of covalent bonds in the molecular structure G or H, μ is the cyclomatic number of G or H, i.e. the number of cycles in the graph, $\mu = M - N + 1$, and the summation goes over all bonds.

An example for the computation of the information operators **U(3M)**, **V(3M)**, **X(3M)**, and **Y(3M)** is presented for the molecular graph of *cis*-1,2-dimethylcyclobutane **1** and *trans*-1,2-dimethylcyclobutane **2**:

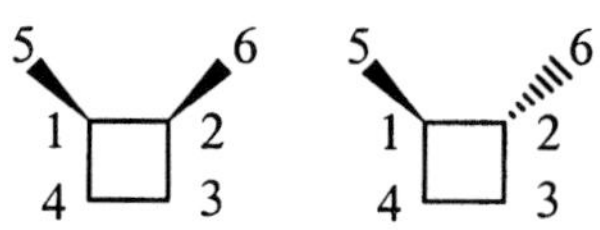

1 **2**

The geometry of the two isomers was optimized with the molecular mechanics method MM+ implemented in HyperChem.[21] The geometrical distance matrix of the carbon skeleton of *cis*-1,2-dimethylcyclobutane **1**, **3D(1**,G), is:

3D(1,*G*)

	1	2	3	4	5	6
1	0.000	1.563	2.205	1.559	1.543	2.648
2	1.563	0.000	1.559	2.205	2.648	1.543
3	2.205	1.559	0.000	1.556	3.370	2.598
4	1.559	2.205	1.556	0.000	2.598	3.370
5	1.543	2.648	3.370	2.598	0.000	2.962
6	2.648	1.543	2.598	3.370	2.962	0.000

The atom sum vector **AS** is computed with formula (10) as the sum of the elements in the column *i*, or row *i*, of the matrix **3D**:

AS(3D,1) = {9.517, 9.517, 11.287, 11.287, 13.122, 13.122}

The information-theory operators **VUinf(3D,***G***)**, **VVinf(3D,***G***)**, **VXinf(3D,***G***)**, and **VYinf(3D,***G***)** are applied to the geometric distance matrix **3D** to compute with formulas (6)-(9) new atom invariants:

VUinf(3D,1) = {2.283, 2.283, 2.257, 2.257, 2.280, 2.280}

VVinf(3D,1) = {28.651, 28.651, 37.210, 37.210, 46.453, 46.453}

VXinf(3D,1) = {21.730, 21.730, 25.477, 25.477, 29.919, 29.919}

VYinf(3D,1) = {9.204, 9.204, 13.991, 13.991, 18.813, 18.813}

The information on geometric distance matrix operators **U(3D)**, **V(3D)**, **X(3D)**, and **Y(3D)** are computed with equations (12)-(15) from the above vectors:

U(3D,1) = 7.916 **V(3D,1)** = 0.534

X(3D,1) = 0.746 **Y(3D,1)** = 1.525

The reciprocal geometric distance matrix **3RD** is computed with equation (5) to give for *cis*-1,2-dimethylcyclobutane **1** the matrix **3RD(1,***G***)**:

3RD(1,G)

	1	2	3	4	5	6
1	0.000	0.640	0.454	0.642	0.648	0.378
2	0.640	0.000	0.642	0.454	0.378	0.648
3	0.454	0.642	0.000	0.643	0.297	0.385
4	0.642	0.454	0.643	0.000	0.385	0.297
5	0.648	0.378	0.297	0.385	0.000	0.338
6	0.378	0.648	0.385	0.297	0.338	0.000

The reciprocal geometric distance matrix **3RD** is the basis for the computation of the information-theory atom operators **VUinf(3RD,**G), **VVinf(3RD,**G), **VXinf(3RD,**G), and **VYinf(3RD,**G) using the corresponding **AS** vector:

AS(3RD,1) = {2.761, 2.761, 2.420, 2.420, 2.045, 2.045}

VUinf(3RD,1) = {2.290, 2.290, 2.262, 2.262, 2.262, 2.262}

VVinf(3RD,1) = {1.755, 1.755, 0.823, 0.823, –0.152, –0.152}

VXinf(3RD,1) = {6.321, 6.321, 5.473, 5.473, 4.626, 4.626}

VYinf(3RD,1) = {–2.276, –2.276, –2.388, –2.388, –2.515, –2.515}

The above vectors of atom invariants are utilized to compute the indices **U(3RD)**, **V(3RD)**, **X(3RD)**, and **Y(3RD)**:

U(3RD,1) = 7.910 **V(3RD,1)** = –1.276

X(3RD,1) = 3.152 **Y(3RD,1)** = 7.655

The geometrical distance matrix of the carbon skeleton of *trans*-1,2-dimethylcyclobutane **2**, **3D(2,**G), is:

3D(2,G)

	1	2	3	4	5	6
1	0.000	1.566	2.211	1.563	1.547	2.613
2	1.566	0.000	1.563	2.211	2.613	1.547
3	2.211	1.563	0.000	1.561	3.352	2.612
4	1.563	2.211	1.561	0.000	2.612	3.352
5	1.547	2.613	3.352	2.612	0.000	3.792
6	2.613	1.547	2.612	3.352	3.792	0.000

The information-theory operators **VUinf(3D,2)**, **VVinf(3D,2)**, **VXinf(3D,2)**, and **VYinf(3D,2)** are computed from the **AS(3D,2)** vector:

AS(3D,2) = {9.500, 9.500, 11.300, 11.300, 13.916, 13.916}

VUinf(3D,2) = {2.285, 2.285, 2.258, 2.258, 2.264, 2.264}

VVinf(3D,2) = {28.568, 28.568, 37.272, 37.272, 50.596, 50.596}

VXinf(3D,2) = {21.708, 21.708, 25.520, 25.520, 31.507, 31.507}

VYinf(3D,2) = {9.145, 9.145, 14.010, 14.010, 21.353, 21.353}

The information on geometric distance matrix operators **U(3D)**, **V(3D)**, **X(3D)**, and **Y(3D)** computed with the above vectors are:

U(3D,2) = 7.920 **V(3D,2)** = 0.527

X(3D,2) = 0.740 **Y(3D,2)** = 1.502

Using equation (1) one obtains the reciprocal geometric distance matrix **3RD** for *trans*-1,2-dimethylcyclobutane **2**:

3RD(2,*G*)

	1	2	3	4	5	6
1	0.000	0.639	0.452	0.640	0.647	0.383
2	0.639	0.000	0.640	0.452	0.383	0.647
3	0.452	0.640	0.000	0.640	0.298	0.383
4	0.640	0.452	0.640	0.000	0.383	0.298
5	0.647	0.383	0.298	0.383	0.000	0.264
6	0.383	0.647	0.383	0.298	0.264	0.000

The above reciprocal geometric distance matrix **3RD** gives the vectors **AS(3RD,2)**, **VUinf(3RD,2)**, **VVinf(3RD,2)**, **VXinf(3RD,2)**, and **VYinf(3RD,2)**:

AS(3RD,2) = {2.760, 2.760, 2.413, 2.413, 1.974, 1.974}

VUinf(3RD,2) = {2.291, 2.291, 2.263, 2.263, 2.245, 2.245}

VVinf(3RD,2) = {1.751, 1.751, 0.805, 0.805, –0.308, –0.308}

VXinf(3RD,2) = {6.322, 6.322, 5.461, 5.461, 4.432, 4.432}

VYinf(3RD,2) = {–2.280, –2.280, –2.393, –2.393, –2.495, –2.495}

The above vectors of atom invariants are utilized to compute the indices **U(3RD)**, **V(3RD)**, **X(3RD)**, and **Y(3RD)**:

U(3RD,2) = 7.917 **V(3RD,2)** = 2.320

X(3RD,2) = 3.178 **Y(3RD,2)** = 7.653

The extension of the **U**, **V**, **X**, and **Y** operators to molecular matrices derived from three-dimensional molecular geometry offers four new families of structural descriptors for QSPR and QSAR models.

4. Topological Electronic Index

The topological electronic index was proposed by Kaliszan[22] to characterize quantitatively the differences of solutes polarity in gas-liquid chromatography:

$$T_1^E = \sum_{\text{all pairs}} \frac{|Q_i - Q_j|}{r_{ij}^2} \qquad (16)$$

where Q_i denotes the partial charge on the ith atom, r_{ij} denotes the distance between ith and jth atoms, and the summation is done over all pairs of atoms in the molecule. CODESSA computes a similar index by considering all bonded atoms:[11]

$$T_2^E = \sum_{\text{all bonds}} \frac{|Q_i - Q_j|}{r_{ij}^2} \qquad (17)$$

where Q_i denotes the partial charge on the ith atom, r_{ij} denotes the distance between ith and jth atoms, and the summation is done over all bonded pairs of atoms in the molecule.

5. Charged Partial Surface Area Descriptors

Charged partial surface area (CPSA)[23] descriptors have been defined by Jurs in terms of the solvent-accessible surface area of each atom and the atomic charge computed from the atomic electronegativity or with a quantum chemistry method. The molecule is considered as an assemble of hard spheres defined by the van der Waals radii of the atoms. The solvent-accessible surface area is traced out by the center of a solvent sphere (usually water) that rolls over the van der Waals surface of the molecule. The CPSA descriptors encode features responsible for polar interactions between molecules. The definitions of these descriptors are presented below:

(1) PPSA-1, partial positive surface area:

$$\text{PPSA-1}=\sum_i SA_i^+ \tag{18}$$

where SA_i^+ is the surface area of the positively charged atom *i*.

(2) PNSA-1, partial negative surface area:

$$\text{PNSA-1}=\sum_i SA_i^- \tag{19}$$

where SA_i^- is the surface area of the negatively charged atom *i*.

(3) PPSA-2, total charge weighted partial positive surface area:

$$\text{PPSA-2}=\sum_i SA_i^+ \sum_i Q_i^+ \tag{20}$$

where Q_i^+ is the partial positive charge of atom *i*, the first summation gives the partial positive surface area, and the second summation gives the total positive charges for the molecule.

(4) PNSA-2, total charge weighted partial negative surface area:

$$\text{PNSA-2}=\sum_i SA_i^- \sum_i Q_i^- \tag{21}$$

where Q_i^- is the partial positive charge of atom *i*, the first summation gives the partial negative surface area, and the second summation gives the total negative charges for the molecule.

(5) PPSA-3, atomic charge weighted partial positive surface area:

$$\text{PPSA-3}=\sum_i SA_i^+ Q_i^+ \tag{22}$$

(6) PNSA-3, atomic charge weighted partial negative surface area:

$$\text{PNSA-3}=\sum_{i} SA_i^- Q_i^- \tag{23}$$

(7) difference in charged partial surface areas:

$$\text{DPSA-1} = \text{PPSA-1} - \text{PNSA-1} \tag{24}$$

$$\text{DPSA-2} = \text{PPSA-2} - \text{PNSA-2} \tag{25}$$

$$\text{DPSA-3} = \text{PPSA-3} - \text{PNSA-3} \tag{26}$$

(8) fractional charged partial surface areas:

$$\text{FPSA-1} = \frac{\text{PPSA-1}}{MSA} \tag{27}$$

$$\text{FPSA-2} = \frac{\text{PPSA-2}}{MSA} \tag{28}$$

$$\text{FPSA-3} = \frac{\text{PPSA-3}}{MSA} \tag{29}$$

$$\text{FNSA-1} = \frac{\text{PNSA-1}}{MSA} \tag{30}$$

$$\text{FNSA-2} = \frac{\text{PNSA-2}}{MSA} \tag{31}$$

$$\text{FNSA-3} = \frac{\text{PNSA-3}}{MSA} \tag{32}$$

where MSA is the molecular surface area computed with the formula:

$$MSA = \sum_{i=1}^{N} SA_i \tag{33}$$

(9) surface weighted charged partial surface areas:

$$\text{WPSA-1} = \frac{\text{PPSA-1} \cdot MSA}{1000} \tag{34}$$

$$\text{WPSA-2} = \frac{\text{PPSA-2} \cdot MSA}{1000} \tag{35}$$

$$\text{WPSA-3} = \frac{\text{PPSA-3} \cdot MSA}{1000} \tag{36}$$

$$\text{WNSA-1} = \frac{\text{PNSA-1} \cdot MSA}{1000} \tag{37}$$

$$\text{WNSA-2} = \frac{\text{PNSA-2} \cdot MSA}{1000} \tag{38}$$

$$\text{WNSA-3} = \frac{\text{PNSA-3} \cdot MSA}{1000} \tag{39}$$

(10) RPCG, relative positive charge:

$$\text{RPCG} = \frac{Q^+_{\max}}{\sum_i SA_i^+} \tag{40}$$

where $Q^+_{\max}$ is the charge of the most positive atom.

(11) RNCG, relative negative charge:

$$\text{RNCG} = \frac{Q^-_{\max}}{\sum_i SA_i^-} \tag{41}$$

where $Q^-_{\max}$ is the charge of the most negative atom.

(12) RPCS, relative positive charged surface area:

$$\text{RPCS} = \text{RPCG} \cdot SA^+_{\max} = \frac{Q^+_{\max} SA^+_{\max}}{\sum_i SA_i^+} \tag{42}$$

where $SA^{+}_{\max}$ is the surface area of the most positive atom.

(13) RNCS, relative negative charged surface area:

$$\mathrm{RNCS} = \mathrm{RNCG} \cdot SA^{-}_{\max} = \frac{Q^{-}_{\max} SA^{-}_{\max}}{\sum_{i} SA^{-}_{i}} \tag{43}$$

where $SA^{-}_{\max}$ is the surface area of the most negative atom.

All the above CPSA descriptors can be computed from the 3D molecular structure using two available programs, ADAPT[24,25] or CODESSA.[11,26-33] CODESSA offers several related descriptors for hydrogen acceptor or donor atoms in a molecule. We present below a selection of these descriptors.

The HASA-1 descriptor is calculated as the sum of exposed surfaces areas of all possible hydrogen acceptor atoms in the molecule:

$$\text{HASA-1} = \sum SA_{a} \tag{44}$$

where SA_a is the surface area of the hydrogen acceptor atom. The following atoms are considered as possible hydrogen acceptors: carbonyl oxygen atoms (except in COOR), hydroxy oxygen atoms, amino nitrogen atoms, aromatic nitrogens, and mercapto sulfur atoms.

The HDSA-2 descriptor is directly related to the hydrogen bonding between the molecules in condensed media. It is calculated according to the following formula:

$$\text{HDSA-2} = \sum \frac{Q_d SA_d^{1/2}}{MSA} \tag{45}$$

where Q_d is the partial charge on the hydrogen bonding donor atom, SA_d denotes the exposed surface area of this atom, and MSA is the total molecular surface area calculated from the van der Waals radii of the atoms. The summation is performed over all possible hydrogen bonding donor sites in the molecule.

The hydrogen-bonding ability of compounds can also be characterized by HDCA-2, the hydrogen bonding donor charged surface area defined with the equation:

$$\text{HDCA-2} = \sum \frac{Q_d SA_d^{1/2}}{MSA^{1/2}} \tag{46}$$

The summation in the formula of HDCA-2 goes over all possible hydrogen bonding donor and acceptor pairs in the molecule. In the computation of HDCA-2 hydrogen atoms attached to carbons connected directly to carbonyl or cyano group are included as possible hydrogen bonding donor centers.

The fractional hydrogen donor surface area FHDSA-2 is defined as:

$$\text{FHDSA-2} = \frac{\text{HDSA-2}}{MSA^{1/2}} \tag{47}$$

The 3D descriptors from this section can be computed either with electrostatic charges computed from the atomic electronegativity or with partial atomic charges computed with a quantum chemistry method.

6. TLSER - Theoretical Linear Solvation Energy Relationship

The linear solvation energy relationship (LSER)[34,35] model was developed by Kamlet, Taft, and co-workers to explain solvent effects on various free energy based properties. The LSER approach contains parameters that measure the solute size, polarity/polarizability, hydrogen bond donating and accepting capacities; this model was applied with success to various QSAR studies, such as the prediction of octanol/water partition coefficients, boiling temperatures, and critical constants. Famini used the LFER philosophy with quantum chemically derived descriptors, and proposed the theoretical linear solvation energy relationship (TLSER) model.[36-38] This model uses a new set of theoretical parameters to correlate a property P:

$$P = a_0 + a_1 V_{\text{mc}} + a_2\pi^* + a_3\varepsilon_\alpha + a_4\varepsilon_\beta + a_5 q^+ + a_6 q^- \tag{48}$$

where V_{mc} is the molecular van der Waals volume, π^* is the polarizability index, ε_α is the covalent acidity index, ε_β is the covalent basicity index, q^+ is the electrostatic acidity index, and q^- is the electrostatic basicity index. The polarizability index is obtained by dividing the molecular polarizability to V_{mc}, q^+ is the magnitude of the most positively charged hydrogen atom in the molecule, and q^- is the magnitude of the most negative atomic partial charge in the molecule. The covalent hydrogen bonding acidity index ε_α is computed with the formula:

$$\varepsilon_\alpha = 0.30 - \frac{\left|E_{\text{LUMO}} - E_{\text{HOMO},w}\right|}{100} \tag{49}$$

where E_{LUMO} is the LUMO energy of the molecule, and $E_{\text{HOMO},w}$ is the HOMO energy of water. The covalent hydrogen bonding basicity index ε_β is:

$$\varepsilon_\beta = 0.30 - \frac{\left|E_{\text{HOMO}} - E_{\text{LUMO},w}\right|}{100} \quad (50)$$

where E_{HOMO} is the HOMO energy of the molecule, and $E_{\text{LUMO},w}$ is the LUMO energy of water. Several QSPR and QSAR applications of the TLSER model were presented in two reviews.[36,37]

7. Quantum Substituent Parameters

Using the extended Hückel theory, Esaki defined new electronic substituent parameters computed from the energy of the single occupied molecular orbital (SOMO).[39] The SOMO resistance of the substituent X is:

$$Re_{\text{SOMO}}(\text{X}) = \exp\left[-c_{\text{SOMO}}^2(\text{X})\right] \quad (51)$$

where c_{SOMO} is the SOMO coefficient of the hybrid orbital which participates in bonding to the parent structure, and X is not hydrogen. For hydrogen a modified formula is employed:

$$Re_{\text{SOMO}}(\text{H}) = 1/\left[\exp c_{\text{SOMO}}^2(\text{H}) - 1\right] \quad (52)$$

The frontier electron current intensity is:

$$I_{\text{SOMO}}(\text{X}) = E_{\text{SOMO}}(\text{X}) / Re_{\text{SOMO}}(\text{X}) \quad (53)$$

where $E_{\text{SOMO}}(\text{X})$ is the energy of the SOMO orbital. Frontier substituent constants are obtained from the above parameters adjusted relative to hydrogen as standard:

$$E(\text{X}) = -10\left[E_{\text{SOMO}}(\text{X}) - E_{\text{SOMO}}(\text{H})\right] \quad (54)$$

$$Re(\text{X}) = 10\left[Re_{\text{SOMO}}(\text{X}) - Re_{\text{SOMO}}(\text{H})\right] \quad (55)$$

$$I(\text{X}) = -10\left[I_{\text{SOMO}}(\text{X}) - I_{\text{SOMO}}(\text{H})\right] \quad (56)$$

Esaki demonstrated the advantage of the new quantum parameters by using them, together with other substituent constants, to develop 45 Hansch-type QSAR models.

8. Frontier Indices for Groups of Atoms

Pires assumed that in the ligand-receptor interaction the frontier orbitals of both the ligand and receptor play an important role and proposed a set of three frontier indices for groups of atoms.[40] Consider a group S composed of M bonded atoms. The group frontier electron density is:

$$G_S^{\mathrm{FED}} = \sum_{i=1}^{M} 2c_{\mathrm{HOMO},i}^2 \tag{57}$$

where $c_{\mathrm{HOMO},i}$ is the coefficient for the highest occupied molecular orbital on the ith atom from the group. The group frontier orbital density is:

$$G_S^{\mathrm{FOD}} = \sum_{i=1}^{M} 2c_{\mathrm{LUMO},i}^2 \tag{58}$$

where $c_{\mathrm{LUMO},i}$ is the coefficient for the lowest unoccupied molecular orbital on the ith atom from the group. A combination of the terms from the above two descriptors gives the group frontier radical density:

$$G_S^{\mathrm{FRD}} = \sum_{i=1}^{M} \left(c_{\mathrm{HOMO},i}^2 + c_{\mathrm{LUMO},i}^2 \right) \tag{59}$$

These three frontier indices computed with the AM1 method were used to model the mutagenic activity of triazenes. Good correlations were obtained when the octanol/water partition coefficient was added to the quantum frontier descriptors.

9. GIPF - General Interaction Properties Function

Politzer proposed the general interaction properties function (GIPF) method for the correlation of physical, chemical, and biological properties with molecular surface descriptors computed from the electrostatic potential.[41-46] The electrostatic potential $V(r)$ created in the space around a molecule by its nuclei and electrons is:

$$V(r) = \sum_{i=1}^{N} \frac{Z_i}{|R_i - r|} - \int \frac{\rho(r')r'}{|r' - r|} \tag{60}$$

where Z_i is the charge on nucleus i, located at R_i, and $\rho(r)$ is the electronic density function. $V(r)$ gives the interaction energy between a positive point charge of unitary magnitude located at r and the unperturbed charge distribution of the molecule. A molecular surface is defined by the 0.001 a.u. contour of the electronic density $\rho(r)$. Politzer found that the hydrogen bond acceptor capability of a molecule is quantitatively related to $V_{\min}$, the most negative potential in space, and $V_{S,\min}$, the most negative surface potential, while the hydrogen bond donor capability is related to the most positive surface potential, $V_{S,\max}$.

The average deviation of the electrostatic potential on the molecular surface is a measure of local polarity:

$$\Pi = \frac{1}{k}\sum_{i=1}^{k}\left|V(r_i) - \overline{V}_S\right| \tag{61}$$

where $V(r_i)$ is the potential at the ith point on the surface and $\overline{V}_S$ is its average value:

$$\overline{V}_S = \frac{1}{k}\sum_{i=1}^{k} V(r_i) \tag{62}$$

It was found that Π is correlated with π^*, the LSER polarity/polarizability index. The variance of the positive regions of electrostatic potential on the molecular surface, $V^+(r)$, is:

$$\sigma_+^2 = \frac{1}{m}\sum_{i=1}^{m}\left[V^+(r_i) - \overline{V}_S^+\right]^2 \tag{63}$$

where $\overline{V}_S^+$ is the average of $V(r)$ on the positive regions of the molecular surface:

$$\overline{V}_S^+ = \frac{1}{m}\sum_{i=1}^{m} V^+(r_i) \tag{64}$$

The variance of the negative regions of electrostatic potential on the molecular surface, $V^-(r)$, is:

$$\sigma_-^2 = \frac{1}{n}\sum_{i=1}^{n}\left[V^-(r_i) - \overline{V}_S^-\right]^2 \tag{65}$$

where $\overline{V}_S^-$ is the average of $V(r)$ on the negative regions of the molecular surface:

$$\overline{V}_S^- = \frac{1}{n}\sum_{i=1}^{n} V^-(r_i) \tag{66}$$

The variance of the electrostatic potential over the molecular surface is:

$$\sigma^2_{tot} = \sigma^2_{+} + \sigma^2_{-} \tag{67}$$

An electrostatic balance term is obtained from the above σ parameters:

$$\upsilon = \frac{\sigma^2_{+}\sigma^2_{-}}{\left[\sigma^2_{tot}\right]^2} \tag{68}$$

The GIPF descriptors, when used in conjunction with a parameter measuring the molecular size (molecular volume or surface area), were effective in correlations with critical constants, boiling temperatures,[45] and octanol/water partition coefficients.[42,43]

10. CoMFA - Comparative Molecular Field Analysis

Although molecular field descriptors where introduced more than 20 years ago, the lack of an efficient statistical algorithm for the analysis of thousands of field variables prevented the widespread use of 3D QSAR models using molecular fields. In 1988 Cramer[47,48] used partial least squares to correlate the molecular field descriptors with biological activities, proposing the now widely used comparative molecular field analysis (CoMFA).[9,10,49] The main steps for the development of a CoMFA model are:

1. A set of molecules is selected by considering only those compounds that interact in a similar manner with the same receptor.
2. The geometry of all molecules in the study set is optimized with molecular mechanics or quantum mechanics methods. Any information regarding the active conformations of the ligands in the actual receptor must be used to optimize the appropriate molecular geometry. For certain molecules several low energy conformations may be considered.
3. All optimized molecules are aligned (superimposed) using some pharmacophore hypothesis. The CoMFA model depends on the molecules alignment and errors in this step can provide 3D QSAR models that have a low predictive power. Several alignment assumptions have to be investigated in order to identify the best model.
4. A subset of molecules is selected to generate the CoMFA virtual receptor model.
5. Atomic partial charges are calculated with an electrostatic (based on electronegativity) or quantum mechanics method for all molecules.
6. The aligned molecules are placed in a box that is larger in all directions than the volume occupied by the superimposed compounds, and the box is partitioned into a grid with points separated by an adjustable distance, usually between 0.5 and 2 Å.

7. A neutral atom, such as a carbon atom, is used as a steric probe to compute the steric field on the grid points. In order to compute the value of the steric field on a certain grid point j, the steric probe is placed in that grid point and the van der Waals interaction energy, $E_{vdW,j}$, is computed with the formula:

$$E_{vdW,j} = \sum_{i=1}^{n} \left(\frac{A_{ij}}{r_{ij}^{12}} - \frac{C_{ij}}{r_{ij}^{6}} \right) \tag{69}$$

where n is the number of atoms in the molecule, r_{ij} is the distance between atom i of the molecule and the grid point j where the probe atom is located, A_{ij} and C_{ij} are constants depending on the types of atom i and steric probe.
8. The electrostatic field values in each grid point are computed by placing a positively or negatively charged atom in the grid point:

$$E_{C,j} = \sum_{j=1}^{n} \frac{q_i q_j}{\varepsilon r_{ij}} \tag{70}$$

where $E_{C,j}$ is the value of the electrostatic field at the grid point j, q_i is the partial charge of atom i in the molecule, q_j is the charge of the probe atom located at the grid point j, and ε is the dielectric constant. The grid points inside the van der Waals molecular surface were excluded from the calculation of the electrostatic field.
9. The values of the steric and electrostatic fields are collected into a QSAR table in order to be correlated with the biological activity values. The resulting matrix, containing thousands of columns corresponding to individual grid points, cannot be correlated with the multilinear regression method. The PLS method uses this data matrix to generate a 3D QSAR. PLS extracts principal component-like vectors (latent variables) from the matrices of independent and dependent variables. This method takes a matrix containing a large number of potentially useful structural descriptors, that can be highly intercorrelated, and offers a correlation using the latent variables. The optimum number of latent variables is determined by cross-validation.
10. The PLS model is used to generate contour maps showing favorable and unfavorable regions for electropositive or electronegative regions, as well as favorable and unfavorable steric regions around the molecules.
11. Predictions for molecules not included in the derivation of the PLS model can be made by computing their steric and electrostatic fields, and by using the grid values into the PLS model.

CoMFA is the most important 3D QSAR model, used in a few hundred drug design studies, mainly to describe the ligand-receptor interactions. However, this method seems to be less appropriate for the correlation of the *in vivo* data. This highly successful model was followed by the introduction of a large number of related 3D QSAR methods.

11. SOMFA - Self-Organizing Molecular Field Analysis

Richards proposed a simplified CoMFA model that generates a 3D QSAR model considering only the first PLS component, the self-organizing molecular field analysis (SOMFA).[50] The most significant steps of the SOMFA algorithm are:

Steps (1)-(6) are identical with those employed for CoMFA.

7. The mean centered activity MCA_k of a molecule k from the calibration set is computed by subtracting the mean activity of all molecules from each molecule's activity, giving a scale where the most active molecules have positive values and the least active molecules have negative values:

$$\mathrm{MCA}_k = \mathrm{A}_k - \mathrm{MA} \quad (71)$$

where A_k is the activity of molecule k and MA is the mean activity of the molecules from the calibration set.

8. For each molecule, the shape field is computed by assigning the value 1 to all grid points situated inside the van der Waals molecular surface and 0 for the outside grid points.
9. The electrostatic potential values at the grid points of each molecule are computed with the formula:

$$\mathrm{ESP}_j = \sum_{i=1}^{n} \frac{q_i}{r_{ij}} \quad (72)$$

where n is the number of atoms in the molecule, q_i is the partial charge of atom i in the molecule, and r_{ij} is the distance between atom i and the grid point j.

10. A self-organizing master grid (SOMG) is generated for each field considered using the grid values of all molecules in the calibration set. For a field f (shape or electrostatic potential) the value of the self-organizing master grid in the grid point $j = j(x,y,z)$, SOMG(f,j), is computed with the formula:

$$\mathrm{SOMG}(f,j) = \sum_{k=1}^{N} f(j)_k \,\mathrm{MCA}_k \quad (73)$$

where the summation goes for all N molecules in the calibration set, and $f(j)_k$ is the value of the field f in the grid point j for compound k.

11. For each molecule k in the calibration or prediction set a SOMFA activity derived from the field f computed in each grid point j is determined for both shape and electrostatic fields:

$$\mathrm{SOA}(f)_k = \sum_{j=1}^{n} f(j)_k \mathrm{SOMG}(f, j) \tag{74}$$

where the summation is performed for all grid points n.

12. The biological activity of the molecule k, BA_k, is computed as a linear combination of the corresponding SOA(f) values for the two molecular fields:

$$\mathrm{BA}_k = c_1 \mathrm{SOA(shape)}_k + (1 - c_1)\mathrm{SOA(electrostatic)}_k \tag{75}$$

where the mixing coefficient c_1 is optimized for each 3D QSAR model.

13. The shape and electrostatic potential self-organizing master grid (SOMG) can generate visual maps of the important features that determine the biological activity.

We have to mention that starting with the same field values for each grid point, the SOMFA model is identical with the CoMFA model computed with only the first PLS component.

12. RSM - Receptor Surface Model

Hahn[51,52] proposed a 3D QSAR model that uses a set of active compounds to generate a virtual receptor model; the virtual receptor is a surface formed by points provided with several properties that are used when calculating interaction energy between a molecule and a surface model. The main steps of the receptor surface model (RSM) are:

Steps (1)-(5) are identical with those employed for CoMFA.

6. A steric surface representing the virtual receptor is generated to enclose the set of aligned molecules. The surface of the virtual receptor is generated by a volumetric field (shape field), characterizing molecular shape, which is produced for each aligned molecule. The shape fields from each individual molecule are combined to produce a final volumetric shape field from which an explicit surface is generated. First, a three-dimensional regularly spaced grid is superposed over the aligned set of molecules; the grid box dimensions are extended several Å in each direction from the coordinates of every molecule. The steric field is computed for each point of the grid, and an isosurface of the field is used to generate the surface of the virtual receptor. Two field functions are used to create the shape of the virtual receptor, namely the van der Waals field

function and the Wyvill field function. Each field source corresponds to an atom. The van der Waals field function generated by the atom i from a molecule is:

$$V(r_{ij})_i = r_{ij} - r_{\mathrm{VDW},i} \tag{76}$$

where r_{ij} is the distance from the atom i and the grid point j and $r_{\mathrm{VDW},i}$ is the van der Waals radius of the atom i. This field function, which is computed for every grid point, has the property that inside the van der Waals volume the value is negative, outside the volume the value is positive, and at the van der Waals surface the value $V(r)$ is zero. If a grid point contains a shape field value computed for a different atom, the smaller of the two values is assigned to that grid point. The Wyvill function is a bounded function that decays completely in a finite distance R:

$$V(r_{ij})_i = -\frac{4r_{ij}^6}{9R^6} + \frac{17r_{ij}^4}{9R^4} - \frac{22r_{ij}^2}{9R^2} + 1 \tag{77}$$

where r_{ij} is the distance from the atom i and the grid point j. A field value is the sum of the field values contributed by each atom; if a grid point is outside of R, its shape field value is not computed. The value of R depends on the atom type, and usually its value is twice the van der Waals radius of the atom i. This function has the properties that $V(0) = 1$, $V(R) = 0$, and $V(R/2) = 1/2$. Using the shape field values the marching cubes isosurface algorithm produces a set of triangulated surface points representing the surface of the virtual receptor. The default grid spacing of 0.5 Å yields an average surface density of 6 points/Å^2. This gives an average distance between neighboring points (points in the same triangle) of about 0.47 Å.

7. After a surface is created, several properties of the virtual receptor associated with each surface point are assigned; these properties include partial charge, electrostatic potential, hydrogen-bonding propensity, and hydrophobicity. These values are used when calculating interaction energy between a molecule and a surface model.
8. A partial atomic charge is assigned to each point from the virtual receptor site. This atomic charge is determined as complementary to the partial charge of any atom in contact with the surface. If a single molecule is used to generate the virtual receptor, each surface point is assigned a charge which is equal to but opposite in sign to the charge of the closest atom in the molecule. If a set of molecules are employed to generate the virtual receptor, each surface point is assigned a charge which is equal and opposite to the average partial atomic charge of the set. The average for a surface point is found by summing the partial atomic charges of the closest atom in each molecule and dividing by the number of molecules. This method assumes that each molecule contributes equally to the description of the virtual receptor.

9. The second property assigned to each surface point is the electrostatic potential, considered to be complementary with that of the ligand. If a single molecule is used to generate the virtual receptor, each surface point is assigned an electrostatic potential value which is equivalent to but opposite in sign to the distance-dependent electrostatic potential at that surface point:

$$\mathrm{ESP}_j = \sum_{i=1}^{n} \frac{q_i q_j}{r_{ij}} \tag{78}$$

where the summation goes over all atoms in the molecule. If a set of molecules are employed to generate the virtual receptor, each surface point is assigned an electrostatic potential which is equal and opposite to the average of the values obtained for all molecules.

10. The third property assigned to each surface point is the hydrogen bond property, corresponding to the tendency of the surface point to be involved in a hydrogen bond. If a hydrogen bond acceptor property would be desirable for a certain surface point a value of 1.0 is assigned to the respective point, while if a hydrogen bond donor hydrogen property would be desirable for a certain surface point a value of –1.0 is assigned to the respective point. Hydrogen bond acceptors are defined as any oxygen or nitrogen atom with a free lone pair of electrons, and hydrogen bond donors are any hydrogens attached to oxygen or nitrogen. The hydrogen bond values are averaged for all molecules, and the resulting surface point values are in the range [–1.0, 1.0].
11. The fourth property assigned to each surface point is the hydrophobicity, with a value of one assigned to points in hydrophobic regions and zero to all other points. A hydrophobic point is a point with a low partial charge (absolute values less than 0.15), a low electrostatic potential (absolute values less than 0.01), and a low hydrogen bond donating or accepting propensity (absolute values less than 0.1).
12. With the virtual receptor model defined in the above steps, the ligand-receptor interaction of a set of molecules is evaluated by computing their interaction energy with the virtual receptor. For a molecule a set of descriptors is obtained by computing the interaction energy between each surface point from the virtual receptor and the atoms in the molecule. These descriptors are stored in a QSAR table together with the biological activity of the investigated molecule.

The total interaction energy contribution of a single atom is computed by summing the individual interaction energies of all valid atom/point pairs. An atom/point pair is valid if the distance between the pair is less than a 6 Å cutoff distance and if the atom is inside the surface with respect to the point. The nonbonded energy between an atom and the surface points is composed of a van der Waals term, an electrostatic term, and a desolvation energy correction term. The van der Waals term is a scaled Lennard-Jones equation:

$$E_{vdW,ij} = K\left[\left(\frac{RA}{r_{ij}}\right)^{12} - 2\left(\frac{RA}{r_{ij}}\right)^{6}\right]D \tag{79}$$

where RA is the hybridization corrected van der Waals radius for the atom, r_{ij} is the distance between the atom i and the surface point j, K is the well depth constant and is set to 0.1 for all van der Waals atom/point interactions, and D is an empirically derived point-density scaling factor, set to 0.01 for the default grid resolution of 0.5 Å and surface point density of 6 points Å^{-2}. RA is computed with the equation:

$$RA = r_{VDW,i} \cdot C_h \tag{80}$$

where $r_{VDW,i}$ is the van der Waals radius of the atom i and C_h is a hybridization correction.

The electrostatic term is a monopole-monopole Coulombic function computed with the equation:

$$E_{C,ij} = 322.1D\frac{q_i q_j}{r_{ij}}S(r_{ij}) \tag{81}$$

where r_{ij} is the distance between the atom i and the grid point j, q_i is the partial charge of the atom i, q_j is the charge of the surface point j, D is the point-density scaling factor used in the computation of E_{vdW}, and $S(r_{ij})$ is an atom-based switching function:

$$S(r_{ij}) = \frac{(r_{off}^2 - r_{ij}^2)^2(r_{off}^2 + 2r_{ij}^2 - 3r_{on}^2)}{(r_{off}^2 - r_{on}^2)^3} \tag{82}$$

where $r_{on} = 7$ Å and $r_{off} = 8$ Å. If $r_{ij} < r_{on}$ then $S(r_{ij}) = 1$.

The desolvation energy term is a penalty function for the presence of polar atoms in hydrophobic regions of the receptor surface model. If the fraction of hydrophobic surface points around a polar atom is greater than 90%, then the desolvation energy term is proportional to the exposed surface area of the polar atom; a value of 0.3 kcal/mol Å^2 is used. The desolvation energy is added to the total energy.

(13) The interactions between a ligand and the virtual receptor are used to compute several structural descriptors. The nonbonded energy terms, i.e. the van der Waals energy E_{VDW}, the electrostatic energy E_C, and their sum E_{total}, representing the sum for all surface points of the respective energy terms, are used as descriptors in MLR equations.

Another descriptor is the intramolecular strain energy of the ligand inside the virtual receptor, E_{inside}. To compute this descriptor, the conformation of the ligand is optimized inside the virtual receptor.

These global descriptor that characterize the ligand-receptor interaction were used to model the binding affinity for corticosteroid binding globulin of 31 steroids, and the inhibition of dopamine β-hydroxylase by 52 1-(substituted-benzyl)imidazole-2(3*H*)-thiones.[52]

The Cerius^2 implementation of the receptor surface model[53] offers a larger population of descriptors for the generation of the 3D QSAR model, by collecting into the QSAR table, for each molecule, the nonbonded energy terms that measure the interaction between that molecule and each surface point *j*, i.e. the van der Waals energy $E_{VDW,j}$ and the electrostatic energy $E_{C,j}$, and their sum $E_{total,j}$. From the large set of several hundreds of parameters, the selection of descriptors for the 3D QSAR model is made with the genetic function approximation (GFA) algorithm.[54-57]

The GFA algorithm generates an initial population of QSAR equations by the random selection of molecular descriptors. The length of the equations is determined by the number of molecular descriptors selected and is allowed to increase or decrease with a certain probability. Each equation is fit to the experimental data using linear least-squares regression techniques, and the 3D QSAR models are ranked according to their lack of fit (LOF), which is an adjusted least-squares error (LSE) statistical index:

$$\mathrm{LOF} = \frac{\mathrm{LSE}}{\left(1 - \frac{c + df}{n}\right)^2} \tag{83}$$

where *c* is the number of basis functions (number of terms in the 3D QSAR equation), *d* is the smoothing parameter, *f* is the total number of structural descriptors contained in all basis functions, and *n* is the number of molecules in the calibration set. The addition of a new descriptor to a 3D QSAR equation may reduce the LSE, but it also increases the values of *c* and *f*, and the LOF index may increase. In this way, the LOF index avoids overfitting of the data by limiting the tendency to add new descriptors and favoring simple, more compact models. The user-defined smoothing parameter *d* controls the growing of the 3D QSAR equations.

The GFA algorithm uses a genetic algorithm to perform the genetic crossover of the best equations and the elimination of the poorer equations. Using pairs of 3D QSAR equations with a low LOF, the genetic algorithm cuts and separates pieces of equations and then recombines the fragments to form new equations. Next, mutation operators are applied randomly in order to increase the diversity of the population. The following probability levels *p* were used for the equation mutation operators:

1. add new term: $p = 0.5$; this mutation increases the diversity in the equation population by randomly adding a new term to a child equation.
2. reduce equation: $p = 0.5$; this mutation operation generates smaller models by eliminating from a child equation the term with the lowest contribution to the model.
3. extend equation: $p = 0.5$; this mutation operation generates larger models by adding to a child equation a new descriptor. Each not yet used descriptor is tested and the algorithm retains the one that has the highest contribution to the model.

The genetic algorithm uses the LOF index to select equations for crossover and survival. With new generations, the equation population evolves to a set of higher quality 3D QSAR models. The output of a GFA calculation consists of a population of 3D QSAR equations that model the relationship between the structural descriptors and the biological activity.

Another modification of the RSM is the comparative receptor surface analysis (CoRSA)[58] that uses the nonbonded energy terms that measure the interaction between a molecule and each surface point j, i.e. the van der Waals energy $E_{VDW,j}$ and the electrostatic energy $E_{C,j}$, and their sum $E_{total,j}$, in a partial least squares data analysis. This 3D QSAR algorithm was used to model the activity of a set of compounds that act as calcium channel agonists for the guinea pig left atrium assay.

13. MOLREF - Molecular Reference

Alsberg proposed a 3D QSAR model, the molecular reference (MOLREF),[59] that compares the structure of test molecules with a reference molecule. The reference may be a representative molecule for the whole set of compounds, or a pseudomolecule that contains all relevant structural characteristics. MOLREF uses a set of descriptors that measure the similarity between each molecule and the reference; subsequently, the relationship between the **X** and **Y** matrices is computed with the PLS method.

The MOLREF algorithm contains the following steps:

1. The geometry of all molecules in the study set is optimized with molecular mechanics or quantum mechanics methods.
2. A compound that contains the relevant structural characteristics for the whole set of compounds is selected as the reference molecule. If such a molecule does not exist a pseudomolecule is generated.
3. All molecules are superimposed over the reference using some pharmacophore hypothesis.
4. Each atom in the reference and model molecules is characterized by the x, y, and z coordinates, van der Waals radius, and atomic charge. Other atomic descriptors can be added if these five parameters are not sufficient to generate a good QSAR model.
5. A model molecule i is selected. For each atom j from the reference find the nearest neighbor atom k from the model molecule. The atomic descriptors of atom k are added to the row i of matrix **X**. If the reference contains n atoms and each atom is characterized by m atomic descriptors, then each row from the matrix **X** has $n \times m$ columns.
6. Repeat step (5) for all model molecules.
7. A 3-D QSAR model is obtained by applying the PLS algorithm to the matrices **X** and **Y**.

MOLREF was used to model the toxicity of 42 benzene derivatives (mainly phenols) against *Daphnia magna*; benzene was employed as the reference, but similar results were obtained when phenol was selected as reference.

14. MOLECULAR SIMILARITY INDICES

The 2D and 3D similarity indices of chemical structures are widely used in searching molecular databases, in pharmacophore identification, and classification of molecules in structure-activity studies.[60-64] Recent applications of these similarity indices as structural descriptors in 3D QSAR offers an efficient way of condensing a large number of field, grid or surface descriptors into a single number.

The molecular similarity may be quantified theoretically by comparing the electron densities, ρ_A and ρ_B, of two molecules A and B, and calculating an index of similarity, R_{AB}, as first introduced by Carbó:[65-68]

$$R_{AB} = \frac{\int \rho_A \rho_B \mathrm{d}v}{\left(\int \rho_A^2 \mathrm{d}v\right)^{1/2} \left(\int \rho_B^2 \mathrm{d}v\right)^{1/2}} \tag{84}$$

where the integrations are considered over all space. Several QSPR and QSAR application of this similarity index were presented in two reviews.[67,68]

Willett revealed that the Carbó index formula computed for a property distributed on a grid surrounding a molecule is essentially equivalent to the Cosine coefficient.[62,64] The Cosine similarity coefficient of two molecules A and B, $C(P)_{AB}$, computed for a property $P = P(j)$ defined in a grid point $j = j(x,y,z)$ is:

$$C(P)_{A,B} = \frac{\sum_{j=1}^{n} P(j)_A P(j)_B}{\left[\sum_{j=1}^{n} P(j)_A^2 \sum_{i=1}^{n} P(j)_B^2\right]^{1/2}} \tag{85}$$

where n is the number of grid points.

Hodgkin and Richards[69] pointed that in tha Carbó index the denominator is a normalizing constant and R_{AB} varies in the range 0 to 1. Such an index of similarity is required to have a value of 1 when the electron density distributions in the two molecules are identical. However, substitution of $\rho_A = a\rho_B$ into the above equation, where a is a constant, gives an index of unity. Thus the Carbó index represents the similarity of the shapes of the density distributions but not of the magnitudes as well.

Although originally proposed as a method of comparing molecules in terms of electron density, Hodgkin and Richards[69] proposed to use the formula of the Carbó index with other quantum properties, such as molecular electrostatic potential (MEP) or molecular electrostatic field (MEF). The use of electrostatic potentials and electrostatic fields is particularly attractive since they are better discriminators than charge and problems can be avoided if only values external to a van der Waals volume of the molecule are considered. The electrostatic potentials and electrostatic fields can be calculated over a grid of points surrounding a molecule.

In an attempt to increase the magnitude sensitivity of similarity calculations, Hodgkin and Richards proposed the Hodgkin index:[69]

$$H_{AB} = \frac{2\int \rho_A \rho_B \mathrm{d}v}{\int \rho_A^2 \mathrm{d}v + \int \rho_B^2 \mathrm{d}v} \tag{86}$$

Analogously with the Carbó index, the Hodgkin index can be used with grid-based properties such as MEP or MEF, when its formula is identical with that of the Dice coefficient, as found by Willett.[62,64] The Dice similarity coefficient of two molecules A and B, $D(P)_{AB}$, computed for a property $P = P(j)$ defined in a grid point $j = j(x,y,z)$ is:

$$D(P)_{A,B} = \frac{2\sum_{j=1}^{n} P(j)_A P(j)_B}{\sum_{j=1}^{n} P(j)_A^2 + \sum_{i=1}^{n} P(j)_B^2} \tag{87}$$

Richards[70] proposed a linear index for the computation of grid-based molecular similarity descriptors:

$$L(P)_{AB} = \frac{1}{n}\sum_{j=1}^{n}\left(1 - \frac{|P(j)_A - P(j)_B|}{\max(|P(j)_A|, |P(j)_B|)}\right) \tag{88}$$

where $\max(|P(j)_A|, |P(j)_B|) = P_{\max}$ equals the larger value of the property P (P_A or P_B) at the grid point j where the similarity is being calculated. A related formula was defined by Good[71] who introduced an exponential similarity index:

$$E(P)_{AB} = \frac{1}{n}\sum_{j=1}^{n}\exp\left(-\frac{|P(j)_A - P(j)_B|}{\max(|P(j)_A|, |P(j)_B|)}\right) \tag{89}$$

So and Karplus[72,73] proposed to encode the 3D chemical structure in molecular similarity matrices computed with the Carbó index. The electrostatic and steric molecular fields were used to generate the similarity matrices, and a genetic neural network was employed to select the relevant descriptors.

15. MIMIC

The MIMIC approach is a molecular-field similarity algorithm for aligning molecules by matching their steric and electrostatic fields.[74] After the alignment of the molecules, two methods can be used to obtain information on feature-based and field-based pharmacophoric patterns. Feature-based pharmacophoric patterns correspond to traditional pharmacophore models and are computed from the contribution of individual atoms to the total similarity. Field-based pharmacophoric patterns are generated by computing the percent contribution to the similarity of individual points in a regular lattice surrounding the molecules; this algorithm identifies steric and electrostatic field-based patterns of similarity onto a 3D grid, van der Waals surface, or solvent-accessible surface. The identification of such patterns is useful in detecting important structural features and pharmacophoric-field patterns that contribute to the bioactivity of the molecules.

MIMIC uses a molecular steric volume (MSV) field that describes the size and shape of a molecule, and a molecular electrostatic potential (MEP) field representing the electrostatic potential of a molecule. A brief description of the most important characteristics of this molecular-field similarity algorithm is provided below. At a point $r = r(x,y,z)$ the MSV field of molecule A is:

$$F_A^{\mathrm{MSV}}(r) = \sum_{i \in A} f_i^{\mathrm{MSV}}(r) \tag{90}$$

where f_i^{MSV} represents the steric volume of atom i and is represented by a Gaussian function located at $R_i = R_i(x_i,y_i,z_i)$, the center of atom i:

$$f_i^{\mathrm{MSV}}(r) = \alpha_i \exp(-\beta_i |r - R_i|^2) \tag{91}$$

where the parameters α_i and β_i are optimized for each atom type. The MEP field of molecule A at a point r is:

$$F_A^{\mathrm{MEP}}(r) = \sum_{i \in A} \frac{q_i}{|r - R_i|} \tag{92}$$

where q_i is the partial charge on atom i located at R_i. A three-Gaussian expansion of the $1/r$ term is used to avoid discontinuity of the function at the nuclei.

For any pair of molecules A and B a similarity measure with respect to the field MF, Z_{AB}^{MF}, is computed with the formula:

$$Z_{AB}^{\mathrm{MF}} = \int F_A^{\mathrm{MF}}(r) F_B^{\mathrm{MF}}(r) \mathrm{d}r \tag{93}$$

A molecular similarity index (MSI) is computed for each pair of molecules A and B using a Cosine coefficient formula:

$$S_{AB}^{\mathrm{MF}} = \frac{Z_{AB}^{\mathrm{MF}}}{\left[Z_{AA}^{\mathrm{MF}} Z_{BB}^{\mathrm{MF}}\right]^{1/2}} \tag{94}$$

The MSI index takes values in the range [0, 1] for the steric field MSV and [–1, 1] for the electrostatic field MEP. The pairwise similarity index for molecules A and B is obtained as a weighted sum of the corresponding MSI values for each field:

$$S_{AB} = \lambda S_{AB}^{\mathrm{MSV}} + (1-\lambda) S_{AB}^{\mathrm{MEP}} \tag{95}$$

where $\lambda = 0.66$, that corresponds to a 2:1 weighting of the steric field compared to the electrostatic field. The determination of the best molecular-field alignment of two molecules A and B requires an exploration of the similarity space of the two molecules. The alignment with the highest similarity for molecules A and B represents a pairwise alignment solution. However, it was found that the optimum alignment for each pair of molecules will not necessarily produce the optimal multi-molecule alignment, leading to inconsistencies when three or more molecules are considered simultaneously. In an experiment involving three non-nucleoside HIV-1 reverse transcriptase inhibitors it was found that the optimum simultaneous three-molecule alignment reproduces the experimental inhibitor alignment. The similarity determined as a simultaneous matching of several molecules is highly important for the development of consistent relative binding orientations of sets of bioactive molecules. The molecular-field similarity of the molecule set $\mathbf{M} = \{A, B, C, \dots\}$ is defined as the average of the pairwise similarities:

$$S_{\mathbf{M}} = \left[\frac{m^2 - m}{2}\right]^{-1} \sum_{I<J} S_{IJ} \tag{96}$$

where m is the number of molecules in set $\mathbf{M}$, and S_{IJ} is the pairwise molecular similarity index for molecules I and J. The solution for the alignment of the m molecules from the set $\mathbf{M}$ is obtained by maximizing the value of the index $S_{\mathbf{M}}$. This equation represents an efficient way of computing the multi-molecule similarity and to compare the pairwise molecule alignments with the multi-molecule optimized results. A pairwise consistency index (PCI) is proposed to measure the quality of combining the pairwise alignments:

$$\mathrm{PCI} = \frac{S_{\mathrm{M}}^{\mathrm{o}}}{S_{\mathrm{M}}} \tag{97}$$

where $S_{\mathrm{M}}^{\mathrm{o}}$ is the multi-molecule similarity computed with Eq. (96) by superposing the m molecules in set **M** according to their optimized pairwise alignments, and S_{M} is the similarity computed from full multi-molecule optimization according to Eq. (96).

After the similarity-based alignment of a set of molecules is finished, two procedures are applied to extract information regarding the principal structural features of the molecules under study. The first procedure identifies pharmacophoric patterns or pharmacophores from atomic similarities computed with the formula:

$$S_{A_i B}^{\mathrm{MF}} = \frac{\int F_{A_i}^{\mathrm{MF}}(r) F_B^{\mathrm{MF}}(r) \mathrm{d}r}{\left[Z_{AA}^{\mathrm{MF}} Z_{BB}^{\mathrm{MF}} \right]^{1/2}} \tag{98}$$

where A_i represents the contribution of the ith atom in molecule A. The total similarity index is defined as the sum of atomic similarities:

$$S_{AB}^{\mathrm{MF}} = \sum_i S_{A_i B}^{\mathrm{MF}} \tag{99}$$

Regions of high atomic similarity in pairwise or multi-molecule alignments represent pharmacophoric patterns that can be more general than those from the classical pharmacophores. Once identified, pharmacophoric patterns can be used to evaluate molecules representing potential novel leads.

The second procedure can be used for the graphical display of molecular similarity fields by computing the percent contribution to the similarity of individual points in a regular lattice surrounding the molecules. The similarity fields can be computed onto a 3D set of grid points into which the aligned molecules are embedded, or onto various molecular surfaces, such as van der Waals or solvent-accessible surfaces. For each grid or molecular surface point r_i a field similarity value is computed with the equation:

$$S_{AB}^{\mathrm{MF}}(r_i) = \frac{F_A^{\mathrm{MF}}(r_i) F_B^{\mathrm{MF}}(r_i)}{\left[\sum_j F_A^{\mathrm{MF}}(r_j) F_A^{\mathrm{MF}}(r_j) \right]^{1/2} \left[\sum_j F_B^{\mathrm{MF}}(r_j) F_B^{\mathrm{MF}}(r_j) \right]^{1/2}} \tag{100}$$

where $F_A^{\mathrm{MF}}(r_i)$ and $F_B^{\mathrm{MF}}(r_i)$ are the molecular field values at the point r_i for molecules A and B, and the summations are carried out over all the grid or surface points. When the summation is carried out over the entire set of points, the above equation gives:

$$S_{AB}^{\mathrm{MF}} = \sum_i S_{AB}^{\mathrm{MF}}(r_i) \tag{101}$$

The percent of the total field-based similarity at each field point is given by the formula:

$$C_{AB}^{\mathrm{MF}}(r_i) = 100\frac{S_{AB}^{\mathrm{MF}}(r_i)}{S_{AB}^{\mathrm{MF}}} \tag{102}$$

The visual recognition of steric and electrostatic similarity patterns can be accomplished with the aid of the graphical representation of $C_{AB}^{\mathrm{MF}}(r_i)$ values at each of the points on a surface surrounding the superposed molecules. Equally well, the structural features that determine the biological activity can be deduced from iso-similarity surfaces computed with $C_{AB}^{\mathrm{MF}}(r_i)$ values.

The MIMIC model was applied to a study involving three non-nucleoside HIV-1 reverse transcriptase inhibitors.

16. Supermolecule Similarity Descriptors

De Benedetti introduced new size, shape and electrostatic similarity descriptors computed from a reference supermolecule.[75-78] The supermolecule, that is an ensemble of the most active and diverse ligands, contains information related to the ligand-receptor complementarity. The calculation of the supermolecule similarity descriptors involves the following steps:

1. The QSAR is developed for a set of molecules that interact with the same receptor, having the same mechanism of action.
2. The geometry of all molecules is optimized with molecular mechanics or quantum mechanics methods.
3. Atomic partial charges are calculated for all molecules with a quantum mechanics method.
4. The supermolecule is generated by the superposition of the most active and structurally most different compounds.
5. A molecule is superimposed on the supermolecule using some pharmacophore hypothesis.
6. The aligned molecule and supermolecule are placed in a box enclosing both of them and extending 3 Å from the larger coordinates value on each Cartesian axis, and the box is partitioned into a grid with points separated by 0.5 Å; the distance between two grid points defines the grid spacing, GS.

7. The van der Waals volumes of the molecule (V_{mol}) and supermolecule (V_{sup}) are computed by counting the number of grid points included within the volume of each of them:

$$V_{mol} = Ngm \times GS^3 \tag{103}$$
$$V_{sup} = Ngs \times GS^3 \tag{104}$$

where Ngm is the number of grid points included within the volume of the molecule, and Ngs is the number of grid points included within the volume of the supermolecule.
8. The intersection volume (V_{in}) is computed by counting the number of grid points falling inside the volumes of both the molecule and supermolecule (Ngc, number of common grid points):

$$V_{in} = Ngc \times GS^3 \tag{105}$$

9. The outer van der Waals volume (V_{out}) of the molecule with respect to the volume of the supermolecule is:

$$V_{out} = Ngo \times GS^3 \tag{106}$$

where Ngo is the number of grid points that belong only to the molecule.
10. Using the above volumes, two normalized indices are computed for the molecule:

$$V_{Dnorm} = (V_{in} - V_{out})/V_{sup} \tag{107}$$

$$V_{in}/V_{mol} \tag{108}$$

11. For each molecule, the indices V_{in}, V_{Dnorm}, and V_{in}/V_{mol} are used as size and shape descriptors in QSAR models.
12. Steps (5)-(11) are repeated for all molecules from the set.
13. The molecular electrostatic potential (MEP) is computed at the intersection of a rectilinear grid which has the same extension and spacing as used for the volume calculations. Each grid point $g = g(x,y,z)$ is uniquely identified by its Cartesian coordinates x, y, and z. A probe atom is placed at each grid point and the MEP values are calculated using atom centered point charges:

$$\mathrm{MEP}_{g,i} = \sum_{j=1}^{na} \frac{q_g q_j}{d_{g,j}} \tag{109}$$

where $\mathrm{MEP}_{g,i}$ is the MEP value in the grid point g for molecule i, q_g is the charge of the probe atom, which is set to 1.0, q_j is the charge of atom j from molecule i, $d_{g,j}$ is the distance between the jth atom and the probe, and na is the number of atoms in the molecule i. In order to avoid singularities the evaluation of MEP is restricted to grid points outside the van der Waals volume of the molecule.

14. At each grid point g the supermolecule MEP ($MEP_{sup,g}$) is calculated as the average MEP values of the molecules that form the supermolecule:

$$MEP_{sup,g} = \frac{1}{nz}\sum_{i=1}^{ns} MEP_{g,i} \tag{110}$$

where ns is the number of molecules that form the supermolecule, and nz is the number of molecules with non-zero $MEP_{g,i}$ values. Whenever the grid point g falls inside the van der Waals volume of one or more molecules from the supermolecule, the summation is averaged only over the remaining molecules with the grid point outside their volumes.

15. The MEP similarity index ($MEP_{sim,i}$) of molecule i with respect to the supermolecule is computed with the Hodgkin similarity index:

$$MEP_{sim,i} = \frac{2\sum_{g=1}^{np} MEP_{sup,g} MEP_{g,i}}{\sum_{g=1}^{np} MEP_{sup,g}^2 + \sum_{g=1}^{np} MEP_{g,i}^2} \tag{111}$$

16. In analogy with the MEP_{sim} index, a surface MEP index (MEP_{sur}) is computed over a set of points distributed on the van der Waals surface of the supermolecule. A gridded sphere is generated around each atom of each molecule from the supermolecule. Each sphere has a radius equal to the van der Waals radius of the corresponding atom. All points falling at the intersection region of any two spheres is discarded, and the remaining grid points are used to compute the MEP_{sur} index for each molecule.

The descriptors V_{in}, V_{Dnorm}, V_{in}/V_{mol}, MEP_{sim}, and MEP_{sur} were used to model pNMS, the cologarithm of the binding affinity constants measured by displacement of the muscarinic antagonist [^{3}H]N-methylscopolamine which labels both high affinity and low affinity states of the receptor, and pOXO-M, the cologarithm of the binding affinity constants measured by displacement of the muscarinic agonist [^{3}H]oxotremorine-M which labels the high affinity agonist state of the receptor.[78]

17. MLP - Molecular Lipophilic Potential

A common assumption in drug design is that the ligand-receptor interactions involve the same intermolecular forces as those acting in the partitioning of a solute between water and an immiscible organic phase, usually *n*-octanol. For these reasons, the logarithm of the *n*-octanol/water partition coefficient, log P, is a widely used QSAR descriptor for the characterization of the molecular hydrophobicity. However, the characterization of the molecular lipophilicity with a single number is not sufficient in 3D QSAR, when the ligand-receptor interactions are investigated. By analogy with the molecular electrostatic potential, a grid-based definition of several types of molecular lipophilic potentials (MLP) were proposed in the literature.[79,80] At a given point in space, the MLP value is the result of the intermolecular interactions encoded by the lipophilicity of all molecular fragments. Therefore, the MLP computation of MLP is based on two components, namely a fragmental system of lipophilicity, and a distance function describing the variation of lipophilicity in space. A general equation of the MLP is:

$$\mathrm{MLP}_j = \sum_{i=1}^{N} f_i F(d_{ij}) \tag{112}$$

where j is a grid point, i is the label of the molecular fragment, N is the total number of fragments in the molecule, f_i is the lipophilic constant of fragment i, F is a distance function, and d_{ij} is the distance between fragment i and grid point j. Unlike the MEP which has a physical significance and which is dependent on the electronic density distribution, an MLP is purely a mathematical tool with no physical existence.

The first MLP field was proposed by Audry, who used a hyperbolic distance function:[81]

$$\mathrm{MLP}_j = \sum_{i=1}^{N} \frac{f_i}{1 + d_{ij}} \tag{113}$$

This MLP definition is based on the assumption that log P can be computed from the hydrophobic constants of certain molecular fragments:

$$\log P = \sum_{i=1}^{N} f_i \tag{114}$$

The values for fragment hydrophobicities can be computed with the Hansch[8,82,83] or Rekker[84-88] systems. However, the calculation of the MLP on the van der Waals surface requires hydrophobic constants defined for atoms not for functional groups. Atomic parameters present several advantages, i.e. for different conformations of the same molecule, the MLP has different values for the relevant space regions. Several atomic hydrophobicity parameters systems were proposed, but the most used are those defined by Broto[89] and Ghose.[90-92] According to these systems, log P for a molecule with N atoms can be expressed as:

$$\log P = \sum_{i=1}^{N} a_i \tag{115}$$

where a_i is the lipophilic contribution of a certain atom type. With a hyperbolic distance function and the atomic system of hydrophobic constants, the MLP in the grid point j is:

$$\mathrm{MLP}_j = \sum_{i=1}^{N} \frac{a_i}{1 + d_{ij}} \tag{116}$$

Using different combinations of distance functions and hydrophobic constants, several other MLP systems were proposed by Furet,[93] Fauchère,[94] Testa,[95] and Rozas.[96,97] For example, the MLP system defined by Testa[79,95] uses the atomic increments of Broto and a modification of the exponential function proposed by Fauchère:

$$\mathrm{MLP}_j = \sum_{i=1}^{N} a_i e^{-d_{ij}/2} \tag{117}$$

In this formula, the distance function is limited by the use of a cut-off of 4 Å to avoid the influence of too-distant atoms.

We have to mention that the intermolecular forces encoded into the MLP field can add important information to the molecular fields usually used in CoMFA or other related 3D QSAR models. As presented in a previous section, the CoMFA analysis reduces the description of ligand-receptor complexes to the intermolecular interactions described by the steric and electrostatic fields. These fields are purely enthalpic, while MLP describes the entropy component of the binding free energy associated with solvation/desolvation of the ligand and receptor.

18. HINT - Hydropathic Interactions

Kellogg introduced a new model for biological interactions, HINT (hydropathic interactions),[98-104] that is based on atom-atom interactions computed with the formula:

$$b_{ij} = a_i S_i a_j S_j f(r_{ij}) \tag{118}$$

where a_i is the hydrophobic atomic constant for atom i, S_i is the solvent-accessible surface area for atom i, a_j is the hydrophobic atomic constant for atom j, S_j is the solvent-accessible surface area for atom j, and $f(r_{ij})$ is a function of the distance between atoms i and j. The distance function usually used is an exponential:

$$f(r_{ij}) = \exp(-r_{ij}) \tag{119}$$

The sum of all ligand-receptor atom-atom interactions defines the total HINT binding score, a descriptor used in 3D QSAR models:

$$B = \sum_{i=1}^{\text{rec}} \sum_{j=1}^{\text{lig}} a_i S_i a_j S_j T_{ij} f(r_{ij}) \tag{120}$$

where atom i belongs to the receptor, atom j belongs to the ligand, T_{ij} is a sign-flip function that discriminates between acid-base interactions, which are favorable, and acid-acid and base-base interactions, which are unfavorable, and r_{ij} is the distance between atoms i and j. The cutoff distance for interactions is 10 Å.

The model proposed by Kellogg can be converted to HINT 3D property maps computed on a grid of points that surround the ligand:[98,104]

$$A_j = \sum_{i=1}^{n} a_i S_i f(r_{ij}) \tag{121}$$

where A_j is the value of the hydropathic field in the grid point j, and the summation goes over all n atoms in the ligand. Together with the MLP fields, HINT 3D maps can be added to the two standard fields from CoMFA. Several experiments show that HINT field represent a significant component of the final CoMFA model whenever hydrophobic interactions are significant in the binding mode, or where membrane transport is encoded in the biological measure.

19. Molecular Surface Lipophilicity

Brickmann[105] proposed an MLP approach particularly designed for mapping local hydrophobicity properties on a solvent-accessible surface of a molecule. He used the atomic hydrophobicity parameters proposed by Ghose[90,91] in the following formula:

$$MLP_j = \frac{\sum_{i=1}^{n} a_i F(d_{ij})}{\sum_{i=1}^{n} F(d_{ij})} \tag{122}$$

where d_{ij} is the distance between atom i and the grid point j, a_i is the lipophilic contribution of a certain atom type, and the summation goes over all n atoms in the molecule. The distance function $F(d_{ij})$ is a Fermi-type function centered on each atom:

$$F(d_{ij}) = \left(1 + e^{a(d_{ij} - d_{\text{cutoff}})}\right)^{-1} \tag{123}$$

This atom-centered function has two adjustable parameters, a and d_{cutoff}, which, for simplicity, are taken to be the same for all atoms. The precise values of these parameters are somewhat arbitrary, but a value of 1.5 was suggested for a, and 4.0 Å for d_{cutoff}. A modified Fermi function was proposed:

$$F(d_{ij}) = \frac{1 + \exp(-a \cdot d_{\text{cutoff}})}{1 + \exp[a(d_{ij} - d_{\text{cutoff}})]} \tag{124}$$

This approach was further elaborated to give a molecular free energy surface density (MOLFESD) approach for a quantitative treatment of hydrophobicity.[106,107]

20. HMLP - Heuristic Molecular Lipophilicity Potential

Du, Arteca, and Mezey proposed the heuristic molecular lipophilicity potential (HMLP),[108] defined on the molecular surfaces from the electrostatic potential and requiring no empirical indices of atomic lipophilicity. This non-empirical, unified lipophilicity and hydrophilicity potential model is computed with the formula:

$$L_i(r_k) = V(r_k)\sum_{\substack{j=1 \\ j\neq i}}^{n} M_j(r_k, R_j, b_j) \tag{125}$$

where $L_i(r_k)$ is the lipophilic potential of atom i computed on the point r_k situated on its exposed surface, $V(r_k)$ is the MEP at point r_k, and the summation is over all atoms in the molecule except atom i. In the screening function $M_j(r_k,R_j,b_j)$ R_j is the nuclear position of atom j, and b_j is the atomic surface-MEP descriptor of atom j:

$$b_j = \sum_{q \in S_j} V(r_q)\Delta s_q \tag{126}$$

where Δs_q is the area element on atom j, and the summation goes over all exposed surface elements of atom j. The atom-based screening function $M_j(r_k,R_j,b_j)$ can be computed with one of the three formulas:

$$M_j(r_k, R_j, b_j) = \frac{r_0^{\gamma}}{b_0}\frac{b_j}{\left\|R_j - r_k\right\|^{\gamma}} = \zeta\frac{b_j}{\left\|R_j - r_k\right\|^{\gamma}} \tag{127}$$

$$M_j(r_k, R_j, b_j) = \frac{b_j}{b_0}\exp\left(-\frac{\left\|R_j - r_k\right\|}{d_0}\right) \tag{128}$$

$$M_j(r_k, R_j, b_j) = \frac{b_j}{|b_j|}\exp\left(-\frac{b_0}{\lambda_0}\frac{\|R_j - r_k\|}{|b_j|}\right)$$
$$= \text{sign}(b_j)\exp\left(-\xi\frac{\|R_j - r_k\|}{|b_j|}\right) \tag{129}$$

In the above three functions (r_0, b_0, γ), (b_0, d_0) and (b_0, λ_0) are parameters. The parameters ζ, γ, ξ, and d_0 have to be optimized in order to obtain good lipophilic and hydrophilic descriptors for QSAR.

The atomic lipophilicity of atom i is defined with the formula:

$$l_i = \sum_{k \in S_i} L_i(r_k)\Delta s_k \tag{130}$$

where the summation is over the exposed surface area S_i of atom i, and Δs_k is the area element associated with the point r_k situated on the exposed surface of atom i. If $l_i > 0$ then atom i is lipophilic, while if $l_i < 0$ then atom i is hydrophilic. The molecular lipophilic index L_M and the molecular hydrophilic index H_M are the sum of the corresponding values for all lipophilic and hydrophilic atoms, respectively:

$$L_M = \sum_{l_i > 0} l_i \tag{131}$$

$$H_M = \sum_{l_i < 0} l_i \tag{132}$$

These two HMLP descriptors were used to model log P values of alkanes, alcohols, amines, and carboxylic acids.

21. CONCLUSIONS

In this review we have presented two important directions of development of 3D QSAR models. The first direction is represented by the new structural descriptors computed from the three-dimensional molecular structure that can be used in a Hansch-like multilinear regression equation or other statistical model. The second direction contains the methods that compute grid descriptors to generate a virtual receptor, and usually use molecular alignment of atoms, pharmacophores, volume, or fields. All these techniques are of essential value whenever the three-dimensional structures of biological receptors and their complexes with the ligands are not known. Important steps in recent developments in 3D QSAR are molecular fields, PLS, molecular similarity indices, genetic and evolutionary algorithms for feature selection.

22. References

1. Kopp, H. Ueber den zusammenhang zwischen der chemischen constitution und einigen physikalischen eigen-schoften bei flüssigen verbindungen. *Ann. Chem. Pharm.* **1844**, *50*, 71-144.
2. Crum-Brown, A.; Frazer, T. On the Connection between Chemical Constitution and Physiological Action. Part 1. On the Physiological Action of the Ammonium Bases, Derived from Strychia, Brucia, Thebaia, Codeia, Morphia and Nicotia. *Trans. Royal Soc. Edinburgh* **1868-1869**, *25*, 257-274.
3. Meyer, H. Zur Theorie der Alkoholnarkose, welche Eigenschaft de Anästhetica bedingt ihre narkotische Wirkung. *Arch. Exp. Pathol. Pharmakol.* **1899**, *42*, 109-118.
4. Overton, C.E. Studien über die Narkose. Zugleich ein Beitrag zur Allgemeine Pharmakologie; Gustav Fisher Verlag: Jena, Germany, 1901.
5. Hansch, C.; Maloney, P.P.; Fujita, T.; Muir, R.M. Correlation of Biological Activity of Phenoxyacetic Acids with Hammett Substituent Constants and Partition Coefficients. *Nature* **1962**, *194*, 178-180.
6. Hansch, C.; Fujita, T. ρ-σ-π Analysis. A Method for the Correlation of Biological Activity and Chemical Structure. *J. Am. Chem. Soc.* **1964**, *86*, 1616-1626.
7. Hansch, C. A Quantitative Approach to Biochemical Structure-Activity Relationships. *Acc. Chem. Res.* **1969**, *2*, 232-239.
8. Fujita, T.; Iwasa, J.; Hansch, C. A New Substituent Constant, π, Derived from Partition Coefficients. *J. Am. Chem. Soc.* **1964**, *86*, 5175-5180.
9. Kubinyi, H. QSAR and 3D QSAR in Drug Design. Part 1: Methodology. *Drug Discovery Today* **1997**, *2*, 457-467.
10. Kubinyi, H. QSAR and 3D QSAR in Drug Design. Part 2: Applications and Problems. *Drug Discovery Today* **1997**, *2*, 538-546.
11. CODESSA 2.13, Semichem, 7204 Mullen, Shawnee, KS 66216, U.S.A., E-mail andy@semichem.com, www http://www.semichem.com.
12. Randić, M. On Characterization of Three-Dimensional Structures. *Int. J. Quantum Chem.: Quantum Biol. Symp.* **1988**, *15*, 201-208.
13. Bogdanov, B.; Nikolić, S.; Trinajstić, N. On the Three-Dimensional Wiener Number. *J. Math. Chem.* **1989**, *3*, 299-309.
14. Randić, M.; Jerman-Blazić, B.; Trinajstić, N. Development of 3-Dimensional Molecular Descriptors. *Comput. Chem.* **1990**, *14*, 237-246.
15. Nikolić, S.; Trinajstić, N.; Mihalić, Z.; Carter, S. On the Geometric-Distance Matrix and the Corresponding Structural Invariants of Molecular Systems. *Chem. Phys. Lett.* **1991**, *179*, 21-28.

16. Diudea, M.V.; Horvath, D.; Graovac, A. Molecular Topology. 15. 3D Distance Matrices and Related Topological Indices. *J. Chem. Inf. Comput. Sci.* **1995**, *35*, 129-135.
17. Randić, M.; Razinger, M. Molecular Topographic Indices. *J. Chem. Inf. Comput. Sci.* **1995**, *35*, 140-147.
18. Randić, M. Molecular Profiles. Novel Geometry-Dependent Molecular Descriptors. *New J. Chem.* **1995**, *19*, 781-791.
19. Balaban, A.T.; Balaban, T.-S. New Vertex Invariants and Topological Indices of Chemical Graphs Based on Information on Distances. *J. Math. Chem.* **1991**, *8*, 383-397.
20. Ivanciuc, O.; Balaban, A.T. Design of Topological Indices. Part 21. Molecular Graph Operators for the Computation of Geometric Structural Descriptors. *Rev. Roum. Chim.* **1999**, *44*, 539-547.
21. HyperChem 5.1, Hypercube, Inc., Florida Science and Technology Park, 1115 N.W. 4th Street Gainesville, Florida 32601, U.S.A., Voice: 352-371-7744, Fax: 352-371-3662, Email info@hyper.com, www http://www.hyper.com.
22. Ośmiałowski, K.; Halkiewicz, J.; Kaliszan, R. Quantum Chemical Parameters in Correlation Analysis of Gas-Liquid Chromatographic Retention Indices of Amines. II. Topological Electronic Index. *J. Chromatogr.* **1986**, *361*, 63-69.
23. Stanton, D.T.; Jurs, P.C. Development and Use of Charged Partial Surface Area Structural Descriptors in Computer-Assisted Quantitative Structure-Property Relationship Studies. *Anal. Chem.* **1990**, *62*, 2323-2329.
24. Stuper, A.J.; Jurs, P.C. ADAPT: A Computer System for Automated Data Analysis Using Pattern Recognition Techniques. *J. Chem. Inf. Comput. Sci.* 1976, 16, 99-105.
25. ADAPT, P.C. Jurs, 152 Davey Lab, Chemistry Department, Penn State University, University Park, PA 16802 U.S.A., Tel: 814-865-3739, E-mail pcj@psu.edu, www http://zeus.chem.psu.edu/ADAPT.html.
26. Murugan, R.; Grendze, M.P.; Toomey, J.E., Jr.; Katritzky, A.R.; Karelson, M.; Lobanov, V.S.; Rachwal, P. Predicting Physical Properties from Molecular Structure *CHEMTECH* **1994**, *24*, 17-23.
27. Katritzky, A.R.; Lobanov, V.S.; Karelson, M. QSPR: The Correlation and Quantitative Prediction of Chemical and Physical Properties from Structure. *Chem. Soc. Rev.* **1995**, 279-287.
28. Karelson, M.; Lobanov, V.S.; Katritzky, A.R. Quantum-Chemical Descriptors in QSAR/QSPR Studies. *Chem. Rev.* **1996**, *96*, 1027-1043.
29. Katritzky, A.R.; Lobanov, V.S.; Karelson, M.; Murugan, R.; Grendze, M.P.; Toomey Jr., J.E. Comprehensive Descriptors for Structural and Statistical Analysis. 1. Correlations Between Structure and Physical Properties of Substituted Pyridines. *Rev. Roum. Chim.* **1996**, *41*, 851-867.
30. Katritzky, A.R.; Mu, L.; Karelson, M. A QSPR Study of the Solubility of Gases and Vapors in Water. *J. Chem. Inf. Comput. Sci.* **1996**, *36*, 1162-1168.
31. Katritzky, A.R.; Wang, Y.; Sild, S.; Tamm, T.; Karelson, M. QSPR Studies on Vapor Pressure, Aqueous Solubility, and the Prediction of Water-Air Partition Coefficients. *J. Chem. Inf. Comput. Sci.* **1998**, *38*, 720-725.

32. Ivanciuc, O.; Ivanciuc, T.; Balaban, A.T. Quantitative Structure-Property Relationship Study of Normal Boiling Points for Halogen-/ Oxygen-/ Sulfur-Containing Organic Compounds Using the CODESSA Program. *Tetrahedron* **1998**, *54*, 9129-9142.
33. Ivanciuc, O.; Ivanciuc, T.; Filip, P.A.; Cabrol-Bass, D. Estimation of the Liquid Viscosity of Organic Compounds with a Quantitative Structure-Property Model. *J. Chem. Inf. Comput. Sci.* **1999**, *39*, 515-524.
34. Kamlet, M.J.; Doherty, R.M.; Abboud, J.-L.M.; Abraham, M.H.; Taft, R.W. Solubility: A New Look. *CHEMTECH* **1986**, *16*, 566-576.
35. Kamlet, M.J.; Doherty, R.M.; Abraham, M.H.; Marcus, Y.; Taft, R.W. Linear Solvation Energy Relationships. 46. An Improved Equation for Correlation and Prediction of Octanol/Water Partition Coefficients of Organic Nonelectrolytes (Including Strong Hydrogen Bond Donor Solutes). *J. Phys. Chem.* **1988**, *92*, 5244-5255.
36. Famini, G.R.; Wilson, L.Y. Using Theoretical Descriptors in Linear Solvation Energy Relationships. In: *Quantitative Treatments of Solute/Solvent Interactions, Theoretical and Computational Chemistry*, Vol. 1; Politzer, P., Murray, J.S., Eds.; Elsevier: Amsterdam, 1994, pp. 213-241.
37. Cramer, C.J.; Famini, G.R.; Lowrey, A.H. Use of Calculated Quantum Chemical Properties as Surrogates for Solvatochromic Parameters in Structure-Activity Relationships. *Acc. Chem. Res.* **1993**, *26*, 599-605.
38. Donovan, W.H.; Famini, G.R. Using Theoretical Descriptions in Structure Activity Relationships: Retention Indices of Sulfur Vesicants and Related Compounds. *J. Chem. Soc. Perkin Trans. 2* **1996**, 83-89.
39. Esaki, T. Quantitative Drug Design Studies. II. Development and Application of New Electronic Substituent Parameters. *J. Pharm. Dyn.* **1980**, *3*, 562-576.
40. Pires, J.M.; Floriano, W.B.; Gaudio, A.C. Extension of the Frontier Reactivity Indices to Groups of Atoms and Application to Quantitative Structure-Activity Relationship Studies. *J. Mol. Struct. (Theochem)* **1997**, *389*, 159-167.
41. Murray, J.S.; Brinck, T.; Grice, M.E.; Politzer, P. Correlations between Molecular Electrostatic Potentials and Some Experimentally-Based Indices of Reactivity. *J. Mol. Struct. (Theochem)* **1992**, *256*, 29-45.
42. Murray, J.S.; Brinck, T.; Politzer, P. Partition Coefficients of Nitroaromatics Expressed in Terms of Their Molecular Surface Areas and Electrostatic Potentials. *J. Phys. Chem.* **1993**, *97*, 13807-13809.
43. Brinck, T.; Murray, J.S.; Politzer, P. Octanol/Water Partition Coefficients Expressed in Terms of Solute Molecular Surface Areas and Electrostatic Potentials. *J. Org. Chem.* **1993**, *58*, 7070-7073.
44. Murray, J.S.; Lane, P.; Brinck, T.; Politzer, P. Relationships between Computed Molecular Properties and Solute-Solvent Interactions in Supercritical Solutions. *J. Phys. Chem.* **1993**, *97*, 5144-5148.
45. Murray, J.S.; Lane, P.; Brinck, T.; Paulsen, K.; Grice, M.E.; Politzer, P. Relationships of Critical Constants and Boiling Points to Computed Molecular Surface Properties. *J. Phys. Chem.* **1993**, *97*, 9369-9373.

46. Murray, J.S.; Brinck, T.; Lane, P.; Paulsen, K.; Politzer, P. Statistically-Based Interaction Indices Derived from Molecular Surface Electrostatic Potentials: A General Interaction Properties Function (GIPF). *J. Mol. Struct. (Theochem)* **1994**, *307*, 55-64
47. Cramer, R.D.; Patterson, D.E.; Bunce, J.D. Comparative Molecular Field Analysis (CoMFA). 1. Effect of Shape on Binding of Steroids to Carrier Proteins. *J. Am. Chem. Soc.* **1988**, *110*, 5959-5967.
48. Clark, M.; Cramer III, R.D.; Jones, D.M.; Patterson, D.E.; Simeroth, P.E.; Comparative Molecular Field Analysis (CoMFA). 2. Toward Its Use with 3D-Structural Databases. *Tetrahedron Comput. Methodol.* **1990**, *3*, 47-59.
49. Kubinyi, H. Comparative Molecular Field Analysis (CoMFA). In: *The Encyclopedia of Computational Chemistry*; Schleyer, P. v. R., Allinger, N. L., Clark, T., Gasteiger, J., Kollman, P. A., Schaefer III, H. F., Schreiner, P. R., Eds.; John Wiley & Sons: Chichester, **1998**, 448-460.
50. Robinson, D.D.; Winn, P.J.; Lyne, P.D.; Richards, W.G. Self-Organizing Molecular Field Analysis: A Tool for Structure-Activity Studies. *J. Med. Chem.* **1999**, *42*, 573-583.
51. Hahn, M. Receptor Surface Models. 1. Definition and Construction. *J. Med. Chem.* **1995**, *38*, 2080-2090.
52. Hahn, M.; Rogers, D. Receptor Surface Models. 2. Application to Quantitative Structure-Activity Relationships Studies. *J. Med. Chem.* **1995**, *38*, 2091-2102.
53. Cerius^2 3.0 QSAR+, Molecular Simulations Inc., 9685 Scranton Road, San Diego, CA 92121-3752, Fax: 619/458-0136, 1997.
54. Rogers, D.; Hopfinger, A.J. Application of Genetic Function Approximation to Quantitative Structure-Activity Relationships and Quantitative Structure-Property Relationships. *J. Chem. Inf. Comput. Sci.* **1994**, *34*, 854-866.
55. Rhyu, K.-B.; Patel, H.C.; Hopfinger, A.J. A 3D-QSAR Study of Anticoccidal Triazines Using Molecular Shape Analysis. *J. Chem. Inf. Comput. Sci.* **1995**, *35*, 771-778.
56. Klein, C.D.P.; Hopfinger, A.J. Pharmacological Activity and Membrane Interactions of Antiarrhytmics: 4D-QSAR/QSPR Analysis. *Pharm. Res.* **1998**, *15*, 303-311.
57. Albuquerque, M.G.; Hopfinger, A.J.; Barreiro, E.J.; de Alencastro, R.B. Four-Dimensional Quantitative Structure-Activity Relationship Analysis of a Series of Interphenylene 7-Oxabicycloheptane Oxazole Thromboxane A_2 Receptor Antagonists. *J. Chem. Inf. Comput. Sci.* **1998**, *38*, 925-938.
58. Ivanciuc, O.; Ivanciuc, T.; Filip, P.A.; Cabrol-Bass, D. Comparative Receptor Surface Analysis (CoRSA) of Calcium Channel Agonist Activity of 1,4-Dihydro-2,6-dimethyl-3-nitro-4-pyridyl-5-pyridinecarboxylates. *Rev. Roum. Chim.* **2000**, *45*, 000-000.
59. Alsberg, B. Molecular Reference (MOLREF): A New Tool in Quantitative Structure-Activity Relationships (QSAR). *Chemom. Intell. Lab. Syst.* 1990, 8, 173-181.
60. Johnson, M.A. A Review and Examination of the Mathematical Spaces Underlying Molecular Similarity Analysis. *J. Math. Chem.* **1989**, *3*, 117-145.

61. Johnson, M.A.; Maggiora, G.M., Eds. *Concepts and Applications of Molecular Similarity*; John Wiley & Sons: New York, 1990.
62. Turner, D.B.; Willett, P.; Ferguson, A.M.; Heritage, T.W. Similarity Searching in Files of Three-Dimensional Structures: Evaluation of Similarity Coefficients and Standardisation Methods for Field-Based Similarity Searching. *SAR QSAR Environ. Res.* **1995**, *3*, 101-130.
63. Skvortsova, M.I.; Baskin, I.I.; Stankevich, I.V.; Palyulin, V.A.; Zefirov, N.S. Molecular Similarity. 1. Analytical Description of the Set of Graph Similarity Measures. *J. Chem. Inf. Comput. Sci.* **1998**, *38*, 785-790.
64. Willett, P.; Barnard, J.M.; Downs, G.M. Chemical Similarity Searching. *J. Chem. Inf. Comput. Sci.* **1998**, *38*, 983-996.
65. Carbó, R.; Leyda, L.; Arnau, M. How Similar Is a Molecule to Another? An Electron Density Measure of the Similarity between Two Molecular Structures. *Int. J. Quantum Chem.* **1980**, *17*, 1185-1189.
66. Carbó, R.; Domingo, L. LCAO-MO Similarity Measures and Taxonomy. *Int. J. Quantum Chem.* **1987**, *32*, 517-545.
67. Carbó, R.; Calabuig, B. Molecular Similarity and Quantum Chemistry. In: *Concepts and Applications of Molecular Similarity*; Johnson, M.A., Maggiora, G.M., Eds.; John Wiley & Sons: New York, 1990, pp. 147-171.
68. Carbó-Dorca, R.; Besalú, E.; Amat, L.; Fradera, X. Quantum Molecular Similarity Measures: Concepts, Definitions, and Applications to Quantitative Structure-Property Relationships. In: *Advances in Molecular Similarity*; Carbó-Dorca, R., Mezey, P.G., Eds.; JAI Press: Greenwich, CT, 1996, Vol 1, pp. 1-42.
69. Hodgkin, E.E.; Richards, W.G. Molecular Similarity Based on Electrostatic Potential and Electric Field. *Int. J. Quantum Chem.: Quantum Biol. Symp.* **1987**, *14*, 105-110.
70. Reynolds, C.A.; Burt, C.; Richards, W.G. A Linear Molecular Similarity Index. *Quant. Struct.-Act. Relat.* **1992**, 11, 34-35.
71. Good, A.C. The Calculation of Molecular Similarity: Alternative Formulas, Data Manipulation and Graphical Display. *J. Mol. Graphics* **1992**, *10*, 144-151.
72. So, S.-S.; Karplus, M. Three-Dimensional Quantitative Structure-Activity Relationships from Molecular Similarity Matrices and Genetic Neural Networks. 1. Method and Validations. *J. Med. Chem.* **1997**, *40*, 4347-4359.
73. So, S.-S.; Karplus, M. Three-Dimensional Quantitative Structure-Activity Relationships from Molecular Similarity Matrices and Genetic Neural Networks. 2. Applications. *J. Med. Chem.* **1997**, *40*, 4360-4371.
74. Mestres, J.; Rohrer, D.C.; Maggiora, G.M. A Molecular-Field-Based Similarity Study of Non-Nucleoside HIV-1 Reverse Transcriptase Inhibitors. *J. Comput.-Aided Mol. Design* **1999**, *13*, 79-93.
75. De Benedetti, P.G.; Cocchi, M.; Menziani, M.C.; Fanelli, F. Theoretical Quantitative Size and Shape Activity and Selectivity Analyses of 5-HT_{1A} Serotonin and α_1-Adrenergic Receptor Ligands. *J. Mol. Struct. (Theochem)* **1994**, *305*, 101-110.

76. Cocchi, M.; Menziani, M.C.; Fanelli, F.; De Benedetti, P.G. Theoretical Quantitative Structure-Activity Relationship Analysis of Congeneric and Non-Congeneric α_1-Adrenoceptor Antagonists: A Chemometric Study. *J. Mol. Struct. (Theochem)* **1995**, *331*, 79-93.
77. De Benedetti, P.G.; Menziani, M.C.; Cocchi, M.; Fanelli, F. Prototropic Molecular Forms and Theoretical Descriptors in QSAR Analysis. *J. Mol. Struct. (Theochem)* **1995**, *333*, 1-17.
78. Cocchi, M.; De Benedetti, P.G. Use of the Supermolecule Approach to Derive Molecular Similarity Descriptors for QSAR Analysis. *J. Mol. Model.* **1998**, *4*, 113-131.
79. Carrupt, P.-A.; Gaillard, P.; Billois, F.; Weber, P.; Testa, B.; Meyer, C.; Pérez, S. The Molecular Lipophilicity Potential (MLP): A New Tool for log *P* Calculations and Docking, and in Comparative Molecular Field Analysis (CoMFA). In: *Lipophilicity in Drug Action and Toxicology*; Pliška, V., Testa, B., van de Waterbeemd, H., Eds.; VCH: Weinheim, 1996, pp. 195-217.
80. Folkers, G.; Merz, A. Hydrophobic Fields in Quantitative Structure-Activity Relationships. In: *Lipophilicity in Drug Action and Toxicology*; Pliška, V., Testa, B., van de Waterbeemd, H., Eds.; VCH: Weinheim, 1996, pp. 219-232.
81. Audry, E.; Dubost, J.P.; Colleter, J.C.; Dallet, P. A New Approach to Structure-Activity Relations: the "Molecular Lipophilicity Potential". *Eur. J. Med. Chem.* **1986**, *21*, 71-72.
82. Hansch, C.; Leo, A.J. *Substituent Constants for Correlation Analysis in Chemistry*; Wiley: New York, 1979.
83. Leo, A.J. Calculating log P_{oct} from Structure. *Chem. Rev.* **1993**, *93*, 1281-1306.
84. Nys, G.G.; Rekker, R.F. Statistical Analysis of a Series of Partition Coefficients with Special Reference to the Predictability of Folding of Drug Molecules. Introduction of Hydrophobic Fragmental Constants (f-Values). *Chim. Ther.* **1973**, *8*, 521-535.
85. Nys, G.G.; Rekker, R.F. The Concept of Hydrophobic Fragmental Constants (f-Values). II. Extension of Its Applicability to the Calculation of Lipophilicities of Aromatic and Hetero-aromatic Structures. *Chim. Ther.* **1974**, *9*, 361-375.
86. Rekker, R.F.; de Kort, H.M. The Hydrophobic Fragmental Constant; An Extension to a 1000 Data Point Set. *Eur. J. Med. Chem.* **1979**, *14*, 479-488.
87. Rekker, R.F.; Mannhold, R. *Calculation of Drug Lipophilicity*; VCH: New York, 1992.
88. Mannhold, R.; Rekker, R.F.; Dross, K.; Bijloo, G.; de Vries, G. The Lipophilic Behaviour of Organic Compounds: 1. An Updating of the Hydrophobic Fragmental Constant Approach. *Quant. Struct.-Act. Relat.* **1998**, *17*, 517-536.
89. Broto, P.; Moreau, G.; Vandycke, C. Molecular Structures: Perception, Autocorrelation Descriptor and SAR Studies. System of Atomic Contributions for the Calculation of the *n*-Octanol/Water Partition Coefficients. *Eur. J. Med. Chem.* **1984**, *19*, 71-78.

90. Ghose, A.R.; Crippen, G.M. Atomic Physicochemical Parameters for Three-Dimensional Structure-Directed Quantitative Structure-Activity Relationships I. Partition Coefficients as a Measure of Hydrophobicity. *J. Comput. Chem.* **1986**, *7*, 565-577.
91. Viswanadhan, V.N.; Ghose, A.K.; Revankar, G.R.; Robins, R.K. Atomic Physicochemical Parameters for Three Dimensional Structure Directed Quantitative Structure-Activity Relationships. 4. Additional Parameters for Hydrophobic and Dispersive Interactions and Their Application for an Automated Superposition of Certain Naturally Occurring Nucleoside Antibiotics. *J. Chem. Inf. Comput. Sci.* **1989**, *29*, 163-172.
92. Ghose, A.K.; Viswanadhan, V.N.; Wendoloski, J.J. Prediction of Hydrophobic (Lipophilic) Properties of Small Organic Molecules Using Fragmental Methods: An Analysis of ALOGP and CLOGP Methods. *J. Phys. Chem. A* **1998**, *102*, 3762-3772.
93. Furet, P.; Sele, A.; Cohen, N.C. 3D Molecular Lipophilicity Potential Profiles: A New Tool in Molecular Modeling. *J. Mol. Graphics* **1988**, *6*, 182-189.
94. Fauchère, J.-L.; Quarendon, P.; Kaetterer, L. Estimating and Representing Hydrophobicity Potential. *J. Mol. Graphics* **1988**, *6*, 203-206.
95. Gaillard, P.; Carrupt, P.-A.; Testa, B.; Boudon, A. Molecular Lipophilicity Potential, a Tool in 3D QSAR: Method and Applications. *J. Comput.-Aided Mol. Design* **1994**, *8*, 83-96.
96. Rozas, I.; Du, Q.; Arteca, G.A. Interrelation between Electrostatic and Lipophilicity Potential on Molecular Surfaces. *J. Mol. Graphics* **1995**, *13*, 98-108.
97. Rozas, I.; Martin, M. Molecular Lipophilic Potential on van der Waals Surfaces as a Tool in the Study of 4-Alkylpyrazoles. *J. Chem. Inf. Comput. Sci.* **1996**, *36*, 872-878.
98. Kellogg, G.E.; Semus, S.F.; Abraham, D.J. HINT: A New Method of Empirical Hydrophobic Field Calculation for CoMFA. *J. Comput.-Aided Mol. Design* **1991**, *5*, 545-552.
99. Kellogg, G.E.; Abraham, D.J. KEY, LOCK, and LOCKSMITH: Complementary Hydropathic Map Predictions of Drug Structure from a Known Receptor-Receptor Structure from Known Drugs. *J. Mol. Graphics* **1992**, *10*, 212-217.
100. Meng, E.C.; Kuntz, I.D.; Abraham, D.J.; Kellogg, G.E. Evaluating Docked Complexes with the HINT Exponential Function and Empirical Atomic Hydrophobicities. *J. Comput.-Aided Mol. Design* **1994**, *8*, 299-306.
101. Wei, D.T.; Meadows, J.C.; Kellogg, G.E. Effects of Entropy on QSAR Equations for HIV-1 Protease: 1. Using Hydropathic Binding Descriptors. 2. Unrestrained Complex Structure Optimizations. *Med. Chem. Res.* **1997**, *7*, 259-270.
102. Kellogg, G.E. Finding Optimum Field Models for 3D QSAR. *Med. Chem. Res.* **1997**, *7*, 417-427.
103. Kellogg, G.E.; Abraham, D.J. Development of Empirical Molecular Interaction Models that Incorporate Hydrophobicity and Hydropathy. The HINT Paradigm. *Analusis*, **1999**, *27*, 19-23.

104. Waller, C.L.; Kellogg, G.E. Adding Chemical Information to CoMFA Models with Alternative 3D QSAR Fields. *Network Science* **1996**, http://www.netsci.org/Science/Compchem/feature10.html.
105. Heiden, W.; Moeckel, G.; Brickmann, J. A New Approach to Analysis and Display of Local Lipophilicity/Hydrophilicity Mapped on Molecular Surfaces. *J. Comput.-Aided Mol. Design* **1993**, *7*, 503-514.
106. Pixner, P.; Heiden, W.; Merx, H.; Moeckel, G.; Möller, A.; Brickmann, J. Empirical Method for the Quantification and Localization of Molecular Hydrophobibity. *J. Chem. Inf. Comput. Sci.* **1994**, *34*, 1309-1319.
107. Brickmann, J.; Jäger, R. The Molecular Free Energy Surface Density (MOLFESD) Approach for a Quantitative Treatment of Hydrophobicity. *Analusis* **1999**, *27*, 15-18.
108. Du, Q.; Arteca, G.A.; Mezey, P.G. Heuristic Lipophilicity Potential for Computer-Aided Rational Drug Design. *J. Comput.-Aided Mol. Design* **1997**, *11*, 503-515.

Chapter 10

VAN DER WAALS MOLECULAR DESCRIPTORS. MINIMAL STERIC DIFFERENCE

Dan Ciubotariu

University of Medicine and Pharmacy, Faculty of Pharmacy, Department of Organic Chemistry, P-ţa Eftimie Murgu No. 2, 1900 Timişoara, ROMANIA

Valentin Gogonea

Squire Booker, 330 South Frear Laboratory, The Pennsylvania State University, University Park, PA. 16802 USA

Mihai Medeleanu

Technical University "Politehnica", Faculty of Chemical Engineering, Department of Organic Chemistry, Str. Bocşa No. 6, 1900 Timişoara, ROMANIA

1. INTRODUCTION

The systems commonly encountered in organic chemistry are of great complexity. The models fashioned to account for them, such as the linear-free energy relationship (LFER), molecular orbital calculations, solvent and isotope studies, thermodynamic and kinetic acidity functions, Brœnsted equation etc., are thus necessarily empirical approximations. A distinction can be made between molecular orbital procedures, in that here one has commences with theory to which experimental data have been applied, while the others have involved initial establishment of empirical laws to which theory is subsequently attached. But in the final analysis, it must be admitted that all involve a blend of theory and empiricism in very similar proportions. However, considerable encouragement is gained from the fact that application of one method to a given problem frequently, if not invariably, corroborates the conclusions reached concerning that system using alternative and essentially independent approaches.

No general theory of the quantitative relationship between molecular structure and molecular properties in organic chemistry (QSPR) or biological activities in medicinal chemistry (QSAR) can reasonably be regarded as satisfactory unless provided a sound basis for predicting and interpreting linear relationships among molecular quantities. A satisfactory theoretical model for linear correlations in organic and/or medicinal chemistry should allow reliable predictions to be made as easily as possible concerning both the circumstances in which correlations should occur (e.g., between which properties and for which compounds) and the magnitudes of the regression coefficients. The concepts used in the model – for example, analysis into electronic (polar and resonance), hydrophobic, and steric effects – should be defined in such a way that knowledge gained through the interpretation of the linear correlations can be readily used in other areas or organic or medicinal chemistry (e.g., in elucidating the reaction mechanisms or receptor-drug molecule interaction).

An important factor to be considered in the development of a model is the degree of parameterization required. An under-parameterized model will fail to predict the existence of certain significant experimentally detectable features in the pattern of (bio)chemical behavior. An over-parameterized model will suggest that a more complex pattern of (bio)chemical behavior exists than is true; the more parameters are involved in a model, the harder it is to apply that model in making predictions. Statistical analyses of experimental data are a valuable guide when searching for the optimum degree of parameterization.[1]

Modern approaches to the design of bioactive molecules such as drugs, insecticides, herbicides, fungicides etc., is based on the quantification of bioactivity as a function of molecular structure (QSAR = **Q**uantitative **S**tructure-**A**ctivity **R**elationship) The concept of receptor site[2] was fundamental for the development of this important field. According to this model biological activity depends on the recognition of a bioactive substrate (effector – E or ligand – L) by a receptor site, followed by binding of the effector to the receptor site, and forming an effector-receptor (E-R) complex. In a similar way are treated the reactivity of organic chemical compounds (rate and/or equilibrium data) for obtaining some insides about the mechanism of organic reactions and the physical properties of these compounds (QSPR – **Q**uantitative **S**tructure-**P**roperty **R**elations). These are generally carried out by means of multiple linear regression (MLR) using a correlation equation of the type:[3]

$$y_n = \beta_1 \cdot x_{n1} + \beta_2 \cdot x_{n2} + \cdots + \beta_p \cdot x_{np} + z_n = (x_{n1}, \ldots, x_{np}) \cdot \boldsymbol{\beta} + z_n \qquad (1.1)$$

where y_n are biological activities or physical properties of organic compounds or rate or equilibrium constants of organic reactions and the matrix $\mathbf{X}=(x_{n1},\ldots,x_{np})$ contains the predictor variables, i.e., the structural parameters φf the compounds from studied series, such as electronic, steric or transport (hydrophobic) parameters or other structural indicators of those molecules, related to the property **Y**.

Linear regression provides estimates and other inferential results for the (statistical) *parameters* $\beta=(\beta_1,\beta_2,\ldots,\beta_p)^T$ in the model (1.1). In this model, the random variable y_n, which represents the *response* for *case* n, n=1,2,...,N, has a *deterministic* part and a *stochastic* part. The deterministic part, $(x_{n1},\ldots,x_{np}) \cdot \beta$, depends upon the parameters β and upon the *predictor* or regressor variables x_{np}, p=1,2,...,P. The stochastic part, represented by the random variable z_n is a *disturbance* that perturbs the response for that case. The superscript ^{T} denotes the transpose of a matrix.

The model for N cases can be written

$$\mathbf{Y} = \mathbf{X}\boldsymbol{\beta} + \mathbf{Z} \tag{1.2}$$

where **Y** is the vector of random variables represented the experimental data we may get, **X** is the N×P matrix of regressor variables, i.e., the molecular structural parameters and/or the physical and chemical properties (especially for QSAR studies) and **Z** is the vector of variables representing the disturbances; one assumes that **Z** is normally distributed. The maximum likelihood estimate $\hat{\boldsymbol{\beta}}$ is the value of $\boldsymbol{\beta}$ which minimizes $S(\boldsymbol{\beta})$:

$$S(\boldsymbol{\beta}) = \|\mathbf{Y} - \mathbf{X}\boldsymbol{\beta}\|^2 = \sum_{n=1}^{N}\left[y_n - \left(\sum_{p=1}^{P} x_{np}\beta_p\right)\right]^2 \tag{1.3}$$

This $\hat{\boldsymbol{\beta}}$ is called the least squares estimate and can be written

$$\boldsymbol{\beta} = \left(\mathbf{X}^T\mathbf{X}\right)^{-1}\mathbf{X}^T\mathbf{Y}$$

Least squares estimates can also be derived using sampling theory or by using a Bayesian approach.[4]

All three of these methods of inference, the likelihood approach, the sampling theory approach, and the Bayesian approach, produce the same point estimates for $\hat{\boldsymbol{\beta}}$ and, also, similar regions of "reasonable" parameter values. In using the least squares estimates one assumes:

(1) The expectation function $\mathbf{X}\boldsymbol{\beta}$ is correct.
(2) The response is expectation function plus disturbance (relation (1.2)).
(3) The disturbance is independent of the expectation function.
(4) Each disturbance is of zero mean and has a normal distribution.
(5) The disturbances are independently distributed and have equal variances.
(For a detailed presentation of MLR models one may consult refs. (3) and (4)).

Our objective in this work is to present surveys of the methods developed by us (van der Waals molecular descriptors) and within the QSAR group of Timişoara (MCD and MTD methods), now available for the quantitative treatment of steric effect in QSPR and QSAR studies.

The recent interest in the van der Waals (vdW) volume and surface affords an adequate reason for introducing vdW molecular descriptors in the treatment of steric effects in analysis of chemical reactivity or in QSAR studies.

Substrate binding to enzyme receptors is intimately tied to spatial requirements and consequently, the analysis of the size and the shape of molecules can help in the search for new structures with enhanced biological activity. Molecular Shape Analysis[5] and Comparative Molecular Field Analysis (CoMFA)[6] are among the most popular methods nowadays for investigating the molecular similarity. Unlike the classical QSAR of Hansch type methods,[7] CoMFA does not require a list of (sub)molecular parameters for each compound included into the calibrating set, but its results cannot be easily expressed in the form of Linear Free Energy Relations of Hammett-Taft type. On the other hand, the molecular volume and surface area are QSAR parameters of Hansch type and belong to the class of van der Waals descriptors, frequently used as molecular parameters by themselves[8] or as a starting point for deriving other QSAR parameters, e.g. lipophilicity/hydrophilicity,[9] surface tension parameters,[10] Weighted Holistic Invariant Molecular (WHIM) descriptors[11] and so on. The purpose of this chapter is also to review in some detail different algorithms for calculating the volume and surface area of molecules and the methods, which are using them as QSAR parameters.

Both numerical and analytical algorithms were devised for the calculation of the volume and surface area of molecules. The numerical algorithms are particularly easy to program but require large amount of memory and CPU time to obtain accurate results, while the analytical algorithms are quite elaborate to code but they are accurate and fast. The concept of molecular volume and surface area found many applications, not only in QSAR, but also in the studies of molecular interactions, especially in relating the bulk properties of substances like crystal packing with molecular structures.[12] The molecular volume is a measure of the space around atomic nuclei filled by electrons[13,14] and is defined geometrically as the combined volume of overlapping spheres centered on the nuclei, similar in shape to a space-filling molecular model. The van der Waals radii are used for the radii of the atomic spheres. The molecular surface area is the area of the surface, which wraps the molecular volume. Exact calculation of the molecular volume and surface area is, however, a formidable task due to multiple overlap of spheres of different radii.

The first methods for the calculation of the molecular volume and surface area used molecular fragments.[13] The additive technique is particularly suited for QSAR because many of its parameters are obtained from molecular fragments (e.g. octanol/water partition coefficients). Recently, Govers and de Voogt proposed a quantum definition of the molecular volume in terms of molecular fragments via electron indices.[15]

Because the volume of overlapping spheres (solvent excluded volume) is a quantity of interest in solution chemistry, attempts were made decades ago to find and analytical expression for it. Thus, Rowlinson performed the first analytical calculation of the volume occupied by three and more overlapping spheres,[16] and used it to give an analytical expression for the triplet radial distribution function $g^{(3)}$ in terms of the intersecting volume of three simultaneously overlapping spheres.[17] But Connolly was the first to obtain a general solution for the analytical computation of the volume and surface area for an ensemble of overlapping spheres with unequal radii.[18] At about the same time, Richmond proposed another method to solve the same problem,[19] this time by analytical integration of surface area obtained from Gauss-Bonnet theorem.[20] Finally, Gibson and

Scheraga obtained an analytical expression of the volume in terms of the inclusion-exclusion principle.[21]

Gavezzotti,[22] Meyer[23] and Ciubotariu *et al.*[24] developed, among others, numerical algorithms for calculating the volume and surface area of overlapping spheres, which use either three dimensional grids or Monte Carlo integration techniques. The grid methods are quite expensive computationally, as a very large number of grid points are necessary to obtain acceptable accuracy. Optimized algorithms were also proposed (based on Lebesgue integral) which eliminate large part of the grid points by focusing the grid near the molecular surface. The method based on the Monte Carlo integration is similar in performance with the grid method. In addition, its results are dependent on the quality of the random number generator. A relative recent review by Mezey[25] gives an account of the methods used to calculate molecular volume and surface area and their use in defining the molecular shape and similarity.

Developing faster algorithms for calculating surface area and volume of molecules, and new QSAR parameters based on them, is still an active area of research in computational chemistry. For example, Chuman *et al.*[26] proposed recently a new method for three-dimensional QSAR analyses of molecular similarity based on the calculation and comparison of Voronoi polyhedra (the Voronoi Field Analysis).[27]

The work described here consists of two types of approaches to the steric fit problem. The first approach consists of developing new parameters to describe different characteristics of the molecular shape and size; this is done by means of vdW molecular indicators. The second approach is based on *minimal steric difference*, a measure for steric misfit who depends not only on molecular shape, but also on the receptor and allows a guess of the shape of the receptor cavity. We present here the following methods:

MSD method – the initial version of minimal steric differences calculated simply as number of nonsuperposable (nonhydrogen) atoms when the molecule is superimposed on the standard molecule, (i.e., the molecule with maximal potency from the series under study) in a low energy conformation allowing maximal superposition;[28,29]

MCD – the minimal nonoverlapping volume when the molecule, characterized by Cartesian coordinates, is superimposed upon the standard molecule which is calculated by use of a Monte Carlo technique;[30,31]

MTD – thc optimization technique, which, starting from the experimental activities of the effectors, allows obtaining the best probable shape of receptor cavity, receptor walls, and steric irrelevant regions; this is a technique with a largely *topological* character.[31-33]

The abbreviations MSD, MCD and MTD will be used also for the values of minimal steric difference calculated by the initial version, by the Monte Carlo technique and, respectively, by the optimization technique.

2. The Nature of Steric Effects

Commonly, the steric (proximity) effects are caused by repulsive forces that appear when the distance between two unbound atoms (or groups of atoms) is smaller than the sum of their vdW radii; this fact produces the unbound compressions and the energy of the entire system increases.[34]

Ingold[35] classifies the steric effects in two ways:

(i) *Primary steric effects* as a result from repulsion between unbound atoms. Such repulsions can only result in an increase in the energy of a group of atoms. If steric repulsions are greater in the Transition State (rate constants) or product (equilibrium constants) than in reactant, the activation energy increases, and one observes a retardation of the reaction compared to a system free of steric effects. If the reverse situation appears, the rate or equilibrium constants will show steric augmentation.

(ii) *Secondary steric effects* involve modeling of polar and resonance effects because of unbound compressions. This variation in the transmission of electrical effects results from twisting the bonds around an active site (an atom or group of atoms at which the observed phenomenon occurs) and the reaction is slowing. They include a change in the solvation of the active site due to steric effects exerted by an adjacent substituent, shielding of the active site from attack by a bulky reagent and variation in the concentration of a reacting conformer due to the steric effect exerted by a substituent.[36]

In medicinal chemistry, the steric effects in the formation of the bioactive substance (ligand – L or effector – E) – receptor (R) site complex (L-R or E-R) are frequently of great importance. In this case, the entire bioactive substance can be the active site.

In order to understand the nature of steric effects in molecular bioactivity we consider the model proposed by McFarland.[37] It involves the following three steps:

1. *The transport step.* The ligand L enters the organism and moves to a receptor site crossing one or more membranes. In this step, the ligand must be transferred from an aqueous phase to a lipid phase, i.e., to the membrane. The process depends upon the difference in intermolecular forces between water and ligand and those between lipid and ligand. From the intermolecular forces, which interfere in the case of a ligand-hydrogen bonding, charge transfer, dipole-dipole, dipole-induced dipole, induced dipole-induced dipole, ion-dipole, ion-induced dipole – only hydrogen bonding and charge transfer interactions can be sensitive to steric effects.

2. *The L-R complex formation.* The ligand L is recognized by the receptor R and a L-R complex is formed. Generally, this complex is held together by intermolecular forces and its formation is reversible (see Figure 1).

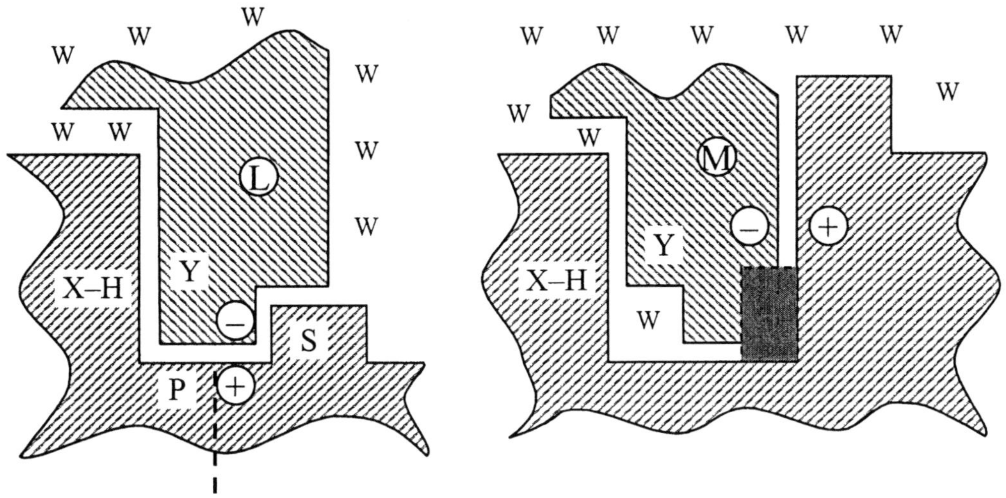

(i) (v)

Figure 1. Interaction of a receptor with (i) a complementary ligand (L) and (v) with another drug molecule (M), called also ligand. P and S are two receptor moieties, W represents a water molecule and Y, HX, -, + are hydrogen bonding and polar groups.

By interaction with the bioactive molecule, the receptor is forced from the lowest energy to the physiologically active conformation (R^*). The L or M molecule binds together two receptor moieties P and S. We consider L complementary to the receptor site, both from the point of view of shape and of intermolecular force types or hydrophobic regions. However, drug-receptor fit for ligand M is not perfect; a water (W) molecule is enclustered in the drug-receptor complex and the position of the S-receptor group is modified by a local conformational transition produced by steric hindrance. The M ligand molecule is not complementary from the point of view of shape. The R-L and R-M interactions imply the hydrophobic interaction of the apolar regions from which water molecules are stripped out by the interaction.

Alternatively, the drug or inhibitor molecule may interact with the inactive lowest-energy conformation preventing the production of the active receptor conformation by interaction with the natural effector (agonic or antagonic actions).[38]

Processes that take place during a L-R interaction are depicted in Figure 1. Various hydration-dehydration processes and conformational changes take place, in addition to the L-R interaction:[33]

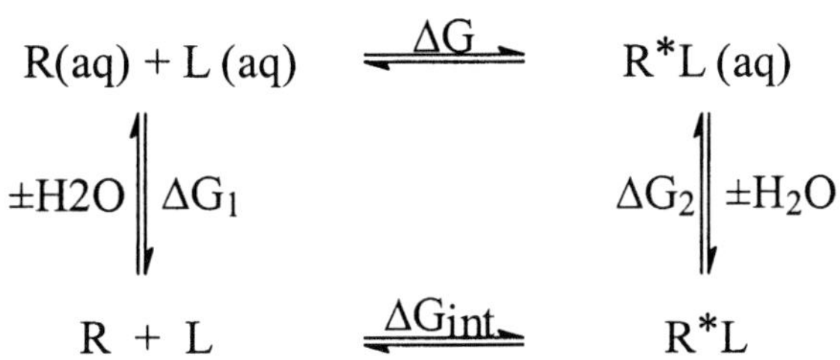

$$\Delta G = \Delta G_{int} - \Delta G_1 + \Delta G_2 \tag{2.1}$$

ΔG_{int} refers to the drug-receptor interaction per se, ΔG_1 and ΔG_2 to hydration processes. Molecular mechanics techniques are quite succesful in predicting molecular conformations (even conformations of peptidic fragments)[39] and they may also be applied for the L-R interaction. One may write:

$$\Delta G_{int} = \Delta U_{R^{*}L} + \Delta U_{conf} - T \cdot \Delta S \tag{2.2}$$

Summation of coulombian, polarisation, van der Waals attractions and repulsions and atom-atom interactions is proposed by the molecular mechanics methods for calculation of the $\Delta U_{R^{*}L}$ interaction energy. The geometry and nature of the dozens of receptor site atoms are to be known. ΔU_{conf} is the conformational energy change from the inactive (R) to active (R^*) conformation. To this, local conformational changes should be added which are forced by steric hindrance of L-molecule groups protruding into receptor walls. Obviously, steric fit effects cannot be dissociated from the hydrophobic and polar attractive attractions.

The point is that a large amount of information is required in order to describe the receptor site features which would allow a calculation of the receptor-drug molecule affinity ΔE.

3. *The chemical reaction step.* The L-R complex may undergo chemical reaction resulting in the appeareance and/or cleavage of covalent bonds. In this step, when it occurs, steric effects should resemble those generally observed for chemical reactivity if the substituent is in close proximity to the centre of reaction. But, in biochemical interactions, the substituents distant from the active site may still exert a steric effect on the fit with the receptor site.

There are several distinct ways for the quantification of steric effects. The first group of parameters was defined from chemical reactivities (E_S-Taft type parameters), vdW radii and molecular geometries (Verloop[40] and our parameters described in Section 5) and from a combination of these sources (Charton[41]). (For an analysis of these steric parameter scales, see Section 4 of this Chapter). A second group is represented by parameters developed by using topological methods; for example molecular connectivity, introduced by Kier and Hall,[42] DARC-PELCO, developed by Dubois and coworkers,[43] and other various topological indices and methods.[44] An alternative to these parameters is the use of overlapping methods such as Minimal Steric Difference – MSD method that contains implicit 3D molecular comparisons, and its improvement – the MTD method, introduced for receptor mapping (see Section 7 of this Chapter), Distance Geometry method,[45] Molecular Shape Analysis – MSA method,[5] Excluded Volume Mapping,[46] etc., and Comparative Molecular Field Analysis – CoMFA method, for developing 3D receptor models,[6] primarily for rigid compounds.[47] Steric parameters may also be obtained from force field calculations.

3. Requirements for a Steric Parameter in Correlation Analysis

The physiological action of drugs is based upon receptor-effector interactions.[48] If drug transport and decay are not rate-limiting and especially if the receptor-drug equilibrium is measured directly, the structure-activity relationship is actually describing the affinity for the active conformation of the receptor as a function of structural features of ligand molecules, expressed explicitly or implicitly by selected physical or structural parameters.[49]

If A_i is the biological response generated by the active compound, the effector E_i (or ligand L_i), one considers $\hat{A}_i$ to be estimated by the following expression:

$$\hat{A}_i = \alpha + \sum_{j=1}^{M} \beta_j \cdot P_{ij}; \quad i = 1,2,\ldots,N; \quad M \geq 1 \tag{3.1}$$

in which $\hat{A}_i$ is the calculated value of A_i and P_{ij} represent structural parameters (also named predictor variables).

The regression coefficients β_j are estimated with the aid of the least square method,

$$\sum_{i=1}^{N} \left(A_i - \hat{A}_i\right)^2 = \text{minimum m} \tag{3.2}$$

and the reliability degree of model (3.1), (called, also, MLR – multiple linear regression) is established using correlation analysis; usually, equations of type (3.1) are characterized by correlation coefficient r, standard deviation s, explained variance EV, confidence limits of model parameters α, β_j, and t-Student and F-Fisher statistics.

Equation (3.1) may be used in one (or several) of the following purposes: pure description, prediction and estimation, extrapolation, estimation of parameters, control and model building.

The MLR model (3.1) requires also the following conditions to be satisfied:

(i) The experimental A_i values must be measured with the same accuracy and precision.

(ii) The values of predictor variables P_j (which codify the physical factors that are responsible of the observed bioactivity A) must be determined with higher precision than that of the dependent variable A

(iii) The regression equation (3.1) must be stable, i.e., small perturbations in the A-values (increase or decrease of A values used to calibrate α and β_j) should not modify strongly the equation.

The predictive power of equation (3.1) is conditioned, besides the above mentioned conditions, also by the size of the domain in the parameter space, explored by the P_j parameters corresponding to the N compounds E_i.

It is usual to speak of hydrophobicity, electronic and steric effects in QSAR for the receptor-drug interaction energy, ΔG (Equation (3.2)). Steric parameters, S, can be used in models of types:

$$\hat{A} = \alpha + \beta_1 \cdot S + \sum \beta_j \cdot P_j \tag{3.3}$$

$$\hat{A} = \alpha + \beta_1 \cdot S + \beta_2 \cdot S^2 + \sum \beta_j \cdot P_j \tag{3.4}$$

with P_j for nonsteric effects (hydrophobic, electronic, etc.). The equation (3.4) allows determining, in principle, the optimal shape and size of effector molecules. Since for several steric parameters the detailed nature of steric interactions they express is not exactly known, one may recommend using alternatively several types of steric constants, increasing thus reliability for the observed correlations. Several successful correlation equations of the type:

$$\hat{A} = \alpha + \beta_1 \cdot \pi + \beta_2 \cdot \sigma + \beta_3 \cdot E_S \tag{3.5}$$

were developed along this line of reasoning, with for the hydrophobicity ($\log P_{octanol}$) of the studied compounds, with σ-Hammett[50] constants for substituents near the "pharmacophoric constellation" as a measure for electronic effects, and with E_S-Taft[51] steric hindrance constants for the same substituents.

The usefulness of steric parameters in correlation analysis models is conditioned by certain fundamental requirements.[52]

Thus, the steric parameter must be a measure of the "size" and "shape" of the substituents or molecules. If the Taft-type parameters estimate the observable steric effect from reactivity data, new extended scales must take into consideration the vectorial nature this effect. The size and shape of molecules and ions depend on the length of the chemical bonds, the value of the valence angles and the dimension of the constituent atoms. The shape of the effector molecules is doubtlessly the main element of most chemical interactions. It is very difficult to quantify this form, i.e., to find appropriate molecular descriptors able to express it. Most procedures are based either on comparing molecules with reference structures, or on sectorising them and defining the sectors by means of geometric distances between certain atoms or by means of Cartesian coordinates.[33,53]

It is very important that steric parameters must be either experimentally determined or calculable for all types of substituents. Obviously, the experimentally measured parameters cannot be estimated for some substituents or molecules that are unstable in the standard reactions used for their definition. In addition, the methods that have been used for extending these scales are unreliable (see Section 4 of this Chapter).

Experimental data from which steric parameters are obtained should be readily and conveniently determined, with high accuracy and precision. One notices that the vdW molecular descriptors fulfill this condition.

The steric parameter must be independent of electrical and hydrophobic (transport) effects. It can be realized that a subset of groups under consideration will show a statistically significant relationship between steric and electrical parameters or between steric and transport parameters, that is, one observes a multicolinearity relation between these parameters. By multicolinearity one understands the existence of functional relations *f* between some of the predictor variables P_j:

$$P_j = f(P_i, \ldots, P_{i+k}), k = 0,1,\ldots \tag{3.6}$$

f being a linear function or, on principle, any other type of function. The main causes that produce multicolinearity are: an over-defined model, sampling techniques and physical constraints in the model or in the true population.[54] In QSAR work multicolinearity is considered nonexistent if the intercorrelation coefficients are low enough, i.e., $r^2(P_k, P_m) \leq 0.400$; an upper limit of 0.400 is considered maximal for r^2 in the case of chance correlation.[55]

4. Taft Parameter and Statistical Analysis of such Types of Steric Descriptors

The first generally successful approach for quantitative treatment of steric effects was deduced by Taft[51] according to a suggestion of Ingold:[35] the polar effects can be neglected in the esterification reactions of aliphatic carboxylic acids with alcohols and in the hydrolysis reactions of esters, as resulted from the low values of ρ, ρ 0. On this basis, Taft defined the steric constant E_S as:

$$E_S = \log\left(\frac{k_X}{k_H}\right)_A \tag{4.1}$$

where k is the rate constant for the acidic hydrolysis (denoted by A) of aliphatic esters (I) or for esterification reactions of carboxylic acids (II) with alcohols (III).

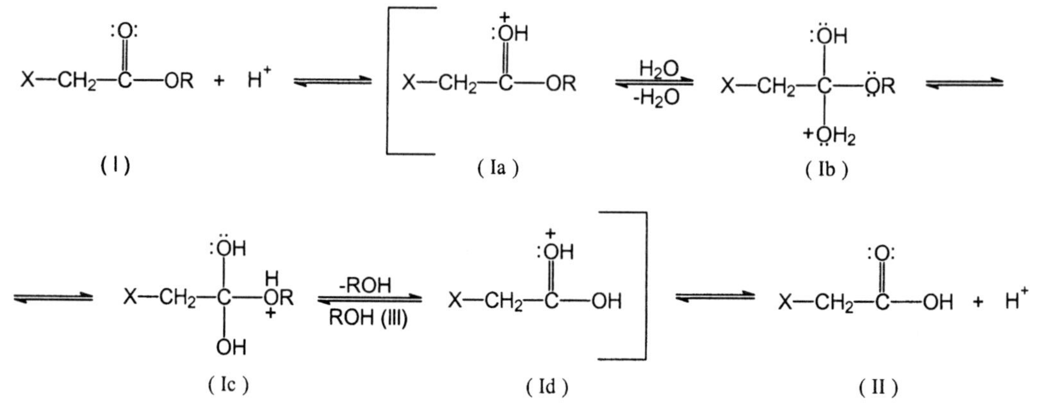

Figure 2. Acid hydrolysis of aliphatic esters

The scale of E_S values was fixed by definition with X=H, that is with methyl (CH_3COOR) as origin ($E_{S,CH_3}=0$). The size of X will affect the transition state for the hydration of (Ia) formed during hydrolysis (or for the nucleophilic addition of (III) to (Id)) and therefore its steric effect will be modeled by E_S. Consequently, bulkier substituents X than H will have $E_{S,XCH_2}<0$, retarding the hydrolysis reaction.

Unfortunately, variations of structure (I) cannot be used to obtain E_S values for many common substituents that are unstable during acid hydrolysis. (i.e. X=CN, OR etc.) Therefore, to overcome this problem and to extend the E_S scale, Kutter and Hansch[56] formulated E_S values for a variety of new substituents via the following correlation equation:

$$E_S = -1.839 \cdot r_{av} + 3.484$$
$$(n = 6; r = 0.996; s = 0.132) \tag{4.2}$$

where r_{av} is the average of the minimum and maximum vdW radii of the substituents estimated according to Charton.[41] This equation, which was established only for symmetrical top substituents such as H, Br, CF_3 or $C(CH_3)_3$, was used to calculate E_S values for a variety of new substituents, but also for unsymmetrical groups like NR_2, OR, SR, NO_2, Ac and Ph.[57] It must be noted that in equation (4.2), only the radius of the first atom has been used to calculate E_S for substituents such as OH, OCH_3, SH, SCH_3 and NH_2. Two values of E_S have been calculated for groups such as NO_2, Ac and C_6H_5, one corresponding to the width and the other to the thickness of the substituents.

The E_S parameter was first successfully introduced in QSAR by Hansch and coworkers[58] for treating steric substituent effects on enzymatic reactions, and has been extensively used (see, for instance, Ref. [59]). However, despite the wide range of applicability, several examples of limitations have also been reported.[57]

Several authors pointed out that E_S is not a purely steric constant. This problem is very interesting because of the following considerations: let us suppose that E_S expresses steric effects (S) with the weight α and electronic effect (E) with a weight β. (The type of E is irrelevant in this context). Thus,

$$E_{S,X} = \alpha \cdot S_X + \beta \cdot E_X \tag{4.3}$$

If X is an electron-withdrawing group it tends to destabilize the Transition State of hydrolysis and X will appear more "voluminous" that it really is. In order to get rid of this deficiency, the "corrected" E_S values were introduced:[57]

E_S^C to eliminate hyperconjugative effects of hydrogen atoms on the α-carbon:

$$E_S^C = E_S + 0.306 \cdot (N_H - 3) \tag{4.4}$$

N_H is the number of α-hydrogen atoms.

E_S^0 to eliminate hyperconjugative effects of both hydrogen and carbon atoms:

$$E_S^0 = E_S + 0.33 \cdot (N_H - 3) + 0.13 \cdot N_C \tag{4.5}$$

In relation (4.5) N_H is the number of (C)–H and N_C is the number of C-C bonds.

E_S^e to eliminate both inductive and conjugative electronic effects. The separations of inductive and resonance effects was used and Equation (4.6) was obtained for CH_2X substituents:

$$E_{S,CH_2X}^e = E_{S,CH_2X} + 1.07 \cdot \boldsymbol{F}_X + 1.05 \cdot \boldsymbol{R}_X \tag{4.6}$$

$\boldsymbol{F}_X$ and $\boldsymbol{R}_X$ are the "orthogonalised" quasi-inductive and quasi-resonant Swain-Lupton constants.[57]

These indices are also limited only to alkyl groups, and there is no convincing evidence that the statistical improvement of the correlation is obtained.

Dubois et al.[60] pointed out that the average procedure used by Taft might introduce errors; consequently, they defined a "revised" Taft steric parameter E_S' based on the acid catalyzed esterification of carboxylic acids (at 40°C) as the reference reaction. The E_S' values thus obtained are similar to E_S except for the bulky substituents. The substituent scale covered by this approach is also limited by the conditions of acid hydrolysis. The values of these parameters (E_S, E_S', E_S^e, E_S^C and E_S^0) for common substituents are summarizes in Table 4.1.

Charton[61] studied the relation between vdW radii r_X^W and $E_{S,X}$ values and established a negligible contribution of inductive (σ_I) and resonance (σ_R) effects. Thus, Charton proposed the following equation:

$$E_{S,X} = \alpha + \beta_1 \cdot \sigma_{I,X} + \beta_2 \cdot \sigma_{R,X} + \Psi \cdot r_X^W \quad (4.7)$$

Because β_i, i=1,2 are usually small, the equation (4.7) becomes:

$$E_{S,X} = \Psi \cdot r_X^W + \alpha$$
$$(\alpha = 0.445; \Psi = -0.412; n = 7; r = 0.915; t = 5,08) \quad (4.8)$$

where n is the number of substituents from correlation series, r and t represent the correlation coefficient and Student statistical test, respectively. According to Charton,[61] this validates the assumption that the E_S parameter is a linear function of vdW radii (but only for substituents of the type CH_2X, CHX_2 and CX_3) and that is independent of electrical effects.

The conclusions generated by models (4.7) and (4.8) have led to definition of the steric parameter υ_X using the following relation:[61]

$$\upsilon_X = r_X^W - r_H^W = r_X^W - 1.20 \quad (4.9)$$

The υ-values for various substituents are determined by a Taft-type methodology, by means of the relation (4.8). Because three values, υ_{mx} (maximum), υ_{mn} (minimum) and υ_{ax} (the vdW radius parallel to the group axis) are the minimum necessary to characterize most substituents, the υ values for many substituents are missing of physical meaning.

Table 4.1 Values of the steric parameters $E_S, E_S^{'}, E_S^{e}, E_S^{C}$ and E_S^{0} for some carbon substituents.[62] (standard substituent: H).

Substituents	$-E_S$	$-E_S^{'}$	$-E_S^{e}$	$-E_S^{C}$	$-E_S^{0}$
1.	2.	3.	4.	5.	6.
H	-1.24	-1.12	-	-	-
Me	0.00	0.00	1.24	1.24	1.24
Et	0.07	0.08	1.31	1.62	1.51
n-Pr	0.36	0.31	1.60	1.91	1.80
i-Pr	0.47	0.48	1.71	2.32	2.09
n-Bu	0.39	0.31	1.63	1.94	1.83
i-Bu	0.93	0.93	2.17	2.48	2.37
t-Bu	1.54	1.43	2.78	3.70	3.38
s-Bu	1.13	1.00	2.37	2.98	2.77
n-Am	0.40	0.31	1.64	1.95	1.84

3-Am	-	0.97	3.22	3.83	-
c-C_SH_{11}	-	-	2.03	2.64	-
c-$C_SH_{11}CH_2$	-	-	2.22	2.53	-
C_SH_S	-	2.31	2.01	-	-
$C_SH_SCH_2$	0.38	0.39	1.61	-	-
F	-	-0.57	0.46	-	-
Cl	-	0.02	0.97	-	-
Br	-	0.22	1.16	-	-
I	-	0.50	1.40	-	-
FCH_2	0.24	0.20	1.48	-	1.81
$ClCH_2$	0.24	0.18	1.48	-	1.81
$BrCH_2$	0.27	0.24	1.51	-	1.84
ICH_2	0.37	0.30	1.61	-	-
F_2CH	0.67	0.32	1.91	-	2.57
Cl_2CH	1.54	0.58	2.78	-	3.44
Br_2CH	1.86	0.76	3.10	-	3.76
F_3C	-	-	2.40	-	3.39
Cl_3C	2.06	1.75	3.30	-	4.29
Br_3C	-	-	3.67	-	4.66
$BrCH_2CH_2$	-	-	2.24	2.55	2.43
ICH_2CH_2	-	-	2.26	2.57	2.44
NC	-	-	0.51	-	-
HO	-	-	0.55	-	-
CH_3O	-	-	0.55	-	-
H_2N	1.28	-	1.01	-	-
O_2N	1.28	-	-	-	-
$HOCH_2$	-	-0.03	1.21	-	1.63
CH_3OCH_2	-	-	1.43	-	1.76

A selection of υ-parameters for several substituents is presented in Table 4.2.

Table 4.2 Values of steric parameter υ for a series of substituents X.[33,62]

X	υ	X	υ	X	υ	X	υ
Me	0.52	C_6H_5[a]	0.57	H	0.00	$ClCH_2CH_2$	0.97
Et	0.56	$C_6H_5CH_2$	0.70	F	0.27	$BrCH_2CH_2$	0.93
Pr	0.68	$C_6H_5CH_2CH_2$	0.70	Cl	0.55	ICH_2CH_2	0.93
i-Pr	0.76	$C_6H_5(Me)CH_2$	0.99	Br	0.65	$MeBr_2C$	1.46
Bu	0.68	MeO	0.36	I	0.78	MeBrCH	0.75
i-Bu	0.98	EtO	0.48	FCH_2	0.62	MeClCH	0.70
sec-Bu	1.02	PrO	0.56	$ClCH_2$	0.60	MeNH	0.39
t-Bu	1.24	HO	0.32	$BrCH_2$	0.64	EtNH	0.59
Am	0.68	NC	0.40	ICH_2	0.67	PrNH	0.64
sec-$BuCH_2$	1.00	H_2N	0.35	F_2CH	0.68	BuNH	0.70
i-$PrCH_2CH_2$	0.68	O_2N[a]	0.35	Cl_2CH	0.81	AmNH	0.50
Et_2CH	1.51	i-PrO	0.75	Br_2CH	0.89	GS	0.60
PhEtCH	1.18	BuO	0.58	I_2CH	0.97	MeS	0.64
F_3C	0.90	i-BuO	0.62	Cl_3C	1.38	CHO	0.50
c-C_6H_{11}	0.87	s-BuO	0.86	Br_3C	1.56	H_2NCO	0.50
c-$C_6H_{11}CH_2$	0.97	t-BuO	1.22	I_3C	1.79	AmO	0.58

The relationship between Taft's E_S and Charton's υ parameter is a linear one, as shown by the following equation:[57]

$$E_S = -2.062(\pm 0.86)\cdot \upsilon - 0.194(\pm 0.10)$$
$$(r = 104; r = 0.978; s = 0.250) \qquad (4.10)$$

But, the statistical quality of the above equation is not so good as expected (see, for example, the confidence limits of statistical model parameters 0.86 and 0.10, respectively, and of standard deviation, s). Beside this, many substituents (CN, I, NO_2, OMe, Br, Cl, NH_2, OR, CF_3, etc.) fit the equation (4.10) rather poorly (s>0,300) as compared to the standard deviation. Hansch and Leo noted that any features that these substituents have in common are not obvious, which simply brings out our lack of understanding of steric effects.[57]

All attempts of extending the scale of steric parameters (E_S and $E_S^{'}$) are based on the generalization of the correlation analysis models developed between these parameters and the vdW radii of the substituents (especially the υ parameters introduced by Charton). Therefore a comparative statistical analysis of these steric parameters must be performed, in order to determine whether they represent samples from the populations with the same statistical structure. The relevant statistics are:[63] the median (m), the mean (μ) and the modal value or the mode (M) of the distributions (the relation between μ, m and m is shown in Figure 3), the Pearson's coefficient of skewness, C_P, the range of the values, their variance and the standard deviation, s.

Let $x_1, x_2, \ldots, x_n$ be a set of steric parameters. The arithmetic mean (usually called just the mean), denoted by μ, is expressed by the following relation:

$$\mu = \frac{\sum_{i=1}^{n} x_i}{n} \tag{4.11}$$

This gives an exact result if we are using all the numbers in the population; otherwise, the mean of the sample gives the best estimate of the mean of the whole population.

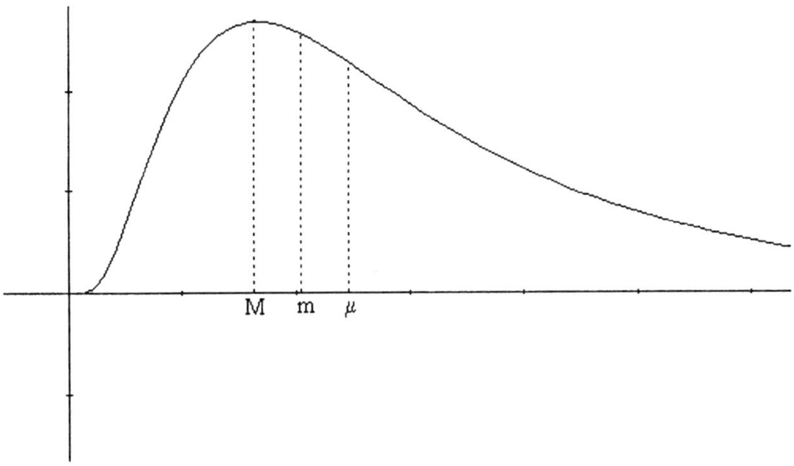

Figure 3 . Relationship between mean, median and mode.

The median (m) is calculated by arranging the n values in either descending or ascending order, and choosing the middle value, that is the $(n+1)/2^{th}$ value in the ordered list. If there is an even number of values, then the average of the middle two values is taken.

Usually, the statistical inferences are based on the mean rather than the median because the median tends to vary more between different samples from the same data than does the mean. It is sometimes useful to compare the values for the mean and median to establish if the data are symmetrical or skewed (lopsided).

The mode (M) is defined as the most frequently occurring value; for discrete data, the following approximation is often used to calculate the mode, M:[63]

$$\mu - M \cong 3 \cdot (\mu - m)$$

Hence

$$M \cong \mu - 3 \cdot (\mu - m) \cong 3m - 2\mu \tag{4.12}$$

The mean and the center of gravity of the distribution coincide, the median bisects the area of the distribution while the mode cuts the highest point on the distribution. If the distribution is symmetrical, the three values – m, μ and M – coincide; otherwise, the distribution is skewed.

The magnitude and the direction of skew (positive, if the skew has longer tail on the right, $C_P>0$ – see Figure 3) are estimated by means of Pearson's coefficient of skewness, C_P:

$$C_P = \frac{3 \cdot (\mu - m)}{s} \tag{4.13}$$

The simplest way of expressing the spread or precision of a set of steric parameters is to quote the range of the numbers, that is the difference between the largest value and the smallest value. But, this quantity is not representative since it only takes account of two values from the set and may be badly distorted by a single abnormal value. A method of avoiding this problem is to use the "inter-quartile range" (DI), i.e. the difference between the values one-quarter and three-quarters down the list in which the values are arranged in ascending order.

A better measure of the spread or precision of the set of steric parameters from Tables 4.1 and 4.2 is given by the variance s^2, and the standard deviation s; for a sample of n terms the best estimate of the population variance is obtained using (n-1) as divisor rather than n,

$$s^2 = \frac{\sum (x_i - \mu)^2}{n-1}; s = \sqrt{s^2} \tag{4.14}$$

because with the divisor n the sample variance s^2 underestimates the variance of the entire population (σ^2). Clearly a large variance or a large standard deviation corresponds to a wide spread of results, and small values for s^2 and s correspond to closely grouped results.

One better measure of precision is called coefficient of variation, C_V, and compares the spread of the measurements with their magnitude:

$$C_V = \frac{s}{\mu} \cdot 100 \tag{4.15}$$

This is arguably a more useful measure of precision than the standard deviation, because it takes into account the magnitude of the numbers. As with the standard deviation, a low value for the coefficient of variation corresponds to high precision while a high value corresponds to low precision (large spread).

A statistical analysis of steric parameters from the Tables 4.1 and 4.2, based on the above statistical characteristics is given in Table 4.3.

The data shown in this table allows a series of interesting inferences.[33,62] Thus, a separation between steric Taft-type parameters and υ-Charton parameter can be made, based on the difference between the corresponding largest and smallest value (the magnitude of the two scales (DV) is different and inter-quartile range (DI), too). The spread of these two sets of steric parameters (s) and the skewness of their distributions (C_P) are also different. The dispersion range around the mean value is twice or even three-fold lower for υ values than for the E_S values. The same effect is observed on the coefficient of variation, C_V. Therefore, the result is that the discrimination ability of the υ-parameters as compared to the E_S for substituents with similar effects, is significantly lower. Moreover, the symmetry of the distribution of υ-values is different from that of the E_S values. For all these reasons, the υ-parameters are not suited for extending the scale of E_S values. The use of υ values and of other parameters based upon r^W values might lead to a leveling of the measured effect, or even to unjustified inversions.

Table 4.3 Statistical analysis of Taft-type parameters ($E_S, E_S^{'}, E_S^{e}, E_S^{C}, E_S^{0}$) and υ-Charton parameter.

Parameters	E_S	$E_S^{'}$	E_S^{W}	E_S^{c}	E_S^{0}	υ
			Values from tables 1 and 2			
m	-0.47	-0.39	-1.60	-2.40	-1.97	0.68
μ	-0.74	-0.63	-1.69	-2.26	-2.35	0.76
M	0.08	0.09	-1.43	-2.68	-1.19	0.53
DV	3.67	3.74	3.67	3.83	4.66	1.79
DI	0.86	0.71	1.65	0.68	1.13	0.35
s	0.81	0.77	0.85	0.91	1.04	0.33
C_P	-1.02	-0.94	-0.30	0.46	-1.11	0.70
C_V	-108.40	-122.20	-50.59	-40.42	-44.36	43.26
			Values for a Standard Set of 11 Substituents			
m	-0.39	-0.31	-1.63	-1.94	-1.83	0.68
μ	-0.40	-0.37	-1.64	-2.00	-1.88	0.71
M	-0.37	-0.19	-1.61	-1.81	-1.74	0.62
DV	2.78	2.55	2.78	3.70	3.38	1.24
DI	0.49	0.51	0.49	0.64	0.58	0.25
s	0.71	0.66	0.71	0.95	0.86	0.32
C_P	-0.04	-0.27	-0.04	-0.20	-0.16	0.27
C_V	-178.20	-178.10	-43.46	-47.16	-45.95	45.01

The E_S-type parameters have relatively similar spreads of values (s) around the mean value (μ). The symmetry of distribution is the same (see C_P from Table 4.3), a surprising but accountable inversion occurring for the E_S^C parameter (Table 4.3, upper half). However, there are significant differences between the substituent structures corresponding to the values of the median (m), mean (μ) and modal value (M). This fact is responsible for the observed differences in using these Taft-type parameters for the correlation of chemical reactivity or bioactivity with molecular structure (MLR studies). The C_V values suggest a possibility of discrimination between the steric effects of substituents by E_S and $E_S^{'}$ parameters twice-fold than for the others. However, from statistical point of view, the scales E_S and $E_S^{'}$ (the values from Table 4.1) represent the samples from the whole populations with very similar means and dispersions. In fact, E_S and $E_S^{'}$ scales code the same type of effect, the practical application conducting to the same results.

5. Van der Waals Molecular Parameters

The modern studies concerning the quantitative structure-properties relationships (QSPR) and those concerning the quantitative structure-activity relationships (QSAR) are focused on the quantification of the molecular structure. This procedure requires a separation of the effects involved in chemical or biological interactions, an independent quantification of these as electronic, steric, hydrophobic, or other types of factors and the quantitative treatment of reactivity or biological activity by means of the correlation analysis models. The use of the extrathermodynamic formalism made the theoretical validation of this approach possible.[64]

The nature of the steric effects is one of the main factors involved in the quantitative treatment of the relations between chemical structure and physical and chemical properties or biological activity. The use of quantum chemistry or molecular mechanics to analyze these effects faces serious difficulties, mainly because of the impossibility to have an exact knowledge of potential energy hypersurfaces. For this reason, empirical models based on correlation analysis are largely used to study the relations between the structure of organic compounds and their properties. The treatment of steric effects in molecular biology is even more complicated because of the limited information concerning the stereochemical characteristics of biological receptors.

In the last years, we have developed some new models for quantitative treatment of steric effects, on the basis of standard or optimized geometry of molecules and the van der Waals space. For this purpose we investigated the way in which the volume and surface of the substituents, as well as different directions in van der Waals molecular space – supposed to be homogeneous and isotropic, are responsible for the steric effects manifested during reactions.

The necessity to define such numerical descriptors, in order to quantify in a proper mode both shape and size of substituents, comes out from the theoretical considerations regarding the nature of steric effects and the practical conditions imposed by such parameters.

5.1. Van der Waals Radii

The distance where attractive forces between the unbound atoms of a molecule, or between atoms of different molecules, are in equilibrium with repulsive forces is known as the van der Waals distance. One may define the van der Waals radius (r^w) as the half of the vdW distance. The van der Waals radii have long been considered a measure of atomic size.

The space occupied by molecules can be described suitable in the approximation of "hard spheres": each atom of the molecule M is represented by an isotropic sphere having the center in the equilibrium position (X_i, Y_i, Z_i) and the radius equal with its van der Waals radius r_i^w. There are several methods to compute the vdW radii.[65] The best extant values of r^W for atoms are those of Bondi,[66] listed in Table 5.1.

Table 5.1 Bondi vdW radii

Atom	**H**	**C**	**O**	**N**	**F**	**Cl**	**Br**	**I**	**S**	**P**
r^W	1.20	1.70	1.52	1.55	1.47	1.75	1.85	1.98	1.80	1.80

These values were obtained from a careful comparison of various types of physical properties and are quite reliable. Unfortunately, values for groups are limited to the methyl group and to the half thickness of the benzene ring.

5.2. Molecular Van der Waals Volume

The molecular van der Waals volume (V^w) is a useful parameter for studying the packing of organic molecules in crystals, the protein folding, and the quantification of bioactivity as a function of molecular structure.[67,68]

A molecular van der Waals envelope, Γ, can be defined in the "hard-spheres" approximation as the external surface resulted from the interaction of all vdW spheres corresponding to the atoms of molecule M. The points (x,y,z) inside the envelope satisfy at least one of the following inequalities:

$$(X_i - x)^2 + (Y_i - y)^2 + (Z_i - z)^2 \le (r_i^w)^2 \qquad i = \overline{1,m} \qquad (5.1)$$

where m represents the number of atoms of M. Consequently, the total volume embedded by the envelope is the molecular vdW volume (V_M^w) of the molecule M.

Let it be a function F=f(x,y,z), continuous in a compact domain M. The integral:

$$I = \iiint_M f(x, y, z) dxdydz \tag{5.2}$$

can be interpreted as a weight, f(x,y,z) being the repartition of density in space M. If we consider the density function $f(x, y, z) \equiv 1$, then the following integral:

$$V^w = \iiint_M dV; \qquad dV = dxdydz \tag{5.3}$$

can be intuitively justified as a volume. This assumption is natural because the properties of molecular vdW space can be considered independent from the nature of the atoms, even in the case when domains of the vdW atomic spheres intersect.

To estimate the integral (5.3), the molecule is inserted into a bounding parallelepiped with the volume V_p. The random points are generated into the parallelepiped, which includes the domain M. If n_t is the total number of generated points and n_s the number of points, which satisfy the inequalities in (5.1), than the van der Waals volume is:

$$V_M^w = \frac{n_s}{n_t} \cdot V_p \tag{5.4}$$

One of the main problems is to find out the volume of the intersection of the spheres, in order to avoid multiple computation of the same volume. One of the approaches is based on the Monte Carlo methods.[24,33,62,64] The accuracy ε of the estimate (5.4) for a given maximum probability is inversely proportional to the square root of the number of trials, or

$$\varepsilon = \frac{1}{2 \cdot \sqrt{\delta \cdot N}} \tag{5.5}$$

This circumstance causes the relatively slow convergence of the Monte Carlo methods. For example, in order to reduce the error of the result 10-fold, the number of trials must be increased 100-fold. If the accuracy of the estimate ε and the guarantee probability 1-δ are given, then from formula (5.5) one derives the necessary number of trials:

$$N = \frac{1}{4\varepsilon\delta^2} \tag{5.6}$$

Taking into consideration the precision and the accuracy of chemical and biological experiments, for ε=0.05 and δ=0.01, the number of necessary points is N=10,000. This makes the Monte Carlo method not difficult to apply, due to the performances of nowadays computers. In order to increase the accuracy of the method the calculus must be repeated at least 10 to 20 times for each volume. The final result, the mean value of these computed volumes, is validated by statistical method.

5.3. Molecular Van der Waals Surface

The van der Waals volume of the envelope Γ, defined in the previous paragraph, can be a measure of the molecules' size. Obviously, this envelope is a surface, and there were methods developed to compute the area of this surface.[23,69,70] Some of them are based on a Monte Carlo method,[70] others on an analytical algorithm.[71] The computed surfaces were especially used to characterize the shape and the similarity of the molecules, their graphical representation,[70,72] etc.

A Monte Carlo algorithm[70] implies the generation of an uniform grid on each sphere of the molecule, followed by the detection of the number of points generated on the surface (n_t) and of those (n_e) that do not satisfy the inequalities in (5.1). For every "hard sphere" i, one computes the outer part of each sphere's surface, S_i^W :

$$S_i^w = \frac{(n_e)_i}{n_t} \cdot 4 \cdot \pi \cdot (r_i^w)^2 \tag{5.7}$$

The final surface is computed as a sum of exterior surface of each sphere, S_i^W :

$$S^w = \sum_{i=1}^{m} S_i^w \tag{5.8}$$

In order to generate a uniform grid, one has to take into account the parametric representation of the sphere in 3D space:

$$\begin{aligned} x &= R \cdot \cos(\varphi) \cdot \sin(\theta) \qquad && \varphi \in [-\pi/2, \pi/2] \\ y &= R \cdot \sin(\varphi) \cdot \sin(\theta) && \theta \in [0, \pi/2] \\ z &= R \cdot \cos(\theta) && \end{aligned} \tag{5.9}$$

where $R=r^w$, and θ and φ are defined in Figure 4:

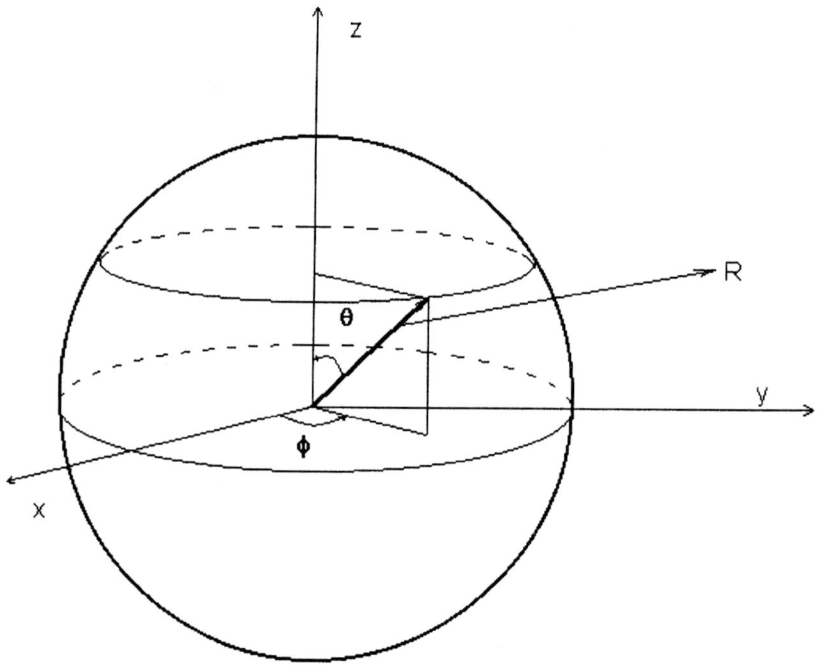

Figure 4. The parametric representation of a sphere in the 3D space.

The uniform grid is set up by means of circles parallel to the xOy plane, with the radius r:

$$r = \sqrt{R^2 - z^2} \tag{5.10}$$

A random selection of $z \in [-R,R]$ and a random selection of φ define a point belonging to the uniform mesh. The following relations give the Cartesian (x,y) coordinates of each point:

$$\begin{aligned} x &= C \cdot \cos(\varphi) \\ y &= C \cdot \sin(\varphi) \\ C &= \sqrt{\left[1 - \left(\frac{z}{R}\right)^2\right]} \end{aligned} \tag{5.11}$$

5.4. Other Van der Waals Parameters

With the van der Waals volume and surface computed, two other parameters can be defined.[73] The first is the ratio between the volume and the surface of the molecule, which has the same dimension as length:[62]

$$L^{W} = \frac{V^{W}}{S^{W}} \tag{5.12}$$

The second one, defined only for acyclic molecules, is named *globularity measure* (G_m) and is given by the relation:[73]

$$G_{m} = \frac{L^{W}}{R_{s}} \tag{5.13}$$

where L^W is defined by relation (5.12) and R_s represents the ratio between the volume and the surface of an equivalent sphere, which surrounds the molecule, with the radius equal to the half of the longest dimension of the parallelepiped that includes the molecule. The above relation cannot be used for cyclic molecules, because the volume of the equivalent sphere includes the internal empty space, which is not included in the van der Waals volume.

These two parameters can be used to describe the shape of the acyclic molecules. The globularity measure decreases with the growth of the linear chains and increases toward unity when the molecule is highly branched or compacted. In Table 5.2 are listed the van der Waals volumes, surfaces, L^W and G_m parameters for C2-C8 alkanes (M represents the methyl group, and the number before M reflects the position of branching). As expected, the longer the chain, the smaller the globularity measure. This measure increases for alkanes such as 2,2- and 2,3-dimethylbutane, 2,2,3-trimethylbutane, trimethylpentanes, ethyl-methylpentanes or tetramethylbutanes.

An useful example that describes the utility of the globularity measure is the case of molecules with long chain, which can have different conformations. For instance, let be the normal C16 alkane, with two conformations presented below (Figure 5 and Figure 6).

Table 5.2 Van der Waals parameters for C2-C8 alkanes

Alkane	V^w	S^w	L^w	G_m
C2	44.205	70.920	0.623	0.653
C3	60.234	93.026	0.647	0.554
C4	77.845	115.315	0.675	0.516
2-M-C3	77.275	114.675	0.674	0.558
C5	94.749	138.127	0.686	0.451
2-M-C4	94.047	136.241	0.690	0.522
22-MM-C3	92.368	135.225	0.683	0.527
C6	110.242	159.338	0.692	0.417
2-M-C5	109.970	158.477	0.694	0.465
3-M-C5	109.676	156.114	0.703	0.453
22-MM-C4	110.161	155.015	0.711	0.537
23-MM-C4	110.215	155.033	0.711	0.496
C7	127.399	181.834	0.701	0.375
2-M-C6	127.317	179.742	0.708	0.429
3-M-C6	126.956	178.780	0.710	0.448
3-E-C5	125.874	176.827	0.712	0.458
22-MM-C5	126.822	176.663	0.718	0.486
33-MM-C5	125.592	174.301	0.721	0.451
24-MM-C5	127.320	178.291	0.714	0.462
23-MM-C5	127.492	174.419	0.731	0.472
223-MMM-C4	126.616	172.912	0.732	0.511
C8	142.613	203.964	0.699	0.347
2-M-C7	143.144	201.813	0.709	0.388
3-M-C7	143.774	200.463	0.717	0.373
4-M-C7	143.925	199.927	0.720	0.401
3-E-C6	141.739	198.490	0.714	0.422
22-MM-C6	142.733	198.900	0.718	0.443
33-MM-C6	142.566	195.458	0.729	0.410
24-MM-C6	144.186	197.986	0.728	0.429
25-MM-C6	143.512	198.892	0.722	0.396
34-MM-C6	142.278	195.908	0.726	0.456
234-MMM-C5	142.593	196.954	0.724	0.465
223-MMM-C5	142.505	193.130	0.738	0.482
233-MMM-C5	141.973	191.844	0.740	0.468
3-E-2-M-C5	142.069	195.215	0.728	0.481
3-E-3-M-C5	142.811	192.962	0.740	0.473
2233-MMMM-C4	142.466	189.633	0.751	0.522

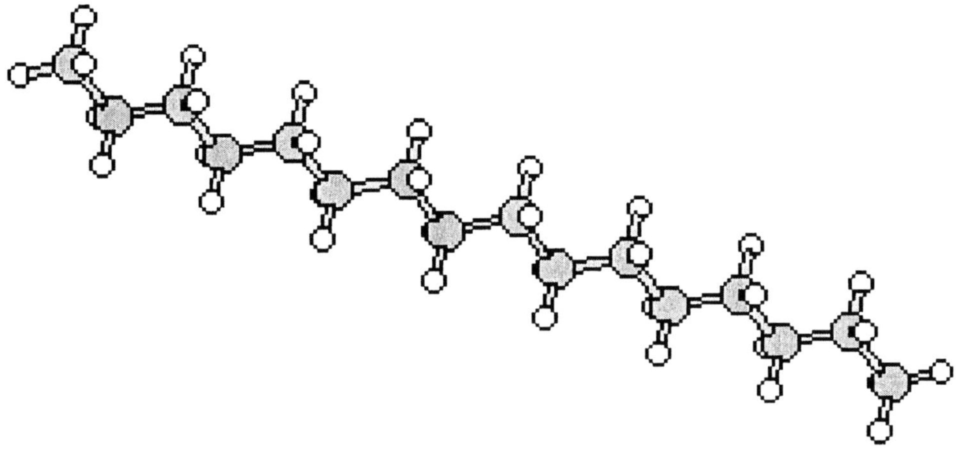

Figure 5. The linear conformation of C16

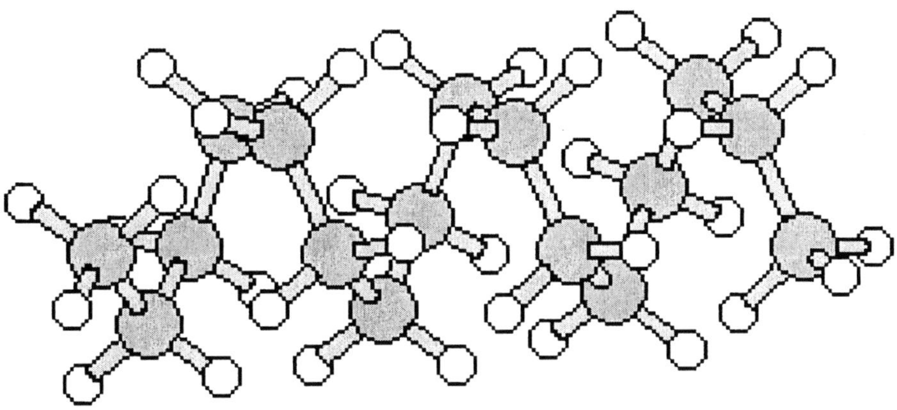

Figure 6. A twisted conformation (all dihedral angles in the chain are set to 30°)

The van der Waals parameters are listed in Table 5.3.

Table 5.3 Van der Waals parameters for two conformations of C16 alkane

Alkane	V^w	S^w	L^w	G_m
C16 normal	283.632	381.516	0.743	0.214
C16 twisted	244.046	249.153	0.980	0.448

5.5. Synthetic Van der Waals Descriptors of Molecular Shape

The shape of molecules (or substituents) is doubtlessly the main element of most chemical interactions. The quantitative treatment of molecular shape, that is the development of appropriate molecular descriptors able to synthesize the characteristics of 3D extension of molecules, is a very difficult problem. Most procedures are based either on comparing molecules with a reference structure, or on dividing them and defining the sectors by means of Euclidean distance between certain atoms or with the aid of Cartesian coordinates of those sectors.

Using a *hard-spheres* model, we developed a series of van der Waals indicators of the shape of the substituents; these are applicable in QSAR analysis (or in mechanistic studies in organic chemistry) as steric parameters. This model allowed the introduction of several synthetic descriptors of molecular shape, which are presented as follows.

(a) A first set of indicators were developed starting from the fact that a substituent can be characterized by the surface of molecular envelope described by equations 5.1 (with the sign "="). One knows that the totality of points whose coordinates satisfy an equation of type:

$$F(x, y, z) = 0 \qquad (5.14)$$

verifying certain initial conditions form a surface.[74] Generally, the surfaces have different shapes depending on the imposed conditions.

In our case, a first condition appears from equation 5.1: the function $F(x, y, z)$ is an algebraic function of second degree. In this case $F(x, y, z)$ represents an algebraic equation of second degree; its general form is:

$$\begin{aligned} &a_{11} \cdot x^2 + 2a_{12} \cdot xy + 2a_{13} \cdot xz + a_{22} \cdot y^2 + 2a_{23} \cdot yz + a_{33} \cdot z^2 + \\ &\quad + 2a_{14} \cdot x + 2a_{24} \cdot y + 2a_{34} \cdot z + a_{44} = 0 \end{aligned} \qquad (5.15)$$

The equation (5.15), in which the first six coefficients are not simultaneously equal to zero, represents a surface of 2nd degree (i.e., a quadric). By a linear mapping of the coordinates (translation-rotation or by their composition) followed by the transformation of principal axis of coordinates, the discussion of 2nd degree algebraic equation can be reduced to the discussion of 2nd degree equation in the form

$$a_{11} \cdot x^2 + a_{22} \cdot y^2 + a_{33} \cdot z^2 + 2a_{14} \cdot x + 2a_{24} \cdot y + 2a_{34} \cdot z + a_{44} = 0 \qquad (5.16)$$

By transformations of coordinates (translation), the Equation (5.16) is simplified and reduced to one of the fifteen equations composed of four terms.[74]

For obvious physical reasons related to spatial extension of substituents, we neglect both singular quadrics and the equations that do not have real solutions – and, therefore, do not represent geometrical figures. From the five non-singular surfaces of 2nd degree which remain and represent geometrical figures (ellipsoid, ellipsoidal and hyperbolic paraboloid, and one-sheet and two-sheet hyperboloid), only the ellipsoid fulfills the physical conditions so that by assimilating the molecule (or substituent) with this geometrical figure, the physical signification of the calculated parameters is maintained.

It is known that the relationship:

$$\frac{x^2}{a^2}+\frac{y^2}{b^2}+\frac{z^2}{c^2}=1 \tag{5.17}$$

represents an ellipsoid, namely a spheroid (or conoid). If $a > b = c$ we have a prolate ellipsoid; if $a = b > c$ we have an oblate ellipsoid of revolution; if $a = b = c$ we have a sphere. In Figure 7 is represented a "hard-spheres" model of a molecule embedded in an ellipsoid (spheroid).

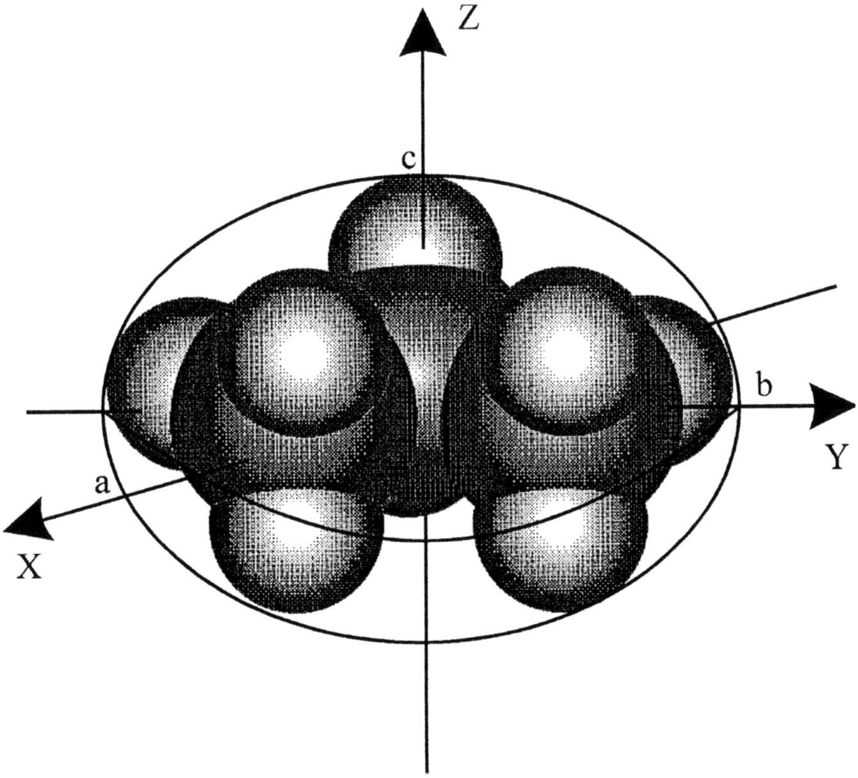

Figure 7. A molecule or substituent assimilated with an ellipsoid

The molecular descriptors of the molecular shape of some substituents are given in Table 5.4. It can be noted that the normal alkyl radicals and other substituents such as CHO, COOH, etc., may be viewed as prolate ellipsoids, whereas the branched radicals (including CX_3, CHX_2, CH_2X) resemble an oblate ellipsoid of revolution.

Table 5.4 Synthetic descriptors of the molecular shape.

X	a	b	c	υ'_V	υ'_S	$(V/S)^W$
Me	1.700	1.983	2.104	0.651	0.691	0.591
Et	2.301	2.459	2.104	0.983	1.113	0.648
n-Pr	2.763	2.705	2.104	1.229	1.457	0.676
i-Pr	2.606	3.104	2.729	1.235	1.465	0.678
n-Bu	3.363	3.166	2.104	1.428	1.718	0.710
i-Bu	2.521	3.104	3.355	1.438	1.735	0.711
s-Bu	2.519	3.735	2.743	1.438	1.742	0.703
t-Bu	2.301	3.110	3.353	1.443	1.757	0.699
n-Am	3.825	3.412	2.104	1.609	1.997	0.723
MeO	2.321	1.983	2.104	0.825	0.911	0.621
EtO	2.921	2.459	2.104	1.107	1.292	0.659
n-PrO	2.681	3.048	2.104	1.338	1.603	0.694
i-PrO	2.921	3.099	2.730	1.335	1.608	0.688
n-BuO	3.984	3.151	2.104	1.523	1.862	0.718
t-BuO	2.921	3.066	3.355	1.525	1.867	0.716
H	1.200	1.200	1.200	0.000	0.000	0.400
F	1.470	1.470	1.470	0.270	0.270	0.489
Cl	1.750	1.750	1.750	0.550	0.550	0.583
Br	1.850	1.850	1.850	0.650	0.650	0.640
I	1.980	1.980	1.980	0.780	0.780	0.659
FCH_2	2.115	1.918	2.350	0.756	0.847	0.596
F_2CH	2.095	1.938	2.554	0.851	0.959	0.616
F_3C	2.336	1.932	2.534	0.928	1.053	0.633
MeNH	2.379	1.973	2.092	0.887	1.003	0.624
EtNH	3.006	2.577	2.104	1.160	1.373	0.662
H_2N	1.567	1.902	1.780	0.496	0.530	0.544
NC	2.205	1.700	1.700	0.672	0.694	0.609
CHO	1.950	2.358	1.700	0.714	0.762	0.607
COOH	2.242	2.628	1.700	0.868	0.959	0.632

(b) Starting from the concept of *packing density* and from the fact that the experimental determination of the cross-section area of a molecule is performed by assimilating it to a sphere,[75] and assuming a maximal packing of molecule spheres, one may consider as a quantitative measure of the steric effect of substituents the υ'_V and υ'_S parameters, defined as follows:

$$\upsilon'_V = r(V) - 1.2 \quad ; \quad r(V) = \left[3V^W/4\pi\right]^{1/3} \tag{5.18}$$

$$\upsilon'_S = r(S) - 1.2 \quad ; \quad r(S) = \left[S^W/4\pi\right]^{1/2} \tag{5.19}$$

where r(V) and r(S) represent the vdW radii equivalent to the calculated vdW volume (V^W) and surface (S^W), respectively (see Section 5.2 and 5.3, respectively) and 1.2Å is the Bondi vdW radius of the hydrogen atom. The values calculated with the relations (5.18) and (5.19) are summarized in Table 5.4.

One may observe from relations (5.18) and (5.19) a formal similarity between these parameters and υ-Charton steric constant. We adopt as a matter of fact this definition, starting from the fact that the steric effect of hydrogen atom can be generally neglected, the packing up of the effector molecule in the receptor site being maximal. In addition, by means of υ'_V and υ'_S parameters one may estimate the validity of semi-empirical extension of E_S-steric scale, with the aid of υ-type (Charton) steric parameter model.

The correlation equations between υ-Charton and υ'_V and υ'_S parameters are systematized in Table 5.5.

One may observe from Table 5.5 the decreasing statistical quality when going from strictly tetrahedral substituents to substituents with other configurations (or conformations). The linear correlation model is without statistical meaning when one considers the substituents having different spatial structures (conformations or configurations). As a matter of fact, we consider that υ-Charton values of substituents, which differ from tetrahedral configuration, have completely less physical signification. Therefore, the model of Charton is an empirical model with restricted applicability.

(c) The ratio V^W/S^W (or S^W/V^W) could also be a measure of the substituent shapes. The relative values of these parameters express the more or less "globular" character (or spherical character) of the given substituent. Because the stereochemical variations affect the volume less than the surface of the substituent envelope, the decrease of V/S value is expected to express the increase of the substituent "globularity" (i.e., for staggered skew n-Bu, V^W/S^W is 0.716, whereas for the intercalated conformer the value of this ratio is 0.705.

Table 5.5 Analysis of physical meaning of υ-Charton parameters by means of the following regression equations: $\upsilon = \alpha + \beta\mu$, $\mu = \upsilon'_V, \upsilon'_S, (V/S)^W$; Y = F, Cl, Br, I; R = alkyl

(a) $\upsilon = \alpha + \beta \cdot \upsilon'_V$

X	R	α	β	s	F	t	EV	n
Y	1.000	0.001	0.999	0.0005	101219	450	1.000	4
Y_3C	1.000	-0.210	1.190	0.001	49010	313	1.000	4
Y_2CH	0.997	0.245	0.504	0.010	79	13	0.991	4
YCH_2	0.697	0.500	0.140	0.020	1	1	0.218	4
$Y\&Y_mC$	0.866	-0.073	0.924	0.199	20	6	0.732	16
R	0.577	0.215	0.458	0.267	13	5	0.321	56

(b) $\upsilon = \alpha + \beta \cdot \upsilon'_S$

X	r	α	β	s	F	t	EV	n
Y	1.000	0.000	1.000	0.000	$\to \infty$	$\to \infty$	1.000	4
Y_3C	1.000	-0.130	0.970	0.003	10742	147	1.000	4
Y_2CH	0.996	0.250	0.440	0.010	68	12	0.989	4
YCH_2	0.702	0.490	0.130	0.020	1	1	0.238	4
$Y\&Y_mC$	0.872	0.007	0.751	0.195	21	6	0.738	16

(c) $\upsilon = \alpha + \beta \cdot (V/S)^W$

X	R	α	β	s	F	t	EV	n
Y	1.000	-1.190	2.990	0.002	6894	117	1.000	4
Y_3C	1.000	-2.650	5.650	0.005	3298	81	≈ 1.000	4
Y_2CH	0.997	-0.560	2.020	0.009	94	14	0.992	4
YCH_2	0.668	0.300	0.510	0.020	> 0	1	0.170	4
$Y\&Y_mC$	0.825	-2.040	4.380	0.225	14	5	0.658	16

n – number of data; r – correlation coefficient; s – standard deviation; EV – explained variance; F, t – Fisher and Student statistics, respectively.

Mention must be made of the fact that these steric parameters have the dimensions of a radius, as υ-Charton parameter. Some values of this parameter for a series of substituents are given in Table 5.4.

5.6. STERIMOL–Type Descriptors: δ, G

The STERIMOL parameters were developed by Verloop et al.[40] in order to obtain more appropriate descriptors of the substituent shape. According to the initial STERIMOL procedure a set of five parameters (L, B_1–B_4), expressed in Å, computed for each substituents extended conformation are enough to describe its shape. The index L represents the length of the substituent, whereas the B_1–B_4 indices measure the "thickness" of that substituent on two orthogonal directions. Afterwards, a new vdW descriptor, denoted B_5, was developed. These parameters represent a powerful tool in describing steric effects and were used in QSAR approaches describing the 3D-character of the biological interactions.

Efforts to extract three-dimensional information regarding drug–(unknown) receptor interaction from measurements of potency are generally centered on the QSAR paradigm, and appropriate characterization of the molecular shape is the major obstacle in the development of a topographical basis for QSAR.

A new set of two parameters (δ,G) of the same type was developed by one of us based on the following assumptions:[62]

(1) The substituents are treated according to the hard-sphere model: an isotropic sphere centered at the equilibrium position of the atomic core and having a radius equal to the vdW radius of the atom represents each atom of the substituent. Consequently, a molecular vdW envelope (relatively impenetrable) may be uniquely defined as the exterior surface of the intersection of the vdW spheres associated with the atoms in the substituent.
(2) The steric behavior of the substituent is due exclusively to the homogenous and isotropic molecular vdW space covered by its vdW envelope.
(3) The steric effect is of a vectorial nature. It is due to the fact that a substituent occupies a certain volume in 3D-space ("space-filling"), relatively impenetrable to external influences.
(4) The substituent shows a rotational symmetry round about the axis linking the contact point of the substituent of parent structure with the van der Waals center of gravity of the substituent.

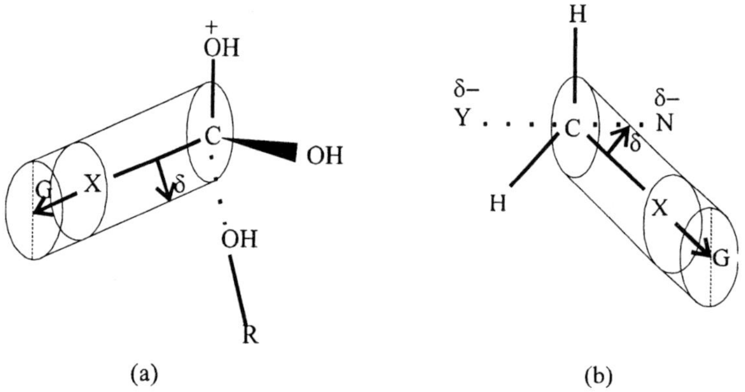

Figure 8. Physical significance of (,G) parameters for the transition states in reactions:
(a) acid hydrolysis of carboxylic acids XCO2H + ROH;
(b) bimolecular nucleophilic substitution, SN2

In the context of the above four considerations, the steric anisotropy of the molecular vdW space is effective in two directions:

(a) the direction of rotational axis – G;
(b) the direction perpendicular to it – δ (see Figure 8).

Some values of the (δ,G)-descriptors for values substituents are summarized in Table 5.6.

Table 5.6 The values of (δ,G) vdW descriptors for some substituents, X.

X	δ_i	G_i	δ_e	G_e	X	δ	G
Et	1.420	4.876	1.625	4.276	Me	1.244	3.400
n-Pr	1.628	5.799	2.187	4.418	FCH_2	1.437	3.474
i-Pr	2.332	4.123	2.748	3.506	$ClCH_2$	1.473	4.387
n-Bu	1.656	7.409	2.121	5.622	$BrCH_2$	1.527	4.688
i-Bu	2.786	4.416	2.234	5.453	ICH_2	1.598	5.059
s-Bu	3.133	3.918	2.689	4.585	F_2CH	1.701	3.379
t-Bu	3.605	3.399	3.593	3.399	Cl_2CH	2.453	3.523
n-Am	1.811	8.318	2.640	5.492	Br_2CH	2.776	3.609
s-BuCH$_2$	3.267	4.589	2.570	5.772	I_2CH	3.265	3.712
i-BuCH$_2$	2.627	5.667	2.113	6.703	F_3C	1.889	3.400
Et$_2$CH	3.617	4.059	3.798	3.835	Cl_3C	3.177	3.400
c-HxCH$_2$	2.553	7.279	2.687	6.928	Br_3C	3.794	3.400
PhCH$_2$	2.334	6.727	2.311	6.771	I_3C	4.668	3.400
Ph(CH$_2$)$_2$	2.106	8.787	2.353	7.868	H_2N	1.055	3.083
Ph(Me)CH	2.600	7.088	2.631	7.252	O_2N	1.604	3.190
Ph(Et)CH	2.991	6.985	3.088	6.653	HO	0.898	3.017
MeO	1.209	4.558	1.303	4.148	CN	0.991	4.410
EtO	1.455	5.608	1.900	4.160	COOH	1.409	4.184

Subscript i refers to intercalated conformer and e to eclipsed conformer.

One may observe the difference between the (δ,G) and the STERIMOL parameters: in the case of (L, B1–B5) steric indices the rotational axes is represented by the direction of the bond that links the atoms of the parent structure and of the substituent. In addition, the δ-value is the radius of a cylinder having a volume equivalent to the vdW volume of the substituent and a generating line, G, which is the length of the substituent on the rotational axis.

Analysis of the δ-parameter for alkyl substituents suggests its possible utility in the quantitative treatment of steric effects in organic reactions (see, for example, the results in Table 5.7).

Table 5.7 Statistical validation of vdW indicators.

Set	p	r	a	b	s	F	t	EV	n
1.	δ_i	0,970	2,00	-0,53	0,09	47,4	9,7	0,930	9
2.	δ_i	0,998	3,51	-1,12	o,o9	*	*	0,992	3
3.	δ_i	0,948	1,58	-0,85	0,34	4,4	3,0	0,848	4
4.	δ_i	0,957	0,18	-0,87	0,33	*	*	0,833	3
5.	δ_i	0,973	-1,31	-1,90	0,54	17,8	6,0	0,929	5
	δ_e	0,930	-1,34	-1,77	0,86	6,4	3,6	0,821	5
6.	δ_i	0,984	0,41	-2,37	0,51	31,0	7,9	0,958	5
	δ_e	0,946	0,40	-2,21	0,93	8,6	4,1	0,861	5
7.	δ_i	0,991	0,30	-2,16	0,35	54,7	10,5	0,976	5
	δ_e	0,963	0,33	-2,04	0,70	12,7	5,1	0,904	5
8.	δ_i	0,982	-1,08	-1,87	0,43	27,7	7,4	0,953	5
	δ_e	0,944	-1,09	-1,74	0,75	8,2	4,0	0,854	5
9.	δ_i	0,999	0,18	-1,57	0,07	169,5	18,4	0,996	4
	δ_e	0,990	-0,06	-1,25	0,17	25,9	7,2	0,992	4
10.	δ_i	0,985	-0,83	-2,03	0,27	16,0	5,7	0,955	4

The δ-parameter was used is structure-reactivity correlations for the reactions in which the steric effects are relevant. We present here the results obtained in the correlation of with alcohols and the hydrolysis reactions of esters (reference reactions for the E_S-Taft quantitative steric model, sets 1–4 from Table 5.7) and, also, of bimolecular nucleophilic substitution, S_N2 (sets 5–10 from Table 5.7).[62,76] See Figure 8 for details on physical significance of (δ,G). We used correlation equations as follows:

$$\log k = \alpha + \beta \cdot \delta \tag{5.20}$$

where k represents the rate constant and α and β are parameters of the linear model (5.20) obtained by means of the least squares methods.

The results reported in Table 5.7 have been obtained for alkyl substituents with ground state geometries. The δ-parameters quantify very well the steric effects and their physical meaning is very clear. The δ-values remain approximately constant when the number of Carbon atoms of the substituents (extended conformations) are increasing, but the δ-values are increasing when the branching degrees are also increasing.

On the other hand, G-parameter representing the length of the substituent in the direction of the rotational axis could be very useful in QSAR studies to detect steric requirements of the (eventually) hydrophobic pockets of the receptor site. Therefore, the quantification of a steric receptor-effector interaction by a set of only two parameters (δ and G) easy calculable may be achieved.

6. Prediction of Octanol/Water Partition Coefficients from First Principles

6.1. Introduction

The biochemical interactions in the living cell occur in both aqueous and hydrophobic media (e.g. coupling to an active site of an enzyme, transport through a biomembrane).[77] In addition, other pharmaco-kinetic properties are related to the difference in solubility of bioactive molecules in aqueous and organic solvents. Hence, it is important to account properly the solute interactions with both aqueous and organic media. The partition of chemical compounds between organic and aqueous phases is often modeled by the octanol/water partition coefficient ($log\ K_{ow}$),[7] because it is assumed that octanol may reflect lipid tissues in living organisms. K_{ow} has been successfully related to bioconcentration factors, soil and sediment sorbtion partition coefficients and to toxicities of organic chemicals towards several aquatic organisms. Direct measurement of K_{ow} through means of the shake-flask procedure yields only reliable data for chemicals with $log\ K_{ow}$ less than 4-5.[78] K_{ow} of more hydrophobic substances can be measured either by the generator-column method or by slow-stirring technique. In addition, to these direct approaches to the determination of K_{ow}, several other methods were employed: (a) calculation based on molecular fragments additivity,[57,79] (b) correlation with capacity factors on reversed-phase HPLC, (c) correlation with molecular descriptors (volume, surface area, molar refraction, parachor, molecular weight),[80] and (d) correlation with molar volume and solvatochromic parameters.

The partitioning of a hydrophobic solute between octanol and water is due to the difference between the interactions that solute is experiencing in water versus octanol. Hence, the relationship between water solubility and K_{ow} (Hansch et al.[57]) has been studied extensively over the last two decades.[81] Examples of such correlation have been published for halogenated benzene, aromatic hydrocarbons, aldehydes, esters and alcohols. However, due to experimental difficulties, few accurate data for compounds with *log* K_{ow} greater than 6 have been reported, which limits the use of such correlation for prediction purposes. The correlation between *log* K_{ow} and molecular volume or surface area is based on the idea that the partitioning of a hydrophobic solute between water and octanol is determined by the difference in solvation free energy in the two media.[81] A large part of the solvation free energy is the free energy of cavity formation, which is related with the size (volume, surface area) and the shape of the molecule,[82] hence for non-polar molecules relationships between size descriptors and solvation free energy seems to be adequate and were used extensively.[71] For polar compounds the solvation free energy depends strongly also on solute-solvent electrostatic interactions. Taft and coworkers have shown that aqueous solubility and octanol/water partition coefficient can be well described by linear correlation with three types of terms which measure cavity size, solute polarity/polarizability and hydrogen bond donor/acceptor character.

6.2. Calculation of Log K_{ow} from the Solvation Free Energies of Octanol and Water

The octanol/water partition coefficient of a solute is related with the free energy of transfer, G_{tr}, from water to octanol as follows:[83]

$$\Delta G_{tr} = G_{so} - G_{sw} = -RT \ln K_{ow} \tag{6.1}$$

where G_{so} and G_{sw} are the solvation free energies of the solute in octanol and water, respectively. R is the gas constant and T the absolute temperature.

The solvation free energy G_s of a solute in an arbitrary solvent can be written as a sum of three terms:[84]

$$G_s = G_c + G_{vdw} + G_{el} \tag{6.2}$$

G_c is the free energy required to build a cavity in solvent, of appropriate size to accommodate the solute, and G_{vdw} and G_{el} are the free energies due to solvent-solute dispersion and electrostatic interactions.[84] The solvent-solute electrostatic interaction free energy contains contributions from solvent polarization due to the electric field generated by solute electronic structure (the reaction field), and solute polarization, i.e. the change in solute electronic structure due to solvent polarization. Solvent polarization is usually accounted for by means of the Poisson-Boltzmann equation (the linear form):[71]

$$\nabla \cdot [\varepsilon(\mathbf{r}) \nabla \phi(\mathbf{r})] - \kappa^2(\mathbf{r}) \phi(\mathbf{r}) = -4\pi\rho(\mathbf{r}) \tag{6.3}$$

where ϕ is the electrostatic potential (due to solute charge density and solvent reaction field) at position **r**, ε solvent dielectric constant, κ the Debye-Hueckel (ionic) parameter and ρ solute charge density. The solvation free energy part due to solvent polarization is obtained from solute electrostatic potential as follows:

$$G_{RF} = \frac{1}{2}\int_V \rho(\mathbf{r})\phi(\mathbf{r})d\mathbf{r} \tag{6.4}$$

Solute polarization can be accounted for effectively only if the solute is described quantum mechanically. In this case, solute polarization free energy is obtained as the difference in solute free energies in gas phase with and without the effect of the reaction field.

The free energies due to cavity formation, G_c, and solvent-solute dispersion interactions, G_{vdw}, can be in principle calculated separately, but it is customary to evaluate their sum (called the non-polar term G_{np}) as a function of solvent-accessible surface area:

$$G_{np} = G_c + G_{vdw} = \sum_i \tau_i A_i \tag{6.5}$$

where A_i is the solvent-accessible surface area, and τ_i the surface tension parameter of atom i. For the evaluation of solvation free energies in water and octanol we used only one surface tension parameter per solvent. The surface tension parameter for water was obtained from the correlation of solvent-accessible surface area of alkanes with their solubility in water. The surface tension parameter for octanol was obtained from the correlation of solvent-accessible surface area of polychlorinated benzenes with their 'experimental' non-polar free energies (obtained from their solvation free energies in octanol).

We exemplify now the calculation of octanol/water partition coefficient from first principles by applying the methodology described above to the calculation of $log\ K_{ow}$ for a set of twelve chlorinated benzene derivatives. The calculations were performed with a program which combines the semiempirical quantum mechanical Hamiltonian AM1 with the Poisson-Boltzmann equation.[85] Table 6.1 shows both experimental (obtained from low stirring data) and calculated octanol/water partition coefficients for chlorinated benzene derivatives. The comparison of the two sets of partition coefficients (calculated and experimental) indicates a good agreement between theory and experiment. Thus, it is now possible to evaluate accurately the partition coefficients from first principle, i.e. from the calculated solvation free energies in octanol and water. The largest deviations from experimental values were found for 1,4-dichlorobenzene (0.244) and hexachlorobenzene (-0.229), which corresponds to a difference in solvation free energy of about 0.3 kcal/mol. This difference is in the range of the average error in calculating solvation free energies for the nowadays state of the art programs, and indicates the accuracy that can be achieved in evaluating partition coefficients too. This 'computational direct' method for the calculation of octanol/water partition coefficients can be refined systematically by improving the methods used to evaluate each term in solvation free energy. Hence, the method can be used not only to obtain higher accuracy in calculating partition coefficients for already know chemical, but it can also be valuable in predicting partition coefficients for novel compounds. Its strength stems from the fact that it takes into account the fine details of molecular structure.

Table 6.1 Octanol/water partition coefficients for polychlorinated benzene derivatives calculated by a combined semiempirical Poisson-Boltzmann equation method.

Compound[1]	Water			Octanol			log K_{ow}	
	G_{el}	G_{np}	G_s	G_{el}	G_{np}[2]	G_s	Calc.[3]	Exp.[4]
benzene	-4.27	2.27	-2.00	-3.49	-1.45	-4.94	2.154	2.186
chlorobenzene	-4.30	2.41	-1.89	-3.46	-2.17	-5.63	2.745	2.898
1,2-dichlorobenzene	-4.28	2.53	-1.76	-3.44	-2.80	-6.24	3.288	3.433
1,3- dichlorobenzene	-3.78	2.55	-1.23	-3.03	-2.89	-5.92	3.439	3.525
1,4- dichlorobenzene	-3.80	2.55	-1.25	-3.05	-2.89	-5.94	3.440	3.444
1,2,3-trichlorobenzene	-3.73	2.65	-1.08	-2.97	-3.42	-6.39	3.895	4.139
1,2,4-trichlorobenzene	-3.29	2.67	-0.63	-2.64	-3.52	-6.16	4.057	4.050
1,3,5-trichlorobenzene	-2.63	2.68	0.05	-2.10	-3.61	-5.71	4.222	4.189
1,2,3,4-tetrahlorobenzene	-2.83	2.77	-0.06	-2.26	-4.05	-6.31	4.583	4.635
1,2,3,5-tetrahlorobenzene	-2.22	2.79	0.57	-1.76	-4.14	-5.90	4.746	4.658
1,2,4,5-tetrahlorobenzene	-2.33	2.79	0.46	-1.86	-4.15	-6.01	4.746	4.604
pentachlorobenzene	-1.42	2.89	1.47	-1.12	-4.66	-5.78	5.322	5.183
hexachlorobenzene	-0.23	2.99	2.76	-0.18	-5.18	-5.36	5.960	5.731

7. Molecular Descriptors Obtained by Overlapping Methods

The Minimal Steric Difference method (abbreviated as MSD) offers a very simple way to express by a single number the molecular shape dissimilarity. The MCD parameter "translates" the topological MSD parameter into the metric context: the molecules are described by Cartesian coordinates and vdW radii of their atoms. The MCD value measures the nonoverlapping volume (in $Å^3$) among two molecules. The Minimal Topological Difference method (abbreviated as MTD) denotes a "hypermolecule optimization" procedure based on the MSD parameter. Actually, MTD is the MSD parameter calculated against a "hypermolecule" as standard.

7.1. MSD – The Original Version of Minimal Steric Difference Method

Steric fit depends, obviously, on the shape of both the biological receptor (R) and the effector molecule (E). Taft-type steric parameters and vdW molecular parameters described in the previous chapters rely only on the shape of the effector molecule. The regression equation will indicate if the receptor prefers large or small values for the corresponding parameter (for example, vdW volume of substituents or molecules, width, length etc. – see Sections (4) and (5) from this chapter); at most the optimal value of these parameters should be indicated.

Minimal steric difference, MSD, depends both on the shape of the effector molecule and of the biological receptor. The fundamental of the MSD method is that the affinity of effectors for a receptor is a linearly decreasing function of the steric misfit of the drug molecule M_i and the receptor cavity, i.e., of the sum of the nonoverlapping volumes of M_i and the cavity.[9] To make use of this concept, one must have a guess for the shape of the receptor cavity and a simple technique to evaluate the nonoverlapping. The MSD values approximate this volume. Thus, if A_i is the biological activity of molecule M_i, the correlation equation for the simple MSD method is:

$$\hat{A}_i = \alpha - \beta \cdot MSD_i \tag{7.1}$$

If other structural parameters P_{1i}, P_{2i},...,P_{mi} are considered, the equation (1) becomes more complicated:

$$\hat{A}_i = \alpha_0 + \alpha_1 \cdot P_{1i} + \alpha_2 \cdot P_{2i} + \cdots + \alpha_m \cdot P_{mi} - \beta \cdot MSD_i \tag{7.2}$$

The receptor site is modeled by a molecular structure of one effector extracted from the data series under study. As reference structure S (which is termed here "standard") one selects generally the molecule of highest activity. The shape of the standard is considered (approximately) complementary to the receptor cavity. One seeks for the maximal superposition of each molecule M_i upon S. Hydrogen atoms are neglected in order to simplify the problem, since their vdW volumes and covalent radii are rather low. Thus, the atom X and the groups XH, XH_2, etc. are considered equivalent.

In order to distinguish between second row atoms and higher rows ones, with larger van der Waals volumes, one can attribute a weight of 1.5 to third row atoms (S, SH, Cl, etc.) and of 2.0 to fourth or higher row atoms. (Br, I, etc.) If a higher row atom is superposed upon a lower row atom, one adds the difference of weights to MSD, but if a higher row atom is superposed upon a trifurcation (for example I on CH of $-CH(CH_3)_2$) one adds to MSD the difference between the weights of the higher period atoms and of the sum of the weights of the trifurcation atom. For example, if a Cl atom is superimposed upon a CH_3 group one adds $|1.5-1| = |1-1.5| = 0.5$ to MSD, and if the iodine atom I is superposed upon the secondary C-atom of an isopropyl group, –

$CH(CH_3)_2$, one adds $|3-2| = |2-3| = 1$ to MSD. One must avoid superimposing pairs of atoms bound by covalent bonds in one molecule (1.2–2.0 Å being the range of length for covalent bonds) upon unbound pairs of atoms of other molecules (the vdW contact distances are in the range 3–4 Å). The MSD parameter is defined as the number of nonsuperposable, non-hydrogen atoms of the two compared molecules.

The small differences in bond lengths and bond angles are neglected, and the various conformations of flexible molecules are considered to be degenerate. If the molecule M_i has several low energy conformations it interacts with the receptor by its conformation which fits the best cavity of the receptor, i.e., one must select the *minimal steric difference.*

A simplified example for calculation of MSD steric parameter is presented in Figure 9.

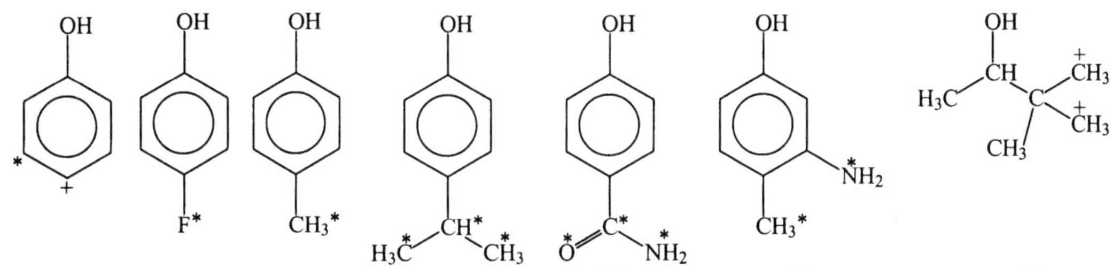

M_1=S M_2 M_3 M_4 M_5 M_6 M_7

Figure 9. Calculation of the MSD steric parameter: illustrative example.

Considering phenol as standard (M_1=S), fot the strucures depicted depicted in Figure 9 the MSD values are: MSD(M_2)=MSD(M_3)=1, MSD(M_4)=MSD(M_5)=3, MSD(M_6)=2, MSD(M_7)=4, and obviously, MSD(M_1)=0.

When tested in correlations,[32] the MSD parameter offered rather modest results. Quite possibly, these results can be justified by the fact that a single number steric parameter does not quantify properly the steric interaction pattern in the context of the "key-in-lock theory". But, the MSD method gives a first inside about the importance of steric fit for a given type of biological activity. One can try different molecules as standards and select the one that yields the highest correlation coefficient, r.

In fact, the MSD parameter is a dissimilarity measure that has a theoretical foundation in one of the pattern recognition (PR) fields, namely *cluster analysis*, and we will prove this in Section 7.4.

7.2. MCD – The 3D-Version of the MSD Method

The Monte Carlo version of minimal steric difference (denoted as MCD) improves the computation of nonoverlapping volumes in the standard-effector superposition, "translating" thus the topological MSD parameter into the (3D) metric context.[86] In order to calculate the MCD, the molecules are described by the Cartesian coordinates and vdW radii of their atoms. The atomic coordinates implicitly specify the way one achieves the superposition: all molecules of the series are represented in the same Cartesian coordinate system.

The mathematical method used in the MCD-technique is the Monte Carlo method.[87] Let us consider the molecules M_S and M_E out of a given series to be used for QSAR, M_S being the standard. M_S consists of N_S atoms of coordinated (X_{Si}, Y_{Si}, Z_{Si}) and vdW radii r_{Si}^{W} (i=1,2,...,N_S) and M_E is composed of N_E atoms of coordinates (X_{Ej}, Y_{Ej}, Z_{Ej}) and their corresponding vdW radii r_{Ej}^{W} (j=1,2,...,N_E). The vdW volumes of these two molecules delimited by the envelopes of M_S and M_E are thus described by the collections of spheres (7.3) and (7.4), respectively.

$$\left(\xi_x - X_{Si}\right)^2 + \left(\xi_y - Y_{Si}\right)^2 + \left(\xi_z - Z_{Si}\right)^2 \le \left(r_{Si}^{W}\right)^2 \qquad (7.3)$$
$$i = 1,2,\ldots, N_S$$

$$\left(\xi_x - X_{Ej}\right)^2 + \left(\xi_y - Y_{Ej}\right)^2 + \left(\xi_z - Z_{Ej}\right)^2 \le \left(r_{Ej}^{W}\right)^2 \qquad (7.4)$$
$$j = 1,2,\ldots, N_E$$

Consequently, the point $P(\xi_x,\xi_y,\xi_z)$ is within the vdW envelope of M_S if it satisfies at least one of equations (7.3), and within that of M_E if it satisfies at least one of equations (7.4).

By definition, the MCD parameter is represented by the total volume of the nonsuperposable vdW envelopes of M_S and M_E. Therefore, the random points $P_k(\xi_{xk},\xi_{yk},\xi_{zk})$ generated in the parallelepiped which embeds the superimposed molecules M_E and M_S fall into the following three categories (see also Figure 10):

(i) $P_k(\xi_{xk},\xi_{yk},\xi_{zk})$, k=1,2,...,$N_N$, belong to a nonoverlapping zone of molecules M_E and M_S if it satisfies one and only one of the relations (7.3) or (7.4), i.e., one single inequality.

(ii) If points $P_k(\xi_{xk},\xi_{yk},\xi_{zk})$, k=1,2,...,$N_O$, satisfy simultaneously the relations (7.3) and (7.4) they fall into a zone in which the vdW envelopes of the two molecules overlap.

(iii) If points $P_k(\xi_{xk},\xi_{yk},\xi_{zk})$, k=1,2,...,$N_{EXT}$, satisfy neither of the equations (7.3) and (7.4) they fall outside the envelopes of both molecules, M_S and M_E.

The total number of generated random points is $N_T = N_N + N_O + N_{EXT}$.

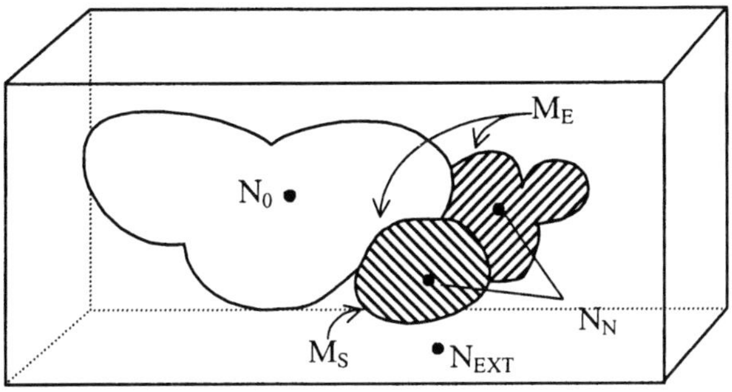

Figure 10. Principle of MCD calculation. The volume of the hatched zone represents MCD. N0 – total number of the overlapping zone of MS and ME; NN – total number of the nonoverlapping zone of MS and ME; NEXT – total number of points outside MS and ME (MS – standard molecule; ME – effector molecule).

For calculating the MCD parameter one generates a sequence of N_T random points uniformly distributed within the parallelepiped which embeds the superimposed vdW of two molecules, the standard M_S and the effector (drug molecule) M_E (see also, Section 5.2). Let V_P be the volume of this parallelepiped. Then, one selects from among the N_T points the N_N random points which are within the vdW envelope of one of the molecule but not within the other one (i.e., the points which satisfy only one single inequality, (7.3) or (7.4)). The MCD value is given by:

$$MCD = \frac{N_N}{N_T} \cdot V_P \tag{7.5}$$

This method was one of the first tentative[86] in formulating 3D-QSAR but its application in QSAR studies was limited to the study of substituent effects in haptenes, in their interaction with the anti-p,p'-azophenyl-azobenzoate antibody and for correlation enzymatic hydrolysis rates of N-glycosidic bonds in nucleosides,[32] with relatively poor results (r=0.680 and r=0.884, respectively). The computational difficulties of the 75's for us explain the abandonment of this idea and its further possible development. A certain similarity exists between MCD and Hopfinger's molecular shape analysis from the 80's.[5]

7.3. MTD – The Actual Improved Minimal Steric Difference Method

The importance of molecular stereochemistry for biological activity was recognized one hundred years ago, by Emil Fisher, with his "lock and key" theory for enzymatic reactions. Nevertheless, molecular stereochemistry has been included only relatively recently into QSAR's. The molecular areas directly involved in receptor-effector interactions are much larger than those involved in organic reactions and cannot be adequately described by the E_S-type constants used for steric effects in organic chemistry.[88] The steric fit depends upon both the shape of the biological receptor and upon that of the effector (drug molecule).

The MTD method, the minimal topological (steric) difference method, allows the description of molecular stereochemistry (of both receptor and effector molecules) by indicating the presence or absence of atoms from the considered M_i molecule (i=1,N) in the vertices of the hypermolecule, **H** (which describes the receptor). The hypermolecule is obtained by an approximately atom-by-atom superposition of the all M_i molecules, neglecting the hydrogen atoms. The hypermolecule **H** can be considered as a topological network in which the vertices correspond to atoms and edges may be viewed as chemical bonds.

During the optimization process, the vertices of **H** are assigned to the receptor cavity, to the receptor walls or to the exterior of cavity, that is the so-called steric irrelevant zone. The degree of steric misfit for the molecule M_i, i.e., the value of MTD_i, is defined as the sum of the number of cavity vertices of **H** unoccupied by M_i and the number of cavity vertices of **H** occupied by M_i. The whole number of **H** (meaning cavity, wall and irrelevant zone) obtained by the optimization procedure makes up a hypothetical steric receptor map.

The actual improved MTD method takes into consideration the (possible) conformational flexibility of the effectors M_i (considering for each M_i multiple low energy conformations) and the series of drugs with some compound for which only threshold bioactivities or their intervals are known. The cross-validation procedure is also used in order to assess the reliability of the obtained results. The method allows the separation of steric factors (measured by MTD_i values) from the others, such as hydrophobic, electrical, etc., that possibly control the biological response. If considerations of chemical, physical or biological nature indicate that the activities are dependent upon the factors $F_1, F_2, \ldots, F_M$ (M<N) expressed by the structural parameters P_{in}(i=1,N; n=1,M), these parameters can also be taken into consideration. The molecular mechanics techniques are used in the superposition process for designing the hypermolecule **H**.

*7.3.1 Description of molecular stereochemistry. The hypermolecule **H***

Let us consider N molecules M_i (i=1,2,...,N) having a common biological property P; this property is known and measurable. It is supposed that the values A_i of the biological activity are measured in the same conditions for all the M_i compounds, with the same accuracy and precision. For extending the applicability of this QSAR method we consider also the cases in which from the N molecules M_i, a part k=1,2,...,K (K<N) should have biological activities A_i less than a maximum value A_{max}, another part n=1,2,...,U (U<N) should have bioactivities A_i greater than a minimum value A_{min} and some of the molecules v=1,2,...,V (V<N) should have their A_i values in the interval [A_m-A_M]. On the basis of the above conditions, we want to obtain a QSAR using the minimal steric difference as a measure of steric misfit of the N effectors with respect to the receptor site. Minimal steric differences are obtained by comparing the shape of each molecule considered with respect to the shape of a hypothetical receptor site (the hypermolecule), with the use of a procedure which will be described later.

One obtains the hypermolecule **H** by approximate atom per atom superposition of the all (N) molecules of the database over the standard molecule (S; see Section 7.1), seeking maximal superposition. Such a superposition procedure is the basis for the description of molecular stereochemistry in the MTD method, and can be described as follows:

(1) The comparative orientation of the molecules to be superimposed is based upon a *pharmacophore model*, which should be regarded as a hypothesis of a three-dimensional chemical pattern shared by a set of compounds interacting at the same site with another molecule. In the absence of any molecular information concerning the receptor, a pharmacophore model once identified, should be regarded as a topographical and chemical-physical specification of the receptor and allows meaningful comparison of congeneric and/or non-congeneric molecules exhibiting the same biological action. For the enzymatic reactions, the "pharmacophore" may be considered as that atomic constellation of the substrate molecule, which is transformed during the reaction. Occasionally, this rule is supplemented with other criteria such as: the reactive groups, or the hydrogen-bonding groups, etc., of each molecule should be superimposed.

Actually, this process is performed interactively using the optimized geometries of the effector molecules, computed with the aid of molecular mechanics force fields[89] or, alternatively, a classical 2D chemical formulas.

Efforts to extract three-dimensional information regarding effector – (unknown) receptor (E–R) interaction from measurements of potency are generally centered on the QSAR domain,[90] and appropriate characterization of the molecular shape is the major obstacle in the development of a topographical basis for QSAR.

The space occupied by a molecule can be conveniently defined in the framework of the hard-sphere approximation: each atom of the molecule is represented by an isotropic sphere centered at the equilibrium position (X_i,Y_i,Z_i) of the atomic nuclei $i=1,2,\ldots,N$ and having a radius equal to the vdW radius r_i^W. Thus, the molecules can be represented in 3D space by Equations (7.3) or (7.4) where (ξ_x,ξ_y,ξ_z) are the locus of points within the molecules.

(2) Once the relative orientation is defined, one superposes the molecules M_i one upon another atom by atom. Consider the molecules M_i, $i=1,2,\ldots,N$, which exhibit the biological activity via a common mode of action, and let M_k, 1 k N, be the most active compound in the database. It follows[33] in agreement with the drug-receptor theory,[91] that M_k is the best available "complementary copy" of the receptor site, including steric features; therefore, it may be considered as *reference structure* (S). Further, as the pharmacophore represents a logical frame of reference for the receptor, meaningful comparison of M_i, $i=1,2,\ldots,N$, with M_k can be achieved by geometrical congruence of M_i over M_k, requiring that the pharmacophore groups occupy approximately the same position. Small differences in bond lengths and bond angles are neglected, but one must not superimpose pairs of atoms linked by covalent bonds in one molecule upon unbound pairs of atoms of other molecules because vdW contact distances (of 3–4 Å) are much larger than covalent bonds (1.2–2 Å).

For each M_i, all conformations within a few RT units above the lowest energy conformation are selected. Since one is usually operating in the absence of any molecular information concerning the receptor, one can only put upper limits on the conformational space accessible to each of the compounds due to possible perturbations from the minimum energy conformation by interaction with the receptor. An ensemble of conformers that sample the conformational hyperspace must consequently represent each compound.

If one is dealing with a congeneric series and assumes a common binding mode, then an obvious frame of reference for comparison of analogs exists. In this case, one can determine all possible positions of atoms or groups (for each sterically allowed conformations) relative to a common reference point.

Comparison of different conformations of non-congeneric molecules for potential similarity requires some definition of criteria. One approach is to allow the chemist to postulate correspondences between functional groups with similar properties based on the available structure-reactivity data and to search for similar three-dimensional arrangements of such functional groups.

The superposition of the N molecules M_i yields a 2D or 3D hypermolecule **H**, in fact a topological (2D or 3D) network. This network consists of **m** vertices, j, corresponding to the approximate position of atoms (in 2D or 3D space) in the superimposed molecules, while the edges can be assimilated to chemical bonds between the atoms. The main purpose of **H** is to reflect the stereochemistry of drug molecules bound to the receptor site.

(3) The entities to be superimposed are second or higher row atoms, X or XH_n groups. The hydrogen atoms are "contracted" into the higher row atoms to which they are bound.

(4) **H** is used as a topological framework for describing the stereochemistry of the drug molecules and of the receptor sites by the vectors $\mathbf{X}=\{x_{ijk}\}$ and $\mathbf{V}=\{v_j\}$, i=1,2,...,N; j=1,2,...,m; k=1,2,...,C_i. The entry x_{ijk} is taken to be 1 if the vertex j of **H** is occupied by a non-hydrogen atom of the molecule i being in conformation k and $x_{ijk} = 0$ if it is not occupied. Alternatively, the vector **X** may contain the corresponding fragmental vdW volumes or hydrophobic constants, MR (molar refraction) or other structural parameters for exhaustive investigation of receptor space.

The stereochemistry of the receptor site is described by the vector **V**, having as elements a ternary parameter v_j (j=1,m), associated to each vertex j; v_j=-1 should correspond to vertices situated in the cavity of the receptor site, v_j=+1 are assigned to the receptor walls, and v_j=0 represent the vertices situated outside of the receptor. Thus, the hypermolecule, which simulates the receptor site in the optimization process, is divided into **m** cells (that can be approximated by the mean values of vdW volumes of the corresponding atoms) by the N molecules M_i that "investigate" the receptor space.

(5) If a molecule M_i has several low energy conformations, it will adopt the one that fits best to the receptor, i.e., that conformation with the lowest MTD value. For a given receptor map represented by the vector **V**, the MTD value for the molecule i, MTD_i, is given by:

$$MTD_{ik} = \left(s + \sum_{j=1}^{m} v_j \cdot x_{ijk} \right); \quad MTD_i = \min_k (MTD_{ik}) \tag{7.6}$$

where m and s stand for the number of **H** vertices, and the number of cavity vertices, respectively.

If the descriptor $\mathbf{X}=\{x_{ijk}\}$ contains other (fragmental) structural parameters, the value of MTD_i is calculated as follows,

$$MTD_{ik} = \left(s + \sum_{j=1}^{m} f_j \cdot v_j \cdot x_{ijk} \right); \quad MTD_i = \min_k (MTD_{ik}) \tag{7.7}$$

where the vector $\mathbf{F}=\{f_j\}$, j=1,m, contains either maximal or minimal values from vector $\mathbf{X}=\{x_{ijk}\}$, and, also, the corresponding mean values. In the MTD procedure, these hypotheses can be tested successively, supposing that the receptor site accommodates maximum, minimum or mean values of atom characteristics from effector molecules.

7.3.2 Significance of the V assignments

The three types of vertex assignments, v_j=-1, 0 or +1, were defined as that vertex belongs to the cavity, to exterior or to the walls of the receptor site. The meaning of these assignments, for the series of considered molecules, is as follows: the occupation of the j vertex produces a beneficial, irrelevant or detrimental effect upon the biological activity. Obviously, this is an approximation; these effects do not necessarily correspond to the location of the j vertex in the cavity, exterior or wall region.[9,Ch.1]

Consider a vertex located in the receptor cavity, but near to the wall boundary. For atoms occupying this vertex, attractive and repulsive effects may be about equal. In this case, it is possible that the optimization procedure will assign a value of v_j=0 to this vertex. Another possible situation appears if a hydrophobic receptor cavity contains a proton donor group near a certain **x** cavity vertex. The assignment of **x** vertex will be v_x=-1 if, in the series under study, this vertex is occupied mostly by proton acceptor atoms. But, if mostly hydrophobic or proton donating atoms occupy the vertex **x**, the resulted assignments will be v_x=0 or even v_x=+1. If the atoms of N molecules occupying this hydrophobic cavity are strongly hydrophobic, v_j=0 assignments will result for most of the cavity vertices.

The usage of other parameters (measuring various chemical or physical effects) together with MTD may change the vertex assignment of hypermolecule **H**. Thus, for a hydrophobic receptor cavity and a series of molecules with predominantly apolar character, the optimization procedure (see the following section) will assign to most cavity vertices the values v_j=-1 if only MTD is used as dependent variable. But, if the hydrophobicity (log P or π, for example) is introduced along with MTD to explain the biological activity, then the values v_j=0 will be assigned to a part of the cavity vertices; the hydrophobic properties of effectors will be the major factor of the attractive E-R interactions.

It is obvious that the original MTD method represents only a crude approximation of the drug-receptor (E-R) interaction. But it is certainly useful, even its topological character. One must be caution with the interpolation of vertex assignments.

The actual improved method realizes (sequentially) the investigation of receptor space from topological (2D), steric (3D), hydrophobic and electronic point of view.

7.3.3 The optimization procedure: mapping of receptor space

The MTD method assumes the equivalence of occupied wall vertices and of unoccupied cavity vertices and the linear decrease with MTD, of the receptor effector (drug) molecule affinity, as the simple MSD method (see Equation (7.1)). Actually, MTD_i = MSD if there are no v_j=0 vertices and if the collection of v_j=-1 vertices is considered as the S standard. From equation (7.6) we see that MTD_{ik} signifies the number of relevant, nonsuperposable atoms of the conformation k of the molecule, and hypermolecule **H**.

The mapping of receptor space for a given series of effectors optimizes[92] the (hypothetical) shape of the biological receptor by using the regressional analysis. The information for the description of the receptor is given as a set of experimental biological activities, A_i, for a N number of molecules M_i. It is supposed that the biological activities are measured in the same conditions for all the M_i compounds, with the same accuracy and precision. Also, if considerations of chemical, physical or biological nature indicate that the activities are dependent upon the factors $F_1, F_2, \ldots, F_M$, quantitatively expressed by the structural parameters P_{ij} (i=1,N; j=1,M), these parameters can also be taken as input values of the optimization procedure.

The structure of the receptor map (denoted here by **V**) obtained on the basis of the hypermolecule **H**, which is constructed by atom per atom superposition of all the molecules, M_i, is described by the vector **V**:

$$\mathbf{V} = \{v_j\}, j = 1, m \tag{7.8}$$

where

$$v_j = \begin{cases} -1 \text{ for the interior of the cavity (beneficial vertices),} \\ 0 \text{ for the steric irrelevant zone (irrelevant vertices),} \\ +1 \text{ for the cavity walls (detrimental vertices).} \end{cases}$$

The steric structure of the M_i molecules is described by the vector $\mathbf{X}=\{x_{ijk}\}$, i=1,N molecules in the data set, j=1,m vertices of **H** and k=1,C_i, when C_i is the number of conformations of molecules M_i, with x_{ijk} as δ Kronecker symbol:

$$x_{ijk} = \begin{cases} 1 \text{ if the molecule } M_i \text{ in conformation k contains a non - hydrogen atom in} \\ \text{ the j vertex of hypermolecule } \mathbf{H}; \\ 0 \text{ if the molecule } M_i \text{ does not occupy the j vertex.} \end{cases}$$

Also, the vector **X** may contain various molecules structural descriptors, which can be used sequentially for investigation of the receptor for conformation k,

$$x_{ijk} = \begin{cases} f_j - \text{a numerical value of structural descriptor of molecule } M_i \\ \qquad \text{corresponding to j vertex of } \mathbf{H} \\ 0 - \text{if the node j of } \mathbf{H} \text{ is not occupied by conformation } M_{ik} \end{cases}$$

The computational procedure implies the evaluation of the steric parameter MTD for each of the M_i molecules, with respect to the receptor map **V** by means of relations (7.6) and/or (7.7), with s defined as

$$s = \sum_{j=1}^{m} |v_j|, \qquad \text{for all } v_j = -1 \tag{7.9}$$

and/or

$$s = \sum_{j=1}^{m} f_j' \tag{7.10}$$

where f_j' are the maximum, minimum or mean values of the structural descriptors of M_i, i=1,N, corresponding to the vertex j of **H**.

One assumes that $\hat{A}_i$ (calculated A_i value) is defined by the following relation:

$$\hat{A}_i = \alpha + \sum_{n=1}^{M} \beta_n \cdot P_{in} - \beta_{M+1} \cdot MTD_i + z_i \tag{7.11}$$

where:

- $\mathbf{z_i}$ signifies a random variable which expresses the degree of non-concordance of the experimental data, A_i, with respect to the linear model (11). Thus, the z_i variables contain the experimental errors and the errors due to the accepted theoretical model. We have seen (in section 1 – Introduction) that the following supposition has been made: Z_i's are uncorrelated random variables with a zero mean value and a σ^2 dispersion.

- α is a constant; due to the inherent experimental errors, it is recommended to assign no physical significance to α.
- β_j, j=1,M+1, represent the regression coefficients. They express the sensitivity of the calculated biological activities, $\hat{A}_i$, with respect to the factors F_n, n=1,M+1. The β_n/β_{n+1} ratio expresses the relative weight of the F_n and F_{n+1} factors if and only if P_{in} and $P_{i(n+1)}$ are measured within the same scale.

Under the conditions specified above, α and β_n (n=1,M+1) of the relation (7.11) are determined by the least square method by minimizing, the sum of squares of the deviations of the calculated values, $\hat{A}_i$, from the experimental values, A_i (see Relation (1.1)). The concordance degree between the used data (A_i, MTD_i and P_{in}; i=1,N) and the theoretical model **V** of the receptor cavity may be evaluated by the correlation coefficient, r.

The $\hat{A}_i$ values depend upon the MTD_i parameter according to the following relation:

$$\hat{A}_i = \alpha + \sum_{n=1}^{M} \beta_n \cdot P_{1n} - \beta_{M+1} \cdot MTD_i \tag{7.12}$$

where M may be zero.

The correlation coefficient (r) has been used the optimization criterion. The fundamental of this method consists in modifying the topography of hypermolecule **H** by moving the cavity vertices to wall and to irrelevant zone, the irrelevant vertices to cavity and wall, and so on, until one obtains the best shape of the analyzed receptor, corresponding to the optimal model (7.12) as measured by correlation coefficient r.

By using the correlation coefficient r, the optimization process tries to estimate the quality of the model (7.12), both the initial ones and those obtained in the following steps:

s1) The initial receptor map (denoted S^0) is derived from **H** using a statistical analysis based on interquartile range.[93]

s2) The shape of the receptor site is changed vertex by vertex, with no restrictions – or, in the connectivity variant is imposed that cavity, wall and irrelevant vertices must form connected graphs, respectively – (using the order j=1,2,...,m) as follows:
(a) if v_j=0, then v_j=–1 and v_j=+1;
(b) if v_j=+1, then v_j=–1 and v_j=0;
(c) if v_j=–1, then v_j=0 and v_j=+1.

s3) One estimates the quality of the new model **V** of the receptor shape for each of the above mentioned cases (a), (b) and (c);

s4) One determines the maximal value of r (r_{max}) from a number of 2·m correlation coefficients and one retains the corresponding map of the receptor S=**V** (r_{max}).

s5) The resulted S map is considered as initial maps and the steps (s2) – (s4) are resumed.

s6) The procedure is stopped when the correlation coefficient obtained at step n, r_m is less than obtained at step n+1, r. The resulted S_n map is termed optimal and denoted by $S^* = \{v_j^*\}\, j = 1, m$. The $v_j^* = -1$ vertices within S^* define the optimal standard and the best shape of receptor is done by the vector $\mathbf{V} = \{v_j^*\}\, j = 1, m$.

It is easy to observe that equation (7.12), for M=0, attributes the whole variance of the observed biological response to MTD parameter and, because the MTD's change during the optimization procedure, the "optimal" MTD value, MTD^*, will code globally the steric and non-steric factors which may control the biological response. One should be aware that, in order to use MTD as a steric parameter, it is mandatory to take into account the non-steric factors that may control the biological response (that is M=1,2,...).

The use of connectivity rules eliminates the appearance of isolated irrelevant vertices and forces all cavity vertices to form a connected graph.

Consideration of several low energy conformations for each molecule was discussed at length in a MTD paper about substituted acetic acid derivatives with auxinic activity.[94] Low energy difference with respect to the one of lowest energy is not large in comparison to the mean thermal energy, kT. In most of the published MTD works, if several low energy conformations are possible for some molecules of the considered series, the MTD value considered for each molecule was checked for being the lowest among those corresponding to the low energy conformations.

The tendency of the MTD-optimization method to yield different optimized receptor maps (local minimums) when beginning with different start map S^0, and, also, to yield maps with interspersed cavity, wall and exterior vertices can be limited by imposing different restrictions on the optimization strategy. For example, we can consider (during the optimization procedure and for the optimized map, S^*) only maps in which all cavity vertices and wall vertices form a unique connected set within the hypermolecule considered as a topological network. Experience with MTD-QSAR's, especially the results obtained for test series, suggest that this limitation is too stringent and that the restriction of a unique connected network, applied to the cavity vertices, gives better results.[CRC,20]

The technique used in MTD to assess predictive ability of a QSAR is cross-validation in which one pretends that one or more of the known experimental values are in fact unknown. The analysis being cross-validated is repeated, excluding the temporarily "unknown" compounds, from the very beginning. The resulting equation is used to predict the experimental measurements for the omitted compound (s), and the resulting individual squared errors of prediction are accumulated. The cross-validation cycle is repeated, leaving out one (or more) different compound(s), until each compound has been excluded and predicted exactly once. The result of cross-validation is the predictive discrepancy sum of squares, sometimes called PRESS (Predictive REsidual Sum of Squares):

$$\mathrm{PRESS} = \sum_{i=1}^{N} \left(A_i - \hat{A}_i\right)^2 \tag{7.13}$$

one chooses the "best" subset regression. This will have a comparatively small predictive sum of squares (PRESS) but not involve too many predictors. The PRESS is a measure of the predictive power of the model with the given complexity for the given data set.

In the actual variant of MTD method we apply the "half leave out" model, that is the half of the data is used to generate the model (7.12) and the other half to validate it,[3] and the PRESS value is transformed in a dimensionless term, called cross-validation coefficient, r_{CV}^2:

$$r_{CV}^2 = 1 - \frac{\mathrm{PRESS}}{\sum \left(A_i - \bar{A}\right)^2} \tag{7.14}$$

The cross-validation coefficient is the complement to the fraction of unexplained variance over the total variance.

Unfortunately, cross-validation results neither offer a guarantee for the validity nor for the non-validity of a model. If there is a high degree of redundancy in the chemical structures of the compounds, the common leave-one-out cross-validation will give results that are too optimistic. Therefore, we use a separation of the data set into two groups, a reciprocally training set and test set of equal size.

7.3.4 Application

We present here an application of the MTD method in a QSAR study for acetylcholinesterase catalyzed hydrolysis rates of a series of 25 acetic acid esters.[95] Conformations were selected according to their energies calculated by the COSMIC modeling program.[96] Information from an X-ray crystallographic study, together with results of conformational energy calculations was used for building up the hypermolecule. We used the molecule computations of conformational energy in order to assess the conformations, which must be considered for the multiconformational MTD method. The multiconformational results have been compared with those of a classical Hansch QSAR. The cross-validation procedure, each containing 50% of the molecules, was also used with two series. The effectors, together with acetylcholinesterase hydrolysis rates $\left(A = \lg {}^{k_{cat}}\!/_{k}\right)$ and structural data are listed in Table 7.1.

Table 7.1 Acetic acid esters, CH_3-COOR, acetylcholinesterase hydrolysis rates[97] and structural parameter.

i	R	A	σ^*	π	$-E_S$	j for x_{ijk}=1
	C_6H_5	6.72	0.60	2.13	0.38	2–6
	$CH_2CH_2C(CH_3)_3$	6.30	0.00	2.98	0.40	4–8
	$CH_2CH_2SC_2H_5$	5.40	0.22	1.95	0.44	5–7, 9
	$CH_2SC_2H_5$	5.35	0.56	1.45	0.44	5–7; 4–6; 5, 6, 8
	$CH_2CH_2CH(CH_3)_2$	5.32	0.00	2.30	0.43	4–7; 4–6, 8; 5–8
	$CH_2CH_2NO_2$	5.20	0.62	1.31	0.40	4–7; 4–6, 8; 5–8
	CH_2CH_2Cl	5.02	0.39	1.39	0.48	5, 6; 6, 10
	CH_2CH CH	4.81	0.55	0.94	0.60	6, 11
	n-C_5H_{11}	4.74	0.00	2.50	0.40	5–7, 9
	n-C_7H_{15}	4.75	0.00	3.50	0.40	5-7, 9, 12, 13
	$(CH_2)_4SC_2H_5$	4.73	0.03	2.95	0.40	5-7, 9, 12, 13
	cyclo-C_6H_{11}	4.71	0.00	2.51	0.98	2–6
	n-C_4H_9	4.72	0.00	2.00	0.40	4-6; 5, 6, 8; 5–7
	n-C_6H_{13}	4.68	0.00	3.00	0.40	5-7, 6, 12
	$(CH_2)_3SC_2H_5$	4.67	0.08	2.45	0.40	5–7, 9, 12
	$CH_2C_6H_5$	4.66	0.25	2.26	0.38	5–7, 10, 14, 15
	$CH_2CH(CH_3)_2$	4.32	0.00	1.80	0.35	5, 6, 10
	$CH_2CH=CH_2$	4.10	0.23	1.23	0.20	5, 6; 6, 10
	n-C_3H_7	3.91	0.00	1.50	0.39	5, 6; 6, 10
	$CH(CH_3)C_2H_5$	3.69	0.00	1.80	0.93	1, 5, 6; 2, 5, 6
	C_2H_5	3.36	0.00	1.00	0.36	6
	CH_3	3.00	0.20	0.50	0.07	–
	$CH(CH_3)_2$	2.72	0.00	1.30	0.93	1, 2; 2, 6
	$C(CH_3)_3$	1.30	0.00	1.98	1.74	1, 2, 6
	$C(CH_3)_2C_2H_5$	1.30	0.00	2.48	1.74	1-3, 6; 1, 2, 5, 6

Järv et al. formulated various regression equations by using π (for hydrophobic effect); they obtained good results ($r>0.950$), but only for series of at most $N=15$ molecules.

We used all the molecules from Table 7.1 to obtain a QSAR with these three parameters. The results are:

$$\hat{A}_i = 3.11(\pm 0.50) + 3.00(\pm 0.68)\cdot \sigma_i^* + 0.97(\pm 0.20)\cdot \pi_i + \\ + 1.94(\pm 0.33)\cdot E_{S(i)} \quad (7.15)$$

$$(N = 25; s = 0.65; F(3,21) = 24.6; r = 0.883; r_{CV}^2 = 0.658)$$

The correlation coefficient r=0.883 is rather modest, but significant. The cross-validation procedure was applied in two different manners. Firstly, we applied the usual leave-one-out and $r_{CV}^2 = 0.658$ was obtained. In the second procedure (more stronger because it avoids chance correlation), the molecules from Table 7.1, listed in decreasing order of experimental activities, A_i, are divided into two series, the ODD one (i=1,3,5,...,25) and EVEN one (i=2,4,6,...,24). Correlation equations were set up, separately, for these two sub-series and the activities $\hat{A}_{i(ODD)}$ were calculated with the correlation equation obtained for the EVEN sub-series and *vice versa*. With this second procedure in which the data series is divided reciprocally into a training set and a test set, was obtained the following cross-validation coefficient: $r_{CV}^2 = 0.577$.

The obtained results (see Equation (7.15)) indicate a strong increasing effect upon enzymatic hydrolysis rates of electron attracting R groups, and also an increasing effect of hydrophobicity. The E_S steric constants have a decreasing effect, the bulky R groups slow down the reaction rates.

In order to build up the hypermolecule **H** (see Figure 13) the internal energies if the conformations k, U_{ik} (i=1,N), will be calculated by means of COSMIC force fields.[23] Because the mean value for the regression coefficient β for MTD is about $\beta \cong -0.7$, corresponding to ~1 kcal/mole per MTD unit,[32] we used an upper limit for U_{ik} of 0.5 kcal/mole above the energy U_{i1} of the lowest energy conformer. In superposing the atoms of molecules upon vertices of the hypermolecule used 0.5 Å as maximal distance between an atom and the position of the vertex upon which it is to be superimposed.

The following considerations are taken into account in order to build-up the hypermolecule **H**:

(a) According to X-ray analysis data of acetylcholinesterase,[98] acetylcholine is, within the receptor cavity, in an all *trans* conformation of the $-O-CH_2-CH_2-N$ moiety, and the rest of the molecule.
(b) The most active compounds (i=1 with R = C_6H_5 and i=2, with R = $CH_2CH_2C(CH_3)_3$, isosteric with acetylcholine; see Table 7.1) will be considered as a basis for the framework of the hypermolecule.
(c) Only low energy conformations (less then 0.5 kcal/mole above the lowest energy conformation) have been considered and unnecessarily introductions of new vertices have been avoided.

The computations of conformational energies were performed with the aid of COSMIC molecular modeling computer package,[96] with D=4.0 for the dielectric constant. Molecular conformations for acetic acid esters with aliphatic R group are presented in Figure 11.

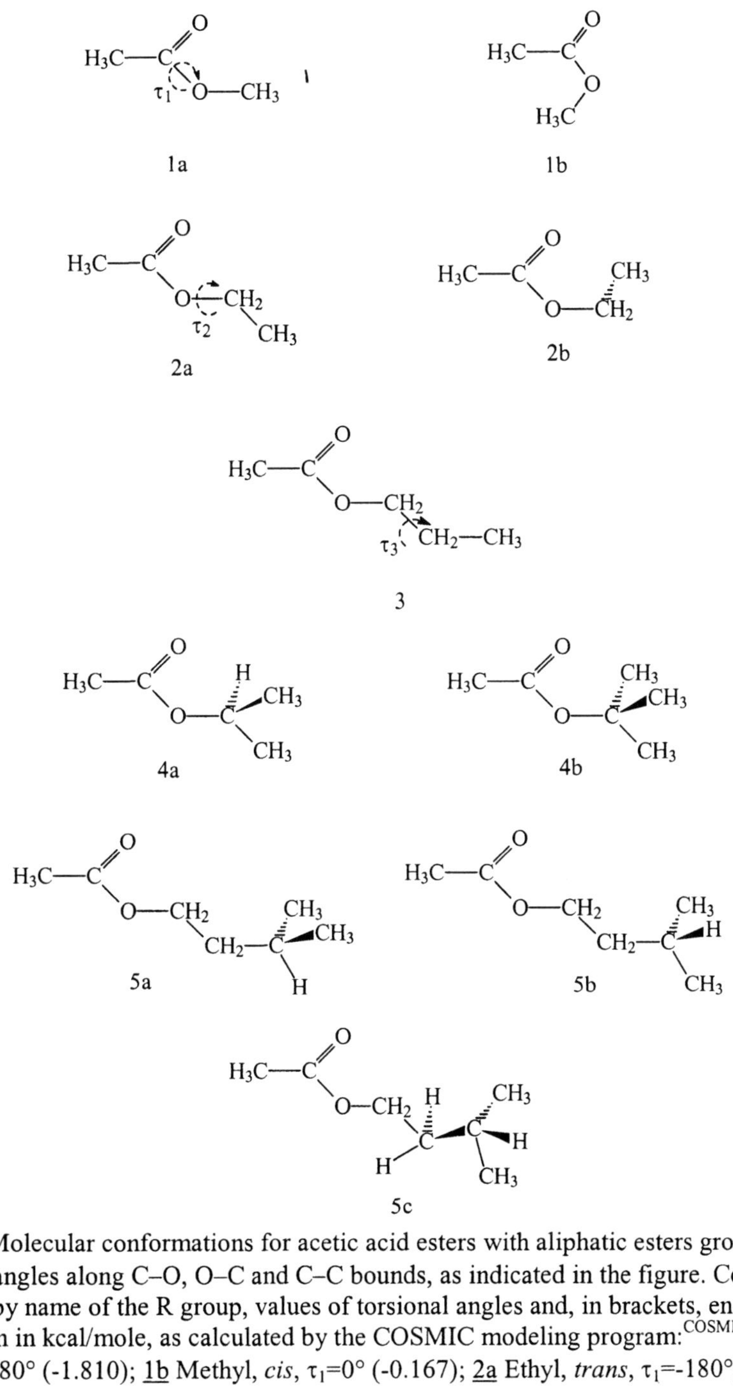

Figure 11. Molecular conformations for acetic acid esters with aliphatic esters group, R; τ_1, τ_2, τ_3-torsional angles along C–O, O–C and C–C bounds, as indicated in the figure. Conformations indicated by name of the R group, values of torsional angles and, in brackets, energy of the conformation in kcal/mole, as calculated by the COSMIC modeling program:[COSMIC] 1a Methyl, *trans*, τ_1=-180° (-1.810); 1b Methyl, *cis*, τ_1=0° (-0.167); 2a Ethyl, *trans*, τ_1=-180°, τ_2=-179.3° (-2.100); 2b Ethyl, *gauche*, τ_1=-180°, τ_2=+72.9° (-1.348); 3 n-Propyl, *trans-trans*, τ_1=τ_2=τ_3=180° (-1.826); 4a i-Propyl, τ_1=1.67.6°, τ_2=72° (-2.850); 4b i-Propyl, τ_2=-192° (-1.587); 5a (3-Methyl)-Butyl, *trans-trans-gauche*, (-2.289); 5b (3-Methyl)-Butyl, *trans-trans-gauche*, (-2.517); 5c (3-Methyl)-Butyl *trans-gauche-trans*, (-2.271).

For the simplest compound, CH_3COOCH_3 (Table 7.1; i=22) the energy barrier between the two conformations **1a** and **1b** (for $\tau_1 = 90°$) is 9.59 kcal/mole; consequently, only conformation **1a** has been considered. For i=21 (R = C_2H_5) the all *trans* conformation **2a** is the most stable one. For i=19 (R = n-C_3H_7), the *trans-trans* conformation **3** ($\tau_2 = \tau_3 = -180°$) is more stable one ($U_{19,1}$=-1.826 kcal/mole) but the *trans-gauche* conformations ($\tau_3 = \pm 61.6°$) are only slightly less stable ($U_{19,2}$=$U_{19,3}$=-1.753 kcal/mole). For i=23 (R = $CH(CH_3)_2$ and i=5 (R = $CH_2CH_2CH(CH_3)_2$) there are several low energy conformations (see **4a**, **4b**, **5a**, **5b**, **5c** from Figure 11). Conformations differing only in rotation of CH_3 groups give small energy variations and are not considered here. As a conclusion, for normal aliphatic chains, all *trans* conformations are favored.

The conformations for R = cyclic groups are presented in Figure 12.

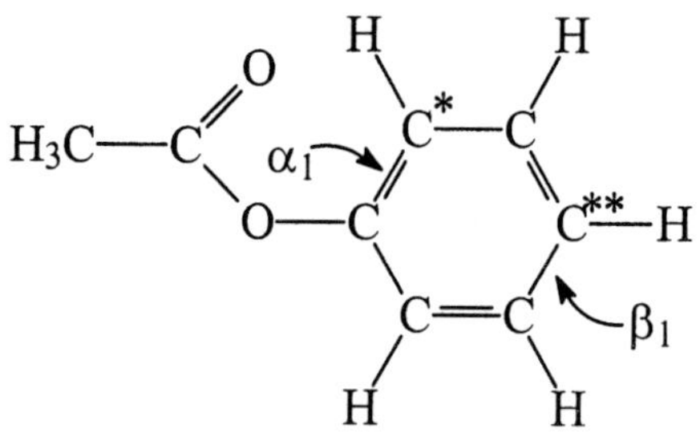

6

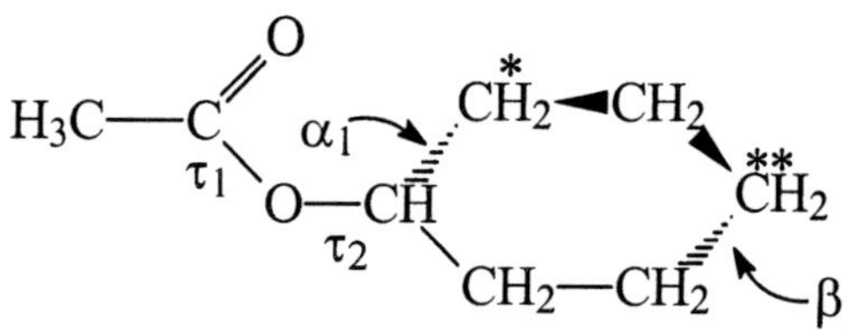

7

Figure 12. Molecular conformations for acetic acid esters with phenyl and cyclohexyl esteric groups. Dihedral angle α – between the acetyl group plane and the phenyl group plane in compound 6, and between the acetyl group plane and the O–C–C* plane in compound 7. Dihedral angle β, for molecule 7, between the lower C–C–C plane of the cyclohexyl ring and the C–C–C* plane of the same ring. For the rest, see legend of Figure 11. Compound 6: Phenyl, α_1=β_2=32.6° (3.209); Compound 7: Cyclohexyl, α_{12}=72°, β_{12}=57.7° (-0.307). Atoms marked with asterisk in the phenyl and cyclohexyl ring, occupy vertex j=2 of the hypermolecule in Figure 13, C^{**}-vertex is j=4.

It is possible to superpose the substituents phenyl (R=C_6H_5) and cyclohexyl (R=C_6H_{11}). If one analyses comparatively the corresponding structures 6 and 7 (see Figure 12), the largest interatomic distances appear for the C atoms marked with one and two asterisks (C^* and C^{**}). The distance between the atoms C^* of structures 6 and 7, respectively, is:

$$d\left(C^* - C^{**}\right) \approx \left(\alpha_{12} - \alpha_1\right)_{rad} \cdot D_{C-C} \cdot \cos 28° \qquad (7.16)$$

When applying formula (7.17) to structures from Figure 12 (with the given data from the figure) one obtains $d\left(C^* - C^{**}\right) \approx 0.92$ Å. A vertex (j=2 in the hypermolecule presented in Figure 13) positioned at the middle of this interatomic distance will be at less than the

0.5Å – interatomic distance limit among the two C^* atoms; these atoms can be superposed upon the vertex. The same is true for the pair of C^{**} atoms; these can be superposed upon another vertex (j=4 in Figure 13).[95]

The hypermolecule resulted from the superposition of all molecules from Table 7.1 is depicted in Figure 13.

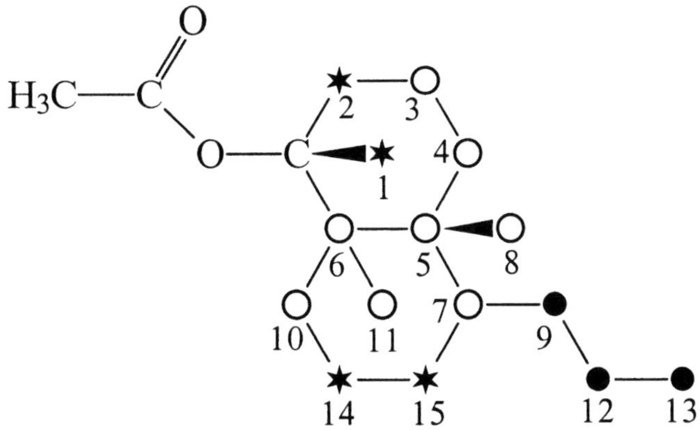

Figure 13. Hypermolecule, vertex (j)-numeration and optimised receptor map, S*, for the molecules of Table 7.1. Vertexes occupied in all molecules are not numbered.
O – cavity vertices (j = -1); ✶ – wall vertices (j = +1); ● – irrelevant vertices (j = 0).

The molecules of the various compounds are superposed such as to have a maximal superposition upon $R=CH_2CH_2C(CH_3)_3$ and $R=C_6H_5$. If more than one conformation fulfills such a requirement, the lowest energy conformation is preferred; other conformations are considered if their energy is not more than 0.5 kcal/mole above the lowest energy one. For example, for $R=C_2H_5$ (i=21), only *trans* conformation, corresponding to occupation of vertex j=6 is considered because the *gauche* conformations with occupation of j=1 or j=2 are 0.7 kcal/mole higher. For $R=C_3H_7$ (i=19), also the *gauche* conformation (τ_2=-180°, τ_3=61.6°), corresponding to occupation of j=6 and j=10 is considered, which is only 0.1 kcal/mole above the *trans-trans* conformation (see 3, Figure 11); it occupies vertices j=5 and j=6. For $R=CH_2CH(CH_3)_2$ (i=17), only the conformation 4a is considered (j=5,6,10 from **H**), because it is easy superposable upon $R=CH_2C_6H_5$ (i=16).

Other conformations, with only slightly higher energies would introduce some unnecessary vertices. For similar reasons we considered a single conformation for longer aliphatic chains, such as $n\text{-}C_6H_{13}$, $n\text{-}C_7H_{15}$ or $(CH_2)_4SC_2H_5$.

Only the σ^* (Taft) electronic constant was considered as a second structural parameter for QSAR study by MTD approach. The start map, S^0, was chosen with vertices j=4–8 as cavity vertices, occupied by $R=CH_2CH_2N^+(CH_3)_3$ in acetylcholine (the natural substrate) and j=1 as wall vertex.

$$S^0 = \begin{cases} j(v=-1): 4-8 \\ j(v=0): 2,3,9-15 \\ j(v=+1): 1 \end{cases} \qquad r_0 = 0.888$$

A rather good explanation for the decreasing order of biological activities, A_i (Table 7.1), is obtained, with r=0.888, if MTD values are considered with respect to S_0 as well as σ^* (electronic Taft constant). The optimized receptor map and correlation equations are:

$$S^* = \begin{cases} j(v=-1): 3-8,10,11 \\ j(v=0): 9,12,13 \\ j(v=+1): 1,2,14,15 \end{cases}$$

$$\begin{aligned} \hat{A}_i &= 8.43(\pm 0.43) + 1.68(\pm 0.46)\cdot\sigma_i^* - 0.75(\pm 0.07)\cdot \mathrm{MTD}_i^* \\ &(N = 25; s = 0.49; F(2,22) = 72.0; r = 0.931; r_{CV}^2 = 0.661) \end{aligned} \tag{7.17}$$

Introduction of π and E_S into the correlation yields to the following regression equation:

$$\begin{aligned} \hat{A}_i &= 7.19(\pm 0.91) + 1.90(\pm 0.52)\cdot\sigma_i^* + 0.26(\pm 0.20)\cdot\pi_i + \\ &+ 0.81(\pm 0.33)\cdot E_{S,i} - 0.55(\pm 0.11)\cdot \mathrm{MTD}_i^* \\ &(N = 25; s = 0.45; F(4,20) = 44.6; r = 0.948) \end{aligned} \tag{7.18}$$

but the coefficient of π (0.26) must be rejected (see Equation (7.18): the confidence limits are ±0.20). If one introduces only the E_S values into the correlation (besides σ^* and MTD^*), the coefficient of this parameter is also rejected from the obtained equation. Thus, equation (7.17) can be considered the best correlation obtained.

For cross-validation the molecules in Table 7.1, ranking into decreasing A_i values, were separated into two subseries, ODD (i=1,3,5,…,25) and EVEN (i=2,4,6,…24). The two inversions i=9/10 and i=12/13 were performed in order to have vertices j=2,12,13 both in the two subseries. The optimized map S^* was used as starting map (S^0) for both subseries. For the ODD subseries, and, respectively, the EVEN subseries one obtains:

$$S_{ODD}^* = \begin{cases} j(v=-1): 3-8,10 \\ j(v=0): 9,12,13 \\ j(v=+1): 1,2 \end{cases}$$

$$\begin{aligned} \hat{A}_{ODD} &= 8.71 + 3.5\cdot\sigma^* - 0.83\cdot \mathrm{MTD}^* \\ &(n = 13; r = 0.971) \end{aligned} \tag{7.19}$$

$$S^{*}_{EVEN} = \begin{cases} j(v=-1): 3-5,7,8,10,11 \\ j(v=0): 6,9,12-14 \\ j(v=+1): 1,2,15 \end{cases}$$

$$\hat{A}_{EVEN} = 8.52 + 0.56\cdot\sigma^{*} - 0.76\cdot MTD^{*} \quad (n=12; r=0.962) \tag{7.20}$$

MTD and Â values were calculated for the molecules from the ODD subseries with S_{EVEN} and equation (7.19), and vice versa. The molecules i=8, the only one in which j=11 is occupied, had to be excluded from cross-validation. The cross-validation result is

$$r^2_{CV} = 0.661; \qquad n = 23 \tag{7.21}$$

which is to be compared with $r^2_{CV} = 0.577$, obtained with the Hansch type equation (7.15). If the usual "leave one out" cross-validation procedure is used for equation (7.17) one obtains $r^2_{CV} = 0.795$ (the corresponding cross-validation coefficient for equation (7.15) is $r^2_{CV} = 0.658$).

The correlation results of this multiconformational MTD study, $r = 0.931$ for a correlation equation with σ^*-Taft and MTD as structural parameters and $r^2_{CV} = 0.661$ for cross-validation coefficient (with explained variance of 0.855 and good statistical test results) as compared to a classical Hansch QSAR with σ^*, π, and E_S as structural parameters (Equation (7.15), explained variance EV=0.747), indicate the success and significant predictive power of the multiconformational MTD method.

The enzyme acetylcholinesterase and its complex with the substrate, acetylcholine, were studied by X-ray analysis at a 2.8Å resolution. Our QSAR study brings nevertheless a significant contribution to the study of this enzymatic reaction. The positive effect of σ^* (i.e., of electron withdrawing esteric R groups) is in agreement with the general nature of this hydrolytic reaction. Details about steric effects are also added to X-ray analysis and the model studies that indicate the binding of the trimethylammonium cation of acetylcholine to an aromatic cavity of the enzyme binding site. The enzyme cavity that accommodates acetylcholine is rather similar in shape to acetylcholine, but somewhat *larger* as indicated by the receptor map in Figure 13.

7.4. SDM – The Similarity/Dissimilarity Measure

The computation of molecular similarity or dissimilarity of chemical bioactive compounds is a very important and fascinating research field for drug designers. Generally, molecules can be described in three distinct ways: (i) by their molecular graphs; (ii) by their atom position, and (iii) by their molecular fields. The quantitative similarity measure can be developed for each of the above molecular characteristics.

7.4.1 Introduction

Molecules of similar biochemical activity often show common 3D shape and size features. Consequently, the characterization of the shape and size of formal molecular bodies and the recognition, description and, ultimately, the numerical evaluation of similarity among molecules are of major importance in modern pharmaceutical research, as well as in pesticide and herbicide chemistry. The analysis of molecular shape and size is an important component of research aimed at the elucidation of drug-receptor interactions and in studies of quantitative structure-activity relationships in contemporary drug design.[33]

Shape and size similarity and complementarity are fundamental principles of biochemistry, relevant to the properties of both stable macromolecular structures and transition structures of biochemical reactions. There is a strong tradition in research efforts towards the quantitative interpretation of chemical properties in terms of structural features of molecules.[4,98] In most physical organic chemistry studies, as well as in most synthesis design, molecular design and QSAR (Quantitative Structure-Activity Relationships) analysis,[32] the concept of structure is usually interpreted in terms of *graphs* depicting formal bonding patterns and structural diagrams which describe the 3D versions of these bonding patterns.

The analysis of shape and size of sequences of molecules with known chemical, biochemical and pharmacological properties in terms of similarity/dissimilarity measures can answer the question of *what* structural features are important for a given effect, even if one does not fully understand *why*. The results of such analysis can be used directly to predict biochemical activity of new molecules.

The aim of this work is to present a new quantitative index that can be used as both similarity and dissimilarity measure for QSAR studies.[98] It was developed starting from minimal steric difference (MSD) parameter by applying the methods of pattern recognition approach. This new structural parameter (denoted by SDM) was applied, with good results, to the study of detoxification process performed in human bodies within P-450 cytochrome by microsomal p-hydroxylation of aniline by alcohols, as described later.

7.4.2 Theory

The idea of measure of similarity comes from cluster analysis, a field of pattern recognition techniques.[4]

Recognition is regarded as a basic attribute of human beings, as well as other living organisms. A pattern is the description of an object. We are performing acts of recognition every instant of our waking lives. But, the problem of pattern recognition may be regarded as one discriminating the input data, not between individual patterns but between populations, via the search for features or invariant attributes among members of a population.

Starting from the study of the pattern recognition capability of human beings and other living organisms one has been developed the theory and techniques for the design of devices capable of performing a given recognition task for a specific application.

The design of an automatic pattern recognition system generally involves several major problem areas. The first one is concerned with the representation of input data, which can be measured from the objects to be recognized. Each measured quantity x_i, i=1,n describes a characteristic of the pattern or object. Thus, a vector X can describe an object (for example, a molecule):

$$\mathbf{X} = \begin{pmatrix} x_1 \\ x_2 \\ \vdots \\ x_n \end{pmatrix} \tag{7.22}$$

The pattern vectors contain all the measured information in the form of real numbers. When the measurements yield information in the form of real numbers, it is often useful to think of a pattern vector as a point $X(x_1,x_2,..,x_n)$ in an n-dimensional Euclidean space. The set of patterns belonging to the same class corresponds to an ensemble of points scattered within some region of the measurement space. (see, for a bidimensional pattern space the Figure 14)

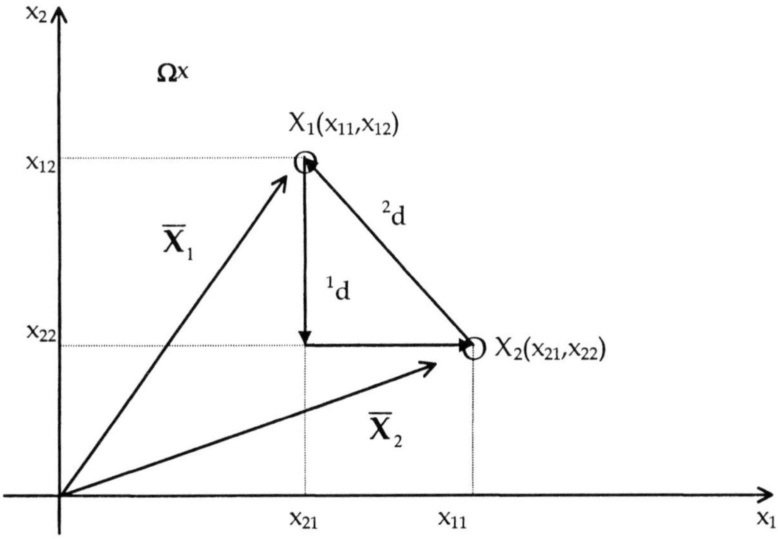

Figure 14. The bidimensional pattern space defined by two characteristics, x_1 and x_2. The patterns ω_1 and ω_2 are represented either by the vectors X_1 and X_2 or by the points $X_1(x_{11},x_{12})$ and $X_2(x_{21},x_{22})$; ${}^2d$ is the Euclidean distance and ${}^1d$ is the Manhattan (City-Block) distance.

The second problem in pattern recognition concerns the extraction of characteristic features or attributes from the received input data and the reduction of the dimensionality of pattern vectors. This is often referred to as preprocessing and feature extraction problem.

The third problem in pattern recognition system design involves the determination of optimum decision procedures, which are needed in the identification and classification process.

When the patterns of a class are vectors whose components are real numbers, a pattern class can be characterized by its clustering properties in the pattern space. The design of a pattern recognition system based on this general concept is guided by the relative geometrical arrangement of the various pattern clusters. If the classes are characterized by the clusters that are far apart, simple recognition schemes such as the minimum-distance classifiers may be successfully employed. Thus, considering M pattern classes $\omega_1, \omega_2,..,\omega_M$ which can be characterized by single prototype patterns $\mathbf{Z}_1,\mathbf{Z}_2,..,\mathbf{Z}_M$, the Euclidean distance between an arbitrary pattern vector **X** and the ith prototype is given by

$$D_i = \|\mathbf{X} - \mathbf{Z}_i\| = \sqrt{(\mathbf{X} - \mathbf{Z}_i)'(\mathbf{X} - \mathbf{Z}_i)} \tag{7.23}$$

where ( )' signifies the transpose vector. A minimum-distance classifier computes the distance from a pattern **X** of unknown classification to the prototype of each class, and assigns the pattern to the class to which it is closest. In other words, **X** is assigned to class ω_i if $D_i < D_j$, for all $j \neq i$.

The ability to determine characteristic prototypes or cluster centers in a given set of data plays a central role in the design of pattern classifiers based on the minimum-distance concept. To define a data cluster, it is necessary to first assigning patterns to the domain of a particular cluster center. The Euclidean distance between two patterns **X** and **Z**, as expressed by relation (7.23), is a measure of their similarity: the smaller the distance, the greater the similarity. *The algorithm developed in this paper for calculating SDM parameter is based on this general concept.*

There are, however, other meaningful distance measures, such as the Mahalanobis distance from **X** to **m**, expressed as follows,

$$D = (\mathbf{X} - \mathbf{m})'\mathbf{C}^{-1}(\mathbf{X} - \mathbf{m}) \tag{7.24}$$

In equation (7.24) **C** is the covariance matrix of a pattern population, **m** is the mean vector, and **X** represents a variable pattern. This is a useful measure of similarity when statistical properties are being explicitly considered.

Measures of similarity are not restricted to distance measures. For example, the following nonmetric similarity function

$$S(\mathbf{X}, \mathbf{Y}) = \frac{\mathbf{X}'\mathbf{Z}}{\|\mathbf{X}\| \cdot \|\mathbf{Z}\|} \tag{7.25}$$

represents the cosine of the angle between the vectors **X** and **Z**. This measure of similarity is useful when cluster regions tend to develop along principal axes, being maximum when **X** and **Y** are oriented in the same direction with respect to the origin.

When the patterns under consideration are binary valued with 0,1 elements, the similarity function of equation (7.25) may be given an interesting non-geometrical interpretation. Thus, if a binary pattern **X** possesses the ith attribute as $x_i=1$, then the term **X'Z** in equation (7.25) is simply the number of attributes shared by **X** and **Y**, while

$$\|\mathbf{X}\| \cdot \|\mathbf{Z}\| = \sqrt{(\mathbf{X}'\mathbf{X})(\mathbf{Z}'\mathbf{Z})}$$

is the geometrical mean of the number of attributes possessed by **X** and the number possessed by **Z**. In this case the similarity function $S(\mathbf{X},\mathbf{Y})$ is, therefore, seen to be a measure of common attributes possessed by the binary vectors **X** and **Y**.

A binary variation of equation (7.25), which has received attention in information retrieval, nosology and taxonomy, is the so-called Tanimoto measure, which is given by

$$S_T(\mathbf{X},\mathbf{Z}) = \frac{\mathbf{X}'\mathbf{Z}}{\mathbf{X}'\mathbf{X} + \mathbf{Z}'\mathbf{Z} - \mathbf{X}'\mathbf{Z}} \tag{7.26}$$

The Tanimoto similarity measure is useful because it extracts only the position of the two patterns which are almost exactly matched but it has an important disadvantage: the tolerance level will be data-dependent and it does not work on very dissimilar molecules.[4]

The similarity measures presented above are typical. But, the following discussion is based on the Euclidean similarity measure given in equation (7.23) because of its simple interpretation in terms of the familiar concept of proximity. However, since the proximity of two patterns is a *relative* measure of similarity, it is usually necessary to establish a threshold in order to define degrees of acceptable similarity in cluster-seeking process. To do this *we consider each bioactive molecule from the series under QSAR study as a cluster prototype, that is the number of molecules represents even the number of clusters and the threshold is given by its corresponding bioactivities (experimentally determined).*

7.4.3 Development of SDM Parameter

Molecular similarity (or dissimilarity) is a term that means different things because when we consider for comparison two or more molecules we may be thinking of their molecular formulas, their molecular graphs, or, in three dimensions (3D), their configurations or conformations, their atom types and atom positions, their van der Waals surfaces or their molecular fields. Therefore, different measures of similarity have to be formulated for each eventual use and almost all of these are used in drug design.[99]

For developing a new method for quantifying on an unique scale both molecular similarity and dissimilarity – the SDM method – we use a 2D description of molecules by means of their molecular graphs characterizing the bonding pattern in the molecules and as similarity measure a modified Tanimoto distance. Thus, we use molecular constitutional formula that can be modeled by a molecular graph (hydrogen-suppressed graph) wherein the points (vertices) symbolize atoms, and the lines (edges) symbolize covalent bonds. But, the expansion of the SDM method into three dimensions can readily be made because we use for superposition the Minimal Steric Difference (MSD) algorithm. In the following we also prove that original MSD method (see Chapter 7.1) offers, in fact, a quantitative measure of topological dissimilarity among bioactive molecules.

The MSD method was introduced as a quantitative measure for steric misfit, taking into account the fact that steric fit depends upon the shape of both the biological receptor and drug molecule, but most steric parameters used in QSAR rely only upon the shape of the drug molecule. The MSD quantity is defined as the number of non-superposable non-hydrogen atoms of the two compared molecules, one of these modeling the shape of receptor cavity. Thus, the molecules ω_i, i=1,2,..,M of the series considered for designing a QSAR were superimposed upon the most active molecule of the series (ω_k), which is termed "standard" and is denoted by S^0. The shape of S_0 is considered (approximately) complementary to the receptor cavity. Obviously, MSD (ω_k=S^0)=0. The method offers a very simple way to express by a single number the molecular shape dissimilarity; in general, MSD (ω_i)>0, i=1,M, i≠k, and the greater MSD is, the higher is the degree of dissimilarity.

The geometrical congruencies of standard *vs.* compared molecule are performed seeking the maximal superposition of the two molecules: small differences in bond lengths and bond angles are neglected, but one must not superimpose pairs of atoms linked by covalent bonds in one molecule (1.2–2.0Å, being the range of length for covalent bonds) upon nonbonded pairs of atoms of other molecules (the van der Waals contact distances are in the range 3–4Å), and the various conformations of flexible molecules are considered to be degenerate.

A basic assumption of the MSD concept is that the drug-receptor affinity is a linearly decreasing function of the steric misfit of the drug molecule, ω_i, and the receptor cavity, i.e. of the sum of the non-overlapping volumes of ω_i and the cavity (approximated by S^0, as described below). The MSD is an approximation of this volume.

The MSD method gives a first inside about the importance of steric fit for a given type of biological activity. One can try different molecules as standards and select the one that yields the highest correlation coefficient, r.

In fact, *the MSD parameter is a dissimilarity measure which has a theoretical foundation in one of the pattern recognition fields (PR), namely* ***cluster analysis****, and we will prove this in the following.*

Clustering is a classification technique for which the semantic of the classification problem is given by similarities between some objects (molecules) usually known by their measurements. Let **ω** be a variable bioactive molecule (the ligands L) defined by N binary variables (x_1, x_2,…,x_N) describing the structural characteristics, in our case constitutional formulae as expressed by the corresponding molecular graph. Let the vector **ω** be an L molecule defined by n binary parameters (x_1, x_2,…,x_N). Let $\Omega=\{\omega_1,\omega_2,\ldots,\omega_M\}$ be the "space" of these molecules **ω** (or points ω). For the sake of simplicity, we consider each L molecule ω_i as a class or a cluster. In the terms of pattern recognition approach *identification* is a mapping ε, which may be not defined on all the ranges of ω:

$$\varepsilon:\omega \rightarrow \Omega$$

or

$$\varepsilon:(x_1,\ldots,x_n) \rightarrow \omega_i$$

Generally, this mapping defines equivalence classes on the space **Ω**. The practical problem is to find a constructive *identification* function (or program or operator) which will perform the above mapping. For our case, we have chosen as *clustering identification operator* the distance function, which is a real valued, symmetric function, obeying three axioms. Let $d(\omega_i,\omega_q)$ be such a function, which we may write d(i,q) if no confusion is possible. This function satisfies the following three axioms:

Reflexivity:	$d(i,j)=0$	(7.27a)
Symmetry:	$d(i,q)=d(q,i)$	(7.27b)
Triangle inequality	$d(i,q)\leq d(i,p)+d(p,q)$	(7.27c)

and induces a metric within the space **Ω**.

As we have seen in the preceding section, a distance is a particular dissimilarity function. Resemblance and dissemblance are terms equivalent to similarity and dissimilarity.

Many dissemblance measures have been proposed between two objects in pattern recognition approach. Among them, we use a particular form of the generalized Minkowski distance,

$$d_{Mk}(i,q) = \left[\sum_{j=1}^{N} \left|x_{ij} - x_{qj}\right|^{1/\lambda}\right]^{\lambda} \qquad (7.28)$$

namely "City block" metric or Manhattan distance, which may be obtained by setting of $\lambda=1$ in equation (7.28).

$$d_{Cb}(i,q) = \sum_{j=1}^{N} w_j\left|x_{ij} - x_{qj}\right| \qquad (7.29)$$

where w_j are the weights. One can easily observe that for $\lambda=2$ one obtains the Euclidean distance.

In general, each parameter x_i, i=1,M may be:[4]

(i) *Quantitative*: x is isomorphic to a real number or to a number represented on a computer;
(ii) *Qualitative*: x may materialize a non-quantitative characteristic (for instance, a color, a name, a bioactive property or quality etc.) for which a complete or partial order may exist on the set {x}, for example, small, medium, large and so on.
(iii) *Binary*: the variable may take two states, usually called 0 or 1. If arithmetic operations are legal on x, they are called *binary quantitative*, otherwise *binary qualitative*.

For the case in which the structural characteristics of molecules ω_i and ω_q are binary encoded the "city block" metric is called Hamming distance d_H. A simplified example for the calculation of this dissimilarity measure by means of the relation (7.30), where all w_j=1, is presented in the Figure 15.

$x=\{x_j\}$:	x_1	x_2	x_3	x_4	x_5
$\omega_i=\{x_{ij}\}$:	0	1	0	1	1
$\omega_q=\{x_{qj}\}$:	1	1	0	1	0
$x_{ij} - x_{qj}$:	-1	0	0	0	1

$d_H(\omega_i,\omega_q) = |-1| + |1| = 2$

Figure 15. The calculation of Hamming distance by means of the relation (7.30); the patterns (i.e. molecules) ω_i and ω_q are described by 5 characteristics $x_1,...,x_5$

In this case the ligands ω_i and ω_k are described by five molecular binary quantitative characteristics $x=\{x_1,\ldots,x_5\}$; for example x_i are indicator variables used in QSAR for quantifying the presence (x_i=1) or the absence (x_i=0) of a given structural feature (e.g., i sometimes refers to hydrogen bond donor or acceptor, the existence of a given group in a given position upon molecular structure, etc.).

One can easily observe from the Figure 15 that the Hamming distance is equal to the number of features that are different in ω_i and ω_q. Thus, let b_i, b_q and b_{iq} be integers such that b_i is equal to the number of occurrences of x_{ij}=1 from ω_i, b_q is equal to the number of occurrences of x_{qj}=1 from ω_q and b_{iq} represents the number of occurrences of x_{ij}=1 ***and*** x_{iq}=1 from both ω_i and ω_q. With these definitions, the relation (11) may be rewritten as

$$d_H(i,q) = b_i + b_q - 2b_{iq} \qquad (7.30)$$

But, if we have a series of bioactive molecules i=1,2,…,q,…,M and ω_q has the highest bioactivity that is it can be considered as standard, and the measurements $\mathbf{x}_i=\{x_j\}$, j=1,N may be interpreted as describing the corresponding molecular (constitutional) graphs of ω_i (i=1,M; i≠q) seeking maximal superposition upon molecular (constitutional) graph of ω_q, then the relation (7.30) defines also the MSD parameters. Therefore, the MSD parameter is, in fact, the Hamming distance between the L-molecules i and the standard molecule, S_0: $d_H(i,q)=MSD(i,q\equiv S_0)$.

A similarity measure τ (or dissimilarity measure λ) gives a numerical value to the notion of closeness (or farness) between two objects X_i, X_q from the initial structured data of their observations.[4] $\tau(X_i,X_q)$ [or $\lambda(X_i,X_q)$] is a real values, symmetric function, whose domain is the set of possible $X\times X$. Usually a high value of τ (or λ) indicates high similarity or closeness (or dissimilarity and farness).

Thus, MSD is a topological dissimilarity measure of ω_i (i=1,M), relative to ω_q as standard S_0. The MSD values are integers; the bigger the value of MSD, the higher the degree of dissimilarity (or lower the degree of similarity). A values of $MSD=d_H$ close to 0 implies a high similarity or closeness and for $MSD(i,q)=d_h(i,q)=0$ we obtain the maximum similarity, i.e. $\omega_i=\omega_q$. The principal disadvantage of this quantitative measure of dissimilarity (or similarity) lies in the fact that is necessary to define an arbitrary threshold from which the MSD values quantifies the dissimilarity. (or similarity) degree.

Therefore, on the basis of Tanimoto distance – see relation (7.26), and MSD idea of realizing superposition of L molecules, as described above, we propose here a new similarity/dissimilarity index (denoted SDM) by normalization of Hamming distance. The new SDM parameter is calculating as follows,

$$SDM(i,q)=\frac{d_H(i,q)}{b_i+b_q-b_{iq}} \tag{7.31}$$

b_i, b_q and b_{iq}, having the same signification as in relation (7.31). From the equations (7.30) and (7.31) we obtain for the SDM the following relation:

$$SDM(i,q)=1-\frac{b_{iq}}{b_i+b_q-b_{iq}} \tag{7.32}$$

Hence, if $d_H=0$, that is $2b_{iq}=b_i+b_q$, the similarity degree is maximum ($\omega_i\equiv\omega_q$ from topological point of view) and, consequently, SDM=0. If $b_{iq}=0$, that is the superposed graphs of molecules ω_i and ω_q have no common vertices, and, then SDM=1 i.e., the degree of dissimilarity among ω_i and ω_k is maximum; clearly, the value of 0.5 is a natural threshold. Therefore, the SDM parameter models these two concepts – similarity/dissimilarity – on the same scale because $SDM\in[0,1]$.

The SDM parameter may be used as structural descriptor in QSAR studies by means of the following correlation equations:

$$A_i=\alpha_0+\alpha_1\cdot SDM_i \tag{7.33}$$

$$A_i=\alpha_0+\alpha_1\cdot SDM_i+\beta_1\cdot\sigma_{i1}+\beta_2\cdot\sigma_{i2}+\ldots \tag{7.34}$$

where σ_1, σ_2, ... stand for other structural parameters.

In the following section, we describe an application of SDM method for QSAR study on inhibition of microsomal p-hydroxylation of aniline by a series of alcohols as L molecules.

7.4.5 Leading example

The SDM method has been applied for QSAR study of a series of saturated alcohols which competitively inhibit microsomal p-hydroxylation of aniline from P-450 cytochrome, a part of the cell's detoxification system in which many foreign substances are oxidized prior to their elimination. The experimental data are from ref.[100]. As bioactivity, A_i, we used the logarithm of reciprocal concentrations (millimolar) that causes 50% inhibition, that is $A_i=\log(1/C_{50}) = pIC_{50}$.

The saturated alcohols analyzed in the present QSAR study together with their inhibitory potency and SDM values as structural descriptor are shown in the Table 7.2.

As standard, S^0, we have chosen n-heptanol (the compound no. 1 from the Table 7.2), the most active compound of this series. For the molecules that can be superimposed in many ways, we selected the conformation that allows maximal superposition upon the standard, i.e., the minimum value of SDM. Thus, we have obtained the hypermolecule **H**, by approximate atom per atom superposition of the all molecules of the database over the S^0. (see Figure 16).

H is used as topological framework for describing each molecule i (involved in the building of **H**) by the vector $\mathbf{X}=\{x_{ij}\}$; x_{ij} is taken to be 1 if the vertex j of **H** is occupied by a non-hydrogen atom of the molecule i, and $x_{ij}=0$ if it is not occupied. The binary descriptor **X**, together with the corresponding SDM values for the 17 alcohols from the Table 7.2 are shown in the Table 7.3.

Table 7.2 Biological activities, experimental $A_i=pIC_{50}=\log(1/C_{50})$ and calculated $\hat{A}$, and corresponding SDM indices for alkyl alcohols which competitively inhibit microsomal p-hydroxylation of aniline

No.	Alcohol	$A = \log IC_{50}$	$\hat{A}_i$ from Eq. (7.35)	SDM
1.	1-heptanol (S_0)	0.68	0.78±0.09	0.000
2.	1-hexanol	0.54	0.49±0.07	0.167
3.	1-pentanol	0.27	0.21±0.05	0.333
4.	2-heptanol	0.25	0.29±0.09	0.286
5.	2-hexanol	0.15	0.04±0.04	0.429
6.	1-butanol	-0.05	-0.08±0.03	0.500
7.	2-pentanol	-0.07	-0.20±0.03	0.571
8.	2-Me-1-butanol	-0.15	-0.20±0.03	0.571
9.	3-Me-1-butanol	-0.19	-0.20±0.03	0.571
10.	2-butanol	-0.35	-0.44±0.04	0.714
11.	3-pentanol	-0.37	-0.50±0.05	0.750
12.	2-Me-1-propanol	-0.39	-0.44±0.04	0.714
13.	3-hexanol	-0.47	-0.29±0.04	0.625
14.	2-propanol	-0.47	-0.69±0.06	0.857
15.	1-propanol	-0.48	-0.36±0.04	0.667
16.	2,2-diMe-1-propanol	-0.67	-0.50±0.05	0.750
17.	2-Me-3-pentanol	-0.89	-0.55±0.05	0.778

Table 7.3 The structural descriptor $X=\{x_{ij}\}$, i=1,17, j=1,13 (see also Figure 16).

No.	x_{ij}/j=	1	2	3	4	5	6	7	8	9	10	11	12	13	SDM
1.	x_{1j}	1	1	1	1	1	1	0	0	0	0	0	0	0	0.000
2.	x_{2j}	1	1	1	1	1	0	0	0	0	0	0	0	0	0.167
3.	x_{3j}	1	1	1	1	0	0	0	0	0	0	0	0	0	0.333
4.	x_{4j}	1	1	1	1	1	0	0	0	0	1	0	0	0	0.286
5.	x_{5j}	1	1	1	1	0	0	0	0	0	1	0	0	0	0.429
6.	x_{6j}	1	1	0	0	0	0	0	1	0	0	0	0	0	0.500
7.	x_{7j}	1	1	1	0	0	0	0	0	0	1	0	0	0	0.571
8.	x_{8j}	1	1	1	0	0	0	1	0	0	0	0	0	0	0.571
9	x_{9j}	1	1	1	0	0	0	0	1	0	0	0	0	0	0.571
10.	x_{10j}	1	1	0	0	0	0	0	0	0	1	0	0	0	0.714
11.	x_{11j}	1	1	0	0	0	0	0	0	0	1	0	0	1	0.750
12.	x_{12j}	1	1	0	0	0	0	1	0	0	0	0	0	0	0.714
13.	x_{13j}	1	1	1	0	0	0	0	0	0	1	0	1	0	0.625
14.	x_{14j}	1	0	0	0	0	0	0	0	0	1	0	0	0	0.857
15.	x_{15j}	1	1	0	0	0	0	0	0	0	0	0	0	0	0.667
16.	x_{16j}	1	1	0	0	0	0	1	0	1	0	0	0	0	0.750
17.	x_{17j}	1	1	0	0	0	0	0	0	1	1	0	1	0	0.778

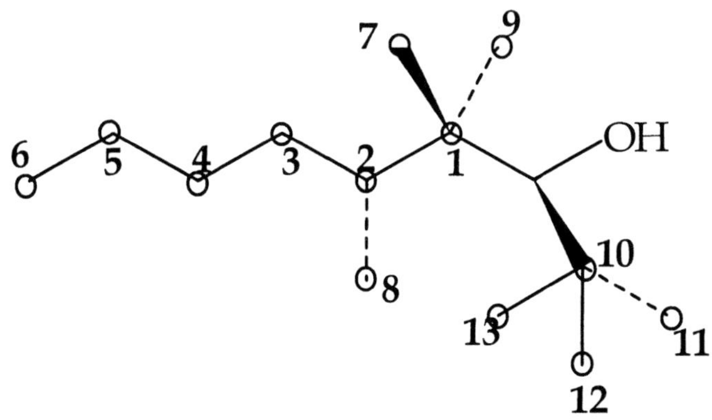

Figure 16. The hypermolecule H obtained by superposition of the alcohols from Table 7.2.

By using the least-squares method, we have obtained the following correlation equation:

$$\frac{A = 0.776(\pm 0.193) - 1.707(\pm 0.327)\text{SDM}; (\text{EV} = 0.892; s = 0.144)}{(t = 8.5; F = 73.0) \quad (t = 11.1; F = 123.7); r = 0.944; r_{CV}^2 = 0.736;} \tag{7.35}$$

where r – correlation coefficient, EV – explained variance, s – standard error, t – Student test, F – Fisher test, r_{CV} – cross-validation coefficient, and (t= , F=) refer to statistical corresponding indicators of the coefficients from equation (7.35), respectively.

The 95% confidence limits for the parameters of the linear model (7.35) (0.776 and 1.707) have also been calculated. They offer important information about the reliability of the model.

Equation (7.35) accounts for about 90% of the variation in the pIC_{50} data, and the standard error of the estimate is only 4% of the range of the pIC_{50} data. The statistical significance of equation (7.35) is very good, as observed of the Fisher's and Student's statistics. The bioactivities, $\hat{A}_i$, predicted by the model (7.35), and the range of variation of each inhibitory activity are also presented in the Table 7.2.

The present QSAR analysis shows that the degree of inhibition of aniline p-hydroxylation by alcohols is greatly influenced by the degree of similarity between them. The negative slope of the line leads to the conclusion that inhibition decreases with the growth of dissimilarity degree between n-heptanol and the other alcohols. As the size or the branching of the alkyl chain are growing, as the molecules tend to be more similar and the inhibitory potency is increasing.

Our QSAR study is in accordance with the results reported for the interaction between cytochrome P-450 and alcohols, which competitively inhibit the microsomal p-hydroxylation of aniline.[100] Thus, the mechanism of interaction between alcohols and the enzymatic receptor can be viewed as a "zipper" mechanism, and it has two stages. The first stage consists in a (possibly hydrogen or dipole–dipole) bond formation between the hydroxyl group of the alcohols and some site of the enzyme. This interaction is responsible for the inhibitory activity of the alcohols. The second stage implies a hydrophobic interaction between the alkyl chain and a hydrophobic zone that is close to the enzyme site involved in the first stage. This stage proceeds step by step for different long chains with conformational flexibility, and it may account for the quantitative differences in activity for the studied alcohols. Thus, the initial interaction from first stage is followed by a series of conformational rearrangements of both alcohol and enzyme, leading to the binding of the remaining segments of the alkyl chain to their appropriate position. This mechanism is strongly supported by the good correlation between experimental values, pIC_{50}, and SDM model (see Equation (7.35)). The decrease of similarity among n-heptanol and the other alcohols from Table 7.3, accompanied by the increase of dissimilarity, also decrease the possibility of interaction with the hydrophobic walls of the (possibly) cleft enzyme site. This situation is realized by smaller chains, the threshold between similarity and dissimilarity being for 2-hexanol (SDM=0.5) when biological activity has still positive value, or by branched alcohols.

7.4.6 Conclusions

SDM method reported in this paper allows quantitative treatment of the topological similarity and dissimilarity between two bioactive molecules on the same scale. The range of variation is from SDM=0, which means the highest similarity, that is the two molecular graphs are identical for any type of atoms, to SDM=1, for which one obtains the lowest similarity, i.e. the highest dissimilarity. In this way, it is not necessary to define an arbitrary threshold between similarity and dissimilarity; the threshold has the value of 0.5.

As a quantitative measure of both topological similarity and dissimilarity, the SDM parameter can be used for QSAR studies. If the correlation equations are statistically validated, it can be used to explain biological interactions in terms of similarity or dissimilarity among bioactive molecules (called also effectors or ligands) and biological receptor or to predict biological activity for unknown compounds.

The potential of SDM method for QSAR studies is revealed by the results obtained in analysis of competitive enzyme inhibition of microsomal p-hydroxylation of aniline by a series of alcohols. Thus, it is evident that the binding of alcohols to cytochrome P-450, which causes the competitive inhibition mentioned above, must take place at the active site of the free enzyme. The size and the degree of the alkyl chains branching of the alcohols, which leads to a higher degree of dissimilarity with respect to the most active compound, n-heptanol, which complementary models the site of biological receptor, account for the quantitative differences in the inhibition. The SDM structural parameter used in our QSAR study adequately describes these quantitative differences. The predictive power of linear model proposed above (Equation (7.35)) is also very good, if one taking into account the difficulty for obtaining the accurate experimental data. The introduction of other structural parameters may improve these results.

The SDM index is also useful for designing test series of bioactive compounds from the general screening procedures, which lead to too many compounds (commonly, more than 10,000 ligand molecules). In this case the molecules, two by two, must be reciprocal dissimilar, for optimization of the information/expenses ratio.

7.5. CoMFA vs. MTD Methods

The Comparative Molecular Field Analysis method[6] (CoMFA) is one of the most appealing and successful QSAR approaches based upon the computation of interaction energies of effectors with a receptor model. A number of applications assess the success of this method. Nevertheless, cross validation results,[6,33] generally r^2 between 0.55 and 0.76, are similar to those of the sensibly less CPU-time consuming Minimal Steric (Topologic) Difference (MTD) method,[95] both with test series and/or cross validation.[95] In our opinion, this is due to the nature of the potential energy function used in the CoMFA method for the effector – receptor affinity equation which make it, in certain respects, equivalent to the MTD method.

Quantitative structure-activity relations (QSAR's), especially those based upon ligand-receptor dissociation constants, are simple, usually linear functions relating structural features of ligand molecules to their receptor affinities. On the other hand, molecular mechanics is successful in predicting geometries and energetic for not too large molecules.[101] Therefore, structure-affinity functions corresponding to QSAR's with good predictive power should be acceptable approximations of force fields, of the type used in molecular mechanics, for the ligand-receptor (L_i-R) interactions.

From the 3D-QSAR methods, the CoMFA method – which actually yields a sort of receptor site model, described by characteristics for the interaction of ligand molecules with a probe atom in various grid locations – is rather successful and has become very popular in last years.[6] Much attention is currently given to the proper use of statistical methods in CoMFA and other QSAR methods (see, for example, ref.[102]), while the relation between these methods and the ligand-receptor interaction mechanism, per se, is somewhat neglected.

The MTD method[29,32] is a rather simple, pre-3D-QSAR approach to molecular stereochemistry. The MTD_L parameter for molecule L is defined as proportional to the steric misfit between L and a hypothetical receptor binding site (unoccupied site volume plus volume of the intersection of the van der Waals envelopes of L and of the walls of the R-site).Actually, the MTD_L values are the result of an optimization process which implicitly includes also other than purely steric effects. The following arguments are valid if steric effects are predominant.

The regression equation for MTD is of the type (if other structural parameters are neglected):

$$A_L = \alpha - \beta \cdot MTD_L \tag{7.36}$$

It is hereby assumed that L-atoms within the R-cavity produce attractive effects, and ones that fall within the (van der Waals envelope of) cavity walls produce repulsive effects; L-atoms which fall within the cavity walls produce R and L deformations, and this part of MTD_L (actually expressed as number of non H atoms) is roughly proportional to the energetic cost of R and L deformations within the R*L complex. If variations in MTD_L are due to variations in the number of L-atoms falling within cavity walls, the relation to terms of equation (2.2) is:

$$2.3RT \cdot \beta \cdot \Delta MTD_L \cong \Delta(U_R^{def} + U_L^{def}) \tag{7.37}$$

With a mean value of $\beta \cong 0.7$, one MTD unit (misfit volume of a fragment such as CH_2, OH, =O etc.) corresponds, for 300°K, to about 1 kcal/mole in ΔG differences.[103]

In the CoMFA method the receptor model is modeled as a lattice of probe atoms, k, with fixed positions. Ligand activity, A_L, is computed as a pondered sum of electrostatic and van der Waals interactions of the probe atom, in each grid position k, with the atoms of L:

$$A_L = \frac{\Delta G}{2.3RT} = a_o + \sum_k \left(b_k U_{kL}^{elst} + c_k U_{kL}^{vdW} \right) \tag{7.38}$$

Terms for hydrophobic interactions are sometimes introduced.

Coefficients a_o, b_k, c_k are obtained, for the studied series of ligands, by the partial least squares (PLS) method. Probe atoms are usually given one $q = +e$ (electron unit) charge and van der Waals characteristics of C-atoms, but other probe atoms are also used.

The b_k-coefficients could be related to the charge q_k of the receptor atom in grid position k; for $D = 1$, $b_k = q_k / 2.3RT$.

Similarly, the c_k-coefficients could be related to van der Waals characteristics of the receptor atom in (or nearby) grid position k. Unfortunately, such an interpretation is not possible because of some unrealistic assumption of force fields used in equation (7.38). Namely, grid positions k are fixed and, for probe atom-L atom interactions below van der Waals contact distances steric repulsive interactions increase the unrealistically high values and a cut-off (usually +30 kcal/mole) is introduced. In van der Waals-type potentials, while attractive minims are small (usually less than 1 kcal/mole), repulsion increases from 0 to the high cut-off value within a range of interatomic distances of only about 0.5 A. Probabilistically, most steric interaction terms will be either very small or equal to the high cut-off value. The resulting picture is rather unrealistic, as steric misfit is circumvented at much lower energy costs (than +30 kcal/mole) by deformation of dihedral angles in both R and L. Similarly, but less stringent, critiques refer also to the calculation of electrostatic terms which, for small inter-distances, require also a cut-off (usually also +30 kcal/mole). The CoMFA interpretation for steric interactions is that an L-atom in vicinity of grid k produces a significant attractive, or repulsive effect (or neither), rather similar to the hypermolecule's vertex attributions to receptor cavity, wall or exterior region. No wonder that CoMFA and MTD seem to yield similar results in cross-validation-like tests ($r^2_{CV} \cong 0.7$).[57,104]

Information concerning structures of R*L-complexes (X-ray crystallography) for related receptors is useful for alignment (superposition) of molecules within the probe atom grid receptor model of CoMFA and within the hypermolecule construction of MTD. With MTD, such information can be used also via the so-called start receptor map and via connectivity restrictions.[32,103]

The discussions above suggest the possibility of relating differences in the dehydration terms of equation (2.2) to differences in hydrophobicity parameters, π_X, and differences in the U_R^{def} and U_L^{def} - deformation energy terms to L and R - site overlap volumes. Our proposal for the CoMFA force field is to use a general equation of the type:

$$A_L = \frac{\Delta G}{2.3RT} = a_o + \sum_k \left(b_k U_{kL}^{elst} + c_k U_{kL}^{ster} + d_k U_{kL}^{hph} \right) \tag{7.39}$$

with the following description of interaction energy terms and cut-off conditions:[105,106]

(i) U_{kL}^{elst} - computed as usual in CoMFA but, for small interatomic distances, with a cut-off value equal to the electrostatic potential at the ligand atom - probe atom van der Waals contact distance.[106]

(ii) U_{kL}^{ster} - considered equal to the overlap of the van der Waals envelopes of the probe atom (in grid position k) and L-molecule. No cut-off condition is necessary.[106]

(iii) U_{kL}^{hph} - equal to the hydrophobic parameter of L-molecule fragments situated at least at van der Waals contact inter-distances and decreasing to zero at larger interatomic distances. This proposal is similar to the HINT-method.

With such interaction energy terms, b_k is proportional to the charge, q_k, of the receptor group situated in (or nearby) the grid position k, c_k - to the rigidity of the receptor site in position k, d_k - to the lipophilic/hydrophilic character of position k. For grid positions which do not contact the L-molecules, $c_k = d_k = 0$. For a proposal to reduce the number of grid points to be considered - see ref. 18. Our proposal for U_{kL}^{ster} eliminates the steep increase, from 0 to 30 kcal/mole within 0.5 A, characteristic for van der Waals - type potentials, which produces certain difficulties within the CoMFA method.[106, 107]

Certain modifications in the PLS procedures, of common use in CoMFA, could be necessary with the new interaction energy terms. Steric interactions per se are repulsive, b_k coefficients should be negative. Ideally, positive c_k - coefficients should signal attractive effects not included in the force field of ΔU (polarization, charge transfer). Receptor sites are usually less polar than water, d_k - coefficients should be positive. Scaling of interaction energy columns should be avoided, as the individual b_k, c_k, d_k - coefficients are to be directly related to structural features of the receptor site. The possibility to use structural data concerning related receptor sites of known structures would be beneficial.

All QSAR methods, even CoMFA, are based on rather poor approximations of the real molecular interaction force fields. The real predictive potencies, as indicated by cross-validation results are usually within $r_{CV}^2 = 0.5$ to 0.75 for both CoMFA, MTD and probably also for Hansch-type QSAR. Of course, predictions with Hansch QSAR's are strongly restricted with respect to variations in molecular stereochemistry, while MTD and especially CoMFA are much less restrictive in this sense. CoMFA has also the advantage of very versatile and user-friendly computer programs.

Our considerations refer to QSAR's based on direct ligand-receptor interaction. They are, probably, valid for most QSAR's, as biological activities are determined, mainly by such interactions and other (transport or drug degradation) phenomena are also based on molecular mechanisms.

In the proposed attempt to relate more directly CoMFA to the underlying molecular processes will prove successful, more information upon structural features of the receptor site could be obtained out of the QSAR results, information useful for drug design, as well as indications concerning the mechanism on which a certain biological activity is based.

8. ACKNOWLEDGEMENTS

We thank very much to our collaborators, Ciprian Ciubotariu and Marian Pasere, for their assistance in the preparation of the manuscript.

9. REFERENCES

1. Godfrey, M. Theoretical Models for Interpolating Linear Correlations in Organic Chemistry, in *Correlation analysis in Chemistry. Recent Advances* Chapman, N.B. and Shorter, J. (Eds.), Plenum Press, New York, 1978, pp. 86-91.
2. Dean, P. M. *Molecular Foundations of Drug-Receptor Interactions*, Cambridge Univ. Press, Cambridge, **1987**, pp.1-11; Mekenyan, O.; Bonchev, D. On the Possible Types of Electronic Drug-Receptor Interactions. *Eur. J. Med. Chem.* **1989**, *24*, 397-409.
3. Draper, N. R.; Smith, H. *Applied Regression Analysis*. Wiley & Sons, Inc., New York, 1981, pp. 25-56.
4. Vancea, R.; Holban, St.; Ciubotariu, D. *Pattern Recognition. Applications*. Edit. Academiei R.S. România, Bucureşti, 1989, pp. 111-139.
5. Hopfinger, A. J. A QSAR Investigation of Dihydrofolate Reductase Inhibition by Baker Triazines Based upon Molecular Shape Analysis. *J. Am. Soc.* **1980**, *120*, 7196-7206.
6. Cramer III, R. D.; Patterson, D. E.; Bunce, J.D. Comparative Molecular Field Analysis (CoMFA). 1. Effect of Shape on Binding of Steroids to Carrier Proteins. *J. Am. Soc.* **1988**, 110, 5959-5967.
7. Hansch, C.; Leo, A. *Exploring QSAR: Fundamentals and Applications in Chemistry and Biology*, American Chemical Society, Washinghton, D.C., 1995, pp. 97-168.
8. (a) Mureşan, S.; Sulea, T.; Ciubotariu, D.; Kurunczi, L.; Simon, Z. Van der Waals Intersection Envelope Volumes as a Possible Basis for Steric Interaction in CoMFA. *Quant. Struct.-Act. Relat.* **1996**, *15*, 31-32; (b) de Brujin, J.; Hermens, J. Relationship Between Octanol/Water Partition Coefficients and Total Molecular Surface Area and Total Molecular Volume of Hydrophobic Organic Chemicals. *Quant. Struct.-Act. Relat,* **1990**, *9*, 11-21.
9. Heiden; W., Moeckel, G.; Brickmann, K. A New Approach to Analysis and Display of Local Lipophilicity/Hydrophilicity Mapped on Molecular Surfaces. *J. Comput.-Aided Mol. Design* **1993**, *7*, 503-514.
10. Hermann, R.B. Modeling Hydrophobic Solvation of Nonspherical Systems: Comparison of Use of Molecular Surface Area with Accesible Surface Area. *J. Comput. Chem.* **1997**, *18*, 115-125.
11. Todeschini, R.; Gramatica, P. 3D-Modelling and Prediction by WHIM Descriptors. Part 5. Theory Development and Chemical Meaning of WHIM Descriptors. *Quant. Struct.-Act. Relat.* **1997**, *16*, 113-119.
12. Desiraju, G. R. *Crystal Engineering, the Design of Organic Solids*, Elsevier, Amsterdam, 1989, pp. 27-62.

13. Bondi, A. J. van der Waals Volumes and Radii. *J. Phys. Chem.* **1964**, *68*, 441-451.
14. Francl, M. M.; Hout Jr., R. F.; Hehre, W. J. Representation of Electron densities. 1. Sphere Fits to Total Electron Density Surfaces. *J. Am. Chem. Soc.* **1984**, *106*, 563-570.
15. Govers, H.; de Voogt, Pim. Calculation of Molecular Volumes from Molecular Fragments via Valence Electron Indices. *Quant. Struct.-Act. Relat.* **1989**, *8*, 11-16.
16. Rowlinson, J. S. The Triplet Distribution Function in a Fluid of Hard Spheres. *Mol. Phys.* **1963,** *6*, 517-524.
17. Pavani, P.; Ranghino, G. A Method to Compute the Volume of a Molecule, *Comput. Chem.* **1982**, *6*, 133-135.
18. (a) Connoly, M. L. Solvent-Accesible Surfaces of Proteins and Nucleic Acids. *Science* **1983**, *221*, 709-713; (b) Connoly, M. L. Computation of Molecular Volume, *J. Am. Chem. Soc.* **1985**, *107*, 1118-1124.
19. Richmond, T. J. Solvent Accesible Surface Area and Excluded Volume in Proteins. Analytical Equations for Overlapping Spheres and Implications for the Hydrophobic Effect. *J. Mol. Biol.* **1984**, *178*, 63-89.
20. do Carmo, M. P. *Differential Geometry of Curves and Surfaces*, Prentice-Hall, Englewood Cliff, 1976, pp. 34-52.
21. Gibbson, K. D.; Scheraga, H. A. Exact Calculation of the Volume and Surface Area of Fused Hard-Spere Molecules with Unequal Atomic Radii. *Mol. Phys.* **1987**, *62*, 1247-1265.
22. Gavezotti, A. The Calculation of Molecular Volumes and the Use of Volume Analysis in the Investigation of Structured Media and of Solid-State Organic Reactivity. *J. Am. Chem. Soc.* **1983**, *105*, 5220-5225.
23. Meyer, A. Y. Molecular Mechanics and Molecular Shape. Part I. van der Waals Descriptors of Simple Molecules. *J. Chem. Soc. Perkin Trans. II* **1985**, 1161-1169.
24. Ciubotariu, D.; Holban, Şt.; Motoc, I. Computation of Molecular van der Waals Volume by means of Monte Carlo Method. *Preprint, Univ. Timişoara, Fac. St. Nat., Ser. Chim.* **1975**; *3*, 1-8; Ciubotariu, D.; Gogonea, V.; Iorga, I.; Deretey, E.; Medeleanu, M.; Mureşan, S.; Bologa, C. New Shape Descriptors for Quantitative Treatment of Steric Effects II The Molecular van der Waals Volume: two Monte Carlo Algorithms. *Chem. Bull. Tech. Univ. (Timişoara)* **1993**, *38*, 63-75.
25. Mezey, P. G. in *Reviews in Computational Chemistry* vol 1, Lipkowitz, K. B.; Boyd, D. B. (Eds.). VCH, Weinheim, 1990, pp. 25-36.
26. Chuman, H.; Karasawa, M.; Fujita, T. A Novel Three-Dimensional QSAR Procedure: Voronoi Field Analysis. *Quant. Struct.-Act. Relat.*, **1998**, *17*, 313-326.
27. Crippen, G. M. Voronoi Binding Site Models. *J.Comput. Chem.*, **1987**, *8*, 943-954.
28. Simon, Z.; Szabadai, Z. Minimal Steric Difference Parameter and the Importance of Steric Fit for Structure-Biological Activity Correlations *Stud. Biophys. (Berlin)*, **1973**, *39*, 123-132.
29. Balaban, A. T.; Chiriac, A.; Moţoc, I.; Simon, Z. (Eds.), *Steric Fit in Quantitative Structure-Activity Relations*.
30. Moţoc, I.; Holban, S.; Ciubotariu, D. Calculation of Minimal Steric Difference Using a Computer. *Preprint, Univ. Timisoara, Ser. Chim.* **1975**, *16,* 1-8.
31. Holban, S.; Vancea, R.; Ciubotariu, D.; Moţoc, I. The MTD/1-Program. The MCD-Program. in *Steric Fit in Quantitative Structure-Activity Relations*. Balaban, A. T.; Chiriac, A.; Moţoc, I.; Simon, Z. (Eds.), Lecture Notes in Chemistry, Vol. 15., Springer-Verlag, Berlin, 1980. pp.119-167.

32. Simon, Z.; Chiriac, A.; Holban, S.; Ciubotariu, D.; Mihalaş, G. I. *Minimum Steric Diference. The MTD method for QSAR Studies*. Research Studies Press (Wiley&Sons Inc., New-York), Letchworth, 1984.
33. Niculescu-Duvaz, I.; Ciubotariu, D.; Simon, Z.; Voiculetz, N. QSAR (SAR) Models and Their Use for Carcinogenic Potency Prediction. in *Modeling of Cancer Genesis and Prevention*. Voiculetz, N.; Balaban, A. T., Niculescu-Duvăz, I.; Simon, Z. CRC Press, Boca Raton, 1991, pp.157-214.
34. Wheland, E. W. *Advanced Organic Chemistry*, 3rd Ed., Wiley, New York, 1960.
35. Ingold, C. K. *Structure and Mechanism in Organic Chemistry*. Cornell Univ. Press, Ithaca, N.Y., 1969, pp. 544-559.
36. Charton, M., The Upsilon Steric Parameter – Definition and Determination. in *Steric Effects in Drug Design*. Charton, M.; Moţoc, I (Eds.). Topics Current Chem No.114, Springer, Berlin, 1983, pp.59-61.
37. McFarland, J. W., ref. cit. in *Progress in Drug Research*. Vol. 15. Jucker, E. (Ed.) Birchäuser, Basel, Stuttgart, 1971, pp. 126-137.
38. Richards, W. E., *Quantum Pharmacology*, 2nd Ed., Butterworths, London, Boston, 1983, pp. 3-18.
39. Momany, F. A.; Drake, L. E.; Aubuchon, J. R. Conformation of Somatostin. *Int. J. Quantum Chem. Quantum Biol. Symp.* **1978**, *5*, 381-387; Loew, G. H.; Burt, S. K. Conformation of Enkephalin and Resemblance to Opiates. *Proc. Natn. Acad. Sci. U. S. A.* **1978**, *75*, 7-19.
40. Verloop, A.; Hoogenstraaten, W.; Tipker, J. Development and Applications of New Steric Parameters in Drug Design. in *Drug Design*, Vol. 7. Ariëns, E. J. (Eds.), Academic Press, New York, 1976, pp. 165-181.
41. Charton, M. The nature of the Ortho Effect. II. Composition of the Taft Steric Parameter. *J. Am. Chem. Soc.* **1969**, *91*, 619-626.
42. Kier, L. B.; Hall, L. H. *Molecular Connectivity in Chemistry and Drug Research*, Academic Press, New York, **1976**.
43. Blankley, C. J. Introduction: Review of QSAR Methodology. in *Quantitative Structure-Activity Relationships of Drugs*, Topliss, J. G. (Ed.), Academic Press, **1983**, pp. 10-12.
44. Diudea, M. V.; Pârv, B. A New centric Connectivity Index (CCI). *MATCH*, **1988**, *23*, 65-87; Diudea, M.V.; Minailiuc, O.M.; Balaban, A.T. Regression Vertex Degrees (New Graph Invariants) and derived Topological Indices. *J. Comput. Chem.*, **1991**, *12*, 527-535; Diudea, M. V.; Ivanciuc, O. *Topologie moleculară*, Compres Cluj-Napoca, 1995.
45. Crippen, G. M.; Havel, T. F.. *Distance Geometry and Molecular Conformation*. Research Studies Press, Ltd (Wiley), New York, 1988, pp. 125-137.
46. Motoc, I.; Marshall, G. R.; Dammkoehler, R. A.; Labanowski, J. Investigation of Receptor Space by Means of Excluded Volume Mapping Method. *Z. Naturforsch.* **1985**, *40*, 1108-1117.
47. Kim, K. H.; Martin, Y. C. Evaluation of Electrostatic and Steric Descriptors for 3D QSAR: The H^+ and CH_3 Probes Using Comparative Molecular Field Analysis (CoMFA) and the Modified Partial Least-Squares Method. in *QSAR: Rational Approaches to the Design of Bioactive Compounds* (Proceedings of the 8th European QSAR Symposium), Silipo, C.; Vittoria, A. (Eds.). Elsevier, Amsterdam, 1991, pp. 151-154.

48. Richards, W. G., *Quantum Pharmacology*, 2nd Ed., Butterworths, London, Boston, 1983, pp. 229-236.
49. Cammarata, A. in *Molecular Orbital Studies In Chemistry and Pharmacology*, Kier, L.B.; Lemant, B. (Eds), Springer, New-York, 1969, pp.156-158.
50. Johnson, C.D. *The Hammett Equation*. Cambridge Univ. Press., Cambridge, 1973; Exner, O. The Hammett Equation – the Present Position. in *Advances in Linear Free Energy Relationships*, Chapman, N.B.; Shorter, J. (Eds.), Plenum Press, London, New York, 1972, pp. 1-70.
51. Taft, R. W., in *Steric Effects in Organic Chemistry*, Newman, M. S. (Ed.), John Wiley&Sons, New York, 1956, pp. 556-557.
52. Charton, M., The Upsilon Steric Parameter – Definition and Determination. in *Steric Effects in Drug Design*. Charton, M.; Motoc, I (Eds.). Topics in Current Chemistry, Vol. 114, Springer, Berlin, 1983, pp. 65-66.
53. Gogonea, V.; Motsenigos, A.; Ciubotariu, D.; Deretey, E.; Chiriac, A; Simon, Z. Molecular Mechanics and Molecular Shape descriptors. 2. Comparative Treatment of Four Methods for Molecular Surface Calculation. *Preprint, University of Timisoara, Ser. Chimie*. **1981**, 1-12.
54. Bard, Y. (Ed.), *The Sampling Distribution*, in *Nonlinear Parameter Estimation*. Academic Press, New York, 1974, pp. 39-46.
55. Topliss, J. G. (Ed.), *Quantitative Structure-Activity Relationships of Drugs*. Academic Press, New York, 1983, pp. 497-504.
56. Hansch, C.; Leo, A.; Taft, R.W. A Survey of Hammett Substituent Constants and Resonance and Field Parameters. *Chem. Rev.* **1991**, *91*, 165-195.
57. Hansch, C.; Leo. A. *Substituent Constants for Correlation Analysis in Chemistry and Biology*. Wiley-Interscience, New York, 1980, pp. 9-12.
58. Hansch, C. Recent Advances in Biochemical QSAR. in *Correlation Analysis in Chemistry. Recent Advances*, Chapman, N. B. and Shorter, J. (Eds.). Plenum Press, New York, 1978, pp. 397-438.
59. Fujita, T.; Iwamura, H. Applications of Various Steric Constants to Quantitative Analysis of Structure-Activity Relationship. in *Steric Effects in Drug Design*. Charton, M.; Motoc, I. (Eds.). Topics Curr. Chem., Vol. 114, Springer, Berlin, 1983, pp. 119-157.
60. McPhee, J.A.; Panaye, A.; Dubois, J.E. Steric Effects–I. A Critical Examination of the Taft Steric Parameter – E_S. Definition of a Revised Broader and Homogeneous Scale. Extension to Highly Congested Alkyl Groups. *Tetrahedron*. **1978**, *34*, 3553-3562.
61. Charton, M. The Upsilon Steric Parameter – Definition and Determination. in *Steric Effects in DrugDesign*, Charton, M.; Motoc, I (Eds). Topics Current Chem. Vol. 114, Springer, Berlin, 1983, pp. 66-75.
62. Ciubotariu, D. *Structure-Reactivity Relationships in the Class of carbonic Derivatives*, PhD Thesis, Polytechnical Institute of Bucharest, Romania, 1987.
63. Lee, J. D.; Lee, T. D. *Statistics and Computer Methods in BASIC*. van Vostrand and Reinhold, New York, 1982, pp. 13-24.
64. Ciubotariu, D.; Deretey, E.; Medeleanu, M.; Gogonea, V.; Iorga, I. New Shape Descriptors for Quatitative Treatment of Steric Effects. I. The Molecular van der Waals Volume. *Chem. Bull. PIT*. **1990**, *35*, 83-98; Muresan, S.; Bologa, C.; Medeleanu, M.; Gogonea, V.; Dragos, D.; Ciubotariu, D. New Shape Descriptors for

Quantitative Treatment of Steric Effects. III Statistical Validation of the Monte Carlo Algorithm MON_CAVE_1, *Chem. Bull. Tech. Univ. (Timişoara)*. **1994**, *39*, 23-33.
65. Charton, M. Van der Waals Radii, in *Steric Effects in Drug Design*, Charton, M. and Moţoc, I (Eds.), Topics Current Chem. Vol. 114, Springer, Berlin, 1983, pp. 60-65.
66. Bartell, L. S., in *Physical Methods in Chemistry*, Weissberger, A.; Rossiter, B. W. Wiley-Interscience, New York, 1972, pp. 125-158.
67. Kitaigorodski, A. I., *Molecular Crystals and Molecules*. Academic Press, New York, 1973.
68. Mezey, P.G. *Shape in Chemistry*, VCH Publishers, Inc., Weinheim, 1993, pp. 92-95.
69. Pearlmann, R. S. *SAREA*. Program QCPE Nr. 413, 1983.
70. Gogonea, V.; Ciubotariu, D.; Deretey, E.; Popescu, M.; Iorga, I.; Medeleanu, M. Surface Area of Organic Molecules: a New Method of Computation. *Rev. Roum. Chim.* **1991**, *36*, 465-471.
71. Gogonea, V. *An Approach to Solvent Effect Modelling by the Combined Scaled-Particle Theory and Dielectric Continuum-Medium Method*, PhD. Thesis, Toyohashi Univ. of Technology, Japan, 1996.
72. Cohen, C. in *Computer Assisted Drug Design*. Olson E.C.; Christoffersen, R.E. (Eds.), ACS Symp. Ser. Vol 112, Washington DC, 1979, pp. 371-382.
73. Medeleanu, M. *Structure-Properties Correlations by Topological Methods*. PhD. Thesis, Univ. "Politehnica", Bucureşti, 1997.
74. Vrânceanu, Gh.; Hangan, Th.; Teleman, C. *Geometrie elementară din punct de vedere modern*. (in romanian). Ed. Tehnică, Bucureşti, 1967, pp. 56-78.
75. Mayer, A. Y.; Farin, D.; Avair, D. Cross-Sectional Areas of Alkanoic Acids. A Comparative Study Applying Fractal Theory of Adsorption and Considerations of Molecular Shape. *J. Am. Chem. Soc.* **1986**, *108*, 7897-7905.
76. Ciubotariu, D.; Mureşan, S.; Gogonea, V.; Medeleanu, M.; Dragoş, D. Classical Hansch Method. Structural Parameters for QSAR. in *Quantitative Structure-Activity Relationship (QSAR). The MTD Method*. Chiriac A.; Ciubotariu D.; Simon Z. (Eds.). MIRTON, Timişoara, 1996, pp. 40-138.
77. Zubay, G. L., *Biochemistry*, McGraw-Hill, London, 1998, pp. 3-26.
78. Kenaga, E. E., Goring, K. A. I., in *Aquatic Toxicity, ASTM STP*. Vol. 707, Eaton, J. G.; Parrish, P.R.; Hendricks, A.C. (Eds.). American Society for Testing and Materials, 1980, pp. 78-115.
79. Rekker, R. F., The Hydrophobic Fragmental Constants, its Derivation and Application: a Means of Characterizing Membrane Systems. Elsevier, Amsterdam, 1977, pp. 73-91.
80. Pearlman, R.S., in *Partition Coefficient, Determination and Estimation*, Dunn, W.J., Block, J.H., Pearlman, R.S. (Eds.), Pergamon, New York, **1986**, pp. 3-20.
81. Pearlman, R. S. in *Physical Chemical Properties of Drugs*. Yalkovsky, S. H.; Sinkula, A. A.; Valvani, S.C. (Eds.). Marcel Dekker, New York, 1980, pp. 321-347.
82. Gogonea, C.; Gogonea, V.; Osawa, E. Thermodynamics of Cavity Formation as a Function of Both Size and Shape of Solute. *The Proceedings of The International Chemical Congress of Pacific Basin Societies*, December 17-22, 1995, Honolulu, Hawaii (USA), 10.PHYS, Abstr. No. 013.
83. Ben-Naim, A. *Solvation Thermodynamics*. Plenum Press, New York, 1987, pp. 189-204.
84. Ben-Naim, A. *Statistical Thermodynamics for Chemists and Biochemists*. Plenum Press, New York, 1992, pp. 51-83.

85. Gogonea, V.; Merz, Jr., K. M. Fully Quantum Mechanical Desctiption of Proteins in Solution. Combining Linear Scaling Quantum Mechanical Methodologies with the Poisson-Boltzmann Equation. *J. Phys. Chem.* **1999**, *103*, 5171-5188.
86. Moţoc, I.; Holban, S.; Ciubotariu, D.; Simon, Z. Calculation of Minimal Steric Difference Using a Computer. *Preprint, Univ. Timişoara, Fac. St. Nat., Ser. Chim.* **1975**, *16*, 1-8; Ciubotariu, D.; Holban, S.; Mihalas, I.; Simon, Z.; Chiriac, A. Computer Programs for the MTD Method. III The MCD Program. *Preprint, Univ. Timişoara, Fac. St. Nat., Ser. Chim.* **1983**, *3*, 1-19.
87. Demidovich, B. P.; Maron, I.A. *Computational Mathematics*. MIR, Moscow, 1987, pp. 649-656.
88. Simon, Z.; Bădilescu, I.; Chiriac, A.; Ciubotariu, D.; Szabadai, Z. Optimized Molecular Shape of Effectors by Minimal Steric Differences. in *Quantitative Structure-Activity Analysis*, Francke, R.; Oehme, P. (Eds.), Akademie Verlag, Berlin, 1978, pp. 161-167.
89. Burkert, U.; Allinger, N.L. *Molecular Mechanics*, American Chemical Society, Washington D.C., 1982.
90. Kubinyi, H. (Ed.), *3D QSAR in Drug Design. Theory, Methods and Applications*, ESCOM, Leiden, 1993.
91. van Rossum, J. M. (Ed.), *Kinetics of Drug Action*, Springer, Berlin, 1977.
92. Ciubotariu, D.; Holban, S.; Mihalas, I.; Simon, Z.; Chiriac, A. Computer Program for the MTD Method. I. The MTDR Method. *Preprint, Univ. of Timişoara, Fac. St. Nat., Ser. Chim.* **1983**, *1*, 1-17; Ciubotariu, D.; Holban, S.; Mihalas, I.; Simon, Z. A. Computer Program for the MTD Method. II. The MTD Program. **1983**, *2,* 1-15.
93. Mureşan, S.; Sulea, T.; Bologa, C.;Ciubotariu, D. QSAR by MTD and MCD Methods and Molecular Modelling Studies on the Mechanism of Inhibition of Microsomal p-Hydroxylation of Aniline by Alcohols, *9th Noordwijkerhout – Camerino Symposion*, May 23-27, 1993, pp. 121-123.
94. Chiriac, A.; Chiriac, V.; Ciubotariu, D.; Holban, S.; Simon, Z. Minimal Steric Difference (MTD) – Study for Flexible Molecules: Substituted Acetic Acid Derivatives with Auxinic Activity, *Eur. J. Med. Chem. – Chim. Ther.* **1983**, *18*, 507-513.
95. Ciubotariu, D.; Deretey, E.; Oprea, T. I.; Sulea, T.; Simon, Z.; Kurunczi, L.; Chiriac, A. Multiconformational Minimal Steric Difference. Structure – Acetylcholinesterase Hydrolysis Rates Relations for Acetic Acid Esters. *Quant. Struct.-Act. Relat.* **1993**, *12*, 367-372.
96. Winter, J. G.; Davis, A.; Saunders, M.R. COSMIC – A New Molecular Mechanics Computer Package. *J. Comput.-Aided Mol. Design* **1987**, *31*, 1-9.
97. Järv, J. G.; Kesvatera, T.; Aaviksaar, K., Inhibition of Microsomal p-Hydroxilation of Aniline by Alcohols. *Eur. J. Biochem.* **1976**, *71*, 525-534.
98. Ciubotariu, D.; Mureşan, S.; Gogonea, V.; Băleanu-Gogonea, C.; Medeleanu, M.; Ciubotariu, C.; M. SDM – A New Similarity/Dissimilarity Measure for QSAR Studies, *Roum. Biotech. Lett.* **1997**, *2*, 114–130.
99. Dean, P.M., Molecular Similarity, in *3D QSAR in Drug Design. Theory, Methods and Applications*. Kubinyi, H. (Ed.). ESCOM, Leiden, 1993, pp. 150-151.
100. Sabljić, A.; Protić-Sabljić, M., Quantitative Structure-Activity Study on the Mechanism of Inhibition of Microsomal p-Hydroxylation of Aniline by Alcohols. *Molec. Pharmacol.* **1983**, *23*, 213-218.

101. Cohen, N. C.; Blaney, J. M.; Humblet, C.; Gund, P.; Barry, D. C., Molecular Modeling Software and Methods for Medicinal Chemistry. *J. Med. Chem.*, **1990**, *33*, 88-95.
102. Clementi, S.; Wold, S., in *Chemometric Methods in Molecular Design*. Methods and Principles in Medicinal Chemistry, vol. VII. Mannhold, R.; Krogsgaard-Larsen, P.; Timmerman, H. (Eds.), VCH, Weinheim, 1995, pp. 590-591.
103. Simon, Z., MTD and Hyperstructure Approach. in *3D QSAR in Drug Design. Theory, Methods and Applications*. Kubinyi, H. (Ed.). ESCOM, Leiden, 1993, pp. 307-319.
104. Thibaout, U.; Folkers, G.; Klebe, G.; Kubinyi, H.; Merz, A.; Rognan, D., Appendix A. Reccommendations for CoMFA. in *3D QSAR in Drug Design. Theory, Methods and Applications*. Kubinyi, H. (Ed.). ESCOM, Leiden, 1993, pp. 711-716.
105. Oprea, T. I.; Ciubotariu, D.; Sulea, T. I.; Simon, Z. Comparison of the Minimal Steric Difference (MTD) and Comparative Molecular Field Analysis (CoMFA) Methods for Analysis of Binding of Binding of Steroids to Carrier Proteins. *Quant. Struct.-Act. Relat.* **1993**, *12*, 21-26.
106. Mureşan, S.; Sulea, T.; Ciubotariu, D.; Kurunczi, L.; Simon, Z. Van der Waals Intersection Envelope Volumes as a Possible Basis for Steric Interaction in CoMFA. *Quant. Struct.-Act. Relat.* **1996**, *15*, 31-32.
107. Cramer III, R.D., De Priest, S.A., Patterson, D.E. and Hecht, P., *The Developing Practice of Comparative Molecular Field Analysis* in *3D QSAR in Drug Design. Theory, Methods and Applications*. Kubinyi, H. (Ed.). ESCOM, Leiden, 1993, pp. 443-485.

Chapter 11

TI-MTD MODEL. APPLICATIONS IN MOLECULAR DESIGN

Ovidiu M. Minailiuc and Mircea V. Diudea
Faculty of Chemistry and Chemical Engineering,
'Babes-Bolyai' University
3400 Cluj, Romania

1. INTRODUCTION

A bioactive molecule interacts with a biological receptor by means of an *effector-receptor complex*, in which the two partners mutually accommodate their structures such that the resulting complex exists sufficiently long for generating a biological response. The structural features of the bioactive molecule, responsible for a given biological activity (i.e. pharmacological profile), are called the *pharmacophore*. It plays an essential role in the recognition process preceding the complex formation. The receptor (i.e. a situs in a biomacromolecule) must contain complementary features to the pharmacophore for the recognition (complexation and ultimately biological response) to occur. In addition to the pharmacophore and its complementary points, the effector and biomacromolecule fix by *areas of nonspecific interaction*, which modulate the biological response.

The relative arrangement of all those atoms in the biomacromolecule (sensitive to the shape, size and chemical identity of the bioactive molecule), interested in the receptor-effector interaction, is called the *receptor map*. Usually the receptor structure is not known. Excepting the fortunate cases in which crystallographic data are available, the receptor map is drawn as complementary to a leading bioactive structure.

Several 2D- and 3D-QSAR approaches[1-12] are performed for modeling the receptor-drug interaction, with ultimate aim the drug design. A quantitative structure-activity relationship (QSAR) correlates the changes in the observed biological activity with the changes in the chemical structure of a series of molecules. Such correlating studies work usually on sets of congeneric structures but, in the last time, non-congeneric and conformationally flexible molecules were considered.[13,14] Refined models using some 3D-databases include MSD,[5,6] MTD,[6-10,15] SIBIS,[16-19] CoMFA,[20-28] Genetic Algorithms.[29] These models are, however, time-consuming particularly because of the huge number of molecular geometries needed to be calculated, for which they clearly require supercomputers.

In this chapter, a variant of MSD-MTD-SIBIS models, called TI-MTD, is presented.

It makes use of graph-theoretical (i.e. topological) molecular descriptors in describing and validating a receptor map.

2. TI – MTD Model

As SIBIS, TI-MTD uses a virtual topological *Receptor Space RS* as a coordinate system. It is a *hypermolecule* constructed by *superimposing* the candidate molecules M_i over the reference molecule M_r. The set of $M_1, M_2, \ldots, M_m$ molecules (i.e. the learning set) is assumed to act by the same mechanism upon the bioreceptor and possess the measured activities $Y_1, Y_2, \ldots, Y_m$. The *lead molecule* M_r is the most active structure within the considered set: $Y_r = \max\ (Y_i;\ i = 1, 2, \ldots, m)$. In words, the lead molecule is considered the best *negative copy* of the bioreceptor.

RS reflects the topology of the space *explored* by the bioactive molecules M_i. It provides a topological basis for some grid-based numerical description of the investigated set of chemical structures.

In construction of *RS*, a *row-vector* X_i of dimension N_R is attached to each candidate M_i

$$\mathbf{X}_i = X_{ij};\quad j = 1,2,\ldots,N_R \tag{1}$$

where N_R represents the number of vertices in *RS*; $X_{ij} = 1$ if the point $j \in RS$ is occupied by an atom (different from the hydrogen) of molecule M_i, and zero if it is empty.

Chemical nature of the points (i.e. atoms) is indicated by a property P_i of atoms $j \in M_i$ (e.g. the Van der Waals volume, molar refraction, the local value of a topological index *TI*, etc.) associated to the above vector

$$P_i X_i = P_{ij} X_{ij} \quad ; \quad j = 1,2,\ldots,N_R \tag{2}$$

With the above notions, the *Receptor Space RS* can be constructed as:

(1) Draw the hypermolecule (i.e. the $[RS]_{init}$) by superimposing the structures M_i over the reference M_r. Consider additional connectivities in $[RS]_{init}$ if the edge resulted by joining points *p* and *q* may represent a covalent bond.
(2) Share $[RS]_{init}$ in three vertex classes :

- points of the receptor cavity (C);
- points of the receptor walls (W) and
- irrelevant points (I)

Basically, the *cavity points* C correspond to the atoms of the reference structure M_r, while the *wall points* W occur in structures M_i, in the zone of their non-overlap over M_r. For convenience, an additional point of I type (i.e. an empty point) is introduced to be bonded with those points in RS whose relevance is tested.

The initial map looks as

$$[RS]_{init} = [C(m_1,...); \quad W(n_1,...); \quad I(p_1,...)] \tag{3}$$

where m, n and p are points belonging to the classes C, W and I, respectively, in $[RS]_{init}$.

(3) Describe numerically the hypermolecule by using some molecular *topological descriptors TD*:

$$\text{TD (Hyp)} = [\text{TD}_C(\text{Hyp}); \text{TD}_W(\text{Hyp}); \text{TD}_I(\text{Hyp})] \tag{4}$$

The candidates M_i are described by using the local values of TI (above calculated for the whole hypermolecule) according to their own $\mathbf{X}_i$ vector:

$$TD_c(i) = \sum_{j \in (c-type)} P_{ij} X_{ij} \tag{5}$$

$$TD_w(i) = \sum_{j \in (w-type)} P_{ij} X_{ij} \tag{6}$$

where P_{ij} and X_{ij} have the meaning above mentioned.

(4) Optimize $[RS]_{init}$ by following the scenario:

(a) calculate the regression (7) within $[RS]_{init}$:

$$Y_{calc}(i) = a + b_1 TD_c(i) + b_2 TD_w(i) + F(i) \tag{7}$$

that provides the correlation coefficient r_0. F is a linear function of non-steric factors (e.g. electronegativities) that may influence the bioactivity.

(b) change the initial attribute of vertices $j \in [RS]_{init}$, (e.g. C changes to W or W changes to C or I) if:

i. eq 7 gives a better correlation index $r_1 \geq r_0 + \Delta r$, where Δr is the desired improvement;

ii. the novel set of C is connected.

(c) an improved map $[RS]_k$ is thus obtained; the attribute changing is iterated until no improvement of the correlation coefficient is recorded.

(d) when the self-consistency is reached, the final optimal map $[RS]_{opt}$ is obtained and the algorithm is canceled.

If condition (*b*(*ii*)) and *F*(*i*) are ignored, the model TI-MTD (and SIBIS, of course) works as a FREE - WILSON bi-parametric variant.[19]

The vertex set of type $C \in [RS]_{opt}$ represents the *most probable molecular profile* complementary to the active center of the bioreceptor and it is reliable for improving the leading structure M_r.

Condition (*b*(*ii*)) imposes the *C* set be connected, that is, a true fragment. This is the reason for which a procedure able to select a desired fragment within a molecular structure was performed. Such a *fragmentation algorithm* will be presented in the next section.

3. Line Graphs

The line graph[30,31] of a graph is a natural concept, independently discovered by many authors. By this reason it was called *interchange graph,*[32] *derivative,*[33] *derived graph,*[34] *edge-to-vertex dual,*[35] *covering graph*[36] or also *adjoint.*[37]

Several properties of line graph were discovered so far.

3.1. Definitions and Properties

The *line graph* $L(G)$ of a given graph G is obtained by representing the lines in $G = L_0$ by points and then joining two such points by a line if the corresponding lines in G are incident to a common point.[38] By repeating this procedure n times, the *iterated line graph* L_n ; $n = 0, 1, 2, \ldots$ (with $L_n(G) = L_1(L_{n-1}(G))$ and $n = 0$ for the original graph, G) is obtained. Figure 1 illustrates the line graphs L_n of G_1 (2-Methylbutane); $n = 0 - 3$, by *edge evolution*.

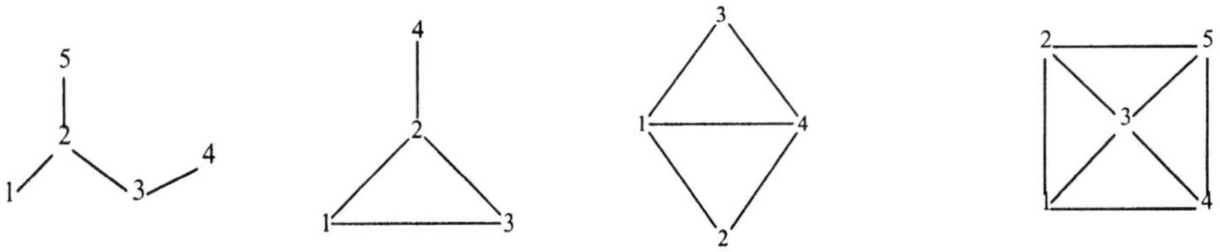

$L_0(G_1)$	$L_1(G_1)$	$L_2(G_1)$	$L_3(G_1)$
1	1 = (1,2)	1 = (1,2)-(2,3)	1 = ((1,2)-(2,3))-((1,2)-(2,5))
2	2 = (2,3)	2 = (1,2)-(2,5)	2 = ((1,2)-(2,3))-((2,3)-(3,4))
3	3 = (2,5)	3 = (2,3)-(3,4)	3 = ((1,2)-(2,3))-((2,3)-(2,5))
4	4 = (3,4)	4 = (2,3)-(2,5)	4 = ((1,2)-(2,5))-((2,3)-(2,5))
5			5 = ((2,3)-(3,4))-((2,3)-(2,5))

Figure 1. The line graphs $L_n(G_1)$; n = 0-3.

The number of vertices, N and edges Q in L_{n+1} is given by relations[39-41]

$$N(L_{n+1}) = Q(L_n) \tag{8}$$

$$Q(L_{n+1}) = -Q(L_n) + (1/2)\sum_{i \in L_n} (k_i)^2 \tag{9}$$

$$Q(L_{n+1}) = \sum_{i \in L_n} \binom{k_i}{2} = \sum_{i \in L_n} k_i(k_i - 1)/2 = B_n \tag{10}$$

where k_i is the vertex degree and B_n - Bertz' s branching index,[41] which is the exact number of edges in the L_{n+1} line graph.

In regular graphs (i.e. graphs with all vertices having the same degree), the number of edges $Q(L_{n+1})$ can be calculated by a recursion, derived from eq 9 or eq 10 by substituting the value for the vertex degree

$$k(L_n) = 2Q(L_n) / N(L_n) = 2Q(L_n) / Q(L_{n-1}) \tag{11}$$

$$Q(L_{n+1}) = -Q(L_n) + 2Q^2(L_n) / Q(L_{n-1}) \tag{12}$$

The number of edges in L_{n+1} can also be expressed as a function of k and N

$$Q(L_{n+1}) = (1/2)\, k(L_{n+1})\, N(L_{n+1}) \tag{13}$$

Since in regular graphs

$$k(L_{n+1}) = 2\,(k(L_n) - 1) \qquad (14)$$

and taking into account eq 8, eq 13 becomes

$$Q(L_{n+1}) = Q(L_n)\,(k(L_n) - 1) \qquad (15)$$

From relations (14) and (15), $k(L_n)$ and $Q(L_n)$ can be expressed in terms of the starting parameters, $k(L_0)$ and $Q(L_0)$

$$k(L_n) = 1 + 2^n k(L_0) - \sum_{e=0}^{n} 2^e = 2^n k(L_0) - 2^{(n+1)} + 2 \qquad (16)$$

$$Q(L_n) = Q(L_0)\prod_{i=0}^{n-1}(k(L_i) - 1) = Q(L_0)\prod_{i=0}^{n-1}(2^i k(L_0) - 2^{(i+1)} + 1) \qquad (17)$$

3.2. Reduced Line Graph

By definition, the line graph $L_1(G)$ provides information on lines (i.e. edges) in G. Each point in $L_2(G)$ corresponds to a fragment of two lines (or three points) in G. Iteratively, a point in $L_n(G)$ will represent a fragment of n lines in the original graph L_0. A natural limit of iteration could be $n = Q(L_0)$ (i.e. the number of lines in G). In such a line graph each point would represent the whole original graph L_0. The above statement is true for any graph except the simple cycles C_N and the star $S_{1,3}$, for which $Q(L_n) = Q(L_0)$ = constant.

The iterated line graphs can be written by *edge evolution*.[42] Figure 2 shows the fragments corresponding to L_3 in the original graph.

$L_3(G_1)$ = (1) ((1, 2) - (2, 3)) - ((1, 2) - (2, 5))
(2) ((1, 2) - (2, 3)) - ((2, 3) - (3, 4))
(3) ((1, 2) - (2, 3)) - ((2, 3) - (2, 5))
(4) ((1, 2) - (2, 5)) - ((2, 3) - (2, 5))
(5) ((2, 3) - (3, 4)) - ((2, 3) - (2, 5))

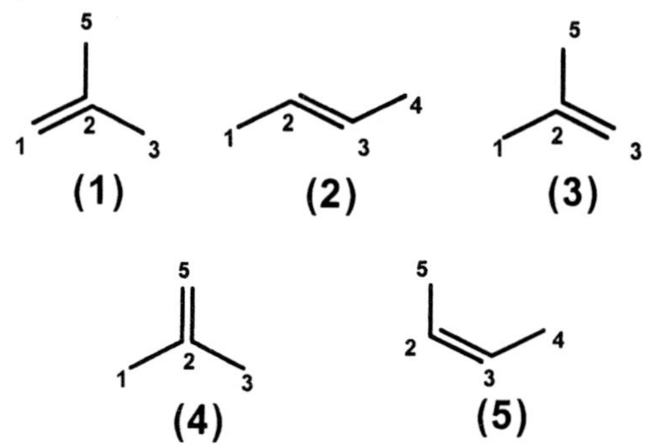

Figure 2. Edge evolution for $L_n(G_1)$; $n = 3$ and the corresponding fragments in $L_0(G_1)$.

From Figure 2 it can be seen that some lines occur twice (boldface):

(1) ((**1, 2**) - (2, 3)) - ((**1, 2**) - (2, 5)) or
(3) ((1, 2) - (**2, 3**)) - ((**2, 3**) - (2, 5))

If the multiplicity of lines is ignored in the iterated line graphs of rank $n \geq 3$ and keeping in mind the procedure for generating a line graph, a *reduced line graph* $R_n(G)$ is obtained.[43] For $L_3(G_1)$ the corresponding $R_n(G_1)$ looks as in Figure 3.

(1) (1, 2) (2, 3) (2, 5)
(2) (1, 2) (2, 3) (3, 4)
(3) (2, 3) (3, 4) (2, 5)

(1) (1, 2) (2, 3) (2, 5)
(2) (1, 2) (2, 3) (3, 4)
(3) (1, 2) (2, 3) (2, 5)
(4) (1, 2) (2, 3) (2, 5)
(5) (2, 3) (3, 4) (2, 5)

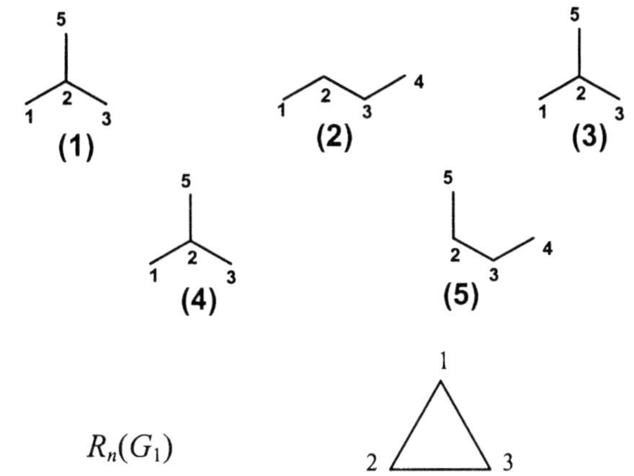

Figure 3. Reduced line graph $R_n(G_1)$; $n = 3$ and the corresponding fragments.

It is easily seen that the resulting fragments consist of three lines, equalling the rank of R_n. It is also seen that the fragments 1, 3 and 4 are identical. By eliminating the *redundant* fragments, (e.g. one of the *points* (1), (3) and (4) in Figure 3) *all the distinct fragments* (consisting of n lines) in G are obtained. Two fragments are called *connected* in R_n if they have n - 1 *common edges*.

The iteration in R_n is cancelled at $n = Q(L_0)$ when the resulting fragment is just the original graph. It is obvious that, in the reduced line graph

$$N(R_{n+1}) \leq Q(R_n) \tag{18}$$

By comparing eqs 8 and 18, on a hand, and L_3 (Figure 1) and R_3 (Figure 3), on the other hand, the difference between L_n and R_n is highlighted.

3.3. The FRAGGEN Algorithm

In a set of congeneric structures, the substituents are linked in various positions of the basic chemical structure (e.g. an aromatic ring). In such a case it is useful to *mark* the docking positions. The FRAGGEN program[43] allows the automatic generation of all fragments or, only of those fragments of a choise docking. The fragments thus generated are stored on disk in the view of optimizing the investigated receptor space RS. Figure 4 illustrates the fragmentation of the structure G_2, with the marked points 1, 2 and 3.

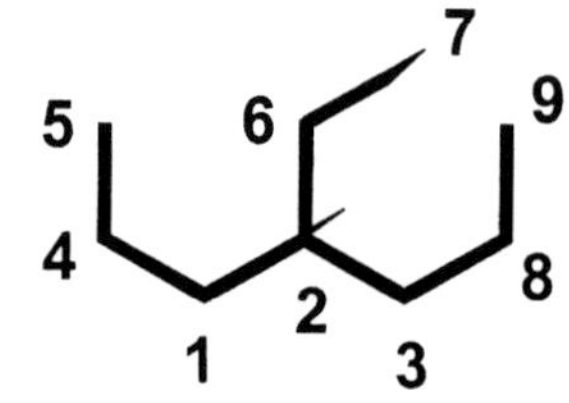

G_2

R_n; n = 6

(1) (1, 2)(1, 4)(2, 3)(2, 6)(3, 8)(4, 5)

(2) (1, 2)(1, 4)(2, 3)(2, 6)(3, 8)(6, 7)

(3) (1, 2)(1, 4)(2, 3)(2, 6)(3, 8)(8, 9)

(4) (1, 2)(1, 4)(2, 3)(2, 6)(4, 5)(6, 7)

(5) (1, 2)(1, 4)(2, 3)(3, 8)(4, 5)(8, 9)

(6) (1, 2)(2, 3)(2, 6)(3, 8)(6, 7)(8, 9)

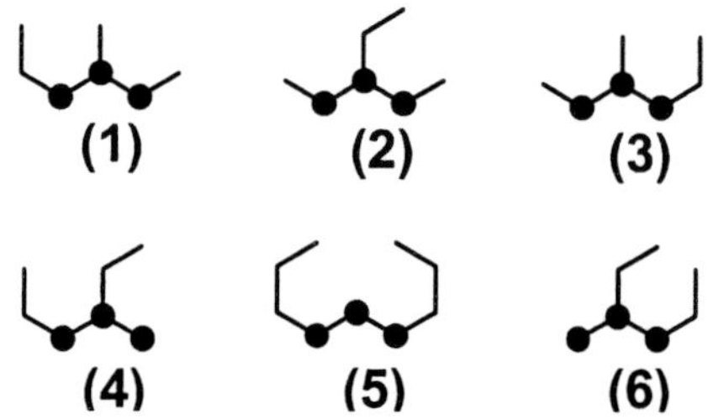

R_n; $n = 7$

(1, 2)(1, 4)(2, 3)(2, 6)(3, 8)(4, 5)(6, 7)

(2) (1, 2)(1, 4)(2, 3)(2, 6)(3, 8)(4, 5)(8, 9)

(3) (1, 2)(1, 4)(2, 3)(2, 6)(3, 8)(6, 7)(8, 9)

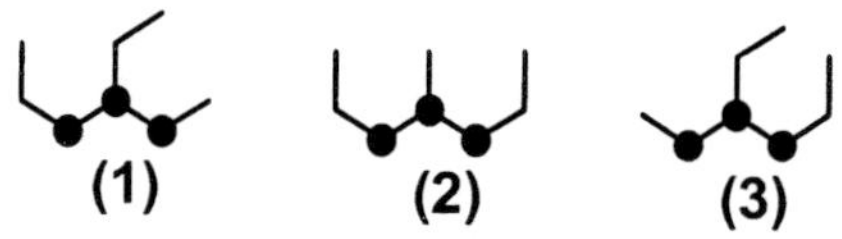

R_n; $n = 8$

(1) (1, 2)(1, 4)(2, 3)(2, 6)(3, 8)(4, 5)(6, 7)(8, 9)

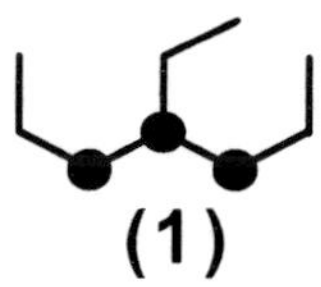

Figure 4. A structure (G_2) and its fragmentation: reduced line graph R_n; n = 6-8.

4. HYPERMOLECULE: ALIGNMENT RULE

The bioreceptor structure is most often unknown. It is believed that, within a set of candidates, the lead structure M_r is most complementary to the receptor situs. The receptor space $[RS]_{init}$ is assimilated to a *hypermolecule Hyp*. It is constructed as a labeled grid (i.e. graph) in a pure topological space, disregarding the bond lengths and angles.

As a preliminary alignment rule, the lead structure M_r is used as template. The candinates M_i are aligned by dockind them to the reference according to a pharmacophore hypothesis or to the maximum common substructure approach. Additional connectivities are consideted if they may represent covalent bonds.

Figure 5 illustrates the docking procedure for the set of trimethoprime congeners[18] (see Table 3, Sect. 6.1)

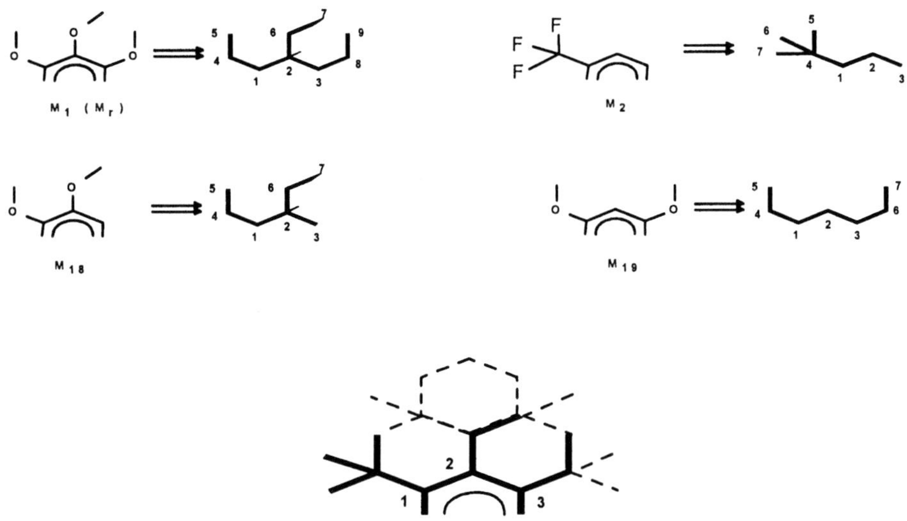

Figure 5. Docking procedure for the trimethoprime congeners.

It is known that the alignment rule is the key input for CoMFA.[20-28] The alignment can be achieved either by manual atom-to-atom mapping technique or by an automatic mapping procedure that analyzes the topological equivalence of each atom of both the reference and the candidate. More elaborated (and more time consuming) molecular field-matching approaches are also used.

In TI-MTD the alignment modes are identified as follows: the maximum number of edges *n* of the M_i structures (or substructures) interested in the interaction with *RS* is taken as the highest rank for generating the iterated reduced line graphs $R_n(Hyp)$ of hypermolecule. The procedure supplies subgraphs consisting of 1, 2,...*n* edges. All distinct subgraphs (of size according to each candidate) *containing the marked docking points*, are selected as *alignement modes* of the series.

The selection of *alignment modes* for M_{14} = 5-(3'-OC_4H_9-benzyl)-2,4-diamino-pyrimidine and a hypothetical M_{xx} = 5-(4'-OC_4H_9-benzyl)-2,4-diamino-pyrimidine (see the set of the trimethoprime congeners,[18] Sect. 5.1) is illustrated in Figure 6. The fosused fragments are 3'-OC_4H_9 and 4'-OC_4H_9. The reduced line graph $R_7(Hyp)$ of hypermolecules I and II, (with marked docking points) is generated thus resulting five substructures of 7 edges (*a, b, c, d* and *e*) for fragment 4'-OC_4H_9 and two ones (*f* and *g*) for 3'-OC_4H_9 . They represent distinct (labeled) subgraphs of the hypermolecule and consequently distinct modes of alignment of the corresponding candidates.

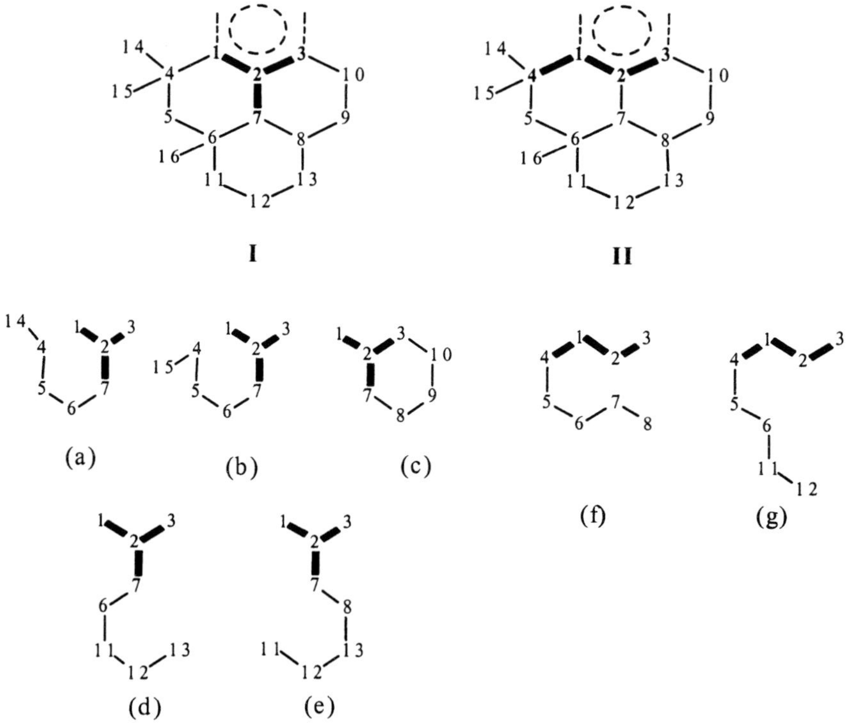

Figure 6. Alignment modes of 4`-$OC_4H_9$ (a –e) and 3`-OC_4H_9 (f, g) fragments within the hypermolecule of trimethoprime congeners.

In the selection of the above substructures (i.e. alignment modes) a highly discriminating *TI* is used as a first criterion. In case of degenerate values of *TI*, permutations in the adjacency matrix are performed, within a routine procedure.[44,45]

The alignment procedure is a *substructure mapping procedure*, useful in any approach requiring structure superposition.

At this point, the TI-MTD algorithm follows the steps 2 to 4. The optimization step 4 is iterated until the self-consistency provides the optimal map $[RS]_{opt}$. The steps 2 to 4 are performed for all alignment modes and the best statistically validated $[RS]_{opt}$ is selected. It represents the *TI-MTD* map that can be used to predict the biological activity of new compounds.

5. PARAMETRIZATION OF TI-MTD

TI-MTD is basically a topological approach. Its ground parameters are topological matrices and/or topological indices.

Any *TI* (locally defined) can be a property P_{ij} in eq 2, or in other words, a parameter of TI-MTD model.

5.1. Connectivity Indices

Among topological indices, frequently used in correlating studies is the Randić index[46] χ, defined by

$$\chi = \sum_{(ij)\in E(G)} (\delta_i \delta_j)^{-1/2} \tag{19}$$

where δ_i *and* δ_j are the degrees of two adjacent vertices. Two extensions of χ index, proposed by Diudea et al.,[47,48] namely *DSI* and *EC* indices, were particularly used in TI-MTD.

DSI[47] is constructed by using some *group electronegativity valences EVG* (defined in Sect. 5.2)

$$DSI_i = \sum_{j(ij)\in E(G)} (EVG_i EGV_j)^{-1/2} \tag{20}$$

$$DSI = \sum_i DSI_i \tag{21}$$

The summation in (20) runs over all *j* vertices adjacent to *i*.

$EC_{P/N}$ were built up by using the *EC* electronegativities[48] (see below)

$$EC_{P/N,i} = \sum_{j(ij)\in E(G)} (EC_i EC_j)^{\pm 1/2} \tag{22}$$

$$EC_{P/N} = \sum_i EC_{P/N,i} \tag{23}$$

The subscript symbol is *P* for +1/2 and *N* for -1/2. Excellent correlations of *DS* and *EC* indices with some physico-chemical and biological properties of aliphatic alcohols, amines and halogeno-derivatives were reported.[47,48] This was a promise for using these descriptors as P_{ij} local parameters in TI-MTD model.

5.2. Electronegativity Valences of Groups

For characterizing the chemical nature of vertices in a molecular graph, Diudea and Silaghi[47] have proposed the *electronegativity valences of groups EVG*

$$ESG_i = (ESA_i\, ESH^{hi})^{1/(1+hi)} \tag{24}$$

$$h_i = (8 - GA_i) - k_i \tag{25}$$

$$EVG_i = (ESG_i)^{1/(1+ki)} \tag{26}$$

where GA_i is the number of column in the Periodic Table for the atom A belonging to the vertex (i.e. group) i. ESA and ESH denote the Sanderson[49] electronegativities for the atom A and hydrogen, respectively. The number of hydrogen atoms attached to the group i is denoted by h_i while k_i stands for the degree of i. When $k_i > (8 - GA_i)$, then $h_i = 0$. In case of multiple bonds $k_i = \sum_j b_{ij}$, with b_{ij} being the conventional bond orders around the vertex i.

Note that these group electronegativities obey the electronegativity equalizing principle within the group i (see eq 24) and per molecule, each group being considered bonded to neighbors with electronegativity 1.[47]

The EVG_i values were used in construction of DS index as well as parameters of TI-MTD model.

The EC valence electronegativities[48] were developed as a variant of EVG parameters. They are based on the idea of modification of covalent radius of an atom by its hybridization state.[50] Such a modification is reflected in the electronegativity values corresponding to the considered state. The following scenario defined the EC parameters:

(i) - covalent radii, relative to carbon atom (0.772 ANG) are calculated by eqs 27-29

$$rc_{ni} = rc_{1i} + \Delta rc_{ni} \tag{27}$$

$$rc_{1i} = r_{1i} / 0.772 \tag{28}$$

$$\Delta rc_{ni} = (r_{ni} - r_{1i}) / 7.72 \tag{29}$$

where : rc is the atomic radius relative to the carbon atom; n is the row and i is the column in the Periodic Table; Δrc stand for the *excess of relative radius*.

(ii) - values EC, for the atoms in the nth row of Periodic Table are calculated by dividing the group electronegativities ESG_i to the mean relative length, mlc, of the bonds around the considered vertex/group i :

$$EC_{ni} = (ESG_{ni} / mlc_{ni}) / EC_C \tag{30}$$

$$EC_C = 2.746 / 1.4996 \tag{31}$$

$$mlc_{ni} = ml_C rc_{ni} \tag{32}$$

EC values are listed in Table 1. They were used in construction of EC indices as well as parameters of TI-MTD model.

Table 1. *EC* Electronegativities

-Br	1.2447	$-NH_2$	1.0644
$-CBr_3$	1.1266	-NO	1.4063
$-CCl_3$	1.1932	$-NO_2$	1.4861
$-CF_3$	1.3260	-O-	1.4634
$-CH_2-$	0.9622	$-OCH_3$	1.1248
$-CH_2Br$	1.0110	-OH	1.2325
$-CH_2Cl$	1.0305	$-P(CH_3)_2$	0.9351
$-CH_2F$	1.0674	-P<	0.8988
$-CH_2I$	0.9744	$-PCH_3-$	0.9314
$-CH_2OH$	1.0228	-PH-	0.9124
$-CH_2SH$	0.9804	$-PH_2$	0.9170
$-CH_3$	0.9575	$-PHCH_3$	0.93053
-CH<	0.9716	-S-	1.1064
$-CH=CH_2$	1.0381	$-SCH_3$	1.0073
-CH=O	1.1596	2PO	0.1222
$-CHBr_2$	1.0672	3P=O	1.3333
$-CHCl_2$	1.1089	=C=	1.1581
$-CHF_2$	1.1897	=CH-	1.0441
$-CHI_2$	0.9914	$=CH_2$	1.0891
$-CI_3$	1.0088	=N-	1.3147
-COOH	1.2220	=NH	1.2474
-Cl	13717	=O	1.6564
-C≡	1.1476	=P-	0.9658
-C≡N	1.2377	=S	1.2523
-F	1.6514	>C<	1.0000
-H	0.9175	>C=	1.0747
-I	1.0262	>C=O	1.2397
$-N(CH_3)_2$	1.0292	$-NHCH_3$	1.0379
-N<	1.2234	≡CH	1.2142
-NH-	1.1021	≡N	1.5288

5.3. Indices Based on Layer Matrices

The most used *TI* within TI-MTD are the indices of *centrality* *C*(*LM*) and *centrocomplexity* *X*(*LM*)[51,52] constructed on some layer matrices.

Indices of centrality[51,52] look for the center of the graph and are defined as

$$C(LM)_i = [\sum_{j=1}^{ecc_i} ([\mathbf{LM}]_{ij})^{j/d}]^{-1} \tag{33}$$

$$C(LM) = \sum_i C(LM)_i \tag{34}$$

where d is a specified topological distance (e.g. d = 10). Most frequently used layer matrices were $\mathbf{L^1W}$ and **LDS**.

Indices of centrocomplexity express the location vs. a vertex of high complexity (eg. a vertex of high degree or a heteroatom).[51] They are defined as

$$X(LM)_i = [\sum_{j=0}^{ecc_i} [\mathbf{LM}]_{ij} 10^{-zj}]^{\pm 1} t_i \tag{35}$$

$$X(LM) = \sum_i X(LM)_i \tag{36}$$

where z denotes the number of bits (of the integer part) of $max([\mathbf{LM}]_{ij})$ in G and t_i is a weighting factor for heteroatom specification. Within TI-MTD model t_i was either EVG_i or EC_i parameters. Matrices $\mathbf{L^1W}$ and **LDS** and the corresponding indices for the graph G_1, are shown in Table 2.

Table 2. Layer Matrices $\mathbf{L^1W}$ and **LDS** as well as C and X Indices (d = 10 and t = 1, respectively) for the Graph G_1.

	$\mathbf{L^1W}$	$C(L^1W)_i$	$X(L^1W)_i$	**LDS**	$C(LDS)_i$	$X(LDS)_i$
1	1 3 3 1	0.2975	1.331	8 5 14 9	0.2082	8.051409
2	3 4 1 0	0.4654	3.410	5 22 9 0	0.3432	5.220900
3	2 4 2 0	0.4353	2.420	6 14 16 0	0.3286	6.141600
4	1 2 3 2	0.2818	1.232	9 6 5 16	0.2052	9.060516
5	1 3 3 1	0.2975	1.331	8 5 14 9	0.2082	8.051409
Global Index:		1.7774	9.724		1.2934	36.525834

These indices showed good sensitivity in discriminating isomeric structures. They were used in studies on intramolecular ordering of subgraphs of various sizes as well as intermolecular ordering.

6. Applications of TI-MTD Model in QSAR and Molecular Design

6.1. Inhibitory Activity of the Trimethoprime Congeners

An application of TI-MTD on a set of trimethoprime (5-(3',4',5'-trimethoxy-benzyl)-2, 4-diaminopyrimidine) congeners[18] (see Table 3) in presented. They show inhibitory activity upon dihydrofolate reductase of *Escherichia coli*.

Figure 7 shows the basic structure of this set while Table 3 lists the substituents for all structures M_i; i = 1,..., 22 along with the observed inhibition constant (as -logK_{app}).

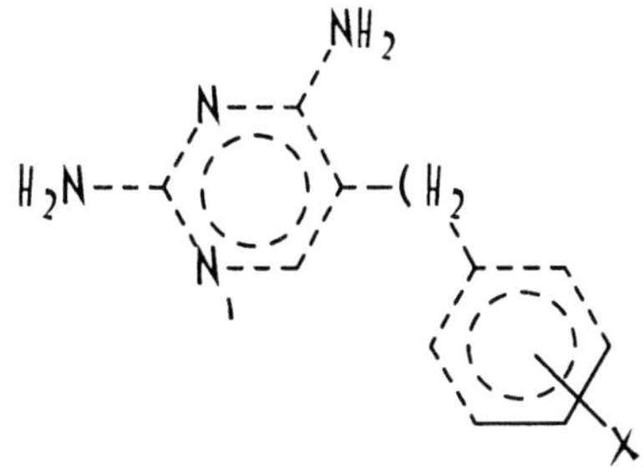

Figure 7. Basic structure of the set of trimethoprime derivatives

Table 3. 5-(Benzyl-Substituted)-2,4-Diaminopyrimidines, Inhibition Constant (as -logK_{app}) and Topological Data for the Active Fragment.

No	X	-logK_{app} logK$_{iapp}$	$DS_{C,S}$*	$DS_{W,S}$*	$DS_{C,N}$*	$EC_{3'}$	$EC_{4'}$
1	3`,4`,5`,-$(OCH_3)_3$	8.87	317	0	252	1.1248	1.1248
2	3`-CF_3	7.02	113	148	82	1.3260	0
3	3`-CH_3	6.70	57	0	52	0.9575	0
4	4`-CH_3	6.48	44	0	34	0	0.9575
5	3`-Cl	6.65	57	0	52	1.3717	0
6	4`-Cl	6.45	44	0	34	0	1.3717
7	3`-F	6.23	57	0	42	1.6514	0
8	4`-F	6.35	44	0	34	0	1.6514
9	H	6.18	0	0	0	0	0
10	4`-$N(CH_3)_2$	6.78	91	47	68	0	1.0292
11	4`-NH_2	6.30	44	0	34	0	1.0644
12	4`-$NHCOCH_3$	6.89	91	124	68	0	1.1021
13	4`-NO_2	6.20	91	47	34	0	1.4861
14	3`-OC_4H_9	6.89	113	230	82	1.4634	0
15	4`-OCF_3	6.57	91	180	51	0	1.4634
16	3`-$OCH_2C_6H_5$	6.99	113	321	82	1.4634	0
17	3`-OCH_3	6.93	113	0	82	1.1248	0
18	3`,4`-$(OCH_3)_2$	7.72	204	0	170	1.1248	1.1248
19	3`,5`-$(OCH_3)_2$	8.38	226	0	184	1.1248	0
20	4`-OCH_3	6.82	91	0	68	0	1.1248
21	3`-OH	6.47	57	0	52	1.2325	0
22	3`,4`-$(OH)_2$	6.46	101	0	76	1.2325	1.2325

* The subscript letters are: C = cavity; W = wall; S = symmetric (hypermolecule); N = non-symmetric.

In building the *hypermolecule*, (i.e. $[RS]_{init}$), the leading structure M_r was taken the trimethoprime, having the substituents 3`,4`,5`-$(OCH_3)_3$. For first, a symmetric $[RS]_{S,init}$, was considers. It is illustrated in Figure 8, a.

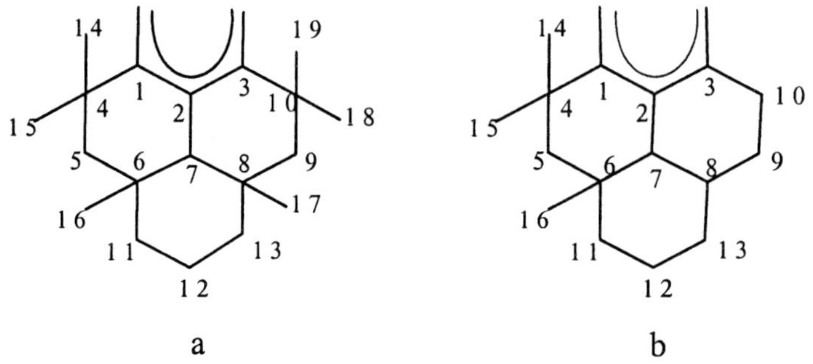

Figure 8. Symmetric (a) and non-symmetric (b) hypermolecules of trimethoprime derivatives

Selected *TI*'s are calculated for the whole hypermolecule and subsequently the descriptors TD_C and TD_w, that represent the predictor variables to be introduced in the regression equation (7).

By the hypermolecule hypothesis, the cavity points (i.e. the *C* subset) are the atoms of the leading structure (i.e. trimethoprime) having the vector $\mathbf{X}_1$ = (0001111011000000000). In words, the *C* set includes the points: 4, 5, 6, 7, 9 and 10 of the hypermolecule (Figure 8, a), while the remainders are considered wall points (i.e. the *W* subset) or irrelevant ones.

The corresponding descriptors *TD*(*i*) for candidates are calculated by summing the local values of the *TI* according to their $\mathbf{X}_i$ vector.

Thus, the cavity descriptor for the reference is

$$TD_C(1) = TI_4 + TI_5 + TI_6 + TI_7 + TI_9 + TI_{10} \tag{37}$$

Analogously one calculates for all candidates *Mi*. For the lead the wall descriptor is $TD_W(1) = 0$, since all its points are considered, by the above hypothesis, entering in the cavity. The descriptors TD_C and TD_W thus obtained are used in the regression analysis.

As *TD*, the distance sum *DS* (i.e. the sum of topological distances from *i* to all other vertices in a molecular graph) was here used. For the trimethoprime set, the descriptors included in Table 3 led to the following regression equation

$$\begin{aligned} Y_{calc} &= 5.9442 + 0.0092 DS_{C,S} - 0.00029 DS_{W,S} \\ n &= 22;\ r = 0.9514;\ s = 0.221;\ F = 90.702 \end{aligned} \tag{38}$$

In eq 38, the coefficient of the wall descriptor is one order of magnitude lower than the coefficient of the cavity descriptor (at the same magnitude of descriptor values). It suggests that, in this case, the wall interaction could be neglected. Indeed, the statistics of the monovariate equation (39) is at least as good as the bivariate regression equation (38)

$$Y_{calc} = 5.9317 + 0.0092 DS_{C,S}$$
$$n = 22;\ r = 0.9506;\ s = 0.217;\ F = 187.635 \quad (39)$$

The good quality of the regression equations (38 and 39) indicates that *DS* is an appropriate topological descriptor. It *encloses* the steric dimension of these molecular structures.

Since for the characterization of the receptor-effector system, the steric factor is, however, not sufficient, the electronegativity valences *EC* (see Sect. 5.2) were introduced as an additional predictor variable. By the viewpoint of electronegativity, the attachment sites of substituents to the benzyl are important. A new regression equation is thus obtained

$$Y_{calc} = 6.2548 + 0.01049 DS_{C,S} - 0.2466 EC_3 - 0.3056 EC_4 + 0.1473 EC_5$$
$$n = 22,\ r = 0.9780,\ s = 0.1584,\ F = 93.69 \quad (40)$$

The *Student test* for EC_5 suggests the possibility of neglecting this variable

$$Y_{calc} = 6.2477 + 0.01124 DS_{C,S} - 0.2807 EC_3 - 0.3374\ EC_4$$
$$n = 22,\ r = 0.9774,\ s = 0.2563,\ F = 128.16 \quad (41)$$

Note that in calculating the above descriptors, in case of large substituents (such as -NO_2, -$NHCOCH_3$, -OCF_3) only the atom attached to the benzyl is considered to be of *C*-type.

The map $[RS]_{S,opt}$ above calculated is based on a symmetric hypermolecule (Figure 8, (a)). It is also conceivable a *non-symmetric hypermolecule* (Figure 8, b). Indeed, in the new hypothesis, the compounds M_3, M_5 and M_7 show a residual value $\Delta = Y_{obs} - Y_{calc}$ lower that in case of symmetric hypermolecule.

With the non-symmetric $[RS]_{N,opt}$, the correlation equation becomes

$$Y_{calc} = -6.288081 + 0.012941 DS_{C,N} - 0.304293 EC_3 - 0.294274\ EC_4$$
$$n = 22,\ r = 0.9931,\ s = 0.086,\ F = 433.20 \quad (42)$$

The statistics of eq 42 are far more improved and it can be used for predicting novel bioactive structures. The plot of Y_{obs} vs Y_{calc} (cf. eq 42) is shown in Figure 9.

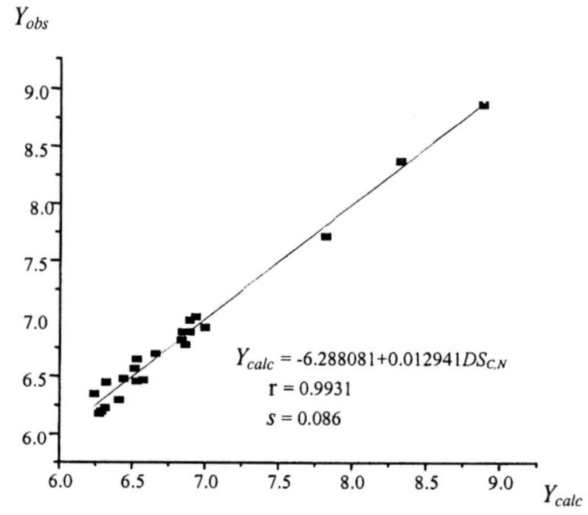

Figure 9. The plot $Y_{obs} = f(Y_{calc})$.

The values Y_{obs}, Y_{calc} as well as the residuals Δ for the whole set of trimethoprime congeners are listed in Table 4.

Table 4. Values Y_{obs}, Y_{calc} and Residuals Δ,(cf. ec 42) in the Set of Trimethoprime Congeners,

M_i	Y_{obs}	Y_{calc}	$\Delta = Y_{obs}-Y_{calc}$
1:	8.8700	8.8803	-0.0103
2:	7.0200	6.9328	0.0872
3:	6.7000	6.6557	0.0443
4:	6.4800	6.4388	0.0412
5:	6.6500	6.5287	0.1213
6:	6.4500	6.3193	0.1307
7:	6.2300	6.3130	-0.0830
8:	6.3500	6.2386	0.1114
9:	6.1800	6.2730	-0.0930
10:	6.7800	6.8602	-0.0802
11:	6.3000	6.4080	-0.1080
12:	6.8900	6.8392	0.0508
13:	6.2000	6.2863	-0.0863
14:	6.8900	6.8907	-0.0007
15:	6.5700	6.5139	0.0561
16:	6.9900	6.8907	0.0993
17:	6.9300	6.9945	-0.0645
18:	7.7200	7.8141	-0.0941
19:	8.3800	8.3207	0.0593
20:	6.8200	6.8326	-0.0126
21:	6.4700	6.5714	-0.1014
22:	6.4600	6.5278	-0.0678

The predicting ability of eq 42 was tested by a *cross validation* (leave 5% out) procedure. The test supplied eq 43

$$`Y_{calc} = -0.00345 + 0.99992\, Y_{cv}$$
$$n = 22,\ r_{cv} = 0.989,\ s = 0.105,\ F = 478.0 \qquad (43)$$

for which the plot $Y_{obs} = f(Y_{cv})$ is shown in Figure 10.

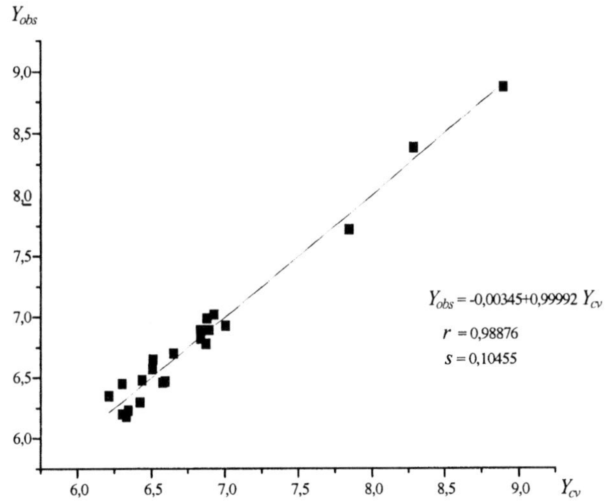

Figure 10. The plot $Y_{obs} = f(Y_{cv})$ cf eq 43.

The good predicting ability of eq 42 allowed to estimate the activity of a *test structure* M_{23}, having the substituents 3`,5`-OCH_3-4`-$O(CH_2)OCH_3$: $Y_{calc} = 8.336$ vs $Y_{obs} = 8.35$, $\Delta = 0.014$. The substituent -$O(CH_2)OCH_3$ is considered a voluminous one and, by this reason, it overlap the cavity set only in position **7** of$[RS]_{N,opt}$, cf Figure 11. Note that this structure was dropped out of the training set.

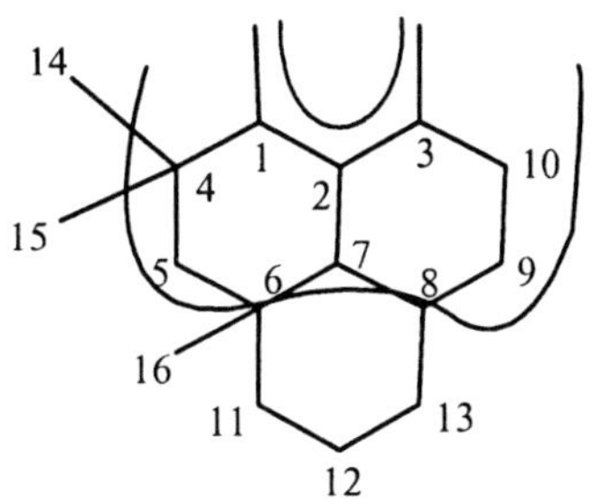

Figure 11. The optimal *RS* map for the trimethoprime series

The parameters used in calculating the activity of the *test structure* M_{23} are: $DS_C = 218$; $EC_3 = 1.1248$; $EC_4 = 1.4634$.

The same eq 42 allowed the prediction of three novel trimethoprime derivatives, for which good activity is expected:

M_{24} (– 3`,4`,5`-($NHCH_3)_3$):	$DS_C = 252$ $EC_3 = 1.0379$ $EC_4 = 1.0379$	$Y_{calc} = 8.92$
M_{25} (– 3`,4`,5`-($SCH_3)_3$):	$DS_C = 252$ $EC_3 = 1.0073$ $EC_4 = 1.0073$	$Y_{calc} = 8.940$
M_{26} (– 4`- $NH_2$ 3`, 5`-($OCH_3)_2$):	$DS_C = 218$ $EC_3 = 1.1248$ $EC_4 = 1.0644$	$Y_{calc} = 8.454$

In comparison to the trimethoprime ($Y_{obs} = 8.87$) the proposed structures appear as promising compounds.

6.2. Activity of 2-Substituted 1, 2, 3-Thiadiazol-5-Sulphonamides

For validating the correlating ability of TI-MTD model, the activity of a set of 2-substituted 1, 2, 3-thiadiazol-5-sulphonamides[53] is further investigated (Figure 12). They show an inhibitory activity upon the *carbonic anhydrase* (a metaloenzyme) higher than that shown by aromatic sulphonamides.

Note that this set was also tested by MTD, MVD and CoMFA approaches.[53]

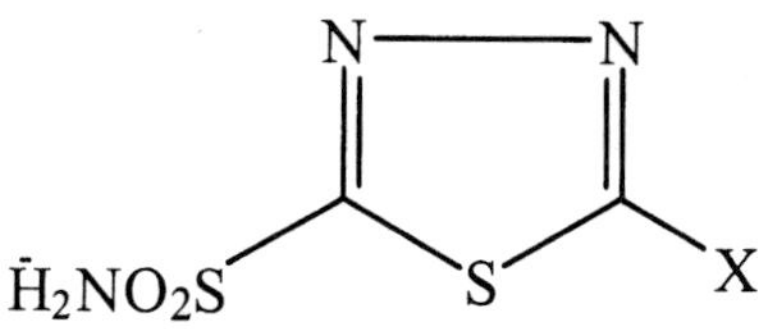

Figure 12. 2-Substituted 1, 2, 3-Thiadiazol-5-Sulphonamides

Table 5 lists the set of 11 tiadiazol-5-sulfonamides along with the observed activity ($Y_{obs} = \log II_{50}$).

Table 5. 2-Substituted 1, 2, 3-Thiadiazol-5-Sulphonamides

No	X	log II_{50}
1	$NHSO_2C_6H_4$-4-$NHCOCH_3$	3.38
2	$NHSO_2C_6H_4$-Cl	3.29
3	$NHSO_2C_6H_5$	3.16
4	$NHCOC_6H_5$	2.95
5	$N(CH_3)COCH_3$	2.66
6	NHC_6H_5	2062
7	$NHCOCH_3$	2.52
8	NHCHO	2.28
9	$NHCH_3$	1.96
10	H	1.90
11	NH_2	1.64

The hypermolecule for the set of 11 tiadiazol-5-sulfonamides is shown in Figure 13.

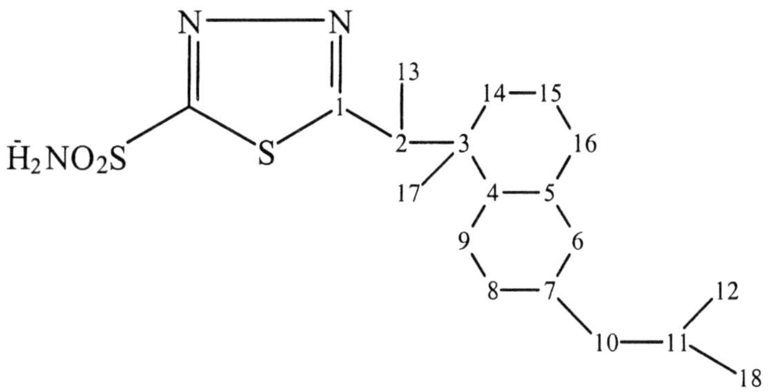

Figure 13. The hypermolecule for the set of 11 tiadiazol-5-sulfonamides

By using *DS* as topological descriptor (see the Sect. 6.1) the following regression equation was obtained

$$Y_{obs} = 1,79877 + 0,00287 DS_C$$
$$n = 11\ r = 0.988;\ s = 0.0943;\ F = 371 \quad (44)$$

The plot $Y_{obs} = f(DS)$ is shown in Figure 14.

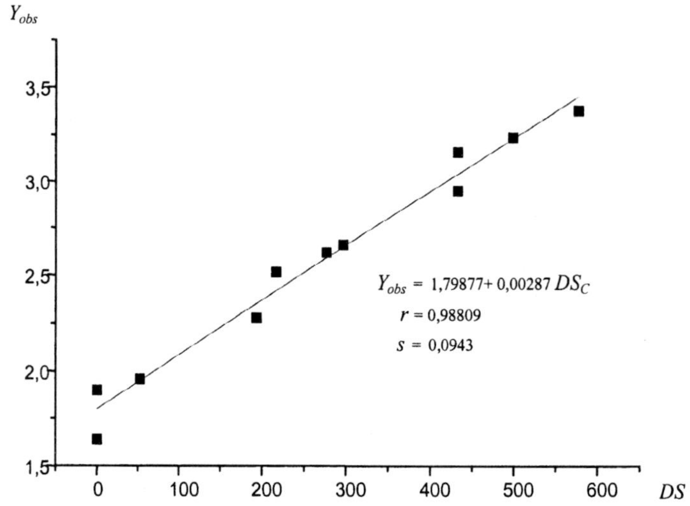

Figure 14. The plot $Y_{obs} = f(DS)$ for the set of 11 tiadiazol-5-sulfonamides.

The *cross validation* test (leave 5% out) performed on eq 44 led to eq 45

$$Y_{obs} = -0.01761 + 1.00387 Y_{cv} \qquad (45)$$
$$n = 11;\ r_{cv} = 0.984;\ s = 0.108;\ F = 280$$

for which the plot $Y_{obs} = f(Y_{cv})$ is shown in Figure 15.

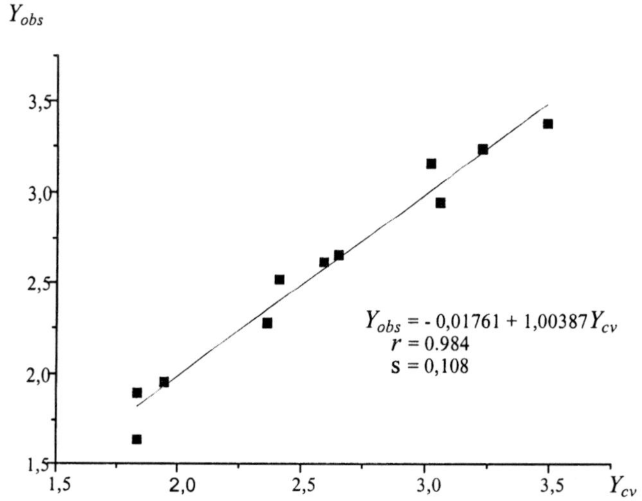

Figure 15. The plot $Y_{obs} = f(Y_{cv})$ for eq 45.

On the above set, the MTD and MVD approaches provided the following results:[53]

$Y_{obs} = 4{,}745 - 0{,}350\ MTD$
$n = 11;\ r = 0.992;\ s = 0{,}078;\ F = 249$ (46)

$Y_{obs} = 4{,}406 - 0{,}013\ MVD$
$n = 11;\ r = 0.993;\ s = 0{,}075;\ F = 272$ (47)

In MVD the volumes are calculated by *Monte Carlo* method. It can be seen that the results of TI-MTD are quite close to those given by approaches using 3D geometries, at a much lower cpu cost.

7. Conclusions

TI-MTD is a 2D topological approach for ligand-receptor interaction description. It provides some grid-descriptors (steric and electrostatic) of such interaction and fine-tunes the model' s statistical quality by changing both the alignment modes and the receptor map until an optimal receptor map is obtained.

The method can be used in predicting novel bioactive structures. An advantage of this topological approach is the relatively reduced computational cost in comparison to the methods using molecular mechanic or quantum calculations. It can be used as a pre-test before investigation by more elaborated procedures. A further comparison of the TI-MTD results with those provided by other 3D-QSAR approaches could be relevant in validation of this method.

8. References

1. Free, S. M.; Wilson, J. W. Mathematical Contribution to Structure-Activity Studies. *J. Med. Chem.* **1964**, *7*, 395-399.
2. Kubinyi, H. Free Wilson Analysis. Theory, Applications and its relationship to Hansch Analysis. *Qant. Struct.-Act. Relat.* **1988**, *7*, 121-133.
3. Hansch, C.; Fujita, T. ρ-σ-π Analysis. A Method for the Correlation of Biological Activity and Chemical Structure. *J. Amer. Chem. Soc.* **1964**, *86*, 1616-1626.
4. Hansch, C.; Leo, A.; Taft, R. W. A Survey of Hammett Substituent Constants and Resonance and Field Parameters. *Chem. Rev.* **1991**, *91*, 165-195.
5. Motoc, I. Holban, S.; Vancea, R.; Simon, Z. Minimal Steric Difference Computed as Nonoverlapping Volumes. Correlations with Enzymatic Hydrolysis of Ribonucleotides, *Studia Biophys.* (*Berlin*), **1977**, *66*, 75-78.
6. Chiriac, A. Ciubotariu, D.; Simon, Z. *Quantitative Structure-Activity Relationships* (*QSAR*). *The MTD Method.* MIRTON, Timisoara, 1996.

7. Simon, Z.; Bohl, M. Structure-Activity Relations in Gestagenic Steroids by the MTD Method. The Case of Hard Molecules and Soft Receptors. *Quant. Struct.-Act. Relat.* **1992**, *11*, 23-28.
8. Comparative Structure-Affinity Relations by MTD for Binding of Cycloadenosine Monophosphate Derivatives to Protein Kinase Receptors. *Quant. Struct.-Act. Relat.* **1994**, *13*, 242-248.
9. Simon, Z.; Chiriac, A.; Holban, S. Steric Fit in QSAR. IV. MTD – Receptor Site Mapping, *Preprint Univ. Timisoara*, **1980**, *4*, 1-50.
10. Balaban, A. T.; Chiriac, A.; Motoc, I.; Simon, Z. *Steric Fit in QSAR* (Lecture Notes in Chemistry, Vol. 15), Springer, Berlin, 1980, Chap. 6.
11. Balaban, A. T. Topological and Stereochemical Molecular Descriptors for Databases Useful in QSAR, Similarity/Dissimilarity and Drug Design, *SAR-QSAR Environ. Res.* **1998**, *8*, 1-21.
12. Balaban, A. T. (Ed.) *From Chemical Topology to Three-Dimensional Geometry*. Plenum Press, New York, 1997.
13. Hurst, T. Flexible 3D Searching: the Direct Tweak Technique, *J. Chem. Inf. Comput. Chem.* **1994**, *34*, 190-196.
14. Willet, P. *Three-Dimensional Chemical Structure Handling*, Research Studies Press-Wiley, Taunton, U. K. 1991.
15. Oprea,T. I.; Ciubotariu D.; Simon, Z. Comparison of the Minimal Steric Difference (MTD) and Comparative Molecular Field Analysis (CoMFA) Methods for Analysis of Binding of Steroids to Carrier Proteins. *Quant. Struct.-Act. Relat.* **1993**, *12*, 21-26.
16. Motoc, I. Biological Receptor Maps.1. Steric Maps. The SIBIS Method. *Quant. Struct.-Act. Relat.* **1984**, *3*, 43-47.
17. Motoc, I.; Marshall, G. R.; Dammkoehler, R. A.; Labanowski, J. Molecular Shape Descriptors. 1. Three-Dimensional Molecular Shape Descriptor. *Z. Naturforsch.* **1985**, *40a*, 1108-1113.
18. Motoc, I.; Marshall, G. R. Molecular Shape Descriptors. 2. Quantitative Structure-Activity Relationships Based Upon Three-Dimensional Molecular Shape Descriptor. *Z. Naturforsch.* **1985**, *40a*, 1114-1120.
19. Motoc, I.; Marshall, G. R.; Labanowski, J. Molecular Shape Descriptors. 3. Steric Mapping of Biological Receptors. *Z. Naturforsch.* **1985**, *40a*, 1121-1127.
20. Cramer R. D. III, Patterson D. E., Bunce J. D.; Comparative Molecular Field Analysis (COMFA). 1. Effect of Shape on Binding of Steroids to Carrier Proteins, *J. Am. Chem. Soc.* **1988**, *110*, 5959-5967.
21. Kellogg G. E.; Semus S. F.; Abraham D. J.; HINT: a New Method of Empirical Hydrophobic Field Calculation for CoMFA. *J. Comput.-Aided Mol. Des.* **1991**, *5*, 545-552.
22. Kim K. H.; Use of the Hydrogen-Bond Potential Function in Comparative Molecular Field Analysis (CoMFA): An extension of CoMFA. *Quant. Struct.-Act. Relat.* **1993**, *12*, 232-238.
23. Waller C.L.; Marshall G. R.; Three-Dimensional Quantitative Structure-Activity Relationship of Angiotensin-Converting Enzyme and Thermolysin Inhibitors. II. A Comparison of CoMFA Models Incorporating Molecular Orbital Fields and

Desolvation Free Energy Based on Active-Analog and Complementary-Receptor-Field Alignment. *J. Med. Chem.* **1993**, *36*, 2390-2403.
24. Muresan, S.; Sulea, T. ; Ciubotariu, D.; Kurunczi, L.; Simon, Z. Van der Waals Intersection Envelope Volumes as a Possible Basis for Steric Interaction in CoMFA, *Quant. Struct.-Act. Relat.* **1996**, *15*, 31-32.
25. Oprea, T. I.; Waller C.L. Theoretical and Practical Aspects of Three Dimensional Quantitative Structure-Activity Relationships. In Reviews in Computational Chemistry, Lipkowitz, K. B. and Boyd, D. B. (Eds.), Wiley, New York, 1997, 11, 127-182.
26. Chuman H.; Karasawa M.; Fujita T.; A Novel Three-Dimensional QSAR Procedure: Voronoi Field Analysis. *Quant. Struct.-Act. Relat.* **1998**, *17*, 313-326.
27. Durst G. L, Comparative Molecular Field Analysis (CoMFA) of Herbicidal Protoporphyrinogen Oxidase Inhibitors using Standard Steric and Electrostatic Fields and an Alternative LUMO Field. *Quant. Struct.-Act. Relat.* **1998**, *17*, 419-426.
28. Pajeva I. L., Wiese M.; A Comparative Molecular Field Analysis of Propafenone-type Modulators of Cancer Multidrug Resistance. *Quant. Struct.-Act. Relat.* **1998**, *17*, 301-312.
29. Devillers, J. (Ed.) *Genetic Algorithms in Molecular Modeling*. Acad. Press, London, 1996.
30. Whitney, H. Congruent Graphs and the Connectivity of Graphs. *Amer. J. Math.* **1932**, *54*, 150-168.
31. Hoffman, A. J. On the Line-Graph of the Complete Bipartite Graph. *Ann. Math. Statist.* **1964**, *35*, 883-885.
32. Ore, O. *Theory of Graphs*. Amer. Math. Soc. Colloq. Publ. 38. Providence, 1962.
33. Sabidussi, G. Graph Derivatives. *Math. Z.* **1961**, *76*, 385-401.
34. Beineke, L. W. Derived Graphs and Digraphs. In *Beiträge zur Graphentheorie*, Sachs, H.; Voss, H. and Walther, H. (Eds.), Teubner, Leipzig, 1968, pp. 17-33.
35. Seshu, S.; Reed, M. *Linear Graphs and Electrical Networks*. Addison-Wesley, Reading, 1961.
36. Kasteleyn, P. W. Graph Theory and Crystal Physics. In *Graph Theory and Theoretical Physics*, Harary, F. (Ed.), Academic Press, London, 1967, pp. 44-110.
37. Menon, V. On Repeated Interchange Graphs. *Amer. Math. Monthly*, **1966**, *13*, 986-989.
38. Harary, F. *Graph Theory*, Addison - Wesley, Reading, M.A., 1969.
39. Diudea, M.V.; Horvath, D.; Bonchev, D. MOLORD Algorithm and Real Number Subgraph Invariants. *Croat. Chem. Acta*, **1995**, *68*, 131-148.
40. Trinajstić, N. *Chemical Graph Theory* : CRC Press: Boca Raton, FL, 1983, Vol.2, Chap. 4.
41. Bertz, S.H. Branching in Graphs and Molecules, *Discr. Appl. Math.* **1988**, *19*, 65-83.
42. Diudea, M. V. ; Ivanciuc, O. Molecular Topology, Comprex, Cluj, 1995 (in Romanian).
43. Minailiuc, M. O. Fragmentation Algorithms and Topological Models. TI-MTD Model. Applications in Molecular design. Ph. D. Thesis, Cluj, Romania, 1999.

44. Razinger, M.; Balasubramanian, K.; Munk, M.E. Graph Automorphism Perception Algorithms in Computer-Enhanced Structure Elucidation. *J. Chem. Inf. Comput. Sci.* **1993**, *33*, 197-201.
45. Bangov, I.P. Graph Isomorphism: A Consequence of the Vertex Equivalence *J. Chem. Inf. Comput. Sci.* **1994**, *34*, 318-324.
46. Randić, M. On Characterization of Molecular Branching, *J. Amer. Chem.Soc.* **1975**, *97*, 6609-6615.
47. Diudea, M. V.; Silaghi-Dumitrescu, I. Valence Group Electronegativity as a Vertex Discriminator, *Rev. Roumaine Chim.* **1989**, *34*, 1175.
48. Diudea, M. V.; Kacso', I. E.; Topan, M. I. A QSPR/QSAR Study by Using New Valence Group Carbon-Related Electronegativities, *Rev. Roum. Chim.* **1996**, *41*, 141-157.
49. Sanderson, R. T. Polar Covalence, Acad. Press, New York, 1983.
50. Allread, A. L.; Rochow, E. G. *J. Inorg. Nucl. Chem.* **1958**, *5*, 264.
51. Diudea, M. V. Layer Matrices in Molecular Graphs, *J. Chem. Inf. Comput. Sci.* **1994**, *34*, 1064-1071.
52. Diudea, M. V.; Topan, M. I.; Graovac, A. Layer Matrix of Walk Degrees, *J. Chem. Inf. Comput. Sci.* **1994**, *34*, 1072-1078.
53. Muresan, S. Contributions to the Development of MTD Method. Applications in QSAR. Ph.D. Thesis, West University Timisoara, 1995, 128-132

Chapter 12

COMPHARM –AUTOMATED COMPARATIVE ANALYSIS OF PHARMACOPHORIC PATTERNS AND DERIVED QSAR APPROACHES, NOVEL TOOLS IN HIGH-THROUGHPUT DRUG DISCOVERY. A PROOF-OF-CONCEPT STUDY APPLIED TO FARNESYL PROTEIN TRANSFERASE INHIBITOR DESIGN.

Dragos Horvath
CEREP MOLECULAR MODELING DEPARTMENT.
128, rue Danton – BP 50601, 92506 Rueil-Malmaison Cedex
E-mail d.horvath@cerep.fr

1. A GENERAL INTRODUCTION TO THE COMFA METHODOLOGY

Comparative Molecular Field Analysis (CoMFA)[1,2,3] is nowadays the most widely used approach[4,5,6] in the evolving field of 3D (geometry-based) Quantitative Structure-Activity Relations (3D-QSAR)[7,8]. In contrast to the physically more rigorous docking[4,5] approaches, that directly monitor the intensity of the site-ligand attractive and repulsive interactions and might even include some empirical evaluations of the binding entropy[11,12,13], CoMFA does not require any knowledge of the three-dimensional structure of the binding site of the targeted biological macromolecule. This approach can be used to extract information relative to the features of an unknown active site, on the basis of a set of ligands of experimentally known affinities with respect to the target macromolecule (receptor or enzyme), the "learning set". Nowadays, the discovery of series of new ligands of novel targets by means of Combinatorial Chemistry[14] and High Throughput Organic Synthesis[15], combined with High Throughput Screening[15] against recombinant targets issued from diverse genomics programs[17] proceeds at a much higher pace than the acquisition rate of 3D-structures of biological macromolecules. Therefore, the importance of CoMFA and related tools[18,19] aimed to infer site-related information on the basis of experimental activity data is expected to increase in the context of "high throughput" drug design.

The CoMFA approach assumes that a spatial alignment of the *bioactive conformers of these ligands* with respect each other, representing the relative positions they would adopt when bound to the active site of the target, can be found. In the absence of any knowledge of the actual binding mode, both the postulated "bioactive" conformers and their relative spatial orientations are obtained on the basis of more or less arbitrary assumptions that will be eventually validated or invalidated by the quality of the derived SAR models. The most widely applied methodologies used to generate the alignment of the bioactive conformers will be briefly discussed below:

- The "manual" atom-to-atom mapping technique[20] requires the medicinal chemist to specify, the pairs of "equivalent" atoms that would, according to his expertise, occupy the same pockets of the site when the corresponding molecules bind. Such a method only applies to small learning sets of rigid analogs that share a common molecular skeleton.
- An automatic[20] atom-to-atom mapping procedure typically analyzes the topological environment of each vertex of both the reference ligand and the current ligand. Pairs of vertices of the current and reference ligand with similar topological neighborhoods will be considered equivalent and used to perform the superposition.
- Molecular field-matching approaches[21] consist in searching for the relative orientation of a current ligand that maximizes the covariance of the intensities of the fields generated, at all the points of the surrounding space, by the ligand and the reference compound respectively. The monitored "molecular fields" may for example[20] represent the interaction energy of the compound with a "probe group". The interaction energy values are monitored in function of the position of the probe, which is successively located at all the points of a three-dimensional grid encompassing all the available ligand structures in their current orientations. In principle, several types of molecular fields, later on generically denoted as $F_t(M;P)$, are simultaneously used in a study. In this notation, "t" stands for the type of the field (e.g. 1=electrostatic potential, 2=van der Waals potential, 3=interaction energy with a molecular probe,...), M denotes the molecule of the learning set generating that field and P stands for the current point (x,y,z) at which the field value is taken. The alignment maximizing the overall degree of match of the ligand and reference fields, as expressed by various field matching indices[22,23,24], offers a better working hypothesis than the somehow arbitrary atom-to-atom mapping approaches, because receptor binding is controlled by the molecular fields and not by topological properties. Unfortunately, molecular field matching is a computationally expensive approach, unless the Gaussian[25,26] approximation of the exact equations describing the force field terms is used to achieve a faster, analytical evaluation of the field matching indices chosen as the

criterion to be maximized. The field matching index values at optimal superimposition defines a similarity[27] score of the two molecules.

- Both atom-to-atom mapping or molecular field-matching approaches can be either performed by a "rigid-body"[28,29] matching algorithm or by a "flexible matching"[28,29] algorithm. The former, fast approach, takes predefined conformers of the two compounds to superimpose and optimizes the specified overlap score in terms of only 3 translational + 3 rotational degrees of freedom describing the relative positions of the two rigid structures. The latter approach can be described as a conformational sampling algorithm[32,33,34] in which the quality criteria of the explored geometries are biased to account for their ability to match a reference geometry.

Given an optimal alignment of the molecules of the learning set with respect to a common reference system, the intensities of the various molecular fields at any point of the space can now be meaningfully compared. Various statistical procedures[35,36,37,38] can be used to select a set of points (P_1, P_2, ...P_n), such that the *activities* A(M) of the molecules M in the learning set can be expressed as a simple (usually linear) function of the *intensities of their different fields at those points*, which represent the *molecular descriptors* of the study:

$$A(M) = \sum_{t}^{\substack{relevant \\ fieldtypes}} \sum_{i}^{\substack{relevant \\ points}} c_{it} F_t(M;P_i) \tag{1}$$

However, monitoring the values of 2-3 different molecular fields at all the points P of a three-dimensional grid with a mesh size of 1-2 Å generates thousands of molecular field descriptors $F_t(M,P)$. Finding the relevant ones, to be used in equation (1), out of such a large number of possible terms, is not a trivial task. Molecular field values at different points P_A and P_B may be correlated: $F_t(M,P_A)=aF_t(M,P_B)+b$ for all the M in the learning set. If this is the case, the model using $F_t(M,P_B)$ would have a comparable predictive power with respect to its learning set, even though the actual ligand-protein interaction happens in P_A. However, it will fail if applied to molecules M' of other structural families, for which $F_t(M',P_A)$ and $F_t(M',P_B)$ are no longer "interchangeable". Such artifacts also blur the interpretation of the CoMFA models, "hiding" the physical reasons that back up the statistical relevance of each of the selected descriptors. An increase of the structural diversity of the compound set used for model calibration triggers a decrease of the number of artifactual inter-descriptor correlations in the set. Significant work was aimed to develop more robust CoMFA methodologies[39,40].

1.1 The Focus of the Present Work: Development, Validation and Testing of ComPharm, a Simplified CoMFA Approach

The development of the ComPharm methodology reported in this paper represents an attempt to translate the classical medicinal chemist's description of molecules in terms of their pharmacophoric groups, into a powerful, fully automated molecular superimposition optimizer, also accounting for conformational flexibility. The goal is to achieve a cost-effective and robust high throughput molecular comparison of large learning set of compounds, as available from combinatorial chemistry[41]-driven drug design experiments. Its possible applications include:

- the refined evaluation of molecular similarity[42] scores of candidates with respect to a reference compound, in the similarity search-driven mining of molecular data bases for analogs of a known lead. Too time-consuming to be directly applied for searching through databases of more than 10^4 candidates, the method was designed to perform a realistic ranking of the remaining candidates in terms of their similarity to the reference, after "filtering" of large data bases by a high-throughput algorithm discarding all the obviously dissimilar compounds. The ComPharm similarity metric represents an objective criterion quantifying the ability of the candidate to mimic the spatial orientation of the pharmacophoric groups of the reference.
- a tool for 3D-QSAR model development. The major difference between CoMFA and ComPharm relies on the divergent definitions of the "molecular fields". The molecular "fields" used in ComPharm reflect *the distribution of the pharmacophoric functional groups in the molecules,* rather than relying on molecule-probe interaction energy calculations. Furthermore, the "grid" points used to probe field intensities in the neighborhood of the overlaid molecules *are bound to the vertices of the molecular graph of the reference structure*, rendering them independent of the conformation and orientation of the reference and keeping their number significantly lower than in CoMFA approaches, where they are typically taken from a 3D-grid spanning the space zone around the molecules.

Farnesyl Protein Transferase (FPT) inhibitors were chosen as a study case to validate all the underlying hypotheses that differentiate ComPharm from the classical CoMFA methods. The present study also addresses some issues related to the feasibility of ComPharm-based QSAR-models involving structurally heterogeneous learning sets, such as:

- ➢ To what extent can a QSAR-model derived on the basis of a structurally homogeneous family be successfully applied to other families of compounds?
- ➢ Knowing that the search for the "optimal" overlay of candidate and reference is a highly complex multidimensional problem, what is the minimal computational effort guaranteeing the discovery of the absolutely optimal superimposition? To

what extent may failure to reach this global optimum affect the quality of the derived QSAR models?

- Can such QSAR-models be derived if some of the candidate molecules present several different, but equally plausible ways to be overlaid on the reference compound? Is there a consistent way to handle such situations in order to eliminate fluctuations induced by molecules in the learning set randomly adopting one particular orientation rather than another one, of comparable overall quality?

The outlined results and conclusions may serve as a general set of rules to follow in order to maximize the chances of avoiding overfitting artifacts when deriving QSAR models. This validation study of the ComPharm approach provides a general insight to the problematic of QSAR development and testing. The problems evidenced in this study are common all the CoMFA approaches and may even be exacerbated by the ones that use full-blown 3D-grids to generate a number of initial descriptors that may exceed by an order of magnitude the number of those provided by the simplified ComPharm method.

2. METHODS

2.1 ComPharm Superimposition Algorithm

2.1.1 Atomic Feature Flags

A rule-based algorithm searches for the putative pharmacophoric centers of a molecule, detecting all the atoms that display one or more of the six considered pharmacophoric features – hydrophobicity (*H*), aromaticity (*AR*), hydrogen bond acceptor (*HBA*) and HB donor (*HBD*) character, as well as the cationic (*POS*) and the anionic (*NEG*) character. For each atom i of a molecule M, atomic feature flags $\gamma_f(i;M)$; f=1…6 are defined according to the following rules:

- $\gamma_f(i;M)=0$ if atom i does not have the pharmacophoric feature f, where f is one of the six above enumerated features
- $\gamma_f(i;M)=1$ if atom i displays the feature f in a solvated molecule at physiological pH. Accordingly, all the aliphatic amino groups are considered to be cations and HB donors, while the anion feature flag is set for carboxylates and the equivalent tetrazole groups, sulfonates, phosphates and phosphonates. Anilines are taken as free bases, e.g. as hydrogen bond acceptors (and donors, if not fully substituted). Nitrogens in heterocycles have the aromatic feature flag set, as well as the HBA flag if they are "pyridine-like", with a free electron pair in an sp^2 orbital or, respectively, the HBD flag if they are "pyrrole-like" and carry a H atom. Amide nitrogens are not considered to be HB acceptors, but are HB donors if bound to a H. Alcoholic and phenolic OH groups are simultaneously HB donors and

acceptors. Sulfur in thiols or thioethers and all the halogen substituents are taken as hydrophobic groups.

- since the previously used binary definition of the presence or absence of a feature is a quite crude representation of the local properties of the molecule, the use of fine-tuned fractional atomic feature flags may represent an important improvement of this methodology. This would however raise the complex problem of the optimal calibration of those values. In the present version of the ComPharm method, the hydrophobic feature flags of aromatic C atoms, as well as the aromatic feature flags of aliphatic groups are empirically set to 0.5, since alkyl and aryl groups may to a certain extent play interchangeable roles in binding. In the case of imidazole rings, for which the protonation status at pH=7 is uncertain and the HB donor and HB acceptor N atoms cannot be discriminated due to ring tautomery, both N atoms are assigned equal HBA and HBD feature flags of 0.5, while the carbon atom C2 is assigned a cationic feature flag of 0.5.
- A pure shape component, not dependent on the nature of the involved atoms, can be simulated by adding a supplementary atomic feature, "existence", to the six ones listed before, such that $\gamma_7(i;M)=1$ for all the atoms of M. *In principle, other supplementary features could be envisaged, and therefore in the following a general mathematical treatment involving a total number of N_f features will be developed. In the current study, however, $N_f=7$, accounting for the six pharmacophoric features and one shape component.*

2.1.2 Definition of the Pharmacophoric Fields

A "pharmacophoric field" can now be associated to each one of the previously enumerated pharmacophoric features, taking the γ values as the formal "charges" or sources of this field, and assuming a Gaussian distance-dependence. The local intensity of the field $F_f(M;P)$ associated to the feature f at the point P in the vicinity of a molecule M can therefore be expressed as:

$$F_f(M;P) = \sum_{i=1}^{N(M)} \gamma_f(i;M)\, e^{-\alpha d^2(i,P)} \tag{2}$$

where N(M) is the total number of atoms in the molecule M, d(i,P) represents the distance between the current atom i and the point P and the exponential factor α represents a fittable parameter of the model. These field terms are smooth and finite functions at any point of space. They are less sensitive to the small artifactual variations of molecular geometry and orientation than the van der Waals fields used in CoMFA, where an offset of a molecular fragment by fractions of an Angstrom may imply dramatic changes of its potentials at a near point.

2.1.3 Molecular Overlap and Similarity Indices Based on the Pharmacophoric Fields

Given a conformer of a reference molecule M, a candidate molecule m will be subjected to *translations* specified by a translation vector (r_x,r_y,r_z) and *rotations* defined by the three Euler angles (ϕ,θ,ξ), starting from the original set of coordinates of its current conformation, in order to superimpose it atop of M. A reasonable criterion to assess the quality of the current superposition of m and M is given by the pairwise degrees of covariance of the intensities of the molecular fields $F_f(M;P)$ and $F_f(m;P)$ in all the points P of space, for each of the considered features f. The Gaussian distance-dependence of the empirical pharmacophoric fields –see equation (2) – has been chosen to allow an easy, analytical evaluation[25,26] of the Carbo[23] or Hodgkin[22] indices. They do, however, present the inconvenient of ignoring the directionality issues characterizing the hydrogen bond donor/acceptor features. The radial symmetry of these functions tends to minimize the distance between the HBA/HBD atoms of the candidate and reference molecules, without including any penalties if the overlapping groups adopt different orientations of their possible H-bonding directions. This problem could be in principle solved by considering "dummy" atoms to define the hydrogen bonding vectors of such groups.

2.1.3.1 Feature Overlap and Similarity Indices

For clarity, it is important to introduce here a distinction between "overlay" and "similarity" indices. Overlay indices quantify the current degree of overlap of two molecules or molecular fields, in function of their current, suboptimal, geometries and relative orientation. The absolute maximum of the considered overlay index with respect to all the degrees of freedom of the molecular superimposition problem, e.g. *the overlay index of the optimal molecular superposition, represents the similarity index.* Overlay indices are functions of molecular conformation and orientation, while similarity indices are intrinsic properties of the two studied molecules and no longer functions of these variables, which are fully specified by the constraint of a maximal overlay index.

In terms of the Hodgkin formalism, *the feature overlay indices $H_f(M,m,\Theta)$* express the degree of "overlap" (covariance) of the fields generated by the atoms of pharmacophoric property f, from M and respectively m, given a relative orientation of m with respect to M defined by the rototranslation vector Θ=(r_x,r_y,r_z,ϕ,θ,ξ).

$$H_f(M,m,\Theta) = \frac{2\sum_{i=1}^{N(M)} \gamma_f(i,M) \sum_{j=1}^{N(m)} \gamma_f(j,m) e^{-\alpha d^2(i,j)}}{\sum_{i=1}^{N(M)} \gamma_f(i,M) \sum_{j=1}^{N(M)} \gamma_f(j,M) e^{-\alpha d^2(i,j)} + \sum_{i=1}^{N(m)} \gamma_f(i,m) \sum_{j=1}^{N(m)} \gamma_f(j,m) e^{-\alpha d^2(i,j)}} \tag{3}$$

Equation (3) can be rewritten in terms of the pharmacophoric field intensities at the points occupied by the atoms:

$$H_f(M,m,\Theta) = \frac{2\sum_{i=1}^{N(M)} \gamma_f(i,M)F_f(m;i)}{\sum_{i=1}^{N(M)} \gamma_f(i,M)F_f(M;i) + \sum_{i=1}^{N(m)} \gamma_f(i,m)F_f(m;i)} \quad (4)$$

The numerator of this fraction features the intensities $F_f(m;i)$ of the pharmacophoric field produced by all the atoms of m at the points i occupied by the atoms of M, dependent on the relative orientation Θ. The denominator is only a function of the field intensities produced by the feature distribution of the molecules at the points occupied by their own atoms, depending only on the conformations of m and M. Introducing a short-cut notation for the sums in equation (4), the expression becomes:

$$H_f(M,m,\Theta) = \frac{2S_f^{\mathrm{int\,er}}(M,m,\Theta)}{S_f^{\mathrm{int\,ra}}(M) + S_f^{\mathrm{int\,ra}}(m)} \quad (5)$$

It can be shown that 1 $H_f(M,m,\Theta)$ 0. This index equals 1 if a conformer of a molecule is effectively superimposed over itself. On the contrary, if a feature f is represented in one and only one of M and m, then $H_f(M,m,\Theta)=0$, irrespectively how the two molecules are oriented. The feature f *must* be represented at least once, in either M or m, or else the H_f index is not defined. At extremely high α values, only the perfectly overlapping atom pairs (i,j) and respectively the diagonal terms (i,i) will have nonzero contributions to the sums in (3), and therefore the index can be interpreted as 2x(the number of pharmacophoric groups of type f that are perfectly superimposed atop of groups of the same type of the other molecule)/(number of groups of type f in M + number of groups of type f in m).

In the particular situation where M is a substructure of m, at the optimal relative orientation which perfectly overlaps the common parts of the molecules, the index $H_f(M,m,\Theta)<1$, as a consequence of the fact that the presence of novel groups representing the feature f in m renders the two molecules dissimilar. Arguably, a similarity metric should be more sensitive to the failure of m to match all the groups that are present in the reference scaffold M and more tolerant to the presence of "orphan" groups in m, which have no equivalent in the reference molecule. Introducing a control parameter λ for the "orphan group penalty" into the Hodgkin index $H_f(M,m,\Theta)$ leads to the definition of an asymmetric[43] (Tversky[44]) overlap coefficient $Q^*_f(M,m,\Theta)$ $Q^*_f(m,M,\Theta)$.

$$Q^*_f(M,m,\Theta) = \frac{2S_f^{\mathrm{int\,er}}(M,m,\Theta)}{(2-\lambda)S_f^{\mathrm{int\,ra}}(M) + \lambda S_f^{\mathrm{int\,ra}}(m)} \quad (6)$$

At λ=1, $Q^*_f(M,m,\Theta)=H_f(M,m,\Theta)$, while at λ=0, $Q^*_f(M,m,\Theta)$ only compares the coverage by m of pharmacophoric groups in M, with respect to the coverage achieved when superimposing M to itself. However, while H_f feature overlap scores are normed and bound between 0 and 1, at zero or low λ values, Q^*_f may exceed 1 if, locally at certain atoms i of M representing the feature f, $F_f(m;i) > F_f(M;i)$:

$$Q^*_f(M,m,\Theta)\Big|_{\lambda=0} = \frac{\sum_{i=1}^{N(M)} \gamma_f(i,M) F_f(m;i)}{\sum_{i=1}^{N(M)} \gamma_f(i,M) F_f(M;i)} \quad (7)$$

An example illustrating such situations would be the replacement of a carbonyl group (HBA) in M by a carboxylate group in m. When overlapping M with itself, the carbonyl group will be perfectly matched and F_{HBA}(M; carbonyl oxygen)=1, the "self term" of this HBA group if no other nearly situated HBA groups exist in M. When superimposing m over M, in the optimal relative position the carbonyl oxygen in M would probably be located at equal distances d=d(i,j1)=d(i,j2) between the two HBA carboxylate oxygens j1 and j2 of m. Since these distances represent only fractions of an Angstrom and the Gaussian factor α will be typically chosen to render the method quite tolerant with respect to distance deviations of this order of magnitude, it is highly probable that F_{HBA}(m; carbonyl oxygen)=$2\exp(-\alpha d^2)>1$. The obtained overlap score Q^*_f would be artificially high, since it was not normed with respect to the self contributions $\sum_{i=1}^{N(m)} \gamma_f(i,m) F_f(m;i)$ in m, accounting for the higher density of HBA groups in this molecule.

The subsequently defined $Q_f(M,m,\Theta)$ is a feature overlap index that allows the introduction of the "orphan penalty" control variable, while being nevertheless bound to the [0,1] range and free of the previously discussed "feature overmatching" artifacts:

$$Q_f(M,m,\Theta) = \frac{2\sum_{i=1}^{N(M)} \gamma_f(i,M)\min\{F_f(m;i), F_f(M;i)\}}{(2-\lambda)\sum_{i=1}^{N(M)} \gamma_f(i,M) F_f(M;i) + \lambda \sum_{i=1}^{N(m)} \gamma_f(i,m) F_f(m;i)} \quad (8)$$

2.1.3.2 The Degrees of Freedom of the ComPharm Superimposition Procedure. Accounting for Conformational Flexibility

For the sake of simplicity, in the previous discussion single conformations have been assumed for both molecules M and m. It is, however, possible to replace the "rototranslation" vector Θ by a more general "superimposition" vector Ω that includes intramolecular degrees of freedom, such as torsional angles χ(r) associated to the rotatable bonds r in both m and M: $\Omega=(r_x, r_y, r_z, \phi, \theta, \xi, \chi_M(1), \ldots,\chi_M(r), \ldots,\chi_m(1), \ldots,\chi_m(r'), \ldots)$. In consequence, the intramolecular sums in the denominators of the previously discussed feature overlap indices - see equations (5) and (6)- would also become functions of Ω. Furthermore, a fully flexible overlapping algorithm would require the definition of an objective function combining the quality of the match with a penalty for unrealistically high internal energies of the conformers described by a given Ω, e.g. it would require a full-blown molecular mechanics energy evaluation for both m and M in parallel to the evaluation of the overlap criteria. On the other hand, if conformational flexibility is ignored and single geometries are submitted to the superimposition algorithm, the probability of failure to achieve a meaningful match increases with the flexibility of m and M.

In ComPharm, a computationally efficient compromise between the two extremes of the fully flexible and the single-geometry rigid-body superimposition was chosen: a rigid-body superimposition algorithm allowing all the possible overlaps between the representatives of predefined families of low-energy conformers of m and M respectively, and selecting the pair of conformers that overlaps best. Replacing the explicit dependence on conformational degrees of freedom with the ability to select the optimal conformer from a set of representative molecular geometries showed to be an effective way of reducing the computational cost of docking calculations[45,13]. In the present work, such families of up to $\nu(M)=40$ low-energy conformers were generated for each molecule M, using the program catConf[34,45,47] from MSI. The superimposition vector of the ComPharm approach includes two integer variables denoting the current ordinal numbers -c(M),c(m)- of the conformations of M and respectively m that should be considered for the current overlap. No penalty for choosing a higher-energy conformer out of the available families, instead of the most stable ones, is included in the scoring function, since first none of the possible choices correspond to physically impossible geometries with intramolecular bad contacts and second, there is no reason to assume that the biologically active conformer corresponds to the one that is most stable in the unbound state.

The success of this conformer enumeration strategy depends on whether both the conformations of m and M that yield an optimal overlap are represented in their respective families. Several conformational sampling programs[13] use intramolecular distance-based diversity criteria to check for the non-redundancy of the resulting family of geometries and would therefore sample only one possible enantiomeric form of a chiral conformation. A binary chirality toggle variable τ was therefore included in the superimposition vector: at $\tau=1$, the algorithm performs a mirroring operation on the coordinates of the selected conformer c(m) prior to proceeding with the superimposition. At $\tau=0$, the coordinates of the conformer are taken as such. The use of the chirality toggle as a degree of freedom of the superimposition is optional and can be turned off when working with chiral products with a well defined and biologically relevant configuration.

A second simplification introduced in ComPharm was to restrain the virtually infinite set of possible translation vectors (r_x, r_y, r_z) to a finite set of translations required to move any atom i of M to the position occupied by any atom j of m, where i and j share at least one of the considered pharmacophoric features. A list of all the possible pairs (i,j) fulfilling the latter condition is constructed by the algorithm, and the integer variable p of the superimposition vector denotes the actual atom pair that is used in the current superimposition attempt. The algorithm then retrieves the corresponding atoms i from m and j from M and their coordinates in the conformations c(m) and c(M), applies a mirroring operation on the coordinates of c(m) if the chirality toggle is set and translates m and M such that both i and j are placed at the origin of the reference system. Eventually, m is rotated with respect to this reference system according to the Euler angles, to obtain the molecular superimposition encoded by the current vector Ω, and with respect to which the feature overlap scores are then evaluated for every $f=1...N_f$.

$$\Omega = \left(p, \tau, c(m), c(M), \phi, \theta, \xi\right) \tag{9}$$

2.1.3.3 Global Molecular Overlay and Similarity Score

It is now straightforward to define the global molecular overlay index O(M,m,Ω) as a weighted average of any of the previously discussed feature overlay indices, where the sum in equation (10) is taken over all the features f' represented in at least one of the molecules m and M:

$$O(M,m,\Omega) = \frac{\sum_{f'} w_{f'} Q_{f'}(M,m,\Omega)}{\sum_{f'} w_{f'}} \tag{10}$$

The feature weighing factors w_f express the relative importance assigned to achieve a good overlap of the pharmacophoric fields of type f. These are tunable parameters of the model, together with the Gaussian coefficient α and the "orphan penalty" coefficient λ. The parameterization scheme used in this work is shown in Table 1 and has been derived in order to maximize the discriminant power in terms of ligand family recognition of a pharmacophoric fingerprint-based similarity metric[41] relying on the same definitions of the pharmacophoric features of the atoms and also including w_f and α as adjustable parameters. Considering a training set designed as a union of small families of ligands of different receptors[48], the parameter space was explored by a Monte Carlo procedure in order to discover a set of w_f and α maximize the performance of the fingerprint-based similarity metric. The quality criterion of the similarity metric has been estimated in terms of its coverage of a maximum of different ligand families within a most diverse subset of compounds, selected on the basis on molecular similarity scores[49]. The weighing factor of the shape contribution w_{shape}, and the orphan penalty λ, which are not parameters of the fingerprint-based similarity metric, were set to 0.2 and 0 respectively.

None of these parameters has been subjected to optimization in order to improve the results of the QSAR studies reported in this work.

The molecular similarity score $\sigma(M,m)$ is defined as the maximal overlap score $O(M,m,\Omega)$ with respect to all the space spanned by the superimposition vector Ω as defined in equation (9). The dissimilarity coefficient or the intermolecular distance $\delta(M,m)=1-\sigma(M,m)$ is the complement of the similarity score.

Table 1: Parameterization scheme of the ComPharm Overlay Scoring Function

Parameter	Value
Hydrophobic groups: w_{HP}	0.41
Aromatic groups: w_{AR}	0.24
HB Acceptors: w_{HBA}	1.00
HB Donors: w_{HBD}	0.78
Cations: w_{POS}	0.68
Anions: w_{NEG}	0.76
Shape contribution: w_{shape}	0.20
exponential factor α	0.32
orphan penalty coeff. λ	0.00

2.1.3.4 Genetic Algorithm-Based Optimization of the Global Molecular Overlay Score used to evaluate the Molecular Similarity Score

Genetic algorithms[50,51] are heuristic methods best suited to search for the absolute optimum of functions of a fixed number of variables, irrespectively of their continuity or derivability. Assimilating the vector of the degrees of freedom $(X_1,X_2,.. X_n)$ to a "chromosome" where each "locus" i encodes a component X_i of the vector, the algorithm emulates an evolution process based on Darwinian selection of the fitter chromosomes against the less fit ones, where the fitness criterion represents the objective function to maximize, in this case $O(M,m,\Omega)$. In order to map the superimposition vector to such a "chromosome", the continuous Euler angle variables were replaced by a series of discrete angle values spanning the required variation range (from 0 to 360° or 180°, respectively) with a constant step of 6°.

First, a population of $N_{pop}=100$ such chromosomes are initialized with random values. Within a current population, the chromosomes are randomly associated to define $N_{pop}/2$ mating pairs (all the chromosomes are allowed to mate) and single-point crossover, mutation and selection operators[52] are applied to build a next generation of fitter chromosomes on the basis of the current ones. N_{pop} "child" chromosomes are generated by the crossovers. A variable number N_{mut} of new chromosomes result from the mutation process of duplicates of the parent chromosomes, in function of the imposed mutation frequency. The fitness function of the new chromosomes are evaluated. Two different evolutionary strategies have been considered in the present work:

The "focussing" strategy consists in letting the totality of N_{pop} parent, and $N_{pop}+N_{mut}$ children chromosomes compete together indiscriminately: the total population of $2N_{pop}+N_{mut}$ individuals is ranked in order of decreasing fitness and the first N_{pop} are conserved, the others discarded. This approach converges very quickly towards a "dominant" family of a locally optimal chromosome and its near neighbors, since the selection process may pass on both parents and the related children to the next generation. The locally fittest chromosome produces offspring that is likely to occupy the top positions in the fitness-related selection list and which at their turn generate only slightly different -therefore quite fit- individuals, until the family eventually occupies the whole "vital space" of N_{pop} chromosomes. Identical "clones" of a chromosome may be generated by a succession of cross-overs and mutations, but they are detected and discarded by the algorithm. The advantage of this strategy is the very rapid convergence and its ability to perform a fine-tuned search around a local maximum. Its main drawback is its likeliness to converge towards suboptimal local maxima. Therefore, as soon as the algorithm detects a stagnation of the evolutionary process (no improvement of fitness during the last 50 generations), the best chromosome is copied to a buffer of locally optimal solutions and the run is restarted with a different initial population, in order to let it converge towards a different local optimum. If, in spite of successive restarts, no improvement of the currently best optimum is reached over typically 250-500 generations, the sampling of local minima is discontinued.

The best N_{pop} chromosomes from the buffer of locally optimal solutions (if less than N_{pop} were stored at the previous step, random chromosomes are added) are then taken as an initial population and evolved according to the "diversity" strategy. This strategy specifically replaces both parents with the two children resulted from their cross-over, if the best of the children is fitter than the best of the parents and discards the children in the opposite case. Similarly, if a mutant chromosome is fitter than the original sequence it came from, it will replace the latter or otherwise will be discarded. The convergence of this strategy towards a minimum is much slower, keeping alternate evolutionary pathways open by preserving the diversity of the population. If evolution stalls for 250-500 generations, the algorithm switches back to focussed evolution, and after fulfillment of the termination criterion for the latter, the best available chromosome Ω^* is used to recreate the corresponding molecular overlay and export the superimposed structures as a molecular data file on disk.

2.2 The Study Case: Farnesyl Protein Transferase (FPT) Inhibitors

Kaminski et. al.[1] have used a training set of 35 polycyclic FPT inhibitors of various potencies (this series will be referred to as "family A" in the present work, its generic structure is shown in Figure 1A, and the most active compound of the series (later on referred to as "A_0", IC_{50}=0.06 μM, shown in Figure 1B) to generate a pharmacophore hypothesis model using Catalyst[54], and subsequently used this hypothesis to query a three-dimensional data base and assess the FPT inhibitory potency of the virtual hits. Among the active virtual hits (with an FPT inhibitory IC_{50}<5 μM), two were found to belong to a class structurally completely different "azole" compounds (Figure 2A,B). Further representatives of this class, although not retrieved by the hypothesis-based query, have consequently been submitted to the FPT inhibition assay. The resulting 37 compounds with measurable IC_{50} values will be referred here as "family B", with the most active representative (later on referred as "B_0"; IC_{50}=0.2 μM) shown in Figure 2C. A subsequent paper by Njoroge et.al.[55] reported 15 new FPT inhibitors based on the structural motif of family A, here referred to as "family A*". A diverse set[55] I of (presumably) inactive compounds with respect to FPT, consisting of 75 known ligands of 14 different enzymes or receptors (not including FPT) has been used in the study in order to monitor the behavior of the QSAR models with respect to other, structurally distinct families. Two subsets I_1 and I_2 of the set I were defined such as to ensure a roughly equal splitting of the subfamilies of ligands of each receptor.

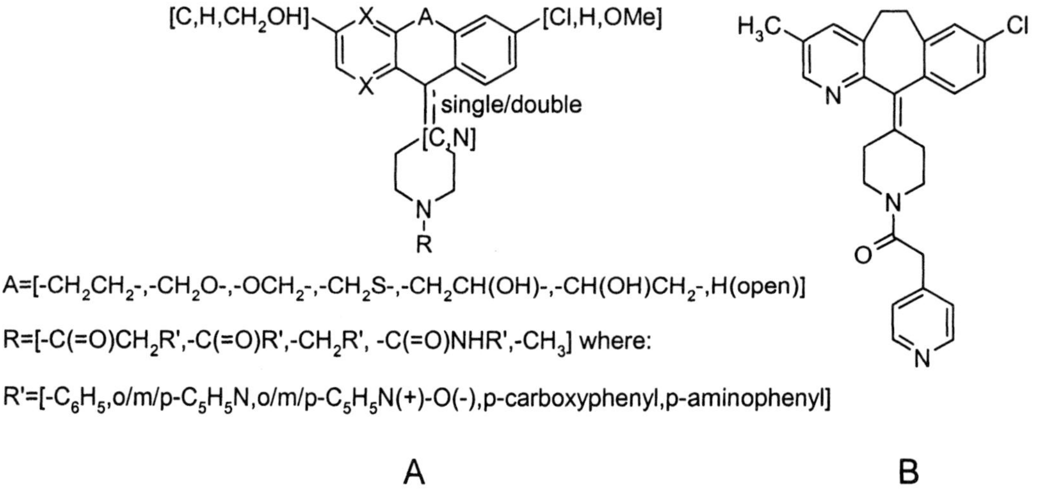

Figure 1. Generic formula (A) and most active compound (B) of the family A of FPT inhibitors.

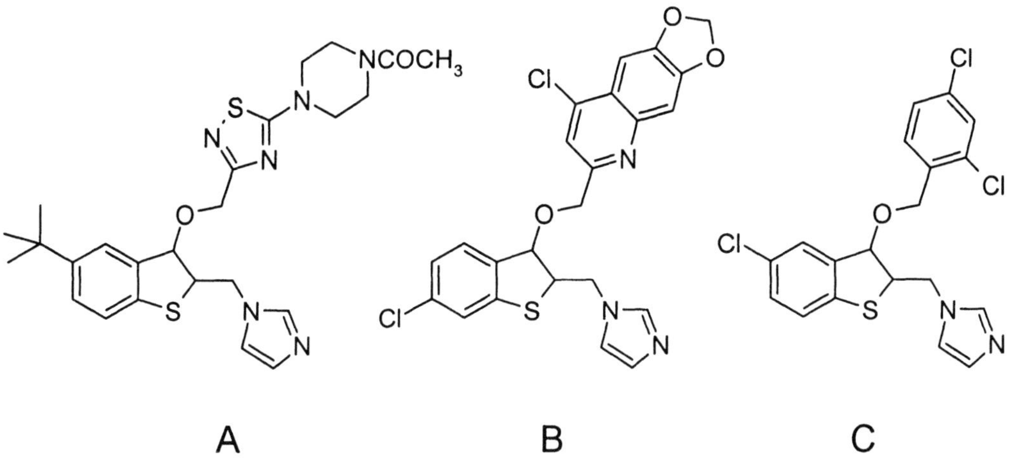

Figure 2. Representatives of "azole" family B: (A) and (B) were active virtual hits found by screening a 3D-molecular database against a Catalyst hypothesis inferred on the basis of family A of inhibitors[53] (C) is the most active representative of family B (IC_{50}=0.2 μM).

2.3 Preliminaries of the QSAR buildup: Generating the Superimposition Models and Deriving ComPharm Descriptors

Ensembles of up to 40 conformers were generated for each of the molecules in families A, A*, B and I, using the catConf[46] software in "best" sampling mode and allowing a strain energy of up to 20 kcal/mol with respect to the lowest-energy conformer. For comparison purposes, both *superimposition models considering the full family of conformers of the reference M*, and *models based only on the lowest-energy conformer of M* were generated. *Given the optimal superimposition vector Ω^*, the pharmacophoric field values -$F_f(m;i)$; $f=1...N_f-1$, as given in equation (2) - generated by the candidate molecule **m** at the points occupied by the atoms **i** of the reference scaffold **M**, form a set of **descriptors of m** relative to the current overlay model. The shape field terms $F_7(m;i)$, not reflecting the pharmacophoric properties of the functional groups of the candidate molecules, are less relevant for QSAR studies and were therefore not exported as molecular descriptors, although they were considered at the superimposition scoring step.*

2.3.1 Reproducibility Study

First, the reproducibility of the ComPharm-driven superimposition results has been assessed, based on a N_{test}=200-fold repeat (with different input random number seeds for the genetic algorithm) of B_0 with respect to (a) the entire family of conformers of A_0, and (b) with respect to the lowest-energy conformer of A_0. The resulting models were sorted in order of decreasing superimposition scores $O(m,M,\Omega^*_r)$, Ω^*_r denoting the optimum found by the superposition run r. The number of the first N_{best} optima that are identical or very close to the global (best-ranked; r=1) one, offers an estimate of the probability of converging towards the global optimum. N_{test}/N_{best} represents an order of magnitude of the number of runs required to provide a reasonable guarantee for the discovery of the global optimum. The difference between an optimum r and the global optimum can be expressed in terms of the correlation coefficient q(1,r) of the pharmacophoric field descriptors $F_f(m;i)\big|_r$, calculated according to the corresponding relative positions of B_0 and A_0, at the space points occupied by the atoms i of the reference A_0:

$$q(1,r)=\frac{2\sum_{f=1}^{N_f}\sum_{i=1}^{N(A_0)}F_f(B_0;i)\big|_1 F_f(B_0;i)\big|_r}{\sum_{f=1}^{N_f}\sum_{i=1}^{N(A_0)}F_f^2(B_0;i)\big|_1+\sum_{f=1}^{N_f}\sum_{i=1}^{N(A_0)}F_f^2(B_0;i)\big|_r} \quad (11)$$

Alternatively, it is interesting to monitor to what extent the use of descriptors from suboptimal superimposition modes may affect the predicted affinity values, given a previously established QSAR model. To this purpose, three preliminary linear relationships, based on pharmacophoric field descriptors build on the basis of only 10 repeated runs per molecule, were established. The activity of B_0 was predicted according to each of the sets of descriptors $F_f(m;i)\big|_r$, monitoring the absolute error between the values obtained from the best and respectively the rth superimposition model.

2.3.2 Build-up of Synthetic Molecular Descriptors on the Basis of the Sampled Superimposition Models.

The synthetic field descriptors[12] integrate information referring to the intensities of the pharmacophoric fields at each vertex of the reference molecule, at given overlay mode, weighted by the assumed relevance of that specific overlay mode. Given the pharmacophoric field descriptor values $F_f(m;i)\big|_r$ corresponding to each of the sampled overlay models r, a synthetic field descriptor is being constructed as a weighted average over all these models r, the descriptors of models with a better overlap score contributing more to the this average:

$$F_f^{\beta}(m;i)=\frac{\sum_r F_f(m;i)\big|_r e^{\beta O(M,m,\Omega^*_r)}}{\sum_r e^{\beta O(M,m,\Omega^*_r)}} \quad (12)$$

The positive "temperature" factor β determines the decrease rate of the participation of a suboptimal model descriptor to the synthetic descriptor, with decreasing overlap score. Selecting very large β values is equivalent to setting the synthetic field descriptor equal to the descriptor of the absolute optimum. At β=0, the relative contributions of the near-optimal solutions to the synthetic descriptors will correspond to their probability of being sampled by the genetic algorithm. As far as the probability of "trapping" the GA in unrealistic, remote-from-optimum, local minima is reasonably low, setting $\beta=0$ (performing a simple average of all the descriptors of the sampled overlay models) may thus be a valid choice.

Several superposition runs of all the candidate molecules (A+B+I), according to the predefined setup of ComPharm parameters (Table 1) and choice of the reference structures have been performed (see **Table 2**). The superimposition of each candidate molecule has been repeatedly run, in order to comply with the conclusions of the reproducibility study. The stability of the synthetic field descriptors has been assessed in terms of the number of runs r and the temperature factor β used for their construction. To this purpose, the F^{β} values have been constructed for all the 162 compounds from this study, using the first 5, the first 10 and the first 30 superimposition runs only, at each of $\beta=(0,5,10,20,50,200)$. At each β value and for each compound, their F^{β} descriptors obtained from 5, 10 and 30 superimposition runs were compared to those build on the basis of 60 runs, using the correlation coefficient(11) as similarity criterion. The worst correlation coefficient with respect to all compounds at given β was taken as measure of the error committed when constructing the synthetic descriptors on the basis of fewer superimposition runs.

2.4 QSAR Models based on ComPharm Pharmacophoric Field Value Descriptors.

For each of the considered sets of synthetic field descriptors, linear QSAR models were built by submitting the activity-descriptor matrix [log(IC_{50}) - non-redundant descriptors], to a GA-driven descriptor selection algorithm, as detailed in the following paragraphs. Whenever the learning set and/or validation set included inactive compounds of the set I, their IC_{50} values were arbitrarily set at 10^4 μM. The models that have been explored in this work are enumerated in **Table 2**, in terms of the reference molecule with respect to which the ComPharm alignment was performed, the learning set (LS) used to calibrate the model, the number of repeated superposition runs and the "temperature" factor β controlling the buildup of the synthetic field descriptor.

Table 2: Studied QSAR models, in function of the reference molecule and learning set. #Runs – number of overlays used to evaluate synthetic descriptors, β - temperature factor, eq(12), $r^2_{XV\text{-}3}$ – best cross-validated coefficient of the models. Reference structures are shown in Figures 1.B (A_0), 2.C(B_0) and 10 (M, N, Q)

Model #	Reference Molecule	#Runs	β	Learning Set	$r^2_{XV\text{-}3}$
1	A_0 – multiple conformers	10	0	A	**0.84**
2,3,4	A_0 – multiple conformers	10	0	randomized(A)	**0.57**
5	A_0 – multiple conformers	10	0	$A+I_1$	**0.92**
6,7,8	A_0 – multiple conformers	10	0	randomized($A+I_1$)	**0.54**
9	A_0 – multiple conformers	10	0	$B+I_2$	**0.87**
10,11,12	A_0 – multiple conformers	10	0	randomized($B+I_2$)	**0.46**
13	A_0 – multiple conformers	10	0	A+A*+B+I	**0.85**
14,15,16	A_0 – multiple conformers	10	0	randomized(A+A*+B+I)	**0.16**
17	A_0 – multiple conformers	10		A+A*+B+I	**0.78**
18,19,20	A_0 – multiple conformers	10		randomized(A+A*+B+I)	**0.33**
21	A_0 – multiple conformers	60	0	A+A*+B+I	**0.87**
22,23,24	A_0 – multiple conformers	60	0	randomized(A+A*+B+I)	**0.22**
25	A_0 – multiple conformers	60	200	A+A*+B+I	**0.86**
26,27,28	A_0 – multiple conformers	60	200	randomized(A+A*+B+I)	**0.29**
29	A_0 –single conformer	10	0	A+A*+B+I	**0.83**
30,31,32	A_0 – single conformer	10	0	randomized(A+A*+B+I)	**0.27**
33	A_0 – single conformer	10		A+A*+B+I	**0.81**
34,35,36	A_0 – single conformer	10		randomized(A+A*+B+I)	**0.37**
37	B_0 – multiple conformers	10	0	A+A*+B+I	**0.85**
38,39,40	B_0 – multiple conformers	10	0	randomized(A+A*+B+I)	**0.27**
41	B_0 – multiple conformers	10	200	A+A*+B+I	**0.83**
42,43,44	B_0 – multiple conformers	10	200	randomized(A+A*+B+I)	**0.28**
45	M – multiple conformers	10	0	A+A*+B+I	**0.84**
46,47,48	M – multiple conformers	10	0	randomized(A+A*+B+I)	**0.19**
49	N – multiple conformers	10	0	A+A*+B+I	**0.82**
50,51,52	N – multiple conformers	10	0	randomized(A+A*+B+I)	**0.19**
53	Q – multiple conformers	10	0	A+A*+B+I	**0.75**
54,55,56	Q – multiple conformers	10	0	randomized(A+A*+B+I)	**0.19**

2.4.1 Discarding Correlated Descriptor Columns

Principal Component Analysis (PCA)[57] is the method of choice to prevent the use of redundant, inter-correlated descriptors in QSAR studies. However, the replacement of the physicochemically meaningful field descriptors with the somewhat obscure eigenvectors in Principal Components (PC) space would significantly affect the interpretability of the model by a scientist. The ability of a human to understand the significance of a QSAR model is a very important quality criterion of such an approach and should not be discarded in favor of mathematical elegance and rigor[58]. In the current work, for each of the considered learning sets, the descriptor columns were clustered, using their linear correlation coefficients as a similarity index. Clusters of descriptors were defined such that any member of a cluster displays a correlation coefficient larger than 0.7 with respect to any other member of the same family. A single representative of each cluster was used in the QSAR buildup process, the others being discarded.

2.4.2 Optimization and Performance Assessment of the QSAR models

The following procedures and statistical indices have been used to search for and evaluate the quality of the ComPharm-descriptor based QSAR models:

- The cross-validated correlation coefficient $r^2_{XV\text{-}3}$ resulting from a 3-step cross-validation procedure (leaving 1/3 of the learning set out at every step) has been chosen as the fitness function to be maximized by the genetic-algorithm based search for the optimal regression model. More details about this linear model building approach were given elsewhere[59]. For each set of input descriptors, the set of all the "descriptor configurations" (e.g. lists of the descriptors entering the current model) visited during the GA run were stored, sorted in order of decreasing $r^2_{XV\text{-}3}$ of the corresponding regression equations.
- While r^2 values are standard quality criteria of linear models, a high r^2 coefficient is not a necessary condition for a QSAR model to be a useful drug design tool. If the most active compounds according to the model do actually display a significant biological activity, using such a model as a selection strategy to decide in which direction to orient the chemical synthesis and biological testing may be of large benefit, regardless on whether or not the predicted activities equaled the measured ones. Therefore, an alternate "optimality criterion" ρ expressing the potential utility of the model in drug discovery has been developed. In absence of any model, in order to retrieve a fraction f of the N_{act} "actives" from a collection of N compounds, it is required to (synthesize and) test a same fraction f of the whole collection. Assuming that a model is used to rank a set of compounds in terms of their predicted affinities and that they will be synthesized and tested in this order, a fraction f_{model} of the whole collection will have to be processed in order to detect a fraction f of active compounds. Among the $N \mathrm{x} f_{model}$ processed compounds, $N_{act} \mathrm{x} f$ $N \mathrm{x} f_{model}$ actives will be retrieved. If the hypothesis that the predicted activities are somehow (not necessarily linearly) correlated to the real activities, then the concentration of actives in the selected

set must be larger than the overall concentration of actives in the entire set, e.g. $(N_{act}xf)/(Nxf_{model})> N_{act}/N$, e.g. $f_{model}<f$ (less effort for screening in order to achieve the discovery of the same number of actives). Accordingly, the enrichment factor of the model can be defined as $E_{model}=f/f_{model}$, so that for a null model (random screening) $E_0=1$. With an ideal model, all the Nxf_{ideal} compounds considered for synthesis and testing will be active, e.g. $N_{act}xf= Nxf_{ideal}$. Therefore, the best enrichment factor that can possibly be obtained is $E_{ideal}=f/f_{ideal} = N/N_{act}$. The potential usefulness of a model can then be situated between the two extremes of the null model and the ideal model, in defining its optimality criterion ρ_{model} according such that $\rho_0=0$ and $\rho_{ideal}=1$. In the current work, the ρ criterion from (13) was taken assuming that the goal of the experiment is to discover f=50% of all the actives from a set of compounds, where "active" molecules are considered to have $IC_{50}<1\mu M$. Accordingly, f_{model} represents the size of the minimal subset of compounds, selected in increasing order of their predicted $\log(IC_{50})$ values, which includes half of all the actives of the set (among some erroneously predicted actives).

$$\rho_{model} = \frac{E_{model} - E_0}{E_{ideal} - E_0} = \frac{f/f_{model} - 1}{N/N_{act} - 1} \qquad (13)$$

2.4.3 Randomization Tests

In order to estimate the likeliness of fortuitous correlations that may occur due to the important number (300) of input descriptors, blind searches for linear models were conducted on the basis of the given descriptor sets, but after having randomly associated each activity value to the descriptor of another molecule. If the used descriptors contain relevant information with respect to the explained biological property, the predictive power of the models associating the correct activity values to the molecular descriptors must be outstandingly larger than the one of spurious correlations found within randomized input sets.

2.4.4 In-depth Analysis of the Predictive Power of Selected QSAR models

In order to evaluate the ability of the models to "recognize" novel families of active compounds, different from the ones used for training, the total population of available compounds was broken down into two structurally distinct data sets. Models trained on the set including family A and half of the inactive compounds ($A+I_1$) were validated against the structurally distinct set including family B and the rest of inactive molecules ($B+I_2$), and vice-versa. For a given LS, a *representative set of linear models* was selected out of the set of visited descriptor configurations scoring a r^2_{xv-3} within 0.2 from the best obtained cross-validated correlation coefficient. These configurations were then classified in function of the number N_{pars} of descriptors entering the corresponding regression models. Within each class with N_{pars} 15, the regression models were then used to predict the activities of the compounds from the validation set, and their predictive power against the latter was compared to the one achieved against their learning sets. Some of the most promising QSAR models will be detailed and discussed.

3. RESULTS & DISCUSSIONS

3.1 General Discussion of the ComPharm Methodology

In classical CoMFA, the field values are taken at well-defined points of a coordinate system bound to the single "bioactive" conformer, such as mesh points of a rectangular grid surrounding this conformer. In ComPharm, each of the candidate molecules may in principle overlap on a different conformer of M - the one that optimally matches one of their geometries. An alignment with respect to a unique external reference system will be achieved only locally, within every subset of candidate molecules that have selected a same conformer of the reference for superimposition. However, in contrast to CoMFA, the grid points at which the molecular field values will be extracted are referred *in terms of the molecular topology of M: these grid points represent the vertices of the molecular graph of the reference compound*, irrespectively of how they are oriented in space. ComPharm tries to avoid the complex problem of the bioactive conformer, *by translating the overlay of m on M into a relationship of equivalence of the vertices of m and M, defined on the basis of the pharmacophoric field values produced by m at the atoms of M.* By comparing the field intensities $F_f(M;i)$ and $F_f(m;i)$ produced by M and respectively by m at an atom i of M, it can be inferred whether a pharmacophoric element of M is:

- "conserved in m", if $F_f(M;i)$ $F_f(m;i)$,
- "absent from m", if $F_f(m;i)$ 0, or,
- "replaced by a pharmacophorically different fragment", if features f exist such that $F_f(M;i) x F_f(m;i)$ 0, but $F_f(M;i)+F_f(m;i)$ 0.

This relationship is however not based on considerations of topological nature, but is conditioned by the set of conformers that can be adopted by every compound. 3D-properties relative to spatial distributions of pharmacophoric centers are mapped onto a 2D-grid defined by the graph of the reference compound. The central working hypothesis of ComPharm is the *assumption that even if the actual conformers used to achieve the optimal overlay do not correspond to the bioactive ones, a meaningful mapping of 3D-features of the candidate onto a geometry-independent 2D-grid can be achieved without loosing the critical information that is required in order to explain the biological activity of a compound.*

If a fragment i of the active compound M is always "conserved" in the active candidates, but "lost" or "replaced" in inactive molecules, then it can be concluded that this fragment is important for activity. The opposite is true if a fragment can be lost or replaced without a sensible loss of activity. In other words, such 2D-maps of the 3D-properties may be directly compared without requiring any initial hypothesis concerning the geometry of the reference used for the alignment.

Obviously, if a single conformer of M is specified, then a meaningful alignment of all the candidate compounds with respect to a common reference system will be achieved, and the vertices of M, at which the field values are taken, will consistently refer to the same spatial coordinates throughout the study. Whenever the bioactive conformer is known, it can be used as such in a ComPharm study.

3.2 Reproducibility of ComPharm Superimposition Models

Unsurprisingly, the superimposition of similar members of a family on the most active representative of the same family, led in most situations to predictable models, in which the corresponding atoms of the common molecular skeleton perfectly overlap. The significant conformational differences between A_0 and its analogs in which the exocyclic double bond was replaced by a single one (see Figure 1) translated to a less than ideal match of such pairs of structures (Figure 3).

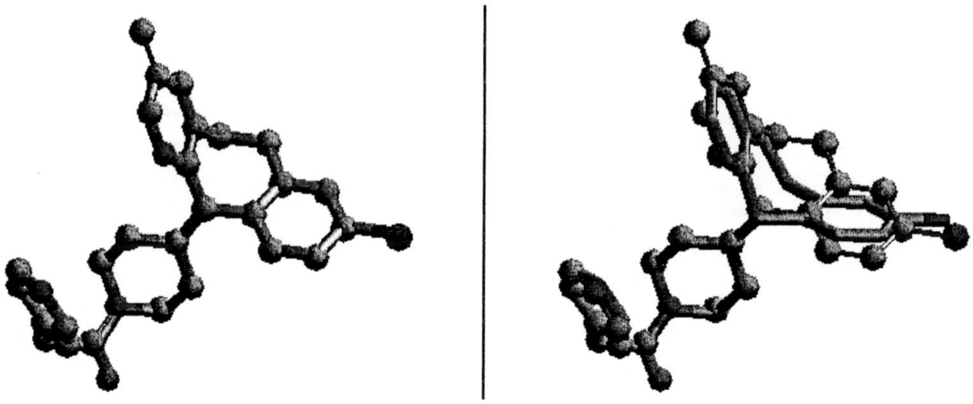

Figure 3. The perfect superimposition of analogs from family A, with a common skeleton (left), is significantly perturbed by a change of the bond order of the exocyclic double bond (right), due to the conformational differences triggered by the change of the hybridization of two central atoms of the candidate molecule: the plane tricyclic system of the saturated candidate is tilted with respect to the one of the reference molecule.

The results of the reproducibility study of the superimposition of B_0 on A_0 are shown in Figure 4, Figure 5 and Figure 6. All the graphs refer to the series of optima that were reached by each of the N_{test}=200 runs, ordered with respect to decreasing optimality criterion, the rank number of each model being given on the X axis (X=1 representing the global optimum):

- The complements of the superimposition score $1\text{-}O(A_0,B_0,\Omega^*_r)$ of the current model r, criterion with respect to which the ranking has been performed, as well as the pharmacophoric field descriptor correlation coefficient q(r,1) defined in equation (11), are shown, for all the 200 sampled local optima, in Figure 4. All the runs reached nearly optimal superimposition score values. When simultaneously accounting for the conformational flexibility of A_0 and B_0, convergence is more difficult to obtain, since the phase space of all the possible solutions significantly increases whit respect to the case when only one, rigid conformer of A is used. Accounting for the flexibility of A_0 allows for the discovery of somehow better optima, e.g. the best-energy conformer used in the single-conformer simulations is not the one that is best mimicked by a conformer of B_0. An important conclusion that can be drawn here is that ComPharm can be successfully used as an accurate molecular similarity metric, a single ComPharm run offering sufficient guarantees that the found optimal overlap score will be close enough to the absolute optimum in order to represent a reasonable estimate of the molecular dissimilarity score $\delta(m,M)$. Larger and more flexible molecule may however require a more important effort in order to obtain an accurate estimate of their similarity score.

- The $q(1,r)$ values for the 20 best local optima are shown in Figure 5. Figure 6 displays the largest absolute deviation $\Delta A(1,r)$ of the activity that would have been predicted from the descriptors corresponding to the rth optimum, with respect to the one obtained on the basis of the best superimposition model. The prediction has been carried out with 3 preliminary linear QSAR models. According to Figure 5, the first 6 best-ranked optima of the runs involving multiple A_0 conformers, and the first 11 optima of the runs based on a single reference geometry, are very close and can be assimilated to the global minimum. Figure 6 confirms that the fluctuation of the descriptor values corresponding to any one of these best overlaps translates into an uncertainty of less than 0.7 log (IC_{50}) units of the evaluated activity values, which is a lower limit of the degree of imprecision that can be expected from empirical QSAR approaches.

It can be seen that the global optimum has been discovered 6 and respectively 11 times in 200 repeated ComPharm runs. For the compounds of the currently used learning and validation sets, more than 30 (using multiconformational models for both m and M) and respectively more than 20 runs (allowing for a single conformer of M) should be required in order to obtain a close-to-one discovery probability of this absolute optimum. Assuming that the superposition of other molecules in the learning set may actually converge even slower, for both the multi- and the monoconformational working hypothesis, 60 successive overlaps of each of the 162 compounds with respect to A_0 have been performed in the present work. A set of 60x162 ComPharm superimposition runs took 143 CPU hours on a single R1000 processor of an Origin200 (SGI), times being slightly reduced when ignoring the conformational flexibility of A_0.

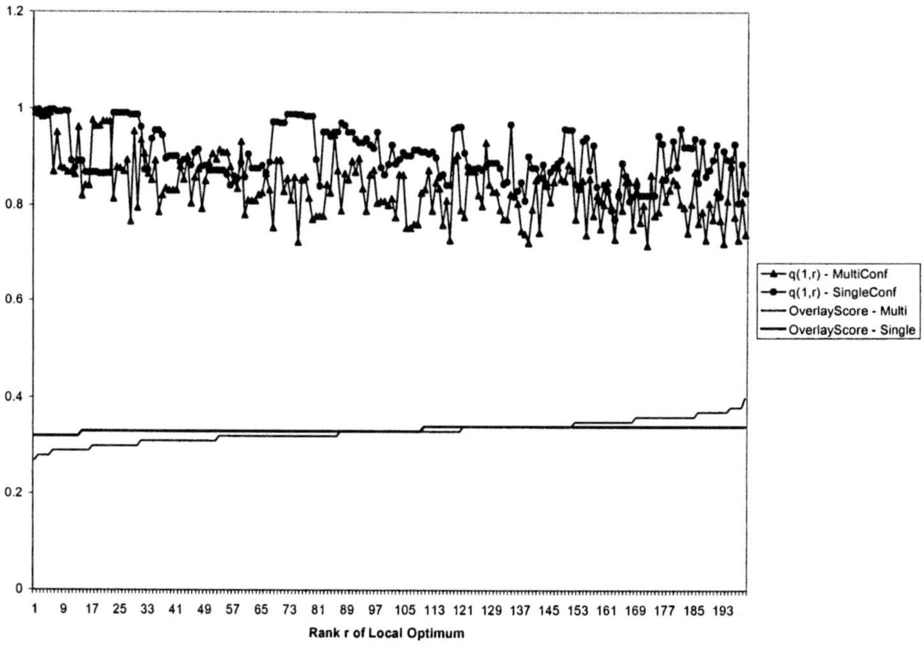

Figure 4. Complements of the overlay scores $1\text{-}O(A_0,B_0,\Omega^*_r)$ and correlation coefficients of the pharmacophoric field descriptors of the best compared to the rth local optimum, obtained from a 200-fold superimposition run of B_0 to A_0 and ranked in function of increasing $1\text{-}O(A_0,B_0,\Omega^*_r)$ values.

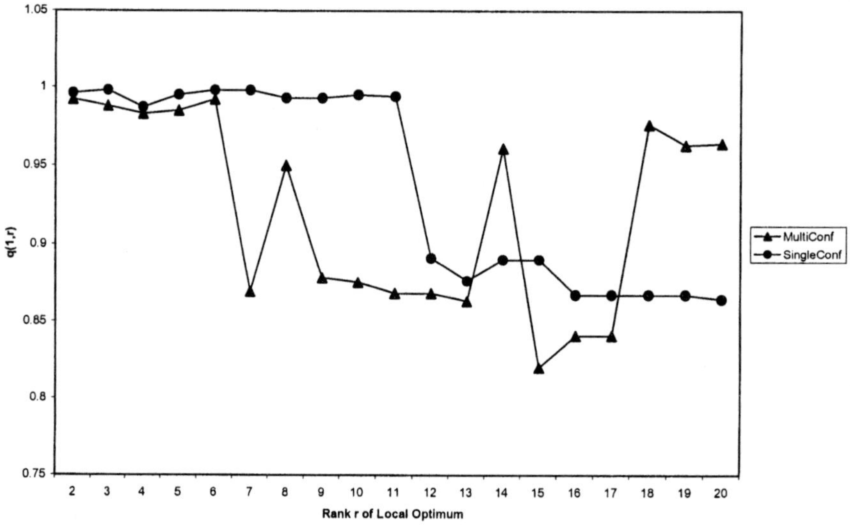

Figure 5. Variation of the correlation coefficients of the pharmacophoric field descriptors of the best compared to the rth local optimum, for the 20 best ranked optima.

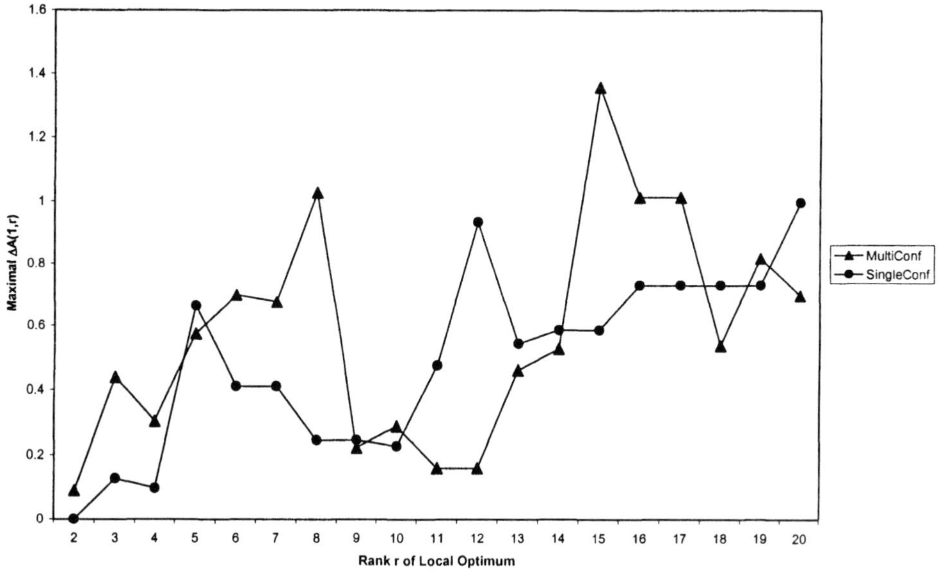

Figure 6. Estimate of the maximal deviation that could be expected in the predicted affinities if descriptors from suboptimal overlay models are used instead of the ones extracted from the absolute superimposition optimum. Deviations on Y represent the worst $\Delta(\log IC_{50})$ fluctuations as obtained with 3 different preliminary linear activity prediction models.

3.3 The Problem of Multiple Near-Optimal Overlay Models

Families of superposition modes were built by clustering of the multiple occurrences of local optima from the set of 200 ComPharm runs based on multiple A_0 conformations. The analysis of the selected representatives of the best four families (Figure 7) reveals that more than one plausible ways to match the pharmacophoric groups of the candidate and reference exist. Differing by as little as 0.03 in terms of the superimposition scores, they nevertheless correspond to radically different intermolecular orientations. The failure to match some pharmacophoric elements can be compensated by a better match elsewhere in the molecule. For example, in the overlay mode shown in the lower right quadrant of Figure 7, the simultaneous match of the two pyridine N atoms of A_0 acting as hydrogen bond acceptors (one by the N atom of the imidazole of B_0, and the other by the ether oxygen of B_0) compensates for the failure to provide a match of the hydrophobic cyclohexylamide moiety of A_0. If the compounds to be overlaid are structurally diverse, situations like the ones described here, with multiple imperfect overlay models of roughly equal overall merit in terms of matching of the potential pharmacophoric points of the reference, are a rule rather than an exception.

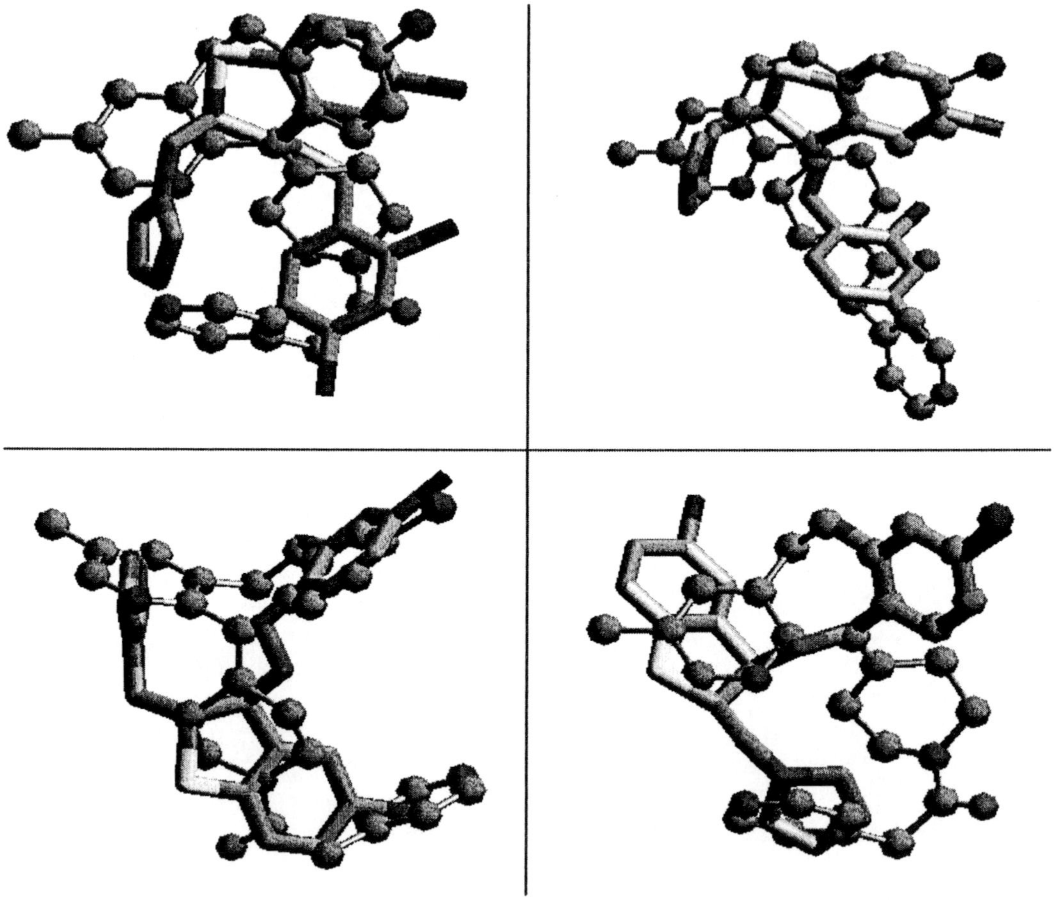

Figure 7. The optimal superimposition model of B_0 (Figure 2) on the best-matching conformer of A_0 (Figure 1), shown in the upper left quadrant, yields a dissimilarity score $\delta(A_0,B_0)=0.28$. This score is not significantly lower than those of next best-ranked suboptimal models (counterclockwise 0.29, 0.30 and 0.31, respectively). However, the corresponding relative alignments of the two compounds significantly differ.

Furthermore, for any close analog B' of B_0, with a slightly different arrangement of the pharmacophoric groups, there is no guarantee that the absolute optimal overlay mode of B' will coincide with that of B_0, rather than with one of the near-optimal overlay models. Therefore, in a QSAR buildup strategy exclusively relying on the absolutely optimal overlay mode of each compound, a minor change of the candidate structure, triggering a minor change of the superposition scores, might nevertheless lead to dramatic differences of the derived sets of pharmacophoric field descriptors. Such artifacts can be avoided by an appropriate choice of the β parameter in equation (12), in order to allow a significant participation of all the near-optimal overlay models to the build-up of the synthetic pharmacophoric field descriptor of the molecule. The elements of the synthetic field descriptor express the average pharmacophoric environment of the candidate "visited" by the probe atoms (of the reference compound) in each of the meaningful candidate-reference overlap modes. If candidate m systematically generates an intense pharmacophoric field of type f at an atom i of the reference, irrespectively of its possible overlay modes, then this pharmacophoric field at point i will be enforced through averaging and conserved in the synthetic descriptors. It is irrelevant whether the source atoms of m of that generate the field at i differ from overlay to overlay. In Figure 7, it can be seen that the aromatic atoms of the tricyclic system of A_0 are always covered by some aromatic atoms of B_0. It is not possible to state which aromatic moiety of B_0 should be considered the equivalent of an aromatic ring of A_0, nor is this issue of paramount importance: the model suggest a high probability that, from point of view of the aromatic pharmacophoric feature, compound B_0 successfully mimics the active reference A. There is a non-negligible probability that the HBA features found in B_0 could successfully match one of the pyridine nitrogens of A_0, but it is unlikely that they represent the equivalent of the carbonyl oxygen of A_0. Since B_0 is a quite potent compound, the latter observation may suggest that the pharmacophoric field descriptors at this carbonyl need not to be entered in the QSAR relationship. If only the absolute overlay optimum (upper left) of Figure 7 would have been taken into consideration, the information that a HBA group of B_0 could replace the pyridine N of the tricyclic system would have been lost.

As evidenced by Figure 8, at low temperature factors β, fewer runs are needed to ensure ensure the convergence of the synthetic field descriptors. At β 50, the synthetic descriptors obtained on the basis of 10 runs only are already highly correlated with the 60-overlay based descriptors. Out of the 162 vectors associated to the considered compounds, the maximal error committed when restricting the sampling to 10 runs was a loss of 8% of the covariance with respect to the corresponding vector build on the basis of 60 runs. At higher temperature factors, however, the synthetic descriptors become more and more dependent on the best overlay optimum currently attained within the number of runs taken for averaging. At β=200, even 30 runs may be not sufficient to ensure the reproducibility of the synthetic descriptors, which may diverge by up to 20% with respect to the ones issued from 60 overlays. It can be concluded that noise, due both to the existence of several near-optimal superposition models and to the convergence problems of the stochastic GA-based overlay algorithm, can be effectively averaged out over few tenths of superimposition runs and without an important bias of the absolutely optimal overlay scores against the near-optimal ones. Therefore, *if the absolutely optimal overlay model is not of a crucial importance for the buildup of QSAR models, reproducible results could be obtained with far less computational effort than suggested in the previous paragraph, which estimated the effort required to ensure the discovery of the absolute overlay optimum of two compounds belonging to structurally different families to 60 or more overlay run repeats.*

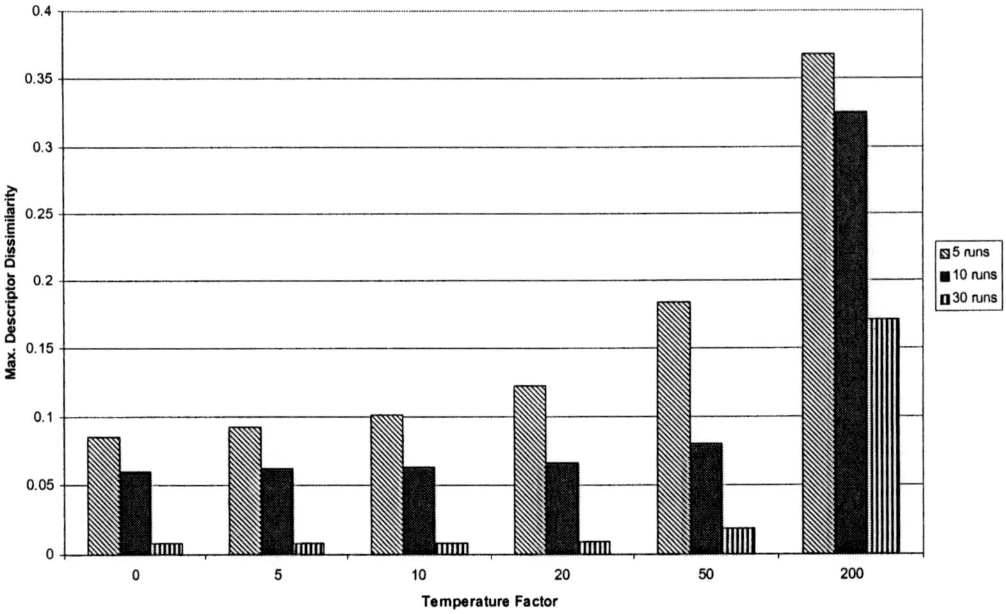

Figure 8. Maximal dissimilarity, - in terms of 1-q; q being defined in equation 3D(11) (12) – between the synthetic descriptor vectors built up on the basis of 5, 10 and respectively 30 overlay runs, and the "reference" descriptors taken as averages over 60 different runs, at given temperature parameter β ,according to equation.

3.4 Significant vs. Spurious Correlations: Results of the Randomization Tests. Impact of the Working Hypotheses at the Basis of Various QSAR Models on their Stability

The use of a cross-validated correlation coefficient $r^2_{XV\text{-}3}$ as fitness function of the GA-based QSAR buildup algorithm, even though significantly increasing the computer effort related to model discovery, is required in order to bias the evolution process in favor of "predictive" models. The existence of such models with the property that, when calibrated on 2/3 of the given LS, they successfully estimate the activities of the 1/3 remaining compounds, is a strong indication that the considered descriptors are actually encoding activity-relevant information. It cannot be precluded that high $r^2_{XV\text{-}3}$ values may be obtained due to another type of overfitting artifacts, resulting from a spurious selection of descriptors that yield a stable model only with respect to the particular cross-validation scheme included in the fitness function.

The maximal expected $r^2_{XV\text{-}3}$ that could be obtained as a result of overfitting artifacts has been estimated by running the QSAR building algorithms with "randomized" activity-descriptor matrices, where the activity values of the compounds were interchanged. The "null" hypothesis assumes that, given the $2^{N_{var}}$ (e.g. 10^{90} possibilities at N_{var}=300!!) different ways to select components out of the N_{var} different pharmacophoric field descriptors representing each of the N_{dat} molecules, it cannot be precluded that at least one of these descriptor selections will, by pure chance, yield a *statistically significant and cross-validated* regression explaining virtually any series of N_{dat} random values – including the actual series of experimental data. Here, the actual number N_{var} of descriptors submitted to QSAR buildup depends on the number of descriptors that have been eliminated because of their strong correlation with respect to other pharmacophoric field contributions (see §2.4.1). The model numbering used in the following paragraphs refers to Table 2.

3.4.1 Models derived on the basis of Family A

The relatively small difference between the $r^2_{XV\text{-}3}$ of the best regression of model 1, based only on the structurally homogeneous family A (N_{dat}=35, N_{vars}=240) and the best quality of spurious correlations found in "randomized" models 2-4, suggests that the models derived form learning set A may suffer from serious overfitting. The 240 descriptors kept after eliminating the redundant ones appear to form a basis set able to explain up to 60% of the variance of any random series of 35 values. Reciprocally, using random vectors of 240 components instead of the pharmacophoric field descriptors might still have lead to a "successful" FPT activity model if the only available experimental data would have been limited to family A. The analogs of A_0 that constitute the learning set A differ by small structural changes affecting various parts of the molecule. They basically represent random modifications and do not provide *a consistent search pattern for an optimal pharmacophoric model*. For example, one of the performed modifications, the deletion of the carbonyl group from A_0, appears to have a dramatic impact on the FPT inhibitory activity (Figure 9). However, the inactivity of the only two available examples without C=O from family A may as well stem from the deletion of the HBA group, as from the apparition of a positive charge on the protonable amino group instead of the neutral amide nitrogen in A_0, from the change in geometry of the cyclohexane ring triggered by change of the hybridization of the N atom, or from the absence, respectively inappropriate orientation of the aromatic ring. Therefore, when adding these two compounds to a LS, the new structure-activity hypotheses that are opened up outnumber the furnished data points against which to confront them. Synthesis and testing of other analogs, exploring different changes of the same region of the lead compound, would be required in order to obtain a sufficiently rich learning set in terms of sampled pharmacophoric configurations. The main difficulty in creating such a set consists in finding the appropriate, chemically feasible transformations that exemplify the desired changes in pharmacophoric patterns. Deletion of the C=O group while avoiding the apparition of the positive charge would imply the replacement of the N atom by a carbon, which leaves the hypothesis of the cyclohexane conformation change still open. Furthermore, local modifications of a pharmacophore element may cause a global change of the pharmacophoric field vectors if they trigger a major change of the overlay modes.

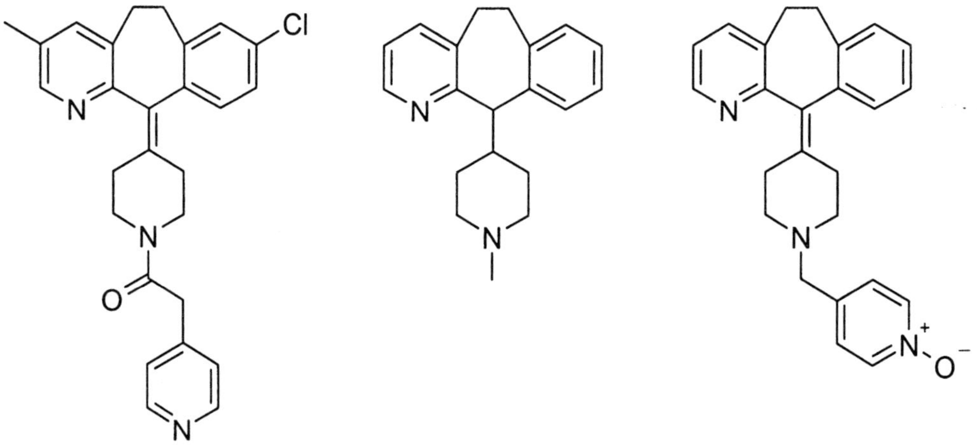

$IC_{50} = 0.06\mu M$ $IC_{50} = 724\mu M$ $Ic_{50} = 1832\mu M$

Figure 9. The only 2 analogs of A_0 (leftmost compound) from family A, in which the carbonyl group has been deleted display a very strong decrease of activity. However, this deletion is also accompanied by other dramatic changes of the pharmacophoric patterns, and therefore it is impossible to predict, using family A as a learning set, whether the HBA character of the carbonyl group is important for binding.

3.4.2 Models derived on the basis of Family A, enriched by inactive compounds

An alternative way to improve the sampling of pharmacophoric configurations without additional synthesis and testing of analogs is to enrich the learning set with a series of inactive molecules. In this work, ligands of receptors and enzymes, other than FPT, have been used to this purpose. By presenting the various pharmacophoric field patterns generated by randomly selected molecules to the activity model, the "background noise" due to fortuitous pharmacophore element matches that do not imply the conservation of the biological activity can be estimated. By discriminating the pharmacophoric field patterns that occur only in actives against those that could be achieved with any randomly chosen compound, the search for the biologically relevant pharmacophore may be significantly enhanced. Model 5, including 50% of the inactive compounds I in the learning set (featuring a total of N_{dat}=72 compounds), scores a high $r^2_{XV\text{-}3}$ value of 0.92 evidencing the ability of the model to easily discriminate between the structurally homogeneous actives of family A and the completely unrelated inactive compounds. Its difference of performance against the corresponding "blind" models using randomized activity data is also improved with respect to the models based on family A alone, even though spurious correlations could account for up to 54% of the total variance of the activity within $A+I_1$.

3.4.3 Models derived on the basis of Family B, enriched by inactive compounds

Model 9 entirely relies on information extracted from the fully automated superimposition of the "azole" set B and a subset of FPT-inactive molecules on a structurally unrelated reference molecule, with respect to which no apparent overlay mode can be postulated. Therefore, in contrast to the learning sets centered on family A, where the validity of the ComPharm overlays could be visually checked against the "expected" superposition modes, the ability of the automated algorithm to find meaningful overlays and provide relevant synthetic descriptors may only be judged in terms of the success of the resulting QSAR models. Intriguingly, with a $r^2_{XV\text{-}3}$ value of 0.87 against only 0.46 scored by the corresponding "blind" models 10-12, model 9 appears to be slightly more robust than model 5, based on the set of roughly equal size ($A+I_1$), but in which the recognition of the active compounds should have been enhanced by their structural relatedness to the reference molecule. ComPharm automated overlays thus appear to be useful in structure-activity relationship elucidation, which is a remarkable fact under the circumstances in which the adjustable parameters controlling the overlay scoring function (Table 1) have been derived on the basis of completely independent considerations, involving a diversity metric unrelated to ComPharm from the point of view of the mathematical formalism, but based on the same definitions of the pharmacophoric features.

3.4.4 Models trained on the totality of available molecules. Impact of the synthetic descriptor buildup strategy on the quality of the resulting regressions

The analysis of the optimal performances of models 13-36 ($N_{dat}=162, N_{vars}=290$) reveals that, in all situations, the maximal quality of the fortuitous correlations between descriptors and randomly assigned activities is significantly lower than the $r^2_{XV\text{-}3}$ values reached when associating the activity values to the proper molecular descriptors. The increase and diversification of the learning set partially lifted the redundancy of pairs of descriptors that seemed to be highly correlated within family A only (compare the significantly larger number of non-redundant terms, $N_{vars}=290$, to $N_{vars}=240$, obtained on the basis of family A alone). The pharmacophoric field descriptors provide significant information relative to the biological activity of the molecules. Furthermore, these results underline the feasibility of a ComPharm-based QSAR study explaining the activities of structurally different compounds on the basis of a unique regression equation, in spite of the fact that the different families did not share any common overlay mode with respect to the reference template.

The most clear-cut results are displayed by model 13, scoring a $r^2_{XV\text{-}3}=0.85$ against a maximal cross-validated coefficient of only 0.16 obtained on the basis of randomized activities. When using an "infinite" β factor, e.g. setting the synthetic descriptors equal to the descriptor of the absolute overlay optimum for each candidate molecule (model 17 vs. models 18-20), it can be seen that the fluctuations affecting the descriptors are on one hand decreasing the ability of the model to explain the experimental activity ($r^2_{XV\text{-}3}$ decreases from 0.85 in model 13 to 0.78 in model 17), while on the other, spurious fitting against the randomized set of activities becomes easier. The noise-reduction within the descriptor sets used in models 13-16, achieved through averaging over near-optimal overlay modes instead of focussing on the absolute overlay optima, has a significant impact on the quality of the models at low numbers of overlays (10).

Extending the number of overlay runs used for descriptor buildup to 60 (models 21-24, at $\beta=0$ and respectively 25-28, at $\beta=200$) shows that the stability of the models based on equal-weight averaging ($\beta=0$) did not significantly differ from what had been observed with the descriptors built from 10 overlay runs only. At high β values, the stability of model 25, comparable to the one of models 21 or 13, could be achieved only at the cost of the extensive sampling of 60 overlay modes. Stable QSAR models based on the pharmacophoric field patterns found in the absolutely optimal overlay configurations can be developed, but at much higher computational effort and – at least within this study case – without offering important gains in quality with respect to the more robust approaches featuring average information relative to all the available suboptimal overlays. In other words, the absolutely optimal overlay models do not appear to provide more relevant input for QSAR models than the suboptimal modes.

The use of a single (lowest-energy, according to catConf[46]) conformation of A_0 in models 29-36, instead of multiple conformers as in 13-20, only slightly decreased the quality of the models, most likely due to certain candidate compounds in the learning set which do not adopt conformations that successfully mimic the considered geometry of A_0. Averaging over all suboptimal overlays (β=0) is reconfirmed as a valid buildup strategy for the synthetic descriptors.

3.4.5 Impact of the choice of the Reference Compound: Models trained on the totality of the molecules, using other reference templates

The success of a model relying on a grid-based sampling of local properties depends on a sufficient grid density, e.g. a sufficiently fine grid step in order to capture all the relevant variations of the monitored field properties, and an appropriate size, ensuring that all the relevant space zones –and, if possible, only the relevant space zones- are covered. From all these points of view, the ComPharm approach choosing an active ligand as reference "grid" presents a number of advantages over regular CoMFA 3D-grids, where, at constant number of grid points, the requirements for grid density and grid coverage are conflicting. In ComPharm, the "resolution" of the grid corresponds to the average interatomic distance (1.5Å) while the size and shape of the spanned space represent the conformational space of a known potent ligand, rather than a "static" and unnecessary large volume arbitrarily defined by a 3D-grid. Problems may however appear for candidate compounds that are much larger than the reference, and therefore unable to map certain of their fragments on the reference grid. They could nevertheless be handled by adding extraneous dummy atoms as novel grid points, and letting the QSAR models "decide" whether or not to penalize the compounds that induce strong pharmacophoric field values at those remote locations. The good results of the previously discussed models suggest that in this case, such supplementary precautions may not be necessary.

The use of B_0 . the most active representative of family B - as a reference, causes a very slight decrease in the quality of the models with respect to their "blind" counterparts – compare models 47-50 to 13-16, and respectively 51-54 to 17-20. With B_0 as reference, the GA-based QSAR model selection is started from an initial set of N_{vars}=238 non-redundant descriptors corresponding to the pharmacophoric field values at the vertices of B_0, compared to the 290 obtained with A_0 as reference.

After ranking the set of inactive compounds I in decreasing order of their similarity score with respect to A_0, the three most similar inactives representing three topologically different families (compounds M, N and Q; see Figure 10), were also successfully used as reference molecules, leading to valid QSAR models. It can therefore be concluded that the template molecule need not to be active, but must present a pharmacophoric pattern that is somehow similar to an active molecule (the ComPharm dissimilarity scores between A_0 and M, N and Q are 0.23, 0.25 and 0.27 respectively). It should at least partially match some of the pharmacophoric elements present in an active compound, since otherwise no meaningful alignments of active compounds could be achieved.

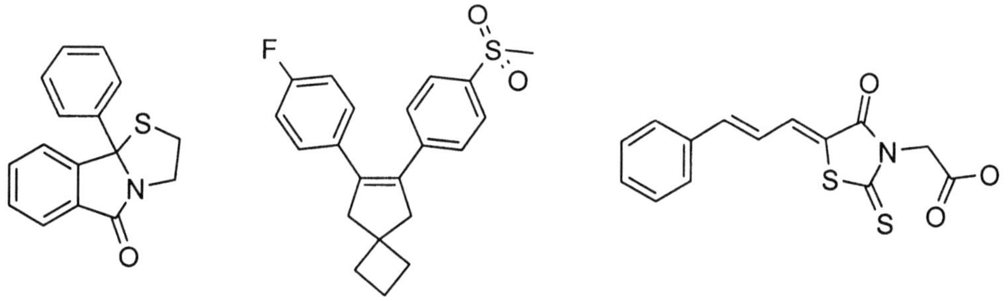

Figure 10. The three compounds from the set of inactive molecules bearing a maximal similarity to A_0.

3.5 In-depth Analysis of QSAR Models

3.5.1 Analysis of the Binding Modes Sampled by Models Calibrated Against the Entire Set of Compounds

As can be seen from Figure 11, thousands of different, relatively successful, activity hypotheses, each representing a unified model explaining the binding of both of the structurally distinct families (A+A*) and B, can be formulated in terms of ComPharm descriptors, provided that all the available compounds are used for training. Even though the complete set of considered compounds (A+A*+B+I) represents a training set of significant size and diversity, the large number of different models with similar predictive powers makes it impossible to single out the "correct", e.g. physically meaningful linear equation including the pharmacophoric elements which are effectively involved in site-ligand interactions. It is incorrect to consider the model with the best $r^2_{XV\text{-}3}$ value as the best approach unless this appears to be the only QSAR equation with an outstandingly high correlation coefficient with respect to all the others. In the current situation, 65 different QSAR models involving between 21 and 26 variables have a $r^2_{XV\text{-}3}$ value within 0.01 from the maximal correlation coefficient that has been found for this data set (0.848). 20 descriptors systematically appear in more than 90% of these best 65 models, but 45 other descriptors occasionally entered some of these equations. The "consensus" equation including only these 20 systematically selected terms displays a $r^2_{XV\text{-}3}$ value of 0.837. However, a $r^2_{XV\text{-}3}$ of 0.748 can be achieved with a linear model involving only 9 descriptors, while an approach with a r^2_{XV-3} of 0.66 may use only 3 descriptors. It is difficult to argue what should be a "best" compromise between a high r^2 value and a low number of variables – definitions of quantitative criteria such as the "lack of fit" (LOF)[60] indices include user-adjustable penalties for additional degrees of freedom of the model.

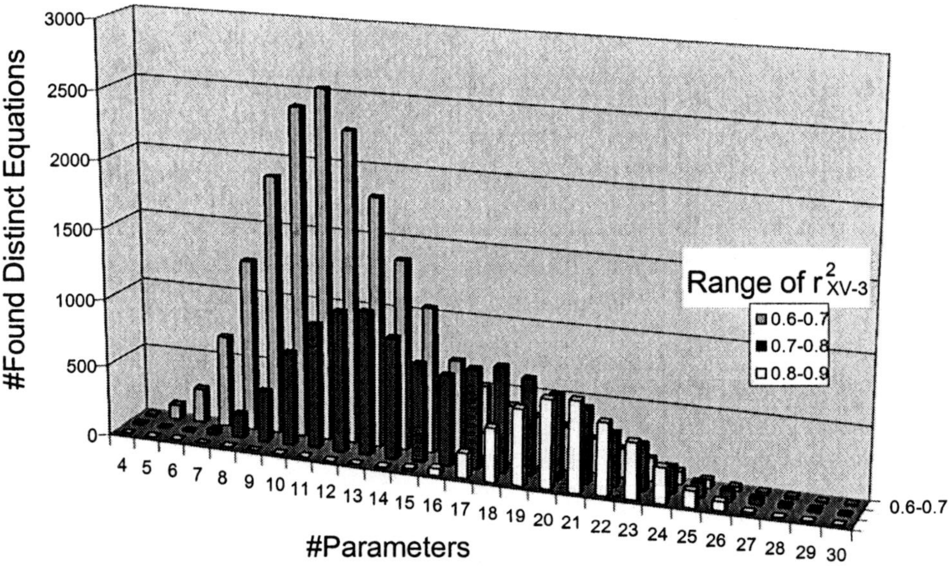

Figure 11. Distribution of the regression models visited by the GA-driven search for the optimal linear model 13 (Table 2), showing on the z-axis the number of distinct equations that were obtained, in terms of the number of involved parameters (on the X-axis) and the range of their r^2_{XV-3} coefficient (three different ranges are color-coded).

Figure 12 compares the previously cited models involving 9 and respectively 3 descriptors (e.g. 10 and respectively 4 degrees of freedom, including the intercept of the linear equation). The key atoms of the reference molecule A_0, designing the locations at which the selected pharmacophoric field descriptors have been taken, are shown as balls. Each such atom is labeled in terms of the type of the associated field descriptor (the pharmacophoric feature abbreviations are those introduced in §2.1.1), followed by the average/maximal contribution of this descriptor to the predicted activity values, over all the compounds of the learning set. Because in this study the pIC_{50} (-log IC_{50}) has been used as activity index, positive values imply that generating a strong pharmacophoric field of that type at the given location of the reference scaffold will decrease the affinity of the compound. The predicted vs. experimental pIC_{50} values according to both QSAR approaches are plotted in a same graph, below the shown pharmacophore models.

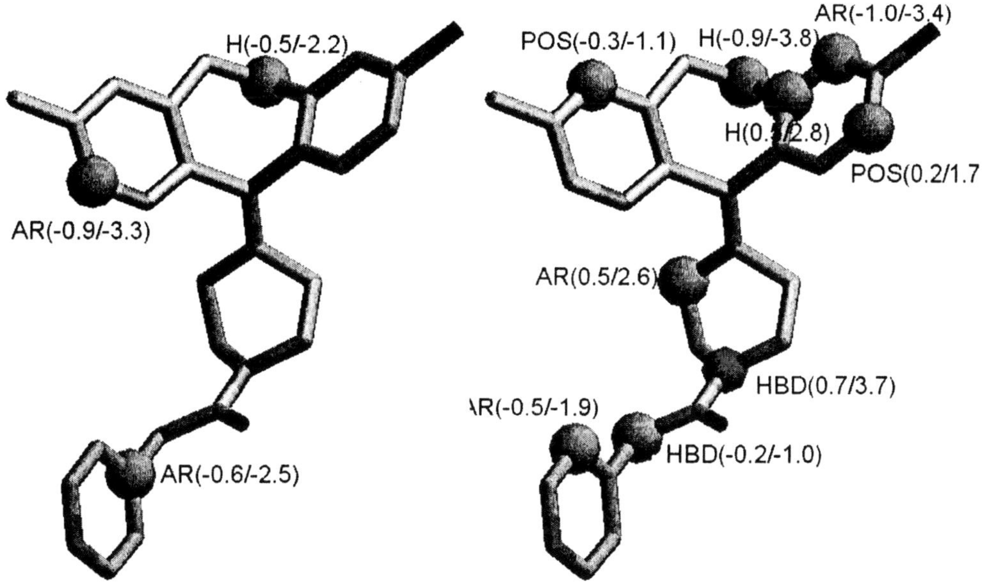

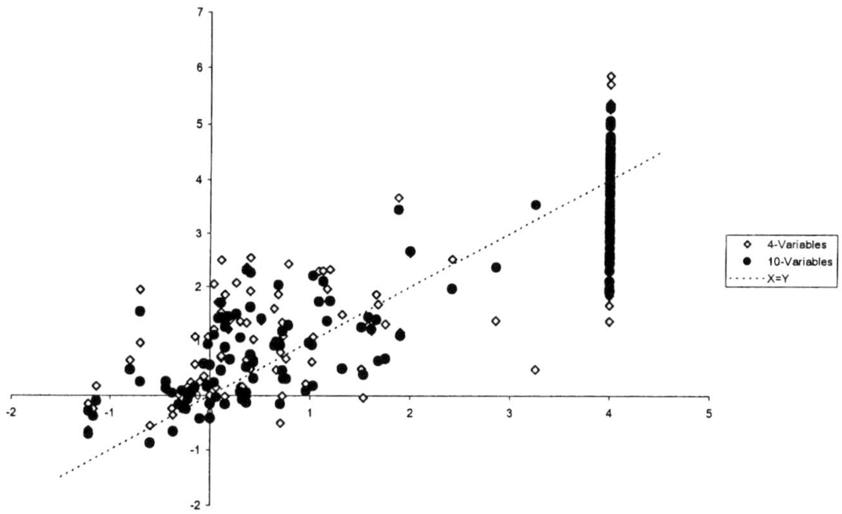

Figure 12. Comparison of two QSAR models with 3 and respectively 9 entered descriptors, visited by the GA-driven search for the optimal linear model 13 (Table 2). See Results section (0) for a detailed description.

The simplest pharmacophore model displaying a significant predictive power with respect to the total set of considered compounds involves only 3 points, predicting that any molecule that can be overlapped to A_0 and will generate significant hydrophobic and respectively aromatic fields at the 3 selected locations will be active against Farnesyl Protein Transferase. *This simple model is sufficient to explain an important part of the observed variance within the set of compounds.* This implies that this 3-point pharmacophore is, on one hand, common to all the active molecules in both families A and B. On the other, and under the assumption that the set I is sufficiently representative sample of "random" molecules, its probability of occurrence within non-binders of FPT appears to be sufficiently low in order to become a useful discrimination criterion between actives and inactives.

Interestingly, the 9-point model includes a related pattern, although it locates one of the two key aromatic centers on the benzene ring, rather than the pyridine ring of the tricyclic system, suggesting that these rings may be equivalent for binding, in spite of the presence of the heteroatom. Again, these 3 points cover the strongest favorable contributions for activity, while most of the other selected features encode weak favorable or unfavorable effects. FPT inhibitors overlapped to the reference molecule should neither possess hydrogen bond donors in the neighborhood of the amide nitrogen of A_0, nor an aromatic group in replacement of the saturated six-membered ring, nor a positive charge next to the benzene ring. However, these supplementary contributions do not account for more than 10% of the experimental variance and their relevance is therefore highly questionable.

3.5.2 The Usefulness of Models Derived on the Basis of A Single Structural Family of Actives, in Predicting the Activity of "Novel" Families of FPT Inhibitors, not used at the Training Step

The development of a QSAR model that would successfully predict the activity of any molecule, irrespectively of its degree of relatedness to the compounds in the training set, is a practically unrealistic goal. Most of the published QSAR approaches apply only to structurally well defined classes, within which the various contributions to the binding affinity that can not be accounted for by the used descriptors are more or less constant. Obviously, a molecular field-based QSAR approach would fail to predict the activity of any molecule displaying a completely different binding mode with respect to any of those encountered in the learning set. If the key interactions occur at points of space that were irrelevant for the binding of all of the training molecules, the corresponding descriptors not could not have entered the model at calibration stage.

The role of a QSAR model is not to postulate the existence of novel binding modes, but to extract a binding mode hypothesis out of the calibration examples, e.g. to evidence a descriptor pattern that occurs only in the active compounds. However, if the class of active compounds is structurally homogeneous and distinct from the non-binders, then QSAR models may spuriously focus on any structural element that is characteristic of that class, whether involved in binding or not, and wrongly infer that any member –and only the members- of that class are active.

Figure 13 represents distribution density plots of the QSAR models derived on the basis of different learning sets and reference scaffold. This bidimensional distribution is taken in function of the number of involved parameters and respectively the difference of predictive power of the model applied to learning and validation set (learning and validation sets were $A+I_1$ and $B+I_2$, respectively). The GA-sampled models with an $r^2_{XV\text{-}3}$ value within 0.2 from the best obtained correlation coefficient were classified in terms of their number of N_{vars} variables (shown on X). The Z-axis of the plot monitors the fraction of N_{vars}-variable equations displaying a loss of predictive power within each of the ranges enumerated on Y. The probability to sample an N_{vars}-variable equation during the GA-run is not apparent in Figure 13, the displayed probabilities being normed with respect to the effective number of models within each class. The "loss of predictive power" was defined as the difference between the optimality criterion ρ(LS) taken on the learning set and respectively ρ(VS) taken on the validation set, reported to the former value:

$$Loss - of - predictive - power = \frac{\rho(LS) - \rho(VS)}{\rho(LS)} \times 100\% \quad (14)$$

Given that the learning and validation sets were chosen such as to represent two structurally unrelated families of molecules, a small loss of predictive power evidences the ability of the model to "discover" novel families of actives, not known at the calibration stage. Several conclusions can be drawn from Figure 13:

- First, the large majority of the explored models *failed* to apply to structurally different families. Even within classes of equations displaying a maximal occurrence of models with low loss of predictive power, no more than an estimated 15% of the models conserved more than 60% of their original predictive power when applied to the structurally distinct validation set. While all the models used to build Figure 13 showed a significant ability to discriminate between the family of actives used for calibration and inactive molecules, very few of these would have predicted the activity of the other family of FPT inhibitors. The original paper[53], reporting the use of a Catalyst hypothesis built on the basis of family A to discover two representatives of family B does not provide any study of the statistical relevance of their model. According to the authors, the other representatives of family B were discovered by means of a substructure search based on the "azole" motif found in the two hits, e.g. had not been recognized by the Catalyst query. Typically, most of the QSAR models studied here are also able to correctly predict the activity of a few members of the validation set, which is however insufficient to ensure a significant optimality coefficient ρ(VS). From this empirical point of view, the fraction of the QSAR models able to "discover" the other family of actives *by hitting at least one of its members* would be much larger that the ones reported to display a low loss of predicted power. As shown in the previous paragraph, ComPharm can be successfully used to derive models that simultaneously explain the activities within the structurally heterogeneous collection A+B+I. However, in a study disposing of experimental data with respect to only one of these families, it would have been difficult to predict which of the multitude of possible models actually applies to other, structurally distinct families, on the basis of statistical criteria exclusively derived on the basis of the learning set.
- The fraction of models preserving their predictive power is seen to be dependent on the reference structure used for the ComPharm overlap of candidates.

Intriguingly, the models trained on $A+I_1$ using A_0 as a reference template (upper left plot) are the ones that display the most striking inability to predict the activity of family B. The overtraining is extreme with this learning set, since the actives of the learning set match very well all the pharmacophoric centers of the template. Therefore, *any* such center may be used to discriminate between actives (for which the perfect match will translate into high field values at that point) and inactives, where the field values will be significantly reduced due to imperfect overlap. Most of the descriptor elements could therefore enter the QSAR model, whether physically relevant for binding or not. The wealth of strongly predictive models that are generated for the LS $A+I_1$ actually represent pattern recognition models (they discriminate between A-like topology and different topologies) and do not evidence the consensus pharmacophore that can be also found in other FPT binders.

- Throughout the studied models, the QSAR models displaying a significant predictive power with respect to the VS are *more likely to be found among the equations involving only few degrees of freedom*. The more parameters a model displays, the higher its chance to represent an overfitting artifact rather than a physically relevant model. *In consequence, none of the models displaying optimal r^2_{XV-3} scores with respect to their learning sets maintained their predictive power with respect to the other families. Therefore, it is impossible to evidence the models of general validity based on criteria relative to the LS only – the use of a structurally distinct VS is absolutely necessary to test its relevance. However, if such a set is not available, the safest choice among all the possible models is the one with a minimal number of degrees of freedom, which nevertheless displays a significant predictive power with respect to the LS.*

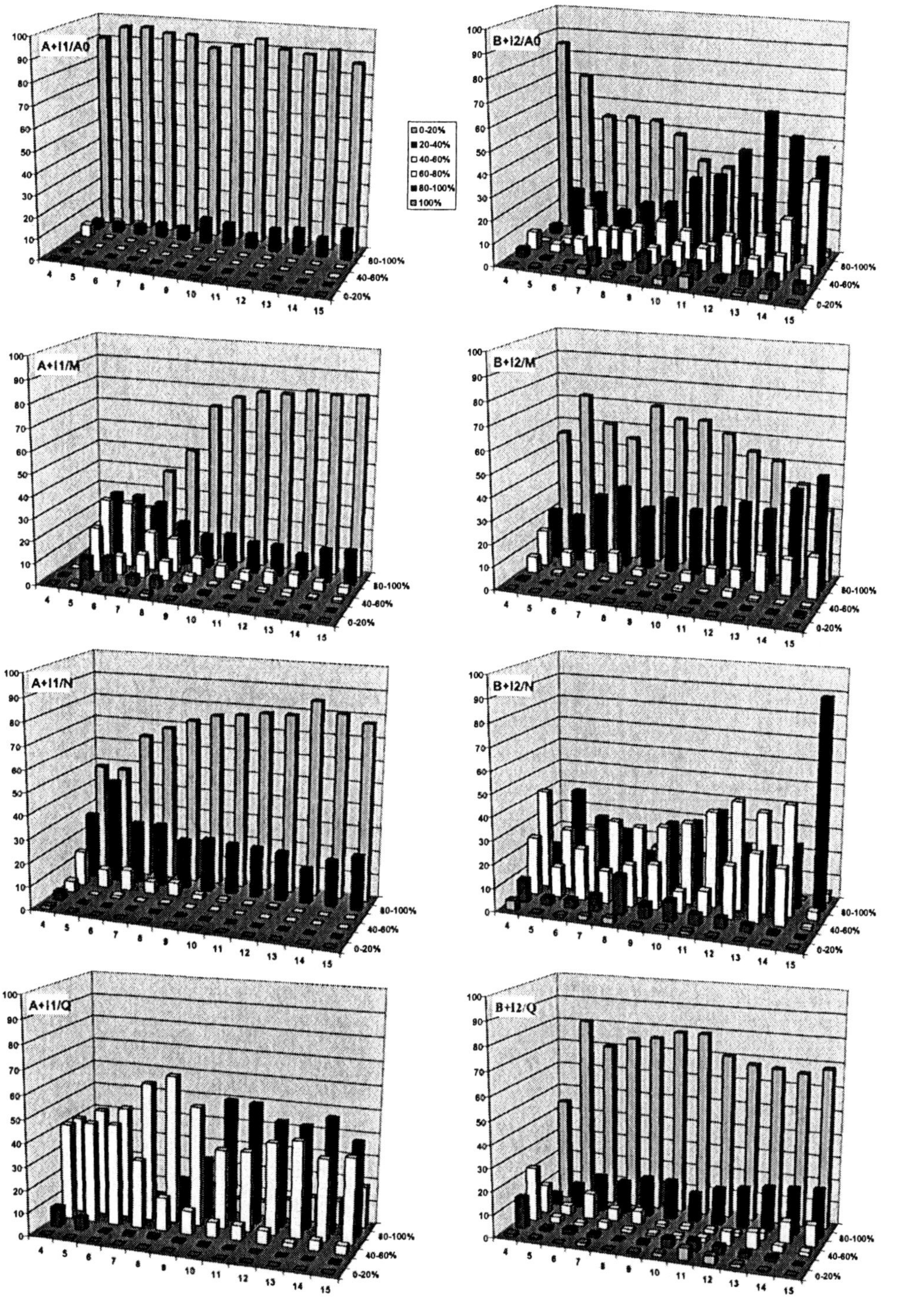

Figure 13. Distribution of the loss of predictive power against validation vs. learning set, as defined in (14). The Z-axis monitors the relative fractions of N(subscript)pars parameter models featuring a predictive power loss that fell within the color-coded classes shown on Y. Left hand graphs were trained on $A+I_1$ and validated on $D+I_2$ the opposite being performed for their right-hand counterparts. Each pair of graphs in a line represent models build on the basis of multiconformational models of the reference structures A_0, M, N and Q, respectively.

4. Conclusions

The ComPharm approach was shown to generate a set of molecular descriptors that can be successfully employed in QSAR models. Compared to the "classical" CoMFA approaches, the advantages of ComPharm reside in its ability to account for multiple overlay models, to circumvent the problem of the choice of the "bioactive" conformer of the reference whenever this is not experimentally determined and to drastically reduce the number of generated descriptors due to a molecular-graph based grid rather than a systematic map of the 3D-space around the threshold. The "pharmacophoric" fields defined as harmonic functions of the distance from the pharmacophoric centers offer a complete description of the spatial distribution of functional groups that are potentially relevant for binding. It was shown that, by including information for possible suboptimal overlay modes into the pharmacophoric field descriptors, the relevance of the latter does not decrease, while the reproducibility of the QSAR approaches dramatically increases as they are no longer dependent on the rare events of reaching the absolutely optimal overlap mode by the stochastic overlay algorithm. The absolutely optimal overlay mode is not the only valid mode to use in molecular field comparison approaches, which is not an astonishing conclusion in the light of the well-known fact that multiple site-ligand orientations may significantly contribute to the binding affinity.

Pharmacophoric field descriptors were proven to be able to explain the affinity of a structurally diverse set of more than 160 Farnesyl Protein Transferase inhibitors and inactive compounds. These results were confirmed against "blind" attempts to build QSAR models with data sets where the affinities were randomly attributed to other compounds of the set. A model involving only 3 pharmacophoric field descriptors has been found to successfully explain 66% of the variance of the activity of the complete set of compounds A+A*+B+I. This model suggests that 2 aromatic rings and a hydrophobic group, arranged such as to generate intense pharmacophoric fields at the positions specified with respect to the reference compound A_0, are sufficient to guarantee the affinity for FPT of small molecules. Such an interpretation is, of course, rather simplistic. Given that the model does not include any excluded volume constraints, it is certain that many inactives may figure among the compounds that satisfy the activity criteria according to this model. Nevertheless, such examples were not available in the current diverse set of compounds, including a representative selection of more than 70 ligands of 14 different biological targets in addition to the FPT ligands. According to the limited knowledge that can be extracted from this learning set, it appears that the occurrence of this tricentric pharmacophore pattern in compounds is strongly correlated with their FPT inhibitory activity. The screening of large virtual data bases against this pattern would reassess its real relevance with respect to the whole Universe of molecules.

It must be kept in mind that applying a QSAR model to search for novel, unrelated compounds represents a key validation of both the quality of the methodology and of the initial learning set, since a QSAR approach may not identify activity patterns never encountered during calibration. A successful QSAR approach should however evidence "hidden" patterns that could not have been understood by a medicinal chemist, e.g. find common features in structurally distinct sets of actives (if their binding mode is similar). The discovery of activity models explaining the IC_{50} values of both compounds of type A and B, and discriminating them against the various subfamilies of inactives I on the basis of a single linear model, can be considered a good example. However, if the calibration has been conducted with respect to a single family (A or B), then the emerging of these common pharmacophoric features was seen to be largely obscured by the overfitting artifacts consisting in the selection of elements characteristic to the specific active family seen at calibration, and not to the family of FPT binders as a whole. While "general" models may be visited by the GA-driven QSAR selection process, it is impossible to predict which equation best applies to structurally unrelated families on the basis of the statistical criteria with respect to the learning set only. According to the results obtained here, the chances to derive an equation of general validity are enhanced when:

- using a reference scaffold that is structurally unrelated to the compounds of the learning set, even if the scaffold molecule itself is not active. Otherwise, the perfect overlap between the scaffold and the active members of the learning set makes that many pharmacophoric elements, whether relevant to binding or not, will be "conserved" in the active structures and "absent" from the inactives, therefore "useful" to discriminate between these two categories. The obtained QSAR model would then actually represent a pattern recognition model, only giving the correct answers within the structural class used for calibration.
- preferentially selecting models with a minimal number of degrees of freedom, among those that display a quite high predictive power with respect to the learning set.

These well-known "rules of the thumb" have been quantitatively illustrated in this work, by analyzing the expectancy to obtain a predictive model in function of the two important aspects.

5. References

1. Cramer, R.D. III; Patterson D.E.; Bunce, J.E.; Comparative Molecular Field Analysis (CoMFA). 1. Effect of Shape on Binding of Steroids to Carrier Proteins, *J. Am. Chem. Soc.*, **1988**, *110*, 5959-5967
2. Klebe, G., Structural Alignment of Molecules, in "3D-QSAR in Drug Design", Kubinyi, H, Ed. ESCOM, Leiden, **1993**, 173-199
3. Oprea, T.I., Waller, C.L., Theoretical and Practical Aspects of Three Dimensional Quantitative Structure-Activity Relationships, in Reviews in Computational Chemistry, K.B. Lipkowitz and D.B. Boyd (Eds.), Wiley, New York, **1997**, *11*, 127-182

4. Cruciani, G.; Watson, K.A.; A Comparative Molecular Field Analysis Using GRID Force-Field and GOLPE Variable Selection Methods in a Study of Inhibitors of Glycogen Phosphorylase b, *J. Med. Chem.*, **1994**, *37*, 2589-2601
5. Huang, Q.; Liu, R.; Zhang, P.; He, X.; McKernan, R.; Gan, T.; Bennet, D.W.; Cook, J.M.; Predictive Models for $GABA_A$/Benzodiazepine Receptor Subtypes: Studies of Quantitative Structure-Activity Relationships for Imidazobenzodiazepines at Five Recombinant $GABA_A$/Benzodiazepine Receptor Subtypes via Comparative Molecular Field Analysis, *J. Med. Chem.*, **1998**, *41*, 4130-4142
6. Wilcox, R.E.; Tseng, T.; Brusniak, M-Y.K.; Ginsburg, B.; Pearlman, R.S.; Teeter, M.; DuRand, C.; Starr, S.; Neve, K.A.; CoMFA-based Prediction of Agonist Activities at Recombinant D_1 vs. D_2 Dopamine Receptors, *J. Med. Chem.*, **1998**, *41*, 4385-4399
7. Chen, X.; Ruskino, A. III; Young, S.S.; Recursive Partitioning Analysis of a Large Structure-Activity Data Set Using Three-Dimensional Descriptors, *J. Chem. Inf. Comp. Sci.,* **1998**, *38*, 112-116
8. Ortiz, A.R.; Pisabarro, M.T.; Gago, F.; Wade, R.C.; Prediction of Drug Binding Affinities by Comparative Binding Energy Analysis, *J. Med. Chem.*, **1995**, *38*, 2681-2691
9. Ajay; Murcko, M.A., Computational Methods to Predict Binding Free Energies in Ligand-Receptor Complexes, *J. Med. Chem.*, **1995**, *38*, 4953-4967
10. Oprea, T.I.; Marshall, G.R., Receptor-Based Prediction of Affinity, *Perspectives in Drug Discovery and Design*, **1998**, *9-11*, 35-65
11. Mammen, M.; Shakhnovich, E.I.; Whitesides, G.M.; Using a Convenient, Quantitative Model for Torsional Entropy to Establish Qualitative Trends for Molecular Processes that Restrict Conformational Freedom, *J. Org. Chem.*, **1998**, *63*, 3168-3175
12. Ercolani, G., Comment on "Using a Convenient, Quantitative Model for Torsional Entropy to Establish Qualitative Trends for Molecular Processes that Restrict Conformational Freedom", *J. Org. Chem.*, **1999**, *64*, 3350-3353
13. Horvath, D., A Virtual Screening Approach Applied to the Search for Trypanothione Reductase Inhibitors, *J. Med. Chem.*, **1997**, *40*, 2412-2423
14. Gallop, M. A.; Barrett, R.W.; Dower, W.J.; Fodor, S.P.A; Gordon, E.M.; Applications of Combinatorial Technologies to Drug Discovery. 1. Background and Peptide Combinatorial Libraries., *J. Med. Chem.*, **1994**, *37*, 1233-1251
15. Gordon, E.M; Barrett, R.W.; Dower, W.J.; Fodor, S.P.A; Gallop, M. A., Applications of Combinatorial Technologies to Drug Discovery. 2. Combinatorial Organic Synthesis, Library Screening Strategies and Future Directions., *J. Med. Chem.*, **1994**, *37*, 1385-1401
16. Molineaux, C.J.; Goodwin, W.; Chai, L.; Zhang, X.; Israel, D.I.; A High-Throughput Functional Assay fo G-Protein-Coupled Receptors: Method for Screening Combinatorial Libraries, in Molecular Diversity and Combinatorial Chemistry, Chaiken, I.M.; Janda, K.D. (Eds), American Chemical Society, Washington **1996**, 273-282

17. Schuler, G.D. *et.al.*, A Gene Map of the Human Genome, *Science*, **1996**, *274*, 540-546
18. Walters, D.E.; Hinds, R.M.; Genetically Evolved Receptor Models (GERM): A Computational Approach to the Construction of Receptor Models, *J. Med. Chem.*, **1994**,*37*, 2527-2536
19. Synder, P.J., Minireceptor Modeling: Intuition, Quantitation and Prediction, Lecture at the Second European Workshop in Drug Design, May 17-24, Siena, Italy; see also Vedani, Zbinden, Snyder, Greenidge, *J. Am. Chem. Soc.*, **1995**, *117*, 4987
20. Cerius^2.Align, Molecular Simulations Inc., San Diego, CA.
21. Kearsley, S.M.; Smith, G.M.; An Alternative Method for the Alignment of Molecular Structures: Maximizing Electrostatic and Steric Overlap., *Tetrahedron Comput. Methodol.*, **1990**, *3*, 615-633
22. Hodgkin, E.E.; Richards, W.G.; Molecular Similarity Based on Electrostatic Potential and Electric Field., *Int. J. Quantum Biol. Symp.*, **1980**, *14*, 105-110
23. Carbo, R.; Leyda, L.; Arnau, M.; An Electron Density Measure of the Similarity between Two Compounds, *Int. J. Quantum Chem.*, **1980**, *17*, 1185-1189
24. Carbo, R.; Domingo, L.; LCAO-MO Similarity Measures and Taxonomy, *Int. J. Quantum Chem.*, **1987**, *32*, 517-545
25. Good, A.C.; Richards, W.G.; Rapid Evaluation of Shape Similarity Using Gaussian Functions, *J. Chem. Inf. Comp. Sci.*, **1993**, *33*, 112-116
26. Good, A.C.; Hodgkin, E.E.; Richards, W.G.; Utilization of Gaussian Functions for Rapid Evaluation of Molecular Similarity, *J. Chem. Inf. Comp. Sci.*, **1992**, *32*, 188-191
27. Clark, M.; Cramer, R.D. III.; Jones, D.M.; Patterson, D.E.; Simeroth, P.E.; Comparative Molecular Field Analysis (CoMFA). 2. Towards its Use with 3D Structural Data Bases., *Tetrahedron Comput. Methodol.*, **1990**, *3*, 47-59
28. Moro, S.; Li, A.-H.; Jacobson, K. A., Molecular Modeling Studies of Human A_3 Adenosine Antagonists: Structural Homology and Receptor Docking, *J. Chem. Inf. Comp. Sci.*, **1998**, *38*, 1239-1248
29. Timoftei, S.; Fabian, W. M. F.; Comparative Molecular Field Analysis of Heterocyclic Monoazo Dye-Fiber Affinities, *J. Chem. Inf. Comp. Sci.*, **1998**, *38*, 1218-1222
30. Payne, A.W.R; Glenn, R.C.; Molecular Recognition using a Binary Genetic Search Algorithm, *J. Mol. Graphics*, **1993**, *9*, 113-130
31. Jones, G.; Willett, P.; Glen, R.C.; Genetic Algorithms in Chemical Structure Handling and Molecular Recognition, in Genetic Algorithms in Molecular Modeling, Devillers, J., Ed. Academic Press, London, **1996**, 211-239
32. Leach, A.R.; An algorithm to identify a molecule's most different conformations, *J. Chem.Inf. Comp. Sci.*, **1994**, *34*, 661-670
33. Leach, A.R.; Prout, K.; Dolata, D.P.; The application of Artificial Intelligence to the Conformational Analysis of Strained Molecules, *J. Comput. Chem.*, **1990**, *11*, 680-693
34. Smellie, A.; Teig, T.S.; Towbin, P.; Poling: Promoting Conformational Variation, *J. Comput. Chem.*, **1995**, *16*, 171-187

35. Leardi, R, Genetic Algorithms in Feature Selection, in Genetic Algorithms in Molecular Modeling, Devillers, J., Ed. Academic Press, London, **1996**, 67-86
36. Kubinyi, H.; Variable Selection in QSAR Studies. I. An Evolutionary Algorithm., *Quant. Struct-Act. Relat.*, **1994**, *13*, 285-294
37. Kubinyi, H.; Variable Selection in QSAR Studies. II. A Highly Efficient Combination of Systematic Search and Evolution., *Quant. Struct-Act. Relat.*, **1994**, *13*, 393-401
38. Glen, W.G.; Dunn, W.J.; Scott, D.R.; Principal Components Analysis and Partial Least Squares Regressions, *Tetrahedron Comput. Technol.;* **1989**, *2*, 349-376
39. Sulea, T.; Oprea, T.I.; Muresan, S.; Chan, S.L.; A Different Method for Steric Field Evaluation in CoMFA Improves Model Robustness, *J. Chem. Inf. Comp. Sci.*, **1997**, *37*, 1162-1170.
40. Pastor, M., Cruciani, G., Clementi, S., Smart Region Definition: A New Way to Improve the Predictive Ability and Interpretability of Three-Dimensional Quantitative Structure-Activity Relationships, *J. Med. Chem.*, **1997**, *40*, 1455-1464
41. Poulain, R., *et. al.*, Work in progress
42. Willett, P.; Barnard, J. M.; Downs, G. M.; Chemical Similarity Searching, *J. Chem. Inf. Comp. Sci.,* **1998**, *38*, 983-996
43. Bradshaw, J.; Introduction to the Tversky Similarity Measure, Presented at Daylight MUG Meeting, Laguna Beach, CA, February 1997, URL http://www.daylight.com/meetings/mug97 /agenda97/Bradshaw/MUG97/tv_tversky.html
44. Tversky, A.; Features of Similaity, *Psychol. Revue*, **1977**, *84*,327-352
45. Vajda, S.; Weng, Z.; Rosenfeld, R.; DeLisi, C.; Effect oof Conformational Flexibility and Solvation on Receptor-Ligand Binding Free Energies, *Biochemistry,* **1994**, *33*, 13977-13988
46. Smellie, A.; Kahn, S.; Teig, S.; Analysis of Conformational Coverage. 1. Validation and Estimation of Coverage, *J. Chem. Inf. Comp. Sci.*, **1995**, *35*, 285-294
47. Smellie, A.; Kahn, S.; Teig, S.; Analysis of Conformational Coverage. 2. Applications of Conformational Models, *J. Chem. Inf. Comp. Sci.*, **1995**, *35*, 295-304
48. Horvath, D. *et. al.*, *Work in Progess*
49. Matter, H., "Selecting Optimally Diverse Compounds from Structure Databases: A Validation Study of Two-Dimensional and Three-Dimensional Molecular Descriptors", *J. Med. Chem.*, **1997**, *40*, 1219-1229
50. Davis, L.; Handbook of Genetic Algorithms, Van Nostrand Rheinhold, New York **1991**
51. Fogel, D.B., Evolutionary Computation. Toward a New Philosophy of Machine Intelligence, IEEE Press, Piscataway **1995**
52. Luke, B.T.; An Overview of Genetic Methods, in Genetic Algorithms in Molecular Modeling, Devillers, J., Ed. Academic Press, London, **1996**, 35-66
53. Kaminski, J.J.; Rane, D.F.; Snow, M.E.; Weber, L.; Rothofsky, M.L.; Anderson, S.D.; Lin, S.L.; Identification of Novel Farnesyl-Protein Transferase Inhibitors Using Three-Dimensional Database Searching Methods, *J. Med. Chem.*, **1997**, *40*, 4103-4112

54. Catalyst v2.1, Molecular Simulations Inc., San Diego, CA
55. Njoroge, F.G.; Vibulbhan, B.; Rane, D.F.; Bishop, W.R.; Petrin, J; Patton, R.; Bryant, M.S.; Chen, K-J.; Nomeir, A.A.; Lin, C-C.; King, I.; Liu, M.; Chen, J.; Lee, S.; Yaremko, B.; Dell, J.; Lipari, P.; Malkowski, M.; Li, Z.; Catino, J.; Doll, R.J.; Girijavallabhan, V.; Ganguly, A.K.; Structure-Activity Relationship of 3-Substituted N-(Pyridinylacetyl)-4-(8-chloro-5,6-dihydro-11H-benzo[5,6]cyclohepta [1,2-b]pyridin-11-ylidene)-piperidine Inhibitors of Farnesyl-Protein Transferase: Design and Synthesis of in Vivo Active Antitumor Compounds, *J. Med. Chem.*, **1997**, *40*, 4290-4301
56. This set can be downloaded from http://www.msi.com/user/consortia /cchem/index.html
57. Everitt, B.S.; Dunn, G.; Applied Multivariate Data Analysis, Oxford University Press, New York **1992**
58. King, R.D., Hirst, J., Sternberg, M.J.E, "Comparison of Artificial Intelligence Methods for Modeling Pharmaceutical QSARs", *Appl. Artificial Intelligence*, **1995**, *9*, 213-233
59. Braban, M.; Pop, I.; Willard, X; Horvath, D., Reactivity Prediction Models Applied to the Selection of Novel Candidate Building Blocks for High Throughput Organic Synthesis of Combinatorial Libraries, *accepted for publication in J. Chem. Inf. Comp. Sci.,* **1999**
60. Friedman, J.H.; Silverman, B.W.; Flexible Parsimonious Smoothing and Additive Modeling, *Technometrics*, **1989**, *31*, 3-39

INDEX

E

F

G

H

I

K

L

M

N

O

P

Q

R

S

T

V

W